Annual Update in Intensive Care and Emergency Medicine 2015

The series *Annual Update in Intensive Care and Emergency Medicine* is the continuation of the series entitled *Yearbook of Intensive Care Medicine* in Europe and *Intensive Care Medicine: Annual Update* in the United States.

Jean-Louis Vincent
Editor

Annual Update in Intensive Care and Emergency Medicine 2015

Springer

Editor
Prof. Jean-Louis Vincent
Université libre de Bruxelles
Dept. of Intensive Care
Erasme Hospital
Brussels, Belgium
jlvincen@ulb.ac.be

ISSN 2191-5709
ISBN 978-3-319-13760-5 ISBN 978-3-319-13761-2 (eBook)
DOI 10.1007/978-3-319-13761-2

Springer Cham Heidelberg New York Dordrecht London

Cover design: WMXDesign GmbH, Heidelberg

Printed on acid-free paper

Springer International Publishing AG Switzerland is part of Springer Science+Business Media
(www.springer.com)

Contents

Part XII Neuromuscular Considerations

Part XIII Rapid Response Teams

Part XIV Data Management

Common Abbreviations

AKI	Acute kidney injury
ARDS	Acute respiratory distress syndrome
BAL	Bronchoalveolar lavage
COPD	Chronic obstructive pulmonary disease
CPR	Cardiopulmonary resuscitation
CT	Computed tomography
CVP	Central venous pressure
DO_2	Oxygen delivery
EKG	Electrocardiogram
EMR	Electronic medical record
FiO_2	Inspired fraction of oxygen
GCS	Glasgow Coma Scale
GFR	Glomerular filtration rate
ICP	Intracranial pressure
ICU	Intensive care unit
IL	Interleukin
INR	International normalized ratio
LV	Left ventricular
MAP	Mean arterial pressure
MRI	Magnetic resonance imaging
NF-κB	Nuclear factor kappa-B
NO	Nitric oxide
OR	Odds ratio
PAC	Pulmonary artery cather
PEEP	Positive end-expiratory pressure
RBC	Red blood cell
RCT	Randomized controlled trial
ROS	Reactive oxygen species
RRT	Renal replacement therapy
RV	Right ventricular
SAPS	Simplified acute physiology score
$ScvO_2$	Central venous oxygen saturation
SOFA	Sequential organ failure assessment
TBI	Traumatic brain injury
TNF	Tumor necrosis factor
VAP	Ventilator-associated pneumonia

Part I
Infections

Early Identification of Ventilator-associated Pneumonia Causative Pathogens: Focus on the Value of Gram-stain Examination

C. Chiurazzi, A. Motos-Galera, and A. Torres

Introduction

Ventilator-associated pneumonia (VAP) is a common nosocomial infection in critically ill patients, associated with increased morbidity and healthcare costs. Early identification of causative pathogens plays a critical role in the administration of appropriate antibiotic therapy and patient outcomes. In particular, in patients with clinical suspicion of VAP, respiratory samples should be obtained promptly to corroborate the provision of effective antibiotic treatment, while avoiding unnecessary antibiotic use that would promote the development of resistance. In this context, the value of the Gram-stain examination, and its potential impact on adequate empiric antibiotic treatment and major outcomes, is still under debate. In this manuscript, we review the most recent evidence on methods for early identification of VAP causative pathogens, with specific focus on Gram-stain examination of respiratory samples, and we highlight potential methodological limitations and future areas of investigation.

Incidence, Etiology and Diagnosis of Ventilator-associated Pneumonia

VAP is the second most common nosocomial infection in patients admitted to intensive care units (ICUs) [1]. VAP occurs in 9–27% of all ventilated patients [2, 3]. However, the incidences of VAP vary considerably among patient populations, e. g., trauma patients or those undergoing cardiac and neurological surgery are at greater risk. Additionally, various comorbidities and co-factors, such as prolonged mechanical ventilation, chronic pulmonary disease, prior use of antibiotics, acute

C. Chiurazzi · A. Motos-Galera · A. Torres ✉
Department of Pulmonary and Critical Care Medicine, Thorax Institute, Hospital Clinic, Barcelona, Spain
e-mail: atorres@clinic.ub.es

J.-L. Vincent (ed.), *Annual Update in Intensive Care and Emergency Medicine 2015*,
DOI 10.1007/978-3-319-13761-2_1

respiratory distress syndrome (ARDS) may increase the risk of VAP. Patients who develop VAP present longer ICU- and hospital stays [4]. As a result, VAP is associated with increased healthcare costs, estimated at around US$ 40,000 per patient who develops VAP [5, 6]. A recent report in VAP patients indicated that the overall attributable mortality was 13%. Nevertheless, mortality rates are inconsistent among studies. Indeed, in a study by Bekaert and collaborators [7], a relatively limited attributable VAP-associated mortality was reported. Importantly, late-onset VAP is often caused by multidrug resistant (MDR) pathogens and is associated with worse outcomes in comparison with VAP that develops early during the course of mechanical ventilation.

VAP is frequently caused by aerobic, Gram-negative pathogens (*Pseudomonas aeruginosa, Acinetobacter baumannii, Klebsiella pneumoniae, Escherichia coli*); the most frequent Gram-positive pathogen is *Staphylococcus aureus*. Underlying diseases may predispose patients to infection with specific organisms. For example, patients with chronic obstructive pulmonary disease (COPD) are often colonized and develop VAP caused by *Haemophilus influenzae, Moraxella catarrhalis* and *P. aeruginosa,* whereas, *Haemophilus spp.* and *Streptococcus pneumoniae* are frequent causative pathogens in trauma patients. *A. baumannii*, *S. aureus*, and *P. aeruginosa* are the most common causative pathogens in ARDS patients. Importantly, VAP is often caused by potentially MDR pathogens, i. e., *P. aeruginosa*, *S. aureus*, *Acinetobacter* spp., *Stenotrophomonas maltophilia, Burkholderia cepacia* and extended-spectrum β-lactamase (ESBL) *K. pneumoniae.* Patients at risk of being colonized by MDR pathogens are extremely varied, commonly present comorbid conditions, are ventilated for longer periods of time and receive antibiotics during the course of their hospitalization. A recent study [8] demonstrated that severity of illness did not affect etiology and risk factors for MDR pathogens. The incidence of MDR pathogens is also closely linked to local factors and varies widely from one institution to another [9].

VAP is commonly suspected in a patient receiving mechanical ventilation for at least 48 hours, who develops new or progressive radiographic infiltrates, and at least two clinical signs of infection, such as fever/hypothermia, leukocytosis/leukopenia and purulent secretions. Other clinical signs may be of some value on a specific case-by-case basis, e. g., worsening gas exchange, increased inflammatory markers. Unfortunately, in critically ill patients, clinical signs of infection have marginal diagnostic specificity/sensitivity. Thus, the Clinical Pulmonary Infection Score (CPIS) is often calculated [10]. The CPIS is based on six clinical assessments (temperature, blood leukocyte count, volume and purulence of tracheal secretions, oxygenation, pulmonary radiographic findings, and semiquantitative culture of tracheal aspirate), each worth between 0 and 2 points. The CPIS showed a good correlation ($r = 0.84$, $p < 0.0001$) with quantitative bacteriology of bronchoalveolar lavage (BAL) samples. Moreover, a value ≥ 6 was the threshold to accurately identify patients with pneumonia.

Importantly, in patients with VAP, the diagnostic strategy should be sensitive enough to identify the greatest number of infected patients and enable early initiation of adequate empiric antibiotic treatment. On the other hand, patients without

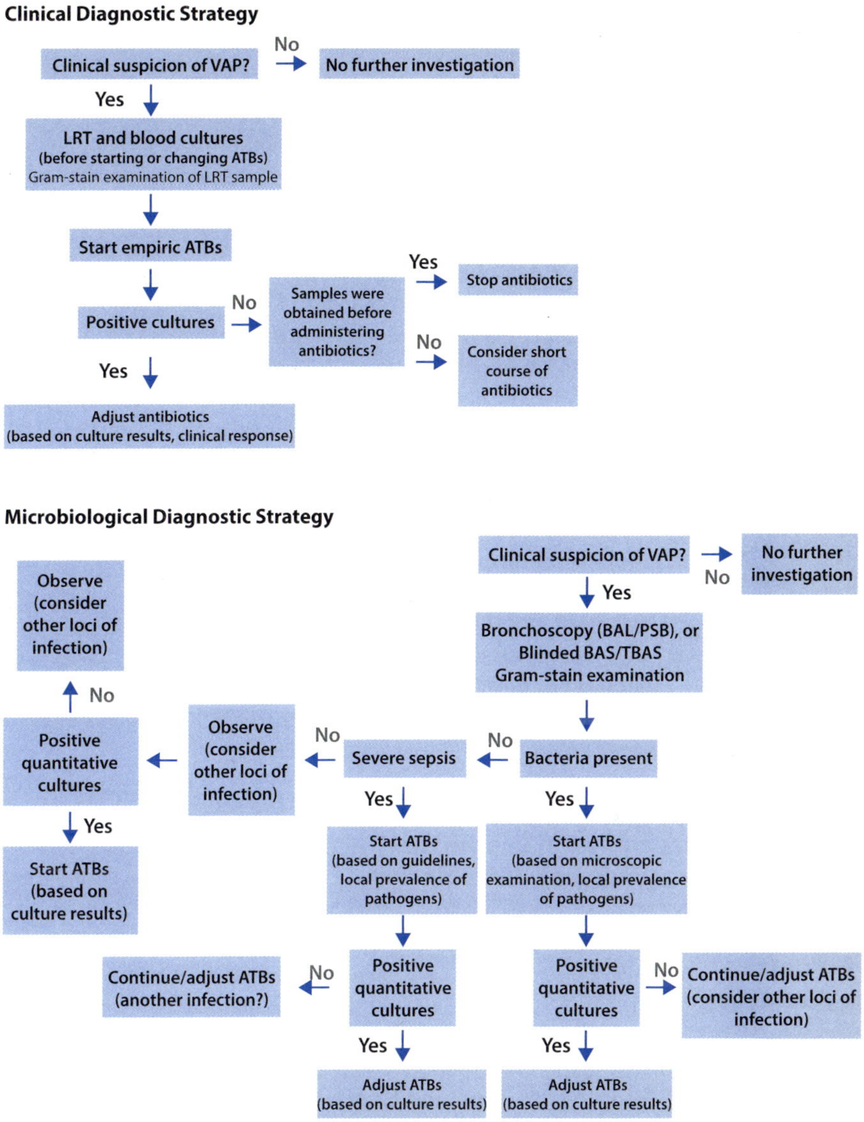

Fig. 1 On the *top*, a proposed clinical strategy for the diagnosis and treatment of ventilator-associated pneumonia (VAP). Gram-stain examination of tracheal secretions can be performed. The main drawback of this strategy is the potential overuse of antibiotics. On the *bottom*, the microbiological strategy for the diagnosis and treatment of VAP. Lower respiratory tract (LRT) samples are obtained through invasive (bronchoalveolar lavage [BAL], protected specimen brush [PSB]) or non-invasive (tracheal aspiration) techniques. Of note, this strategy has high specificity for the diagnosis of VAP, but lower sensitivity compared to the clinical strategy. BAS: bronchial aspirate; ATB: antibiotic; TBAS: tracheobronchial aspirate

infection should be discriminated to avoid overtreatment with antimicrobial drugs, and selection of MDR microorganisms.

In a patient with clinical suspicion of VAP, two diagnostic algorithms can be used following clinical suspicion of nosocomial pneumonia (Fig. 1). The clinical approach recommends treating every patient with suspicion of having a pulmonary infection with new antibiotics. Samples of respiratory secretions, such as endotracheal aspirate (ETA), should be obtained before the initiation of antibiotic treatment. In this strategy, the selection of appropriate empirical therapy is based on risk factors and local resistance patterns. The etiology of pneumonia is defined by semi-quantitative cultures of ETA or sputum, with potential Gram-stain examination of the sample. Antimicrobial therapy is adjusted according to culture results or clinical response. This clinical strategy provides antimicrobial treatment to the majority of the patients. The main drawback is that the high sensitivity of semi-quantitative cultures of tracheal aspirates may lead to antibiotic overtreatment.

The bacteriological strategy is based on the results of quantitative cultures of lower respiratory tract secretions. Samples can be obtained using ETA, BAL or protected specimen brush (PSB). Specific threshold cut-offs for each test (10^5–10^6 CFU/mL for ETA, 10^4 CFU/mL for BAL, and 10^3 CFU/mL for PSB) are applied to discriminate between colonizing microorganisms and those producing infection. Ideally, Gram-stain examination of these samples can be performed to improve early adequacy of antibiotic treatment. The bacteriological strategy attempts to identify patients with true VAP, reduce overuse of antibiotics and improve outcomes. Yet, false negative results may be obtained using this strategy, which leads to delayed antibiotic treatment and worse outcomes.

The Importance of Rapid Diagnostic Techniques for Ventilator-associated Pneumonia

Early diagnosis and initiation of appropriate antibiotic therapy for VAP is associated with improved outcomes; conversely, delayed or inappropriate administration of targeted antibiotic therapy is associated with increased mortality. In particular, inadequate therapy during the first 48 hours following clinical suspicion of VAP is associated with a 3-fold increase in mortality (91%), in comparison with patients appropriately treated (38%) [11]. The importance of a prompt microbiological diagnosis of VAP is aimed not only at optimizing antimicrobial treatment, but also at narrowing or de-escalating the initial empiric treatment, as soon as antimicrobial susceptibility data are available.

The main limitation in the use of standard microbiology cultures for the diagnosis of VAP and guiding empiric therapy is that the results are not available for 48 hours. Thus, several alternative techniques to microbial cultures have been developed to achieve a more rapid and accurate diagnosis of VAP (Table 1).

In this context, the Gram-stain examination of respiratory samples, described in the following paragraphs, can promptly provide information regarding the type of microorganisms and the purulency of the biomaterial (defined as ≥ 25 neutrophils

Table 1 Diagnostic methods for the identification of ventilator-associated pneumonia causative pathogens

Method	Required time to generate results	Advantages	Drawbacks
Bacterial culture	48–72 h	Diagnostic gold standard Quantitative analysis Assessment of antibiotic susceptibility Identification of bacterial species	Time to identify causative pathogen of an infection is overly long
Gram-stain	1 h	Rapid test Inexpensive test Direct analysis of clinical samples	Expertise required Considerable colonization is needed to identify causative pathogens Qualitative analysis No information on antibiotic susceptibility No identification of bacterial species
Nucleic acid-based amplification method (i. e., multiplex real-time PCR)	1 h	Direct analysis of clinical samples Multiple causative pathogens are tested Assessment of antibiotic susceptibility	Expensive Lack of clinical validation
Mass spectrometry (MS) (e. g., matrix-assisted laser desorption ionization time-of-fly (MALDI-TOF)	1–2 minutes, after standard bacterial culture	Identification of bacterial species Identification of bacterial toxins Assessment of antibiotic susceptibility	Reduced reliability during poly-microbial colonization Analysis performed only after standard culture
Electrospray ionization (ESI MS)	4–6 h	Direct analysis of clinical samples Semi-quantitative analysis	High risk of contamination (open work platform) Expensive test Reduced reliability during poly-microbial colonization

PCR: polymerase chain reaction.

and ≤ 10 squamous epithelial cells per low power field) [2]. As an alternative, new molecular-based methods for early identification of respiratory pathogens have been developed. Similar to the Gram-stain examination, molecular methods are aimed at identifying the causative agent of infection in a timely manner [12]; yet, these novel techniques can also determine antimicrobial susceptibility profiles. Molecular diagnostic techniques simultaneously target a wide range of bacterial species and resistance genes through polymerase chain reaction (PCR) amplification of nucleic acid. The technique most frequently applied is multiplex real-time PCR and detection through arrays, such as two dimensional micro-chips or three-dimensional beads and dye-labeled probes. More recently, rapid detection and identification of pathogens directly from clinical specimens can be performed with the use of matrix-assisted laser desorption ionization time-of-fly (MALDI-TOF) and PCR-electroSpray ionization mass spectrometry (PCR/ESI-MS) systems, which rely, however, on the use of expensive operating systems [13].

Some of the main advantages with use of molecular diagnostic techniques are the rapid results and the possibility to detect very low quantities of target sequences irrespective of pathogen viability or concomitant use of antibiotics. Additionally, these techniques also target specific sequences related to antimicrobial resistance and improve detection of microorganisms that are difficult to culture using conventional methods [14]. The main limitations are potential contamination, overlap among genetic sequences of different pathogens, lack of validation of some assays, complex interpretation of the results, and increased costs [12]. Finally, the majority of these systems only provide qualitative results, and it is difficult to distinguish between colonizers and invasive pathogens [13].

Gram-stain Examination of Respiratory Samples: Methodological Notes

Gram-stain examination is a technique applied to cluster bacterial species into two groups – Gram-positive and Gram-negative – based on specific features of their cell wall. The Gram-stain procedure begins by placing a very thin layer of respiratory sample onto a glass slide. The sample should be air-dried rather than heated, because the heat distorts bacterial and cell morphology. The sample is then stained with crystal violet and iodine. The length of time that crystal violet and iodine are left on the smear is not critical. A minimal 10-second stain with these reagents is sufficient. A decolorizing agent, such as ethanol or acetone, is then applied briefly, and the solution is rinsed across the smear. Gram-positive bacteria retain the crystal violet and iodine, because their thick cell wall comprises peptidoglycan. Conversely, a thinner cell-wall layer characterizes Gram-negative pathogens; thus, the stains are diffused from the bacteria with the use of ethanol. Finally, a counterstain, such as a red dye, safranin or fuchsin, is applied for at least 30 seconds to allow staining of Gram-negative bacteria and a clear distinction from Gram-positive microorganisms.

Upon microscopic examination, Gram-positive bacteria appear purple-blue; whereas, Gram-negative microorganisms are reddish (Fig. 2). Several other bacterial features may help in the correct identification of pathogens. In particular, the bacterial shape, e.g. cocci, rods, fusiform, narrows the range of potential causative pathogens. In addition, the presence and quantification of inflammatory cells increases the likelihood of an ongoing infection. Finally, the presence of oropharyngeal squamous epithelial cells corroborates contamination of the sample with saliva. Ideally, squamous epithelial cells should be less than 1% of all cells present in the field of view [15].

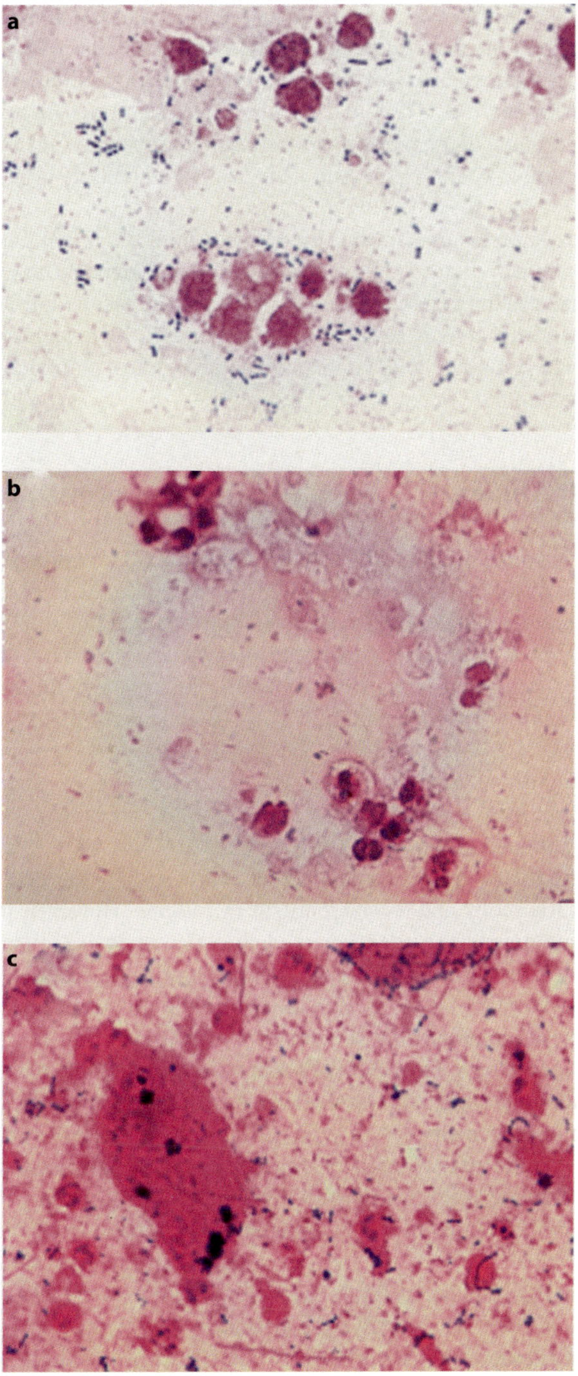

Fig. 2 Gram-stain images. **a** Gram-stain appearance of bronchoalveolar aspirate showing *Streptococcus pneumoniae* and *Haemophilus influenzae*. **b** Gram-stain appearance of bronchoalveolar aspirate showing Gram-negative bacilli and some intracellular bacteria. **c** Gram stain appearance of tracheal aspirate showing *Nocardia*. (1000 × magnification, Nikon Eclipse 50i Microscopy, Nikon digital sight- NIS Elements). Micrographs were kindly provided by Dr. Puig, Microbiology Department, Hospital Clinic, Barcelona, Spain

Gram-stain is a very rapid tool in the diagnosis of VAP and provides useful information on etiology; indeed, results may be ready within an hour. Additionally, the test is inexpensive to perform in comparison with newer molecular tests. A recent meta-analysis [16] found no difference in Gram-stain results in patients undergoing antibiotic therapy and those without therapy. Thus, in comparison with standard microbiology cultures, Gram-stain is not significantly influenced by ongoing antibiotic therapy.

Nevertheless, several limitations should be highlighted. First of all, the Gram-stain technique requires considerable experience to adequately assess the samples and provide reliable results. Additionally, considerable colonization of the sample is needed – at least 10^5 organisms per milliliter – to identify pathogens on microscopy [17]. Finally, the technique does not quantify pathogens and does not provide any information on bacterial viability.

The Value of Gram-stain in Ventilator-associated Pneumonia

Given the rapid results and the valuable interpretation of respiratory samples using Gram-stain, there has been considerable interest in recent years on the role of this technique in the diagnosis of VAP, as detailed in Table 2.

In a recent meta-analysis, O'Horo and colleagues pooled data from 24 studies published from 1994 to 2008; the primary aim was to determine the value of Gram-stain examination in the diagnosis of patients with clinical suspicion of VAP [16]. Additionally, the possible role of Gram-stain examination in guiding empiric therapy was assessed. The meta-analysis included a total of 3,148 respiratory samples obtained through BAL, mini-BAL, ETA and PSB. Gram-stain examination was associated with a sensitivity of 0.79 and specificity of 0.74. Additionally, there was fair agreement (κ 0.54) between bacteria identified through microscopy and those identified by culture. However, it is important to emphasize that among the studies included in the analysis, several did not report antibiotic use; furthermore, the studied populations, the methods used to obtain respiratory specimens and the Gram-stain examination were highly heterogeneous. Based on these limitations, the authors concluded that Gram-stain examination should not be recommended to guide early antimicrobial therapy; nevertheless Gram-stain examination was slightly more sensitive in the diagnosis of VAP caused by Gram-positive bacteria; finally, Gram-stain results had a very high negative predictive value.

In the last two decades, several key studies assessed the role of Gram-stain examination in the diagnosis of VAP. In a study published by Blot et al. in 2000 [18], ETA and PSB samples were concomitantly obtained from 91 suspected cases of VAP to evaluate concordance between Gram-stain and microbiology results. The sensitivity and specificity of Gram-stain examination in the diagnosis of microbiologically-confirmed pneumonia were, respectively, 91% and 64% for ETA and 70% and 96% for samples obtained through PSB. Thus, the authors proposed a diagnostic algorithm based on three possible combinations: 1) When Gram-stain examination of ETA samples is negative, VAP is highly improbable and therapy should be delayed

Table 2 Studies assessing the value of Gram-stain examination in the diagnosis of microbiologically-confirmed ventilator-associated pneumonia

Study	Year	Number of samples	Collection Methods	Study Design	Main results vs. bacterial identification through standard cultures
Allaouchiche et al. [23]	1996	163	BAL	Prospective cohort study	Se 92, Sp 76.5, PPV 69, NPV 91, κ 0.44
Allaouchiche et al. [24]	1999	146	BAL	Prospective cohort study	Se 90.2, Sp 73.7, PPV 64.8, NPV 93.3, κ 0.586
Blot et al. [18]	2000	91	BAL/ETA	Prospective cohort study	ETA: Se 89, Sp 56, PPV 53, NPV 90 PTC: Se 74, Sp 97, PPV 93, NPV 87
Duflo et al. [25]	2001	116	Mini-BAL	Prospective cohort study	Se 76.2, Sp 100, PPV 100, NPV 75.4, κ 0.73
Davis et al. [26]	2005	155	BAL	Retrospective chart review	GP: Se 87, Sp 59, PPV 68, NPV 83 GN: Se 73, Sp 49, PPV 78, NPV 42
Kopelman [27]	2006	227	BAL	Retrospective chart review	GP: Se 79.7, Sp 65.6 %, PPV 47.7 %, NPP 89.2 % GN: Se 67.0%, Sp 73.6 %, PPV 68.9 %, NPV 71.8 %
Veinstein et al. [19]	2006	78	PTC/ETA	Multicenter prospective trial	Se 83, Sp 74, PPV 79, NPV 79 (combining the two techniques)
Albert et al. [21]	2008	705	BAL/ETA	Retrospective analysis of multicenter randomized control trial	Se 74, Sp 72, PPV 75, NPV 70, κ 0.36
Goldberg et al. [28]	2008	309	BAL	Prospective trial	Se 90, Sp 67, PPV 45, NPV 96
O'Horo et al. [16]	2012	3141	BAL/PTC/ETA	Meta-analysis	Se 79, Sp 74, PPV 40, NPV 90
Gottesman et al. [22]	2014	115	ETA	Prospective cohort study	GP: Se 90.47, Sp 82, PPV 57, NPV 97 GN: Se 69.6, Sp 77, PPV 97, NPV 20 Sterile culture: Se 50, Sp 79, PPV 13, NPV 96 κ 0.54

Se: sensitivity (%); Sp: specificity (%); PPV: positive predictive value (%); NPV: negative predictive value (%); BAL: bronchoalveolar lavage; ETA: endotracheal aspirate; GP: Gram-positive; GN: Gram-negative; PTC: plugged telescoping catheter; κ: kappa statistic.

until microbiology results become available; 2) when Gram-stain examination of PSB samples is positive, VAP is probable and antibiotic therapy should be promptly administered and later readjusted based on microbiology results; finally, 3) when Gram-stain examination of PSB samples is negative, but Gram-stain examination of ETA is positive, diagnosis of VAP should be confirmed from standard microbiology results; antibiotic therapy should be initiated only in patients with severe signs of infection. In a later report by the same group [19], the value of concomitant Gram-stain evaluation of PSB and ETA samples was reassessed and the aforementioned diagnostic algorithm validated. Seventy-six patients with clinical suspicion of VAP were enrolled into the trial. The diagnostic algorithm allowed early appropriate antibiotic therapy in 83% of the patients with microbiologically confirmed pneumonia, and 74% of those without confirmed infection. The rate of appropriate diagnosis and therapy using this algorithm was significantly higher compared with a strategy based on the CPIS (80 vs. 50%, $p<0.001$). Thus, it seems that combining Gram-stain examination of the distal airways (PSB) with microbiological confirmation of VAP could help guide initial antibiotic therapy, particularly when severe signs of infection are also taken into account. Nevertheless, further larger studies are needed to confirm these findings, particularly, in patients with greater VAP severity.

In 2006, the Canadian Critical Care Trials group published a study on 740 patients included in a randomized trial to compare two diagnostic strategies of VAP (BAL with quantitative culture of the BAL fluid or ETA with non-quantitative culture of the aspirate) [20]. In a subsequent analysis of these patients [21], investigators retrospectively examined the correlation between Gram-stain examination of respiratory samples and microbiology results. They found a very poor association, both in the analysis of ETA and BAL samples, and warned about the risks associated with withholding antibiotic therapy based on Gram-stain results. Nevertheless, similar to the results by O'Horo et al. [16], they found a high negative predictive value associated with Gram-positive microorganisms (93%). Thus, it would be reasonable to stop empiric therapy against Gram-positive bacteria when Gram-stain examination yields negative results and no previous history of methicillin-resistant *S. aureus* is confirmed.

The most recent prospective clinical trial [22] that assessed the diagnostic efficacy of Gram-stain examination, specifically focused on the negative predictive value of this technique in the context of *S. aureus* VAP. Gottesman et al. [22] enrolled 114 patients with clinical suspicion of VAP, excluding patients with a recent change in antibiotic therapy in the previous 48 hours. Interestingly, Gram-stain sensitivity was 90.5% for Gram-positive cocci, 69.6% for Gram-negative rods and 50% for negative cultures; whereas, specificity was 82.5, 77.8 and 79%, respectively. In agreement with previous publications, these authors reported a high negative predictive values for Gram-positive cocci (97%) as well as for negative culture (96%), but a low negative predictive value for Gram-negative rods (20%). Finally, the positive predictive values for Gram-positive pathogens, negative results and Gram-negative microorganisms were 57, 97 and 13%, respectively. Although this study had a few limitations – single center study, lack of power due to only 21 cases of *S.*

aureus VAP – it was confirmed that the absence of Gram-positive bacteria on early microscopic examination has a high negative predictive value and could help avoid unnecessary antibiotics against these pathogens.

Conclusion

In conclusion, the use and validity of Gram-stain examination in the diagnosis of VAP is still highly debated. A few studies in particular support its use, specifically in patients at risk of Gram-positive colonization, when samples from distal airways are obtained and concomitant standard microbiology techniques are applied. Nevertheless, further studies are needed to corroborate the value of this "old" technique, particularly now that several alternative molecular methods for early diagnosis of VAP are being developed. Importantly, identifying the causative agent of infection in a timely manner and determining its antimicrobial susceptibility profile is pivotal in the management of VAP patients. Conventional microbiology methods are overly long for optimal patient care and potentially increase risks for development of MDR pathogens. Development and validation of molecular diagnostic techniques and a reappraisal of Gram-stain examination within a multi-tiered diagnostic approach should be a primary focus to improve patient care.

References

1. Hunter JD (2012) Ventilator associated pneumonia. BMJ 344:e3325
2. American Thoracic Society and Infectious Diseases Society of America (2005) Guidelines for the management of adults with hospital-acquired, ventilator-associated, and healthcare-associated pneumonia. Am J Respir Crit Care Med 171:388–416
3. Fagon JY, Chastre J (2003) Diagnosis and treatment of nosocomial pneumonia in ALI/ARDS patients. Eur Respir J Suppl 42:83
4. Rello J, Ollendorf DA, Oster G et al (2002) Epidemiology and outcomes of ventilator-associated pneumonia in a large US database. Chest 122:2115–2121
5. Warren DK, Shukla SJ, Olsen MA et al (2003) Outcome and attributable cost of ventilator-associated pneumonia among intensive care unit patients in a suburban medical center. Crit Care Med 31:1312–1317
6. Zimlichman E, Henderson D, Tamir O et al (2013) Health care-associated infections: a meta-analysis of costs and financial impact on the US health care system. JAMA Intern Med 173:2039–2046
7. Bekaert M, Timsit JF, Vansteelandt S et al (2011) Attributable mortality of ventilator-associated pneumonia: a reappraisal using causal analysis. Am J Respir Crit Care Med 184:1133–1139
8. Di Pasquale M, Ferrer M, Esperatti M et al (2014) Assessment of severity of ICU-acquired pneumonia and association with etiology. Crit Care Med 42:303–312
9. Rello J, Sa-Borges M, Correa H, Leal SR, Baraibar J (1999) Variations in etiology of ventilator-associated pneumonia across four treatment sites: implications for antimicrobial prescribing practices. Am J Respir Crit Care Med 160:608–613
10. Pugin J, Auckenthaler R, Mili N, Janssens JP, Lew PD, Suter PM (1991) Diagnosis of ventilator-associated pneumonia by bacteriologic analysis of bronchoscopic and nonbronchoscopic "blind" bronchoalveolar lavage fluid. Am Rev Respir Dis 143:1121–1129

11. Luna CM, Vujacich P, Niederman MS et al (1997) Impact of BAL data on the therapy and outcome of ventilator-associated pneumonia. Chest 111:676–685
12. Mothershed EA, Whitney AM (2006) Nucleic acid-based methods for the detection of bacterial pathogens: present and future considerations for the clinical laboratory. Clin Chim Acta 363:206–220
13. Lung M, Codina G (2012) Molecular diagnosis in HAP/VAP. Curr Opin Crit Care 18:487–494
14. Bhat N, O'Brien KL, Karron RA, Driscoll AJ, Murdoch DR (2012) Use and evaluation of molecular diagnostics for pneumonia etiology studies. Clin Infect Dis 54(Suppl 2):S153–S158
15. Bouza E, Torres MV, Burillo A (2005) The contribution of the microbiology laboratory to the diagnosis of ventilator-associated pneumonia. Enferm Infecc Microbiol Clin 23(Suppl 3):2–9
16. O'Horo JC, Thompson D, Safdar N (2012) Is the gram stain useful in the microbiologic diagnosis of VAP? A meta-analysis. Clin Infect Dis 55:551–561
17. Brooks GF, Carroll KC, Butel JS, Morse SA, Mietzner TA (2007) Jawetz, Melnick, & Adelberg's Medical Microbiology. McGraw Hill, New York
18. Blot F, Raynard B, Chachaty E, Tancrede C, Antoun S, Nitenberg G (2000) Value of gram stain examination of lower respiratory tract secretions for early diagnosis of nosocomial pneumonia. Am J Respir Crit Care Med 162:1731–1737
19. Veinstein A, Brun-Buisson C, Derrode N et al (2006) Validation of an algorithm based on direct examination of specimens in suspected ventilator-associated pneumonia. Intensive Care Med 32:676–683
20. Canadian Critical Care Trials Group (2006) A randomized trial of diagnostic techniques for ventilator-associated pneumonia. N Engl J Med 355:2619–2630
21. Albert M, Friedrich JO, Adhikari NK, Day AG, Verdant C, Heyland DK (2008) Utility of Gram-stain in the clinical management of suspected ventilator-associated pneumonia. Secondary analysis of a multicenter randomized trial. J Crit Care 23:74–81
22. Gottesman T, Yossepowitch O, Lerner E et al (2014) The accuracy of Gram-stain of respiratory specimens in excluding Staphylococcus aureus in ventilator-associated pneumonia. J Crit Care 29:739–742
23. Allaouchiche B, Jaumain H, Dumontet C, Motin J (1996) Early diagnosis of ventilator-associated pneumonia. Is it possible to define a cutoff value of infected cells in BAL fluid? Chest 110:1558–1565
24. Allaouchiche B, Jaumain H, Chassard D, Bouletreau P (1999) Gram-stain of bronchoalveolar lavage fluid in the early diagnosis of ventilator-associated pneumonia. Br J Anaesth 83:845–849
25. Duflo F, Allaouchiche B, Debon R, Bordet F, Chassard D (2001) An evaluation of the Gram-stain in protected bronchoalveolar lavage fluid for the early diagnosis of ventilator-associated pneumonia. Anesth Analg 92:442–447
26. Davis KA, Eckert MJ, Reed RL et al (2005) Ventilator-associated pneumonia in injured patients: do you trust your Gram's stain? J Trauma 58:462–466
27. Kopelman TR (2006) Can empiric broad-spectrum antibiotics for ventilator-associated pneumonia be narrowed based on Gram's stain results of bronchoalveolar lavage fluid. Am J Surg 192:812–816
28. Goldberg AE, Malhotra AK, Riaz OJ et al (2008) Predictive value of broncho-alveolar lavage fluid Gram's stain in the diagnosis of ventilator-associated pneumonia: a prospective study. J Trauma 65:871–876

Central Line-associated Bloodstream Infections: A Critical Look at the Role and Research of Quality Improvement Interventions and Strategies

K. Blot, D. Vogelaers, and S. Blot

Introduction

Central venous catheters (CVC) are ubiquitous in the intensive care unit (ICU). Central lines are necessary for infusion, withdrawal of blood, or hemodynamic monitoring. Unfortunately, use of these devices predisposes to the development of central line-associated bloodstream infections (CLABSI). Approximately half of the patients admitted to the ICU require a CVC [1], and these catheters account for the majority of CLABSIs [2]. In the USA, up to 5 million CVCs are inserted each year and approximately 200,000 patients reportedly develop a CLABSI; the number of deaths attributable to these infections has been estimated at 25,000 (12.5%), equating to 0.5% of CVC insertions [3]. The 2009 Extended Prevalence of Infection in Intensive Care (EPIC II) study reported that, of 13,796 adult patients, 7,087 (51%) were classified as infected on the day of the study; BSIs accounted for 15% of these infections, however, this percentage includes BSIs of unknown origin (not related to an infection at another site, including intravascular-access devices) and secondary BSIs (related to an infection with the same organism at another site). CLABSIs were responsible for 4.7% of all ICU infections [4]. A 2011 systematic review calculated that CLABSIs were associated with the highest number of preventable deaths and associated costs compared to other healthcare-associated infections [5].

CLABSIs have been shown to cause additional patient morbidity, leading to longer ICU length of stay (LOS) and increased hospital costs [6]. These infections can lead to metastatic infection, severe sepsis and multiple organ failure (MOF). Published estimates of extra hospital costs attributable to CLABSI vary: $6,005–9,738 [7], €13,585 [6], $25,849–$29,156 [8], and $34,508–$56,000 [9]. Total yearly costs to the US healthcare system range between $300 million and $2 billion [10]. Reported attributable catheter-related BSI mortality ranges from 0–35% [9]

K. Blot ✉ · D. Vogelaers · S. Blot
Faculty of Medicine and Health Sciences, Ghent University, Ghent, Belgium
e-mail: koen.blot@ugent.be

J.-L. Vincent (ed.), *Annual Update in Intensive Care and Emergency Medicine 2015*,
DOI 10.1007/978-3-319-13761-2_2

and 4–20% [8]. However, the attributable impact of these infections on mortality is still debated [2, 11].

There are four ways in which a catheter tip can become contaminated [1].

1. Skin microorganisms migrate along the external surface of the catheter tract and colonize the catheter tip.
2. The catheter or catheter hub is contaminated by contact with hands, fluids or devices. Organisms subsequently migrate along the internal surface towards the catheter tip.
3. Microorganisms from another focus of infection may hematogenously colonize the catheter.
4. Direct infusate contamination.

Colonization of the catheter tip may then lead to bloodstream infection. Routes 1 and 2 constitute the vast majority of CLABSIs and are the focus of preventive interventions [2].

Quality Improvement Interventions

Despite the presence of evidence-based interventions, a quality gap exists between evidence and practice [9]. Quality improvement strategies improve reliability of care by making the implementation of best practice easier to achieve. In this fashion, the quality gap towards a zero infection rate can be envisaged [10]. An estimated 65–70% of CLABSI cases are preventable with current evidence-based strategies. If best practices in infection control were applied in all US hospitals, the estimated number of preventable deaths and associated costs range from 5,520–20,239 lives and $960 million to $18.2 billion annually. Due to their preventable nature, Medicare has stopped providing reimbursement for treatment of CLABSIs [5].

As part of the 100,000 Lives Campaign, implemented from January 2005 through June 2006, the Institute of Healthcare Improvement (IHI) offered nationwide hospital support to reduce morbidity and mortality in American healthcare. Among other steps, the IHI campaign encouraged use of central line bundles to prevent catheter-related BSIs. Bundles were defined as a structured way of improving processes of care and patient outcomes. Each bundle consists of a small, straightforward set of practices that have been recommended to decrease CLABSIs when performed collectively [12–14]. The IHI central line bundle includes five evidence-based preventive interventions: Use of hand hygiene, maximal sterile barriers upon catheter insertion, chlorhexidine skin antisepsis, optimal catheter site selection (with avoidance of the femoral vein), and daily review of line necessity with prompt removal of unnecessary lines. This bundle can be combined or used as a checklist to facilitate compliance to prevention measures during catheter insertion and maintenance.

In addition to encouraging use of the aforementioned preventive interventions, the 2011 CDC guidelines emphasize education and training of healthcare personnel, use of bundled strategies, and documenting and reporting rates of compliance with

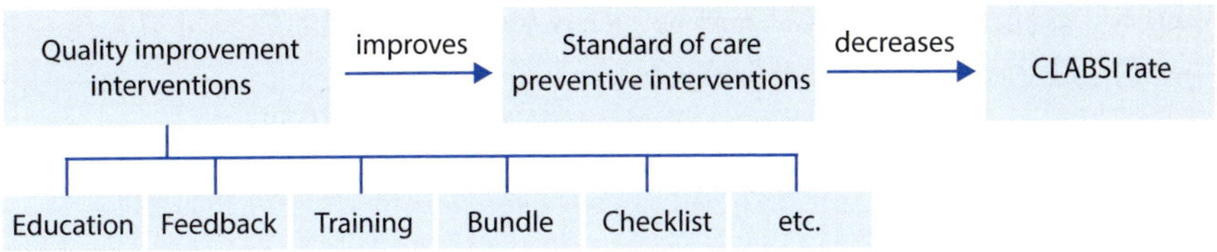

Fig. 1 Quality improvement interventions and impact on baseline standard of care. CLABSI: central line-associated blood stream infection

bundle components as benchmarks for quality assurance and performance improvement. Use of antiseptic/antibiotic impregnated short-term CVCs and chlorhexidine impregnated sponge dressings are encouraged if the infection rate is not decreasing despite adherence to other strategies. The guidelines conclude by stating that interventions to improve reliability of care should focus on rendering the implementation of best practice easier to achieve [2].

Quality improvement interventions are distinct from preventive ones insofar that they improve compliance with the standard of care, which consists of an ICU's baseline care item processes (Fig. 1).

Methods of Quality Improvement

A recent systematic review and meta-analysis of studies using quality improvement initiatives to prevent CLABSIs classified the various interventions that were introduced in adult ICUs [15]. The result was a diverse list of methods for improving compliance with preventive interventions during CVC insertion and maintenance (Table 1).

These interventions focused on different areas for improvement. Certain initiatives were actively implemented to enforce change in process adherence. Such examples include the use of bundles and checklists, surveillance of compliance, and nurse empowerment to stop and redo CVC procedures when a bundle care item was incorrectly applied or forgotten. Other methods aimed to increase best practice implementation through designation of leaders to facilitate introduction of new initiatives, introduction of care process aids (procedure flowcharts or algorithms and daily goals lists), pre-packaged materials with all supplies necessary to insert or maintain a CVC (pre-packaged cart or CVC kits), infrastructure changes (facility renovations and installation of hand-rub dispensers), or organizational changes (leader designation, staffing of extra personnel and assistance or supervision in central line insertion). Other more passive interventions focused on knowledge transmission included education and training of personnel, and feedback of CLABSI or preventive item compliance rates.

Table 1 Classification of quality improvement interventions

Quality improvement intervention	Definition and examples
Enforcement of prevention measure adherence	
Bundle	A short list of IHI prevention measures for CVC insertion and/or maintenance
Checklist	Checklist of bundled care item prevention measures
Empowerment to stop procedure	Nurses are empowered to halt and restart CVC insertion care or maintenance when a prevention measure is not implemented correctly to ensure optimal catheter care
Surveillance: compliance-monitoring	Nurses supervise CVC insertion or maintenance prevention measures
Facilitation of best practice implementation	
Leader designation	A leader is designated to facilitate implementation of quality improvement intervention
Pre-packaging of CVC materials	Use of a CVC cart or kit stocked with all supplies necessary to insert or maintain a central line
Infrastructure changes	Changes to hospital infrastructure to facilitate adherence to prevention measures
Organizational changes	Increased staffing to decrease the patient-to-nurse ratio, provide compliance surveillance, or assistance in central line insertion
Information transfer	
Education	Teaching lectures or tests transmitting theoretical knowledge concerning CLABSI
Training	Training sessions for aseptic CVC insertion and maintenance
Feedback	Reporting of CLABSI or care item compliance rates to ICU personnel during team rounds or through posters

Adapted from [15]. CLABSI: central line-associated bloodstream infection; CVC: central venous catheter; IHI: Institute for Healthcare Improvement.

Research of Interventions

Recent research has focused on the prevention of CLABSI through quality improvement interventions, meant to increase compliance to evidence-based preventive measures. Two systematic reviews were unable to conclusively decide which initiatives should be recommended for widespread implementation [10,16]. Two meta-analyses assessed the effect of quality improvement initiatives on the CLABSI rate in interrupted time-series study designs. There was no decrease in overall infection rates when combining the results of the six included studies, with individual trials reporting rate increases and decreases [17]. However, another meta-analysis identified different trials by employing different inclusion criteria and demonstrated similar CLABSI rate decreases for 41 before-after and six interrupted time series study design trials [15]. Subgroup analysis of the before-after trials identified a significantly stronger CLABSI rate decrease (odds ratio 0.34 vs. 0.45) among trials implementing bundle and/or checklist interventions. The interrupted time series studies demonstrated a decrease at 3 months post-intervention. This overall intervention effect was not sustained over longer follow-up periods, possibly reflecting the presence of a Hawthorne effect. This phenomenon, defined as the alteration of behavior by the subjects of a study due to their awareness of being observed, complicates the interpretation of trials assessing the utility of quality improvement initiatives. However, the short-term effect of quality improvement interventions might as well be explained by a timely increased awareness of the problem. It is well known that initiatives in infection prevention and control need rehearsal to keep the team alert.

Issues in Quality Improvement Research

There are inherent factors that complicate the measurement of hospital-acquired infection rates. CLABSI rates fluctuate naturally throughout the year. Sudden increases can occur during epidemic infectious outbreaks, defined as an unusual increase above the baseline rate of a specific infection or infecting organism. Contrarily, observed CLABSI rate decreases, certainly in the case of high baseline CLABSI rates, can be due to regression to the mean. Regression toward the mean is a term used to describe the phenomenon in which extreme values for parameters (such as a disproportionately high infection rate) will spontaneously return to their average (lower) values over time [10]. This is relevant when hospital units decide to implement and study interventions due to a perceived sudden infection rate increase. A spontaneous return toward the average infection rate could be misinterpreted as a result of the studied intervention. Such phenomena complicate the interpretation of simple before-after studies because these study designs lack the multiple data points necessary to identify these influential factors. Interrupted time series studies provide at least three data points before and after a well-defined intervention implementation period. Analysis of interrupted time series study designs through time series regression detects whether an intervention has an effect greater than the underlying baseline trend by comparing baseline and post-intervention infection rate slopes [18]. However, this precludes the analysis of quality improvement studies implementing interventions in a step-wise manner, a technique of gradual introduction of interventions for which there is evidence of efficacy [19], since these study designs require the designation of a well-defined point in time at which the initiative begins.

Other confounding factors complicate the study of quality improvement interventions for the prevention of hospital-acquired infections. Measuring adherence to prevention measures, such as hand hygiene, offers perspective on whether an infection rate decrease is due to a successful increase in compliance as a direct result of the quality improvement intervention. Nonetheless, this does not avoid the Hawthorne phenomenon, but rather affirms its presence. Blinding of personnel to the intervention is difficult, since the quality improvement explicitly aims to change healthcare personnel practice standards. Likewise, randomization of interventions aimed at improving awareness and adherence to prevention measures is unattainable within a hospital unit due to communication and spread of awareness between personnel. Crossover study designs that aim to introduce and later negate interventions between two study periods would have difficulty correcting for the wash-over effect of increased prevention measure compliance between periods.

Furthermore, implementation of quality improvement interventions to improve compliance to care items to change CLABSI risk exposure, such as the IHI care bundle item 'daily review of central line necessity with prompt removal of unnecessary catheters', confound study results. Measurements of CLABSI require adjustment for risk exposure, hence the reporting of BSIs as a rate per 1,000 central line days. Nevertheless, this adjustment does not properly account for changes in the device-utilization rate (equal to number of catheter-days divided by number of patient-days). Not all catheter days are equal in terms of risk exposure. Interventions to decrease central line usage within an ICU can lead to the selection of a post-intervention cohort of central line patients with longer average duration of catheterization, since patients who were previously treated with short-term central line usage are now managed without, leading to their exclusion from the study population [20]. Additionally, since CDC definitions for central line days do not account for the presence of multiple catheters per patient, a risk adjustment is not feasible. Although statistically equivalent, a catheter-day from days 1–2 contains less infection risk than days 14–15 due to microbial biofilm development and accumulating gaps in prevention measure adherence. The calculation of a post-intervention CLABSI rate with a selection of central line patients with longer duration of catheterization could overestimate the infection rate, thereby underestimating the impact of the quality improvement intervention. Likewise, changes in device-utilization rates leading to increased central line use, associated with decreases in mean catheterization duration, could overestimate the impact of implemented initiatives.

In a recent meta-analysis, it was revealed that, of studies reporting central line and patient days, the device-utilization rate both increased and decreased between pre- and post-intervention periods, regardless of whether the study introduced the care bundle item 'daily review of line necessity' [15]. Furthermore, the majority of these studies did not report nor adjust for this difference in device-utilization rates. To help assess the impact on the CLABSI rates, the mean duration of catheterization should be reported in turn. However, since many studies calculate the average catheterization duration by dividing central line days (a CDC definition that does not take into account the presence of multiple catheters per patient) by the number of inserted central line catheters, this value is likewise difficult to interpret.

The aforementioned confounding factors in research, and clinical heterogeneity between studies, such as differing baseline standards of care and different quality improvement interventions, make it difficult to extrapolate results from research to practice. Even with excellent internal validity in a high-quality study, i. e., low level of within-study bias, the question remains as to whether the results achieved in one ICU with a specific quality improvement intervention can be extrapolated to another with a different baseline standard of care. Because quality improvement initiatives increase compliance to preventive measures, the external validity of trial results,

i. e., the applicability of the results to other ICU settings, is largely dependent on the similarity of the baseline standard of care between hospital units. Making this comparison is complicated by the sheer number of applicable preventive interventions, as recommended by recent guidelines [2], such that adherence to all items cannot realistically be fully measured.

Applying Quality Improvement Strategies

Considering the current evidence for the efficacy of quality improvement for the prevention of CLABSI, notwithstanding the limitations associated with this type of research, the next question that poses itself is how these interventions can be optimally implemented in ICUs. Understanding the requirements of successful adaptation of interventions in varying hospital settings is essential [21]. Several studies have already studied the impact of strategies for the implementation of quality improvement initiatives.

One study chose to adopt a pro-active approach to eliminating CRBSI through what they called a 'root cause analysis team'. Through continuous monitoring, Shannon et al. aimed to avert increases in infection rates through reactionary preventive interventions targeting the cause of measured spikes of infections [22]. This approach was supported through use of an improvement system: Perfecting Patient Care (PPC). The PPC methods entail five steps for quality improvement: (i) Establish the true dimension of the current problem and establish zero as the goal; (ii) observe the actual work to find opportunities to standardize processes and stabilize systems; (iii) move quickly from retrospective data to actionable, real-time data analyzed and acted on immediately with every symptomatic patient; (iv) solve problems one by one as close to the time and place of occurrence as possible; and (v) provide continuous education in both process improvement and technique for new and rotating staff members. These steps were adapted and implemented as five initiatives: Chart review of patients with central lines, observation of line placement and maintenance, real-time investigation of individual infections, developing counter-measures, and continuous learning. These new processes were implemented over a 90-day period and led to a reduction in CLABSI rates (10.5 to 1.2 CLABSI per 1,000 catheter days) despite an increased use of central lines and number of catheter days.

Other studies described related methods to guide the process of implementing quality improvement strategies. In a quality improvement study, 70% of surveyed hospitals reported having a procedure for conducting root cause analysis [23]. Another used corporate process-improvement Six Sigma methods to minimize variability or defects in their catheter-related BSI prevention procedures. The Six Sigma methodology ascribes causes of defects (increases in infection rates) to the six 'M's: Mother nature, manpower, measurement, materials, methods, and machines. Five of these factors were respectively defined as patient factors, personnel factors, culture technique, catheter issues, and sterile training/technique. These factors were discussed at regular ICU meetings with the medical ICU director, nursing staff, resident physicians, infection control staff and facilitation personnel versed in Six Sigma methodology. Different healthcare personnel ascribed different factors to be the cause of a higher infection rate. For each factor, a list of areas for improvement was made. Quality improvement interventions were introduced in a stepwise fashion to tackle these issues, beginning with simple and progressing into complex process changes. These initiatives were supplemented with the use of an action plan depicting what was being changed, why it was being changed, and when. This led to a reduction in the infection rate from 11 to 1.7 CLABSI per 1000 catheter days over a period of two years [24].

Another method is the Comprehensive Unit-Based Safety Program, which aims to improve patient safety culture through eight steps: Measurement of the patient safety climate through surveys, staff education on the science of safety, identification of staff's safety concerns, adoption of a unit by a senior executive that meets monthly with the team, implementation of three improvement interventions, documentation of the results, online sharing of the safety stories, and finally re-measurement of the safety culture through surveys [25]. Multiple studies have documented success in decreasing CLABSI rates with this quality improvement strategy [21, 26–28].

Three studies implemented their quality improvement strategies using a plan-do-study-act (PDSA) model for improvement [23, 29, 30]. The PDSA cycle is a four-step plan, which consists of planning processes, implementing them, studying the results, and subsequently analyzing the processes to correct for gaps between actual and planned results. One study described the barriers and issues identified through the PDSA cycle [29]. Small tests of change could encounter resistance with groups outside the ICU and halt process improvement. Thus the status quo remained due to a lack of facilitated cooperation across hospital groups. Furthermore, during collaborative site visits, a platform introduced for teams to air issues with hospital leadership, a bias was noted towards discussion and presentation of successes rather than barriers to quality improvement. Other barriers that were identified included finding a consistent time for team rounds and getting physicians to attend. Physician participation was hindered by time constraints and competing demands. Although they perceived designation of physician champions to be a crucial initiative to the success of the collaborative, few had training or interest in team-based or system-level quality improvement concepts. Nurses were perceived to be the most enthusiastic participants; however, professional boundaries could lead to objections. For instance, at some sites, introduction of the nursing central line checklist was met with resistance because they considered surveillance of physician process adherence not to be part of their job responsibilities. However, the most burdensome challenge proved to be the increase in workload associated with the collection, management and reporting of data.

Quality improvement interventions themselves can be used as methods to identify barriers for change. One study implemented a central line checklist for the IHI care bundle items and discovered a low compliance with the item 'maximal sterile barrier precautions'. Not surprisingly, the analysis revealed that CLABSI was more likely to develop in patients in whom maximal sterile barrier precautions were not utilized and when central lines were inserted by non-intensivists [31]. Such results provide an indication of areas for improvement through stepwise introduction of new interventions.

Conclusion

Optimal quality improvement measures for the prevention of CLABSIs remain important due to the preventable nature of these infections, their associated morbidity, mortality, and economic costs due to increased length of hospitalization and resource use. Research of quality improvement interventions will continue to be hampered by the inability to comply with the requirements for high-quality research, such as personnel and patient blinding or treatment randomization. Considering these inherent limitations, there remains evidence for the beneficial impact of quality improvement interventions. However, extrapolating the achieved results in one ICU to another remains difficult due to differing baseline standard of care practices. Proper intervention implementation requires an understanding of the requirements for successful adaptation. Introduction of quality improvement interventions can be achieved through multifaceted strategies such as Six Sigma, Comprehensive Unit-based Safety Program, and PDSA, which aim to gradually introduce initiatives while identifying specific barriers.

References

1. Mermel LA (2000) Prevention of intravascular catheter-related infections. Ann Intern Med 132:391–402
2. O'Grady NP, Alexander M, Burns LA et al (2011) Guidelines for the prevention of intravascular catheter-related infections. Clin Infect Dis 52(162):193
3. Hockenhull JC, Dwan K, Boland A et al (2008) The clinical effectiveness and cost-effectiveness of central venous catheters treated with anti-infective agents in preventing bloodstream infections: a systematic review and economic evaluation. Health Technol Assess 12:iii–iv (xi–xii, 1–154)
4. Vincent JL, Rello J, Marshall J et al (2009) International study of the prevalence and outcomes of infection in intensive care units. JAMA 302:2323–2329
5. Umscheid CA, Mitchell MD, Doshi JA, Agarwal R, Williams K, Brennan PJ (2011) Estimating the proportion of healthcare-associated infections that are reasonably preventable and the related mortality and costs. Infect Control Hosp Epidemiol 32:101–114
6. Blot SI, Depuydt P, Annemans L et al (2005) Clinical and economic outcomes in critically ill patients with nosocomial catheter-related bloodstream infections. Clin Infect Dis 41:1591–1598
7. Saint S, Veenstra DL, Lipsky BA (2000) The clinical and economic consequences of nosocomial central venous catheter-related infection: are antimicrobial catheters useful? Infect Control Hosp Epidemiol 21:375–380
8. Scott RD II (2009) The direct medical costs of healthcare-associated infections in u.s. hospitals and the benefits of prevention. http://www.cdc.gov/hai/pdfs/hai/scott_costpaper.pdf
9. Berenholtz SM, Lipsett PA, Pronovost PJ et al (2004) Eliminating catheter-related bloodstream infections in the intensive care unit. Crit Care Med 32:2014–2020

10. Ranji SR, Shetty K, Posley KA et al (2007) Vol 6: Prevention of Healthcare–Associated Infections) Closing the Quality Gap: A Critical Analysis of Quality Improvement Strategies, Agency for Healthcare Research and Quality, Rockville
11. Eggimann P, Sax H, Pittet D (2004) Catheter-related infections. Microb Infect 6:1033–1042
12. Timsit JF, Laupland KB (2012) Update on bloodstream infections in ICUs. Curr Opin Crit Care 18:479–486
13. Venkatram S, Rachmale S, Kanna B (2010) Study of device use adjusted rates in health care-associated infections after implementation of 'bundles' in a closed-model medical intensive care unit. J Crit Care 25:174 e11–174 e18
14. Richardson J, Tjoelker R (2012) Beyond the central line-associated bloodstream infection bundle: the value of the clinical nurse specialist in continuing evidence-based practice changes. Clin Nurse Spec 26:205–211
15. Blot K, Bergs J, Vogelaers D, Blot S, Vandijck D (2014) Prevention of central line-associated bloodstream infections through quality improvement interventions: a systematic review and meta-analysis. Clin Infect Dis 59:96–105
16. Safdar NAC (2008) Educational interventions for prevention of healthcare-associated infection: A systematic review. Crit Care Med 36:933–940
17. Flodgren G, Conterno LO, Mayhew A, Omar O, Pereira CR, Shepperd S (2013) Interventions to improve professional adherence to guidelines for prevention of device-related infections. Cochrane Database Syst Rev 3:CD006559
18. Eccles M, Grimshaw J, Campbell M, Ramsay C (2003) Research designs for studies evaluating the effectiveness of change and improvement strategies. Qual Saf Health Care 12:47–52
19. Prior M, Guerin M, Grimmer-Somers K (2008) The effectiveness of clinical guideline implementation strategies – a synthesis of systematic review findings. J Eval Clin Pract 14:888–897
20. Longmate AG, Ellis KS, Boyle L et al (2011) Elimination of central-venous-catheter-related bloodstream infections from the intensive care unit. BMJ Qual Saf 20:174–180
21. Palomar M, Álvarez-Lerma F, Riera A et al (2013) Impact of a national multimodal intervention to prevent catheter-related bloodstream infection in the ICU: the Spanish experience. Crit Care Med 41:2364–2372
22. Shannon RP, Frndak D, Grunden N et al (2006) Using real-time problem solving to eliminate central line infections. Jt Comm J Qual Patient Saf 32:479–487
23. Koll BS, Straub TA, Jalon MS et al (2008) The CLABs collaborative: a regionwide effort to improve the quality of care in hospitals. Jt Comm J Qual Patient Saf 34:713–723
24. Frankel HL, Crede WB, Topal JE et al (2005) Use of corporate Six Sigma performance-improvement strategies to reduce incidence of catheter-related bloodstream infections in a surgical ICU. J Am Coll Surg 201:349–358
25. Pronovost P, Weast B, Rosenstein B et al (2005) Implementing and validating a comprehensive unit-based safety program. J Patient Saf 1:33–40
26. Pronovost P, Needham D, Berenholtz S et al (2006) An intervention to decrease catheter-related bloodstream infections in the ICU. N Engl J Med 355:2725–2732
27. DePalo VA, McNicoll L, Cornell M et al (2010) The Rhode Island ICU collaborative: a model for reducing central line-associated bloodstream infection and ventilator-associated pneumonia statewide. Qual Saf Health Care 19:555–561
28. Watson SR, George C, Martin M et al (2009) Preventing central line-associated bloodstream infections and improving safety culture: a statewide experience. Jt Comm J Qual Patient Saf 35:593–597
29. Bonello RS, Fletcher CE, Becker WK et al (2008) An intensive care unit quality improvement collaborative in nine Department of Veterans Affairs hospitals: reducing ventilator-associated pneumonia and catheter-related bloodstream infection rates. Jt Comm J Qual Patient Saf 34:639–645
30. Render ML, Hasselbeck R, Freyberg RW et al (2011) Reduction of central line infections in Veterans Administration intensive care units: an observational cohort using a central infrastructure to support learning and improvement. BMJ Qual Saf 20:725–732
31. Tang HJ, Lin HL, Lin YH, Leung PO, Chuang YC, Lai CC (2014) The impact of central line insertion bundle on central line-associated bloodstream infection. BMC Infect Dis 14:356

Clostridium difficile Infection

M. H. Wilcox, M. J. G. T. Vehreschild, and C. E. Nord

Introduction

Clostridium difficile is a Gram-positive, anaerobic, spore-producing anaerobe [1] responsible for approximately 50–70% of gastrointestinal infections in hospitalized patients [2, 3]. An episode of *C. difficile* infection (CDI) is defined as a clinical picture compatible with CDI (i. e., diarrhea, ileus and toxic megacolon) with microbiological evidence of *C. difficile* (ideally free *C. difficile* toxins) in stool, without reasonable evidence of another cause of diarrhea, or identification of pseudomembranous colitis during endoscopy, after colectomy or on autopsy [4, 5]. Life-threatening cases are associated with severe colitis and shock, and can require intensive care unit (ICU) admission and colectomy [4, 6].

CDI is increasingly recognized as a leading public health threat. European surveillance data indicate that CDI rates among hospitalized patients have increased in many countries [2] and that approximately one in ten cases of CDI cause – or contribute to – ICU admission or death, or lead to colectomy [6]. The infection significantly prolongs hospitalization, and total length of hospital stay in studies was on average 15 days [7]. In the US, the incidence of CDI among hospitalized adults almost doubled from 2001 to 2010, to 8.2 discharges per 1,000 total adult discharges [8]. Indeed, *C. difficile* is the most common pathogen isolated from patients with healthcare-associated infections in the US [3], causing an estimated

M. H. Wilcox ✉
Department of Medical Microbiology, Leeds Teaching Hospitals and Leeds Institute of Biomedical and Clinical Sciences, Faculty of Medicine and Health, University of Leeds, Leeds, UK
e-mail: mark.wilcox@leedsth.nhs.uk

M. J. G. T. Vehreschild
1st Department of Internal Medicine, German Centre for Infection Research (DZIF), University Hospital of Cologne, Cologne, Germany

C. E. Nord
Division of Clinical Microbiology, Department of Laboratory Medicine, Karolinska Institute, Karolinska University Hospital Huddinge, Stockholm, Sweden

J.-L. Vincent (ed.), *Annual Update in Intensive Care and Emergency Medicine 2015*,
DOI 10.1007/978-3-319-13761-2_3

250,000 infections and 14,000 deaths a year [9]. CDI is regarded by the Centers for Disease Control and Prevention (CDC) as one of its top three 'urgent' (antibiotic resistant) threats [9].

An understanding of current knowledge and guidelines on CDI is essential for intensivists both to manage patients admitted to ICU facilities with, or as a result of, CDI and because critically ill patients are at risk of developing the infection while in the ICU.

Epidemiology and Outcomes

Data on the epidemiology of CDI in ICU patients are limited and heterogeneous. Mixing data from patients with CDI that results in ICU admission, as opposed to CDI that begins after a patient has entered the ICU, contributes to this heterogeneity. Retrospective cohort studies in various types of ICU have typically found that approximately 0.5–5% of patients acquire CDI during an ICU stay [10–17]. In France, for example, 512/5260 (9.7%) patients admitted to three ICUs had diarrhea and were tested for CDI. Of these, 69 patients (13.5% of tested patients and 1.3% of all admitted patients) had CDI; 68.1% of CDI cases were ICU-acquired [12].

Crude ICU or in-hospital mortality rates among ICU patients with CDI are typically around 21–31% [10, 11, 12, 16, 18]. Generally, 30-day or in-hospital mortality typically reaches 33–40% among patients who undergo emergency surgery for fulminant CDI [19, 20]. Studies in hospitalized patients (not ICU-specific) clearly show that CDI increases the risk of 30-day mortality by approximately 2 or 2.5-fold [5, 21]. For example, a recent very large study of 6,522 inpatient diarrhea episodes showed an approximate doubling of 30-day mortality in CDI cases (defined according to the presence of toxin in fecal samples) versus controls (odds ratio 1.61; 95% confidence intervals 1.12–2.31; $p=0.0101$) [5]. The attributable contribution of CDI to mortality risk specifically in critically ill patients is less clear and studies have not shown a significant effect after adjusting for confounding factors [12, 13, 18]. However, CDI has been shown to independently extend hospital or ICU stay [12, 13, 18]. A key feature of CDI is recurrence of symptoms, which is reported in ~20–25% of patients treated with metronidazole or vancomycin [22, 23]. The CDI recurrence rate was 47% lower in patients given fidaxomicin versus vancomycin in studies [22]. However, recurrence in critically ill patients has not yet been studied in great detail.

Pathogenesis and Risk Factors

CDI results from transmission of *C. difficile* spores by the fecal-oral route. Infection control measures employed in relation to CDI focus on preventing infection transmission from symptomatic patients with CDI (see below). However, recent research has revealed that, outside of an outbreak setting, the majority of CDI cases cannot be linked to earlier cases using whole genome sequencing of isolates [24]. This finding highlights the potential importance of other sources of *C. difficile*, possibly asymptomatic patients or environmental reservoirs, in the transmission of infection.

Ingested spores pass through the stomach and into the upper intestine, where they germinate into vegetative cells. The vegetative cells proliferate in the colon, a process facilitated when the normal gut microbiota are altered by antibiotics. *C. difficile* produces two enterotoxins, known as toxins A and B, the principal virulence factors in CDI. Studies in recent years have demonstrated that these toxins trigger not only various inflammatory processes and cell death locally [25], but also a comprehensive systemic inflammatory response [26]. Notably, excess mortality correlates with changes in inflammatory biomarkers that are specific to particular *C. difficile* genotypes, implicating the host inflammatory pathways as a major influence on poor outcome [27]. A third *C. difficile* toxin, known as binary toxin, has also been identified, although its clinical significance is still unclear [28]. Virulence also appears to be determined by other non-toxin factors that modulate germination, sporulation and colonization, and by the effect of the microbiota on colonic metabolite levels [25, 29].

Studies into CDI risk factors have generally been heterogeneous in terms of their methods and quality [30] and there are few data specific to ICU patients.

Primary Infection

The two main risk factors for CDI are exposure to antibiotics and exposure to *C. difficile* in the hospital setting [1]. Most antibiotic classes have been implicated, but fluoroquinolones and third-generation cephalosporins are associated with higher risk, including in ICU patients [16]. CDI is particularly common in elderly patients [6]. Other important risk factors include multiple co-morbidities, frailty, immunosuppression and gastrointestinal surgery [1]. Gastric acid suppression for stress ulcer prevention, especially with proton pump inhibitors (PPI), also increases the risk of CDI in ICU patients [16, 17]. In one recent study in critically ill medical patients, PPIs increased the risk of CDI by an odds ratio of 3.1 (1.11–8.74) in a multivariate analysis, compared with ratios of <2 for all antibiotic classes [16]. However, it should be cautioned that the microbiological definition of CDI in this retrospective study was not optimized. Speculation that elemental, non-residue enteral feeds could predispose patients to CDI [31] is supported by recent evidence of an independent effect of nasogastric tube use [32]. Evidence suggests that patients receiving prolonged mechanical ventilation are at a high risk of CDI: 5.3% of such adults were discharged with a concomitant diagnosis of CDI in one large study [33].

Severe/Complicated Infection and Mortality

Severe/complicated CDI and mortality (not limited to ICU patients), typically associated with leukocytosis, is seen more commonly in the elderly, those with multiple co-morbidities, and/or patients with renal failure or hypoalbuminemia [1, 4, 30].

Infection by hypervirulent ribotypes (e.g., 027 and 078) is also associated with increased mortality risk [27, 30]. Although ribotype epidemiology has been relatively well characterized in some regions (especially Europe and North America) relatively few data are available from other areas. Regional variations are often marked, suggesting that clonal expansion/transmission of particular strain(s) drives local epidemiology. Clinical risk factor scores are in development [34], and these will become more germane as the treatment options for CDI increase.

Diagnosis of CDI within the ICU is itself a strong predictor of a complicated disease course [34]. However, few data exist on risk factors for severe/complicated CDI or mortality specifically in ICU patients, and there is no validated score to aid treatment stratification. Risk factors associated with mortality among ICU patients with CDI, determined via multivariate analyses, have variously included advanced age, septic shock, ward-to-ICU transfer, increasing Acute Physiology and Chronic Health Evaluation (APACHE) score, end-stage liver disease, and length of hospital stay prior to CDI [18, 35, 36]. In addition, male sex, rising C-reactive protein (CRP) levels and previous exposure to fluoroquinolones have been independently associated with severe CDI in the ICU [14]. Additional risk factors for poor outcomes identified by univariate analyses include immunosuppression, high Logistic Organ Dysfunction Score, high McCabe score [12], hypoalbuminemia, history of corticosteroid prescription, prolonged ICU stay, high Sequential Organ Failure Assessment (SOFA) score at the time of CDI diagnosis, and high Simplified Acute Physiology Score (SAPS II) [37].

Recurrence

Generally, the main risk factors for CDI recurrence include older age, continued use of antibiotics after CDI diagnosis, co-morbid diseases, possibly use of PPIs, strain type and initial disease severity [4, 30, 38]. However, these factors have not been well studied specifically in ICU patients.

Diagnosis

CDI remains under-diagnosed, in part owing to low clinical suspicion among healthcare staff and low laboratory testing rates [2, 39]. Rapid and accurate diagnosis is important, however, to avoid delays in appropriate therapy and to reduce empirical therapy [40]. Laboratory testing should be performed on loose stool samples in patients with typical signs and symptoms (usually unexplained diarrhea) of CDI to confirm the diagnosis [1, 4]. All patients who are immunosuppressed (as a result of malignancy, chemotherapy, corticosteroid therapy, organ transplantation or cirrhosis) should be tested if they develop diarrhea [1]. Routine screening for *C. difficile* in hospitalized patients without diarrhea is not recommended [1].

Advances in recent years have resulted in an array of different types of laboratory tests for *C. difficile*. These can be categorized as: (1) Tests to detect *C. difficile* toxins, i.e., cell culture cytotoxicity assay and enzyme immunoassays (EIA) or membrane immunoassays for toxins A/B, or glutamate dehydrogenase (GDH); (2) toxigenic culture of *C. difficile*; and (3) nucleic acid amplification tests (NAAT), such as polymerase chain reaction (PCR) for the genes that code for *C. difficile* toxins [1, 4]. The best standard test has not been established. European guidelines recommend the use of a two or three-stage algorithm in which a positive sensitive screening test is followed by use of a more specific test [4, 41]. Recent evidence that presence of *C. difficile* toxin in the stool predicts mortality from CDI [5] implies that testing algorithms should certainly include toxin testing. Moreover, there is good evidence that use of PCR tests alone leads to over-diagnosis of CDI, principally because these highly sensitive tests will detect colonization by a toxigenic strain in some patients with diarrhea who do not have true infection [5].

Treatment

Updated guidelines for specific therapy for CDI, based on disease severity, have recently been published in Europe [4, 42] and North America [1]. The response to CDI treatment should be monitored on a daily basis to detect patients who fail to respond or have worsening symptoms. Treatment response is defined as a reduction in stool frequency or an improvement in stool consistency, together with improvements in markers of disease severity and no new signs of severe disease [4].

Supportive Measures

Supportive measures recommended for patients with CDI include fluid resuscitation and electrolyte replacement. Anti-motility therapy should be avoided in acute CDI, PPI use should be reviewed, and unnecessary antimicrobial therapy discontinued [1, 4]. In the absence of ileus or significant abdominal distention, oral or enteral feeding should be continued [1]. Fecal collection systems can be useful in critically ill patients with diarrhea, including that caused by CDI [43].

Mild-moderate CDI

Patients with mild CDI may not need specific antibiotic therapy against *C. difficile* [4, 42]. In non-epidemic situations, in which a mild CDI case is clearly induced by antibiotics, it may be acceptable to stop the inducing antibiotic and closely observe the clinical response for 24–48 h [4]. European guidelines recommend 10 days of metronidazole (500 mg three times daily [TID]), vancomycin (125 mg four times daily [QID]) or fidaxomicin (200 mg twice daily [BID]) for initial episodes of non-severe CDI (Table 1) [4]. It is noted that fidaxomicin was not associated with a reduced rate of recurrent CDI due to PCR ribotype 027 as opposed

Table 1 Overview of therapeutic regimens for *Clostridium difficile* infection (CDI) according to European Society of Clinical Microbiology and Infectious Diseases guidelines. Adapted from [4]

Severity	Antibiotic treatment	Non-antibiotic regimens
Non-severe	Metronidazole 500 mg oral TID 10 days (A-I) Vancomycin 125 mg oral QID 10 days (B-I) Fidaxomicin 200 mg oral BID 10 days (B-I)	Stop inducing antibiotics + 48 hours clinical observation (C-II) Immunotherapy with human MAb (C-I) or immune whey (C-II) Recommendation against use of probiotics (D-I) or toxin binding (D-I)
First recurrence (or risk of recurrence)	Vancomycin 125 mg oral QID 10 days (B-I) Fidaxomicin 200 mg oral BID 10 days (B-I) Metronidazole 500 mg oral TID 10 days (C-I)	
Multiple recurrences	Pulse/taper therapy oral vancomycin (B-II) Fidaxomicin 200 mg oral BID 10 days (B-II) Vancomycin 125 mg oral QID 10 days (C-II) Recommendation against metronidazole 500 mg oral TID for 10 days (D-II)	Fecal transplant (with oral antibiotic treatment) (A-I) Recommendation against use of probiotics (D-I) or immune whey (D-I)
Severe disease or complicated course[1]	Vancomycin 125 mg oral QID 10 days (A-I)[2] Fidaxomicin 200 mg oral BID 10 days (B-I)[3] Recommendation against metronidazole 500 mg oral TID for 10 days (D-I)	
Oral treatment not possible	Non-severe CDI: Metronidazole 500 mg i.v. TID 10 days (A-II) Severe CDI: Metronidazole 500 mg i.v. TID 10 days (A-II) + vancomycin 500 mg QID enteral 10 days (B-III) Tigecycline 50 mg i.v. BID 14 days (C-III)	

1. Surgical therapy not included in this overview. 2. Increasing the oral vancomycin dosage up to 500 mg QID for 10 days can be considered. 3. There is no evidence that supports the use of fidaxomicin in life-threatening CDI (D-III)

Strength of recommendation: A, strongly supports a recommendation for use; B, moderately supports a recommendation for use; C, marginally supports a recommendation for use; D, recommendation against use. Numerals indicate quality of evidence; please see source for details.

Other abbreviations: BID, twice daily; MAb, monoclonal antibody; QID, four times daily; TID, three times daily.

* This recommendation predated publication of a pooled analysis of data from two phase 3 clinical trials, in which three factors were strongly associated with clinical success: Vancomycin treatment, treatment-naive status, and mild or moderate CDI severity [23].

to non-027 ribotypes [22]. US and English guidelines recommend metronidazole for mild-to-moderate CDI [1, 42]. Recent data have questioned the relative efficacy of metronidazole in comparison with vancomycin. In a pooled analysis of data from two phase 3 clinical trials, three factors were strongly associated with clinical success: Vancomycin treatment, treatment-naive status, and mild or moderate CDI severity [23].

European guidelines recommend metronidazole, vancomycin or fidaxomicin for a first CDI recurrence and for patients at risk of recurrence [4], although it is probably prudent to avoid metronidazole given increasing evidence of its lower efficacy [23]. Vancomycin and fidaxomicin are recommended in Europe for multiple recurrences [4]. Fecal microbiota transplantation (FMT), in combination with oral antibiotic treatment, is strongly recommended for multiple recurrent CDI episodes unresponsive to repeated antibiotic treatment [4]. US guidelines recommend pulsed vancomycin for a second recurrence and that FMT should be considered in the case of a third recurrence [1]. In general, guidelines recommend against the use of probiotics or toxin binding agents for treatment of any severity of CDI [4].

Severe or Complicated CDI

Vancomycin and fidaxomicin are recommended in Europe for severe infection [4]. The dose of vancomycin can be increased in life-threatening infection (500 mg QID). These guidelines caution that there is no evidence to support the use of fidaxomicin in life-threatening CDI [4]. In England, national guidelines recommend that fidaxomicin should be considered for patients with severe CDI who are considered at high risk of recurrence (elderly, multiple co-morbidities, or concomitant antibiotic therapy) and for those with recurrent CDI of any severity [42]. If oral therapy for severe CDI is not possible, it is recommended that intravenous (i.v.) metronidazole (500 mg TID) should be combined with vancomycin (500 mg QID for 10 days) administered either by intracolonic retention enema, oro- or nasogastric tube. Intravenous tigecycline (50 mg BID for 14 days) may be an alternative [4], although it does not have a licensed indication for CDI treatment.

US guidelines recommend oral vancomycin for severe CDI, defined as the presence of hypoalbuminemia plus either leukocytosis or abdominal tenderness [1]. Severe and complicated CDI is defined as that necessitating ICU admission, or with various signs of shock and severe disease. In these circumstances, oral vancomycin (125 mg QID) plus i.v. metronidazole (500 mg TID) is recommended in the absence of significant abdominal distension. Vancomycin delivered orally (500 mg QID) and by enema (500 mg QID) plus i.v. metronidazole is recommended when there is ileus or toxic colon and/or significant abdominal distension [1].

Surgery

Surgery (usually total colectomy with ileostomy) is indicated when there is perforation of the colon or systemic inflammation and a deteriorating clinical condition not responding to antibiotic therapy (including toxic megacolon, an acute abdomen and severe ileus) [4]. A future alternative to colectomy may be diverting loop ileostomy and colonic lavage [44], combined with intracolonic antegrade vancomycin and i.v. metronidazole [4].

Infection Control and Prevention

Infection control measures are mandatory following a diagnosis of CDI [4]. Recommended measures include hand hygiene (with soap and water instead of alcohol hand rubs), protective clothing, sporicidal decontamination of the hospital environment and the use of dedicated patient care equipment for infected patients, with appropriate disinfection [1, 45, 46] (Table 2). More widely, hospital-based infection control programs, including antibiotic stewardship programs, can help to decrease the incidence of CDI but are beyond the scope of this review.

Table 2 Key measures recommended for *Clostridium difficile* infection (CDI) control and prevention [45, 46]

Isolation precautions	Single room or cohorts, designated staff, designated toilet or commode
Hand hygiene	Use of gloves and meticulous hand washing with soap and water
Protective clothing	Gloves, gowns, aprons should be worn
Environmental cleaning	Regular disinfection using sporicidal agents
Medical equipment	Dedicated devices for single patients, sporicidal disinfection, disposable materials where possible
Outbreaks: specific measures include	All measures reinforced Closure and environmental cleaning if transmission continues, as appropriate Molecular typing of isolates to elucidate epidemiology
Other	Prompt *C. difficile* testing of patients with unexplained diarrhea, according to guidelines Antibiotic stewardship (emphasis on avoiding use of high-risk agents, e. g., cephalosporins and fluoroquinolones) Education of healthcare workers and visitors Surveillance of CDI

Conclusion

Critically ill patients in the ICU typically have multiple risk factors for the acquisition of CDI. Accordingly, all healthcare staff in the ICU should be aware of the risk of CDI. Crucially, all patients with unexplained diarrhea in the ICU should be tested promptly for CDI using optimized laboratory assays. Supportive care and specific therapy should be provided in patients with suspected or diagnosed CDI according to current guidelines. Rigorous, multifaceted infection control measures are vital to prevent the onward spread of infection.

Acknowledgements

The authors are members of the CDI Europe expert group, which is supported by Astellas Pharma EMEA (Chertsey, UK). Astellas Pharma EMEA supported and funded the development of this chapter, with medical writing support provided by Lee Baker (Interel, London, UK).

References

1. Surawicz CM, Brandt LJ, Binion DG et al (2013) Guidelines for diagnosis, treatment, and prevention of Clostridium difficile infections. Am J Gastroenterol 108:478–498
2. European Centre for Disease Prevention (2013) Point prevalence survey of healthcare-associated infections and antimicrobial use in European acute care hospitals. Stockholm, ECDC. http://www.ecdc.europa.eu/en/publications/Publications/healthcare-associated-infections-antimicrobial-use-PPS.pdf. Accessed 17 October 2014
3. Magill SS, Edwards JR, Bamberg W et al (2014) Multistate point-prevalence survey of health care-associated infections. N Engl J Med 370:1198–1208
4. Debast SB, Bauer MP, Kuijper EJ (2014) European Society of Clinical Microbiology and Infectious Diseases (ESCMID): update of the treatment guidance document for Clostridium difficile infection (CDI). Clin Microbiol Infect 20(Suppl 2):1–26
5. Planche TD, Davies KA, Coen PG et al (2013) Differences in outcome according to Clostridium difficile testing method: a prospective multicentre diagnostic validation study of C difficile infection. Lancet Infect Dis 13:936–945
6. Bauer MP, Notermans DW, van Benthem BH et al (2011) Clostridium difficile infection in Europe: a hospital-based survey. Lancet 377:63–73
7. Wiegand PN, Nathwani D, Wilcox MH, Stephens J, Shelbaya A, Haider S (2012) Clinical and economic burden of hospital onset health care facility acquired Clostridium difficile infection in Europe: a systematic review. J Hops Infect 81:1–14
8. Reveles KR, Lee GC, Boyd NK, Frei CR (2014) The rise in Clostridium difficile infection incidence among hospitalized adults in the United States: 2001–2010. Am J Infect Control 42:1028–1032
9. Centres for Disease Control and Prevention (2013) Antibiotic resistance threats in the United States, 2013. CDC. http://www.cdc.gov/drugresistance/threat-report-2013/pdf/ar-threats-2013. Accessed 17 October 2014
10. Ang CW, Heyes G, Morrison P, Carr B (2008) The acquisition and outcome of ICU-acquired Clostridium difficile infection in a single centre in the UK. J Infect 57:435–440
11. Musa SA, Moran C, Thomson SJ et al (2011) Clostridium difficile-associated disease acquired in the cardiothoracic intensive care unit. J Cardiothorac Vasc Anesth 25:263–267

12. Zahar JR, Schwebel C, Adrie C et al (2012) Outcome of ICU patients with Clostridium difficile infection. Crit Care 16:R215
13. Dodek PM, Norena M, Ayas NT, Romney M, Wong H (2013) Length of stay and mortality due to Clostridium difficile infection acquired in the intensive care unit. J Crit Care 28:335–340
14. Khanafer N, Touré A, Chambrier C (2013) Predictors of Clostridium difficile infection severity in patients hospitalised in medical intensive care. World J Gastroenterol 19:8034–8041
15. Tripathy S, Nair P, Rothburn M (2013) Clostridium difficile associated disease in a neurointensive care unit. Front Neurol 4:82
16. Buendgens L, Bruensing J, Matthes M et al (2014) Administration of proton pump inhibitors in critically ill medical patients is associated with increased risk of developing Clostridium difficile-associated diarrhea. J Crit Care 29:696.e11–696.e15
17. MacLaren R, Reynolds PM, Allen RR (2014) Histamine-2 receptor antagonists vs proton pump inhibitors on gastrointestinal tract hemorrhage and infectious complications in the intensive care unit. JAMA Intern Med 174:564–574
18. Micek ST, Schramm G, Morrow L et al (2013) Clostridium difficile infection: a multicenter study of epidemiology and outcomes in mechanically ventilated patients. Crit Care Med 41:1968–1975
19. Bhangu A, Nepogodiev D, Gupta A, Torrance A, Singh P, West Midlands Research Collaborative (2012) Systematic review and meta-analysis of outcomes following emergency surgery for Clostridium difficile colitis. Br J Surg 99:1501–1513
20. Lee DY, Chung EL, Guend H, Whelan RL, Wedderburn RV, Rose KM (2014) Predictors of mortality after emergency colectomy for Clostridium difficile colitis: An analysis of ACS-NSQIP. Ann Surg 259:148–156
21. Hensgens MP, Goorhuis A, Dekkers OM, van Benthem BH, Kuijper EJ (2013) All-cause and disease-specific mortality in hospitalized patients with Clostridium difficile infection: a multicenter cohort study. Clin Infect Dis 56:1108–1116
22. Mullane KM, Gorbach S (2011) Fidaxomicin: first-in-class macrocyclic antibiotic. Expert Rev Anti Infect Ther 9:767–777
23. Johnson S, Louie TJ, Gerding DN et al (2014) Vancomycin, metronidazole, or tolevamer for Clostridium difficile infection: results from two multinational, randomized, controlled trials. Clin Infect Dis 59:345–354
24. Eyre DW, Cule ML, Wilson DJ et al (2013) Diverse sources of C. difficile infection identified on whole-genome sequencing. N Engl J Med 369:1195–1205
25. Peniche AG, Savidge TC, Dann SM (2013) Recent insights into Clostridium difficile pathogenesis. Curr Opin Infect Dis 26:447–453
26. Rao K, Erb-Downward JR, Walk ST et al (2014) The systemic inflammatory response to Clostridium difficile infection. PLoS One 9:e92578
27. Walker AS, Eyre DW, Wyllie DH et al (2013) Relationship between bacterial strain type, host biomarkers, and mortality in Clostridium difficile infection. Clin Infect Dis 56:1589–1600
28. Gerding DN, Johnson S, Rupnik M, Aktories K (2014) Clostridium difficile binary toxin CDT: mechanism, epidemiology, and potential clinical importance. Gut Microbes 5:15–27
29. Vedantam G, Clark A, Chu M, McQuade R, Mallozzi M, Viswanathan VK (2012) Clostridium difficile infection: toxins and non-toxin virulence factors, and their contributions to disease establishment and host response. Gut Microbes 3:121–134
30. Abou Chakra CN, Pepin J, Sirard S, Valiquette L (2014) Risk factors for recurrence, complications and mortality in Clostridium difficile infection: a systematic review. PLoS One 2014 9:e98400
31. O'Keefe SJ (2010) Tube feeding, the microbiota, and Clostridium difficile infection. World J Gastroenterol 16:139–142
32. Huang H, Wu S, Chen R et al (2014) Risk factors of Clostridium difficile infections among patients in a university hospital in Shanghai, China. Anaerobe 30 C:65–69
33. Zilberberg MD, Nathanson BH, Sadigov S, Higgins TL, Kollef MH, Shorr AF (2009) Epidemiology and outcomes of Clostridium difficile-associated disease among patients on prolonged acute mechanical ventilation. Chest 136:752–758

34. Hensgens MP, Dekkers OM, Goorhuis A, Lecessie S, Kuijper EJ (2014) Predicting a complicated course of Clostridium difficile infection at the bedside. Clin Microbiol Infect 20:O301–O308
35. Kenneally C, Rosini JM, Skrupky LP et al (2007) Analysis of 30-day mortality for Clostridium difficile-associated disease in the ICU setting. Chest 132:418–424
36. Zilberberg MD, Shorr AF, Micek ST, Doherty JA, Kollef MH (2009) Clostridium difficile-associated disease and mortality among the elderly critically ill. Crit Care Med 37:2583–2589
37. Sabau L, Meybeck A, Gois J et al (2014) Clostridium difficile colitis acquired in the intensive care unit: outcome and prognostic factors. Infection 42:23–30
38. Zilberberg MD, Reske K, Olsen M, Yan Y, Dubberke ER (2014) Development and validation of a recurrent Clostridium difficile risk-prediction model. J Hosp Med 9:418–423
39. Davies KA, Davis GL, Longshaw CM et al (2014) Second report from the EUropean, multicentre, prospective bi-annual point prevalence study of Clostridium difficile Infection in hospitalised patients with Diarrhoea (EUCLID). Presented at 24th European Congress on Clinical Microbiology and Infectious Diseases, Barcelona, 10–13 May 2014. (Abstract P0753)
40. Barbut F, Surgers L, Eckert C et al (2014) Does a rapid diagnosis of Clostridium difficile infection impact on quality of patient management? Clin Microbiol Infect 20:136–144
41. Crobach MJ, Dekkers OM, Wilcox MH, Kuijper EJ (2009) European Society of Clinical Microbiology and Infectious Diseases (ESCMID): data review and recommendations for diagnosing Clostridium difficile-infection (CDI). Clin Microbiol Infect 15:1053–1066
42. Public Health England (2013) Updated guidance on the management and treatment of Clostridium difficile infection. London; PHE. https://www.gov.uk/government/uploads/system/uploads/attachment_data/file/321891/Clostridium_difficile_management_and_treatment.pdf. Accessed 17 October 2014
43. Beitz JM (2006) Fecal incontinence in acutely and critically ill patients: options in management. Ostomy Wound Manage 52:56–58, 60, 62–66
44. Neal MD, Alverdy JC, Hall DE, Simmons RL, Zuckerbraun BS (2011) Diverting loop ileostomy and colonic lavage: an alternative to total abdominal colectomy for the treatment of severe, complicated Clostridium difficile associated disease. Ann Surg 254:423–427
45. Vonberg RP, Kuijper EJ, Wilcox MH et al (2008) Infection control measures to limit the spread of Clostridium difficile. Clin Microbiol Infect 14(Suppl 5):2–20
46. Dubberke ER, Carling P, Carrico R et al (2014) Strategies to prevent Clostridium difficile infections in acute care hospitals: 2014 Update. Infect Control Hosp Epidemiol 35:628–645

Viral Sepsis

P. Amin and V. Amin

Introduction

Viruses are the smallest infective agents currently known to affect humans and animals. The virus has a centrally situated nucleic acid, which is encased within a capsid consisting of a protein core. Viruses are obligatory intracellular microorganisms that live inside cells, using components of the nucleic acid and protein generating system of the host to replicate and trigger cell destruction leading to diseases. Alternatively, the host's defense mechanisms lead to cell destruction in an attempt to clear cells infected by the viruses. The nucleic acid is RNA or DNA, which may be single-stranded or double-stranded [1]. The pathophysiology of viral infections may be attributed to the degeneration and cellular necrosis of the infected cells, leading to local and systemic inflammatory responses. The body's defense mechanisms include phagocytosis, humoral and cell-mediated responses and the production of interferons [2]. Interferons prevent the local spread of viruses, whereas antibodies prevent viremia, ensure long-term immunity and sensitize infected cells to be destroyed by T-cells and macrophages [3, 4]. Cell-mediated immunity leads to an increase in cytotoxic cells that then release lymphokines, including interferon.

Epidemiology

Most of the infective viruses are constantly present in human or animal reservoirs; under certain conditions they are then transmitted to susceptible individuals. During epidemics, such as influenza, measles, mumps, severe acute respiratory syndrome (SARS), a large proportion of the susceptible community is affected by aerosol transmission [5]. Antigenic drift is the reason underlying the epidemic spread of

P. Amin ✉ · V. Amin
Bombay Hospital Institute of Medical Sciences, Mumbai, India
e-mail: pravinramin@gmail.com

J.-L. Vincent (ed.), *Annual Update in Intensive Care and Emergency Medicine 2015*,
DOI 10.1007/978-3-319-13761-2_4

variation in structure, leading to different subtypes (e. g., influenza virus) [6]. An epidemic is said to occur when the number of cases is in excess of the expected number for that population based on past experience. When multiple continents are involved, the disease is said to be a pandemic, e. g., human immunodeficiency virus (HIV).

There are two major forms of transmission by which viruses can be classified: Viruses that stay within a single species and viruses that alternately infect different host species [7]. There are a few exclusions, such as rabies and influenza viruses, which spread across species. Animal reservoirs are an important source of transmission for diseases like rabies, arboviruses and certain hemorrhagic viruses. Humans are an important pool of chronic carriers of viruses, such as hepatitis B virus (HBV), HIV and some herpesviruses [8–10].

Certain host factors predispose the individual to increased severity of that infection (e. g., smoking and respiratory syncytial virus [RSV] infections; alcohol and hepatitis; development of paralytic poliomyelitis in exercised limbs; reactivation of Epstein-Barr virus (EBV) may be a risk factor for developing lymphoma).

Method of Transmission

Respiratory This is the most common route of transmission in viral illnesses. The virus may be present in saliva or respiratory secretions and may spread by a bite as in rabies, or by kissing as with EBV, or may be spread as an aerosol, e. g., influenza and measles. Hantavirus may spread by aerosols formed from the urine of rodents in the soil. Viruses that spread by the aerosol route clearly increase the risk of spread to health care workers and other indoor patients.

Gastrointestinal This is the second most common mode of spread of viral infections. The major enteric viruses are coxsackie, echo, rotaviruses, poliomyelitis, Norwalk viruses, hepatitis A, E and sometimes B.

Personal Contact Some of the viruses that are thought to be transmitted by aerosol or from gastrointestinal sources may actually spread by personal contact. The recent epidemic of Ebola virus, which is known to be highly infective, has spread to healthcare workers and other patients, as body fluids are highly infective in this illness.

Skin This is another important portal of entry of viruses, but need not necessarily be through intact skin. Virus may enter the body by bites, as in rabies, arboviruses in mosquito or tick bites, or by needlestick injury or blood transfusions, e. g., in HIV or hepatitis B and C. The skin also serves as a portal of exit from ruptured skin vesicles disseminating the disease to the community, e. g., small pox, chicken pox, herpes simplex virus (HSV).

Genital Viruses that are transmitted both heterosexually and homosexually include HSV, HIV, HBV, and cytomegalovirus (CMV). These viruses are spread not only sexually, but also to babies during passage through the cervical canal. Some of the above viruses, including rubella and varicella, may lead to intra-uterine infection through trans-placental transmission.

Arthropod Borne Mosquito, ticks and flies may transmit viruses like Dengue, yellow fever, and Crimean-Congo hemorrhagic fever (CCHF).

Nosocomial Infection About 5% of nosocomial infections may be due to viral infections; however, the incidence may be underestimated because of difficulty in diagnosis and limitations in the availability of diagnostic tools. These viruses include the respiratory viruses (e. g., HSV, CMV), hepatitis virus (e. g., HBV and hepatitis C virus [HCV]), enteric viruses (e. g., rotavirus) and picornavirus. There is a potential 0.3% risk of transmitting HIV to other patients and healthcare workers. Cases of slow virus Creutzfeldt-Jakob disease have occurred following corneal transplantation. Ebola and Marburg viruses have also been transmitted as nosocomial infections. The most frequently studied virus implicated in nosocomial spread is RSV in the pediatric ward, neonatal intensive care unit (ICU) and adult ICU.

Incubation Period

Viruses that have short incubation periods of 2 to 5 days, usually affect the respiratory system. Infections that spread by the hematogenous route to distal organs like the brain may take 2–3 weeks. Incubation periods in HIV infection may be spread over a few months. Viruses like the rabies virus, which spreads through the nerves, may have an incubation period of as little as 2 weeks to as much as a year. Knowledge of the incubation period is important to determine the infectivity of the microbe. The extent of infectivity depends on the preservation of the virus and its exodus to the environment.

The Immune System

The immune system plays a major role in the defense mechanism and pathophysiology of the disease caused by viruses. The primary host defenses against virus infection are physical/chemical barriers to infection and the immune system [11]. Virus infection in humans usually evokes two types of immune response. The initial rapid-onset ‘innate’ response against the virus involves the synthesis of proteins, namely interferons, and the stimulation of ‘natural killer (NK)’ lymphocytes [12, 13]. In some cases, the innate response may be enough to prevent a wide spread infection. However, if the infection evolves beyond the first few rounds of viral replication, the ‘adaptive immune response’ comes into play [14]. The adaptive immune response itself has two components: The humoral response and the cell-mediated response. Both of these components of the adaptive immune response result in the production of long lasting memory cells that provides immunity to successive infections by same virus. These extremely precise cell-surface detecting receptors detect the antigen or certain viral proteins specific to that virus [4]. This process leads to an immunological memory, which then forms the origin for vaccination [3]. The innate immune system provides universal host protection from infectious diseases. It identifies the presence of pathogens using numerous methods of detection. The major targets of innate immune recognition are viral nucleic acids. Generally, the innate immune system detects structural features of viral RNA and DNA that are distinct from the host nucleic acid [15, 16].

Detection of viral pathogens by the innate immune system has two major consequences: First, it leads to the induction of the innate antiviral mechanisms, most of which are mediated primarily by interferons. Subsequently, it leads to the activation of the adaptive immune response, which can offer a more directed, antigen-specific, and long-term antiviral immunity. The primary aim of the body's defense mechanism is to eradicate the infected cells. This is accomplished by cell-intrinsic mechanisms that are brought about by type-I interferons in the infected cells. It can also be implemented by cytotoxic lymphocytes, such as NK cells and CD8 T cells [17]. Prevention of entry of the virus into the host cell is an important protection process. Neutralizing antibodies primarily carry this out. Other methods that interfere with viral replication, gene expression and exit from the infected cells vary depending on the virus and the host. Acute phase proteins and the complement system play an active role in innate immune response. Leukocytes, including neutrophils, monocytes, macrophages, dendritic cells, NK cells and NK T cells, are the principal innate immune cell types that respond to viral infection [14]. C-type lectins on their cell surface recognize viral protein or nucleic acid content and, in the case of NK and NK T cells, changes on the cell surfaces of infected cells [18]. These cells enter tissues invaded by these microorganisms from the plasma through the action of cytokines that are released during infection. The adaptive immune system displays two distinct cell types: B and T lymphocytes. On exposure to a virus, B-lymphocytes stimulate the release of a soluble form of antibody able to bind the circulating virions, effectively leading to eradication of the virus. An antiviral B-lymphocyte response is effectively sensitive in preventing or limiting reinfection and forms the basis of vaccination against specific viruses [19].

Viruses are essentially intracellular organisms that reproduce within cells of the infected host and use the cellular constituents to produce the next generation virions. This process of replication can take place rapidly or slowly over time. This progression over a time frame determines the rapidity of evolution of illness. In acute viral infections, the multiplication of the virus and the host response will result in eradicating the virus and clearing the infection or if the infection is overwhelming will lead to the severe sepsis or death of the host. The tissue injury caused by viruses at the site of infection is due to the cytotoxic injury of virus multiplication and the host's immune response to infection. In chronic infection, the time frame of virus multiplication in the host is usually assessed in weeks, months, or even years, with the host immune response spanning over prolonged periods. Viruses causing chronic and lasting infection have developed processes to subdue or alter the immune response whereby these viruses persist in the patient. The immune responses encountered both in acute and chronic viral infections can lead to tissue injury. The classic example of chronic viral infection leading to immune-mediated tissue destruction over years is hepatitis C cirrhosis. These immune responses, seen in a host of viral infections, may be responsible for the associated autoimmune diseases associated with certain viruses [20].

T-lymphocytes and cell-mediated immunity are concerned with virus-infected cells rather than free virus. Virus-immune T lymphocytes recognize viral antigens in association with self-major histocompatibility complex (MHC) class I glycoproteins [21]. These T lymphocytes perform key regulatory functions of the immune system. Through these T-cell receptors, the CD4 and CD8 molecules participate in an immune response leading to an interaction with antigen presenting cells, release of cytokines, proliferation of a host of cells with cytolytic destruction of target cells [22]. A major development is the understanding of the structure and functioning of the MHC, the T-cell receptor and cell surface components, such as CD3, CD4, and lymphocyte function-associated antigen-1.

Classification of Viruses

Viruses are divided into two large groups (Table 1)
- RNA containing viruses.
- DNA containing viruses.

Baltimore Classification

In this classification, viruses are divided into seven groups based on their nucleic acid and m-RNA production.
- Double stranded (ds)-DNA viruses.
- Single stranded (ss)-DNA viruses.
- ds-RNA viruses.
- ss-RNA viruses with positive strands (positive polarity).
- ss-RNA viruses with negative strands (negative polarity).
- ss-RNA viruses associated with the reverse transcriptase enzyme.
- ds-DNA viruses associated with the reverse transcriptase enzyme.

Poxviruses

Orthopox: smallpox virus (variola), vaccinia virus, cowpox virus, and monkeypox virus.
Para pox: orf virus, pseudocowpox, bovine papular stomatitis virus.
Yabapox: Tanapox virus, Yaba monkey tumor virus.
Mollusc pox: molluscum contagiosum virus.

Papovavirus

Papillomavirus, polyomavirus, various neoplasms in mammals.

Hepadnaviruses

A family of enveloped, ds-DNA viruses, including HBV.

Herpesviridae

At least five species of herpesviridae are extremely widespread among humans: HSV-1 and HSV-2 (both of which can cause orolabial herpes and genital herpes), varicella zoster virus (VZV, which causes chicken-pox and shingles), EBV virus (which causes mononucleosis), and CMV.

Adenoviruses

These cause a wide range of illnesses, from mild respiratory infections in young children to life-threatening multi-organ disease in people with a weakened immune system.

Papillomaviridae

Non-enveloped DNA virus, collectively known as papillomaviruses. Causes small benign tumors, known as papillomas or warts (e. g., human papillomavirus [HPV] 1, HPV6 or HPV11). Papillomas caused by some types, however, such as HPV 16 and 18, carry a risk of becoming cancerous.

Table 1 Classification of viruses

ds-DNA viruses associated with the reverse transcriptase enzyme	ds-DNA	ss-DNA	ds-RNA	ss-RNA(−) with transcriptase enzyme	ss-RNA(+)	ss-RNA with reverse transcriptase enzyme
Hepatitis B (HBV) only	Pox-viridae	Parvo-viridae	Reo-viridae	Orthomyxo-viridae	Picorna-viridae	Retro viruses
	Papova-viridae			Paramyxo-viridae	Calici-viridae	
	Hepadna-viridae			Rhabdo-viridae	Astro-viridae	
	Herpes-viridae			Filo-viridae	Corona-viridae	
	Adeno-viridae			Arena-viridae	Flavi-viridae	
	Papilloma viridae			Bunya-viridae	Toga-viridae	

ds: double stranded; ss: single stranded.

Parvoviridae

Parvovirus B19 causes a childhood exanthem (erythema infectiosum).

Reoviridae

A family of viruses that can affect the gastrointestinal system (such as rotavirus) and respiratory tract.

Orthomyxoviruses

A family of RNA viruses that includes influenzavirus A, influenzavirus B, influenzavirus C. These viruses cause influenza in vertebrates, including birds (avian influenza), humans, and other mammals.

Paramyxoviruses

Includes mumps virus, measles virus, RSV, parainfluenza virus and human metapneumovirus, which is the major cause of bronchiolitis croup and pneumonia in infants and children.

Rhabdoviridae

Rhabdoviruses carry their genetic material in the form of negative-sense ss-RNA. Rhabdoviruses include rabies virus and vesicular stomatitis virus (VSV).

Filoviridae

Filamentous infectious viral particles (virions), encode their genome in the form of negative-sense ss-RNA. Two members of the family that are commonly known are Ebola virus and Marburg virus causing viral hemorrhagic fevers.

Arenavirus

Lymphocytic choriomeningitis virus infection can cause aseptic meningitis. Hemorrhagic fever syndromes are derived from infections by viruses, such as Lassa virus.

Bunyaviridae

A family of negative-stranded, enveloped RNA viruses. Although generally found in arthropods or rodents, certain viruses in this family occasionally infect humans. *Bunyaviridae* are vector-borne viruses. With the exception of hantaviruses, transmission occurs via an arthropod vector (sandfly, mosquito or tick). Hantaviruses are transmitted through contact with mice feces. Human infections with certain bunyaviridae, like CCHF virus, are associated with high levels of morbidity and mortality.

Picornavirus

Picornaviruses are non-enveloped, positive-stranded RNA viruses. The diseases they cause are varied, ranging from acute 'common-cold'-like illnesses to polio.

Caliciviridae

A family of viruses with ss-RNA. Transmission of caliciviruses is generally by the fecal-oral route but can also be via the respiratory route. Calicivirus infections commonly cause acute gastroenteritis (e. g., the Norwalk virus).

Astrovirus

The *Astroviridae* comprise a third family of non-enveloped viruses the genome of which is composed of plus-sense ss-RNA. Astroviruses are now recognized as a cause of gastroenteritis in children and adults.

Coronaviridae

A family of enveloped, positive-stranded RNA viruses. Coronaviruses are transmitted by the fecal-oral route or by aerosols of respiratory secretions. Although most diseases are mild, sometimes they can cause more severe situations in humans, such as, for example, the infection of the respiratory tract known as SARS.

Flaviviridae

A family of viruses that are primarily spread through arthropod vectors (mainly ticks and mosquitoes). Major diseases caused by the *Flaviviridae* family include: Dengue fever, Japanese encephalitis, Kyasanur Forest disease, Murray Valley encephalitis, St. Louis encephalitis, tick-borne encephalitis, West Nile encephalitis, yellow fever, HCV Infection.

Togaviridae

A family of viruses, including the following genera: Genus *Alphavirus,* type species, *Sindbis virus*, Eastern equine encephalitis virus, Western equine encephalitis virus, Venezuelan equine encephalitis virus, Ross River virus, O'nyong 'nyong virus, Chikungunya, Semliki Forest virus; genus *Rubivirus,* type species *Rubella virus*.

Retroviridae

A family of enveloped viruses that replicate in a host cell through the process of reverse transcription, e. g., HIV.

Viral Diagnostic Methods

Viral testing is now essential in the management of patients with infections. Multiple test methods continue to be used and molecular tests are up-and-coming as a leading technology. A number of molecular assays are either in use or are in the process of being developed for *in vitro* diagnosis [23]. For the diagnosis of acute viral infections, the samples are usually collected from the site of disease (e. g., cerebrospinal fluid [CSF] in viral meningitis). Viral culture is technically difficult as viruses are labile and may not survive the process of transfer. Samples may be sent for serological tests, viral antigens and nucleic acid testing. Immunofluorescence is another technique used to determine viral activity [24].Viral diagnostic techniques are shown in Box 1.

Box 1. Techniques Used in Diagnostic Virology

- Cell culture
- Antigen detection
  - Fluorescent antibody staining
  - Immunoperoxidase antibody staining
  - Enzyme immunoassay
- Nucleic acid detection
  - Polymerase chain reaction
  - Other nucleic acid amplification methods
- Electron microscopy
- Cytology
- Histology
  - Immunohistochemistry
  - In situ hybridization
- Serology

From [67] with permission.

Identification in Cell Culture

Virus growth in cell culture often produces a distinctive cytopathic effect (CPE) that can provide a presumptive identification, but CPE is not specific (i. e., many viruses cause it). If the virus does not produce a CPE, its presence can be detected by:

1. hemadsorption
2. interference with formation of a CPE by a second virus;
3. a decrease in acid production by infected, dying cells. This can be detected visually by a color change in the phenol red (a pH indicator) in the culture medium.

Definitive identification of the virus grown in cell culture is made by complement fixation, hemagglutination inhibition, and neutralization of CPE. Other tests, such as fluorescent antibody, radioimmunoassay, ELISA and immunoelectron microscopy are also used in certain circumstances.

Microscopic Identification

1. Inclusion bodies – developed by aggregates of virus particles – can be demonstrated in the nucleus or cytoplasm of infected cells. These non-specific inclusion bodies are seen in the nucleus, in certain herpes viruses and the Negri bodies seen in the cytoplasm of cells in patients with rabies virus infection.

2. In cases of RSV, measles and herpes multinucleated giant cells may be seen.
3. Fluorescent antibody staining of cells in culture can provide definitive diagnosis.
4. Electron microscopy can detect virus particles that have specific morphology and size, e. g., Ebola virus.

Serologic Studies

1. The detection of IgM may be an indicator of current infection.
2. The detection of IgG is more an indicator of past infection rather than current infection.

A four-fold rise in antibody titer in the convalescent serum sample compared with the acute sample may help in making the diagnosis.

Detection of Viral Antigens and Nucleic Acids

The presence of viral proteins, such as p24 of HIV, HBV surface antigen and NS1 antigen for Dengue are regularly used in diagnosis. The presence of viral DNA or RNA is increasingly used to confirm viral infections. Using labeled probes to determine viral load, assay of CMV and HIV RNA has ensured specific and rapid diagnosis of certain viral illnesses.

Serious Community-Acquired Viral Infections

Viral infections cause many community-acquired infections, particularly serious respiratory viral infections. Among the causes of serious community-acquired pneumonia requiring hospital admission, viruses account for 15–40% of all cases in which the underlying etiology is known [25].

Viruses that invade through the airway can be grouped as follows:

1. Upper airway infections
   - Viruses that limit their action to the epithelial surface: Common cold viruses (human rhinoviruses, Coxsackie A and echoviruses) and mild cases of influenza and parainfluenza. These viruses have mild clinical presentation with a generally favorable course and outcome.
   - Viruses that invade the epithelium and spread to other parts of the body: Viruses producing measles, mumps, rubella, herpes viruses (HSV, VZV], EBV and some cases of CMV [26].
2. Lower airway infections and pneumonias

   These form the most common serious respiratory disorders in immunocompetent adults – 'febrile respiratory illnesses'. The viruses included in this group are myxoviruses (including the different types associated with influenza A, B and C), adenoviruses (23 different types, of which 18 have been isolated in humans), parainfluenza viruses, and pneumonic conditions caused by HSV, VZV, EBV and CMV [26].

Influenza

The seasonal 'flu' virus is an RNA virus with three known subtypes (A, B and C) belonging to the family *Orthomyxoviridae*. These viruses have considerable genetic variability and have a capacity to cause epidemics and pandemics. Typically infection manifests as self-limiting upper airway disease presenting with fever, chills, malaise, headache, muscle pain and non-productive cough that lasts for 3 or 4 days. A very small proportion of infections can lead to complications, such as bacterial pneumonia, sepsis and acute respiratory distress syndrome (ARDS). Influenza virus is transmitted via the aerial route and hence is responsible for large epidemics. The virulence and antigenicity of the virus, the immune condition of the host, and the environment all interact, conditioning person- to-person transmission of the disease [27].

Diagnosis is based on clinical manifestations and tests, such as antigen determination tests, nucleic acid tests, polymerase chain reaction (PCR) amplification or viral cultures. Treatment consists of neuraminidase inhibitors (oseltamivir and zanamivir), which are preferred to amantadine and rimantadine because of resistance.

Extracorporeal membrane oxygenation (ECMO) is a potential modality of therapy in patients with influenza and severe ARDS, which has been associated with encouraging results. In a study in New Zealand and Australia, ECMO-treated patients with influenza A(H1N1)-associated ARDS were often young adults with severe hypoxemia and had an overall survival rate greater than 70% [28]. This method was applied in Europe [29], the United States [30], South America [31], Canada [32] and Asia [33] as the H1N1 pandemic spread. In H1N1 patients, survival rates ranged from 56 to 79% across the centers, independent of the applied strategy of mechanical ventilation.

Respiratory Syncytial Virus and Parainfluenza Virus

These are RNA viruses with structural similarities and belong to the same family, *Paramyxoviridae*. They share features relating to epidemiology, pathogenesis and clinical manifestations. Both these microorganisms cause serious disease, particularly in elderly patients or individuals with high risk of serious respiratory infection (e. g., COPD, cystic fibrosis, post-lung transplant). Clinically, these infections present as a febrile illness with bronchospasm, bronchiolitis, pneumonia, and may progress to ARDS [34]. Transmission is via fomites or infected secretions. Diagnosis is based on clinical signs, antigenic detection tests, viral isolation and PCR. Treatment consists of supportive measures, the administration of bronchodilators, corticosteroids, and the use of nebulized ribavirin in high-risk patients. Mortality rate is close to 10% in elderly individuals [34].

Coronavirus-SARS (SARS-CoV)

The SARS virus is an RNA virus. It was first described after an outbreak in Asia in 2003. It exhibits a biphasic clinical course with prodromic manifestations (fever, chills, muscle pain, nausea, headache). It usually progresses within about 7–8 days to respiratory distress with severe hypoxemia (in 45% of the cases) respiratory failure and ARDS (in 20%) [35]. Transmission is via droplets, the aerial route and by contact. PCR, immunofluorescence, viral cultures and enzyme-linked immunosorbent assay (ELISA) establish diagnosis. Treatment is fundamentally supportive. Steroids have been tried with questionable efficacy. Mortality rate is about 11%.

Other Respiratory Viruses

Adenoviruses can cause lower airway disease. Infections may rarely progress to pneumonia that can deteriorate towards ARDS. Extrapulmonary symptoms include gastritis, hepatitis, meningitis, and hemorrhagic cystitis. Diagnosis is established by PCR and viral cultures. Transmission is via droplets and contact. Treatment is supportive; cidofovir and ganciclovir appear to have activity *in vitro*.

Hantavirus produces two different clinical conditions: Hemorrhagic fever with renal failure syndrome (HFRS) and hantavirus cardiopulmonary syndrome (HCPS). The clinical picture is characterized by prodromic manifestations (fever, chills, muscle pain, abdominal pain), rapid progression towards respiratory failure, ARDS, coagulopathy and shock. Transmission is through contact with urine or excrement from infected mice. Diagnosis is based on serological tests. Treatment is supportive and the administration of ribavirin in HFRS (not effective in HCPS) [26].

Viral Encephalitis

Acute viral encephalitis can be caused by a number of viruses (Box 2) but the most important is herpes simplex encephalitis (HSE). The outcome of any central nervous system (CNS) viral infection is dependent on the immune status of the host and the virulence of the infecting virus. In immunocompromised patients (e. g., acquired immunodeficiency disease [AIDS], bone marrow and solid organ transplants) one can encounter varicella and CMV infections [36].

Box 2. Causes of Viral Encephalitis

Herpes simplex virus (HSV-1, HSV-2)

Other herpes viruses – varicella-zoster virus (VZV), cytomegalovirus (CMV), Epstein-Barr virus (EBV), human herpes virus 6 (HHV6)

Adenoviruses, influenza A

Enteroviruses, poliovirus, measles, mumps and rubella viruses

Rabies

Arboviruses, e. g., Japanese B encephalitis, West Nile encephalitis virus, tick-borne encephalitis viruses

Bunyaviruses e. g., La Crosse strain of California virus

Reoviruses e. g., Colorado tick fever virus

From [36] with permission.

Presentation of acute encephalitis may include a history of headache, fever, neurological signs, seizures. Other diagnostic signs include CSF pleocytosis, focal abnormalities seen on electroencephalogram (EEG) and changes seen on either computed tomography (CT) or magnetic resonance imaging (MRI). PCR has a specificity of about 95% to detect HSV-1 [37, 38].

General management includes the treatment of raised intracranial pressure (ICP) with intravenous mannitol and/or steroids, control of seizures with appropriate anticonvulsants and correction of fluid and electrolyte imbalances. Acyclovir treatment should be started as soon as a diagnosis of HSE is considered. Intravenous acyclovir at a dose of 10 mg/kg three times daily should be continued for at least 14 days [37].

Arthropod-Borne Viruses

Arthropod-borne viruses (arboviruses) are viruses that can be transmitted to man by arthropod vectors [39]. Arboviruses are mostly RNA viruses that belong to four families: *Flaviviridae* (e. g., yellow fever, Dengue, Japanese encephalitis); *Bunyaviridae* (e. g., Sandfly fever, Rift Valley fever, CCHF); *Reoviridae* (e. g., Colorado Tick virus); and *Togaviridae* (e. g., Eastern equine encephalitis [EEE], Western equine encephalitis [WEE]). They have a similar mode of transmission, through the bite of bloodsucking arthropods (mosquitoes, ticks, midges, and sandflies).

Arthropod-borne viruses and non-arthropod borne viruses can be categorized into arboviral encephalitides and viral hemorrhagic fever.

Arboviral Encephalitides

Chikungunya

Chikungunya (CHIKV) is an alphavirus of the family *Togaviridae,* transmitted principally by the *Aedes aegypti* mosquito. Clinical presentation includes sudden onset of high fever (> 102 °F), severe poly-arthralgia, headache, myalgia, back pain, rash (~ 50% of cases) [40]. Symptoms typically resolve within 7–10 days. The joint pain and stiffness may last longer. Complications include:

- *CNS*: Meningoencephalitis, encephalopathy, seizures, Guillain-Barré syndrome, paresis, palsies, and neuropathy.
- *Ocular:* Optic neuritis, iridocyclitis, episcleritis, retinitis and uveitis
- *Renal:* Nephritis and acute renal failure
- *Other:* Bleeding dyscrasias, pneumonia, respiratory failure, hepatitis, pancreatitis, syndrome of inappropriate secretion of antidiuretic hormone (SIADH) and hypoadrenalism.

Infections with CHIKV are confirmed by the detection of the virus, viral RNA, or CHIKV-specific antibodies in patient samples. Treatment is symptomatic and supportive.

Japanese encephalitis virus

Japanese encephalitis virus (JEV) is an ss-RNA virus that belongs to the genus *Flavivirus* and is closely related to West Nile and Saint-Louis encephalitis viruses. The *Culex* mosquito transmits the virus and it is the most common vaccine-preventable cause of encephalitis in Asia. Among patients who develop clinical symptoms, the incubation period is 5–15 days. Clinical features consist of acute encephalitis, acute flaccid paralysis, similar to poliomyelitis, status epilepticus, increased ICP, and brainstem herniation. About 20–30% of patients die, and 30–50% of survivors have neurologic or psychiatric sequelae [41, 42]. There is no specific antiviral treatment for Japanese encephalitis; therapy consists of supportive care and management of complications.

Viral Hemorrhagic Fever

Viral hemorrhagic fever refers to a group of illnesses that are caused by several distinct families of viruses (Fig. 1). It is typically a combination of endothelial dysfunction causing a capillary leak syndrome and a bleeding diathesis, caused by thrombocytopenia and disseminated intravascular coagulation (DIC) [43]. Viruses that cause viral hemorrhagic fever are present globally and manifest symptoms pertaining to the virus in that geographic area. Viral hemorrhagic fevers continue to pose a major threat in most world regions today.

Ebola Virus Disease

Ebola virus disease, formerly known as Ebola hemorrhagic fever, is a severe, often fatal illness in humans. Ebola and Marburg viruses are non-segmented, negative-sense, ss-RNA viruses that resemble rhabdoviruses and paramyxoviruses in their genome organization and replication mechanisms [44].

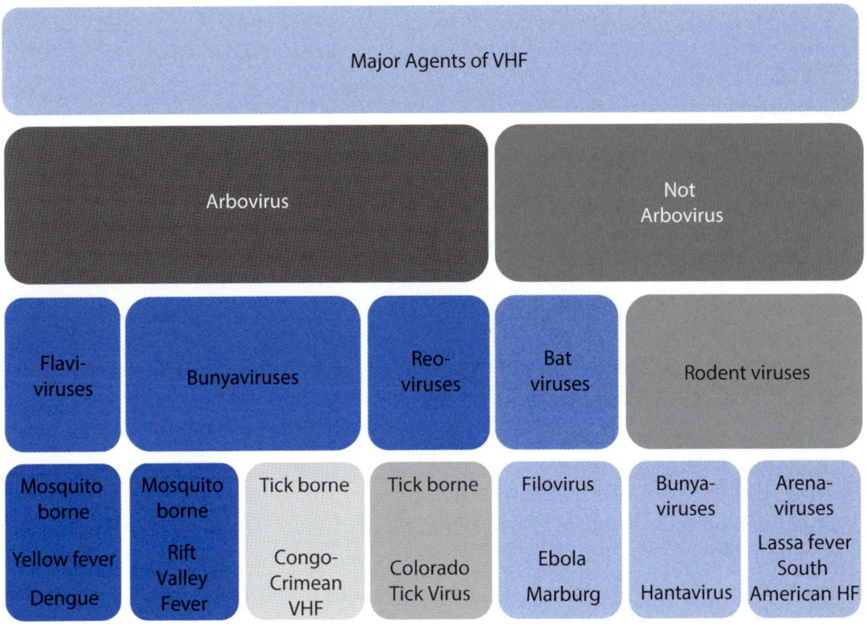

Fig. 1 Agents of viral hemorrhagic fever (VHF). Togaviruses are not included as they do not cause viral hemorrhagic fever. From [43] with permission

Ebola virus is subdivided into five species: Bundibugyo ebolavirus, Zaire ebolavirus, Reston ebolavirus, Sudan ebolavirus, Tai Forest ebolavirus.

Ebola virus causes severe hemorrhagic fever with up to 90% mortality. Ebola virus disease outbreaks occur primarily in remote villages in Central and West Africa, near tropical rainforests [45]. Transmission of the disease generally results from contact with blood, secretions or tissues from patients or infected animals. In Africa, infection has been documented through the handling of infected chimpanzees, gorillas, fruit bats, monkeys, antelope and porcupines found ill or dead in the rainforest. Ebola virus disease can then spread in the community through human-to-human transmission, with infection resulting from direct contact with blood, secretions, organs or other body fluids of infected people, and indirect contact with environments contaminated with such fluids. The incubation period is 2 to 21 days.

Ebola virus disease is characterized by a severe febrile illness, with profound gastrointestinal manifestations, and is complicated by intravascular volume depletion, shock, electrolyte abnormalities and organ dysfunction. Both internal and external bleeding occur due to coagulopathy [46].

Diagnosis is performed by antibody-capture ELISA, antigen detection tests, serum neutralization test, reverse transcriptase PCR (RT-PCR) assay, electron microscopy and virus isolation by cell culture. Samples from patients are an extreme biohazard risk; testing should be conducted under maximum biological containment conditions [46].

Treatment for Ebola virus disease is mainly supportive and involves a combination of fluid resuscitation, administration of analgesics and standard nursing measures. There are currently no specific antiviral drugs for the treatment of Ebola virus disease.

Dengue

Dengue virus is a member of the Flaviviridae family composed of ss-RNA. It is transmitted by *Aedes aegypti* mosquitoes. It has four serotypes (DEN-1, 2, 3, 4). Dengue virus infections cause a spectrum of illnesses ranging from asymptomatic to Dengue fever, Dengue hemorrhagic fever, and Dengue shock syndrome [47] (Table 2). While Dengue fever is a self-limiting febrile illness, Dengue hemorrhagic fever is often characterized by prominent hemorrhagic manifestations associated with increased vascular permeability. The incubation period is typically 4–7 days.

After the incubation period, the illness begins abruptly and, in patients with moderate to severe disease, is followed by three phases: Febrile, critical, recovery (Fig. 2). Dengue fever is characterized by the sudden onset of fever and other non-specific symptoms, such as headache, flushed face. During the first 24–48 h, a petechial rash or maculopapular rash can frequently be seen during the period of defervescence. The fever may continue for 5–7 days. Hemorrhagic complications may also appear, such as bleeding from the gums, nosebleeds, and bruising. Mortality from Dengue fever is low, whereas mortality from Dengue hemorrhagic fever is fairly high. Spontaneous bleeding, plasma leakage, fever, and thrombocytopenia characterize Dengue hemorrhagic fever. Dengue shock syndrome is the most severe

Table 2 Dengue clinical syndromes. From [68] with permission

DHF grade	Duration of fever, d	Hemorrhage	Thrombocytopenia: platelets/mm^3	Increased vascular permeability
I	$>2, \leq 7$	Positive tourniquet test only	$\leq$ 100,000	Plasma leakage[a]
II	$>2, \leq 7$	Spontaneous bleeding[b]	$\leq$ 100,000	Plasma leakage[a]
III (DSS)	$>2, \leq 7$	Positive tourniquet test and/or spontaneous bleeding[b]	$\leq$ 100,000	Plasma leakage[a] and circulatory failure with pulse pressure $\leq$ 20 mmHg or hypotension for age
IV (DSS)	$>2, \leq 7$	Positive tourniquet test and/or spontaneous bleeding[b]	$\leq$ 100,000	Plasma leakage[a] and profound shock with undetectable pulse and blood pressure

[a] As demonstrated by any of the following: elevation of the admission hematocrit to $\geq$ 20% above the expected mean for age, sex, and population; reduction of the hematocrit to $\geq$ 20% of the baseline value after fluid resuscitation; and clinical signs of plasma leakage, such as pleural effusion or ascites.

[b] For example, skin petechiae, bruising, or mucosal/gastrointestinal bleeding.

DHF: Dengue hemorrhagic fever.

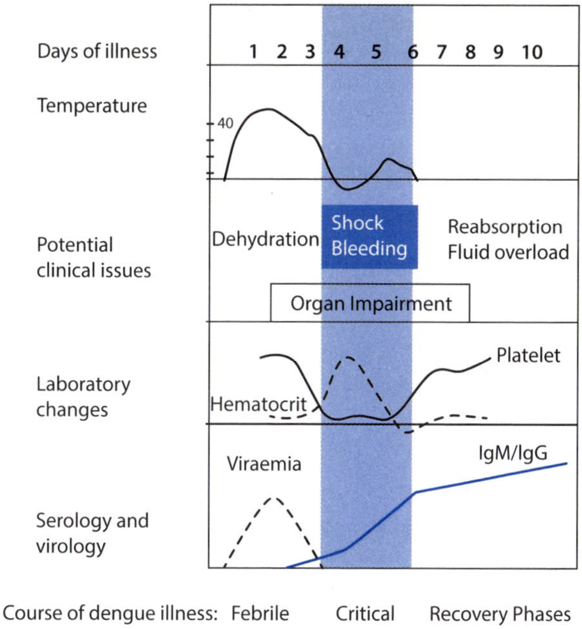

Fig. 2 The course of Dengue illness. IgM: immunoglobulin M; IgG: immunoglobulin G. Temperature is given in degrees Celsius (°C). From [69] with permission

form of Dengue hemorrhagic fever and is characterized by the presence of all four Dengue hemorrhagic fever clinical manifestations (increased vascular permeability, thrombocytopenia, fever lasting two to seven days, hemorrhagic tendency) and circulatory failure [48].

Laboratory abnormalities include thrombocytopenia, leukocytopenia, and increased levels of hepatic aminotransferase. Serological detection is based on IgM-capture ELISA and IgG ELISA or a hemagglutination inhibition test, detection of the genomic sequence by RT-PCR or viral isolation [49].

There are no specific antivirals that can be used in Dengue syndrome. However, supportive care, paracetamol and other analgesics and antipyretics can be used to treat the fever. During episodes of Dengue hemorrhagic fever/Dengue shock syndrome, patients will need comprehensive ICU care with intensive algorithm-based fluid therapy (Fig. 3), vasopressors, and mechanical ventilation.

Crimean-Congo Hemorrhagic Fever

The CCHF virus is a *Nairovirus* in the *Bunyaviridae* family and causes severe disease in human beings, with a reported mortality rate of 3–30%. Human beings become infected through tick bites. CCHF virus circulates in an enzootic tick–vertebrate–tick cycle, and the virus causes no disease in animals [50]. CCHF virus has been detected in the sera of horses, donkeys, goats, cattle, sheep, and pigs in various regions of Europe, Asia, and Africa. Birds may have a role in the transportation of CCHF virus-infected ticks between different countries. The major at-risk groups are farmers living in endemic areas. Hospital healthcare workers are at serious risk:

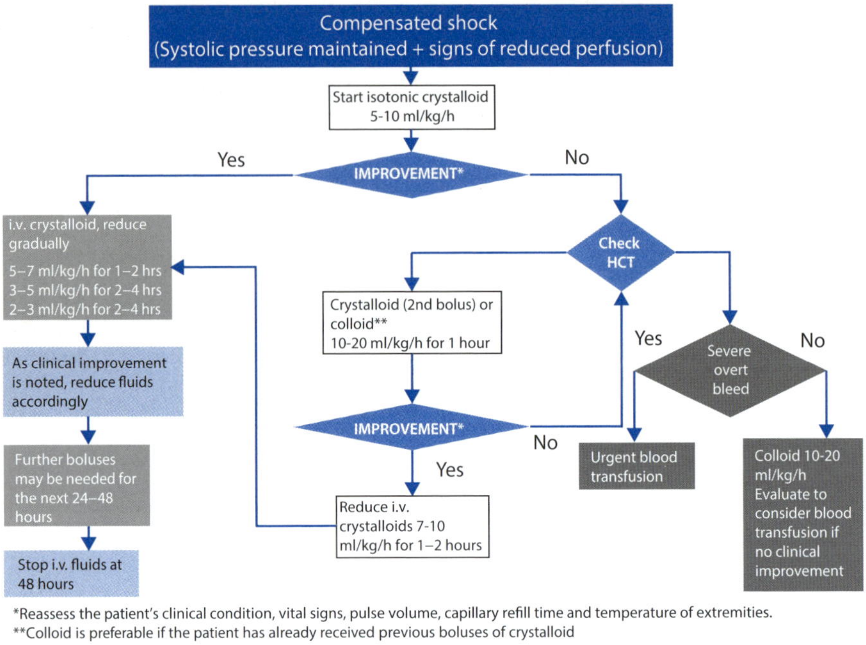

Fig. 3 Algorithm for fluid management of compensated shock in adults. i.v.: intravenous; HCT: hematocrit; ↑: increased; ↓: decreased. From [69] with permission

8.7% of healthcare workers who were exposed to infected blood and 33% of those who had a needlestick injury developed the disease.

Laboratory methods include virus isolation, serological assays, and molecular assays. Immunofluorescence assays (IFAs) using specific monoclonal antibodies may enable virus visualization under microscopy.

The antiviral drug, ribavirin, is currently used in the treatment of CCHF. Patients need to be aggressively fluid resuscitated. Replacement therapy with blood components is the basis of management in severe CCHF. Suspected and diagnosed patients with CCHF should be isolated [51].

Hospital-Based Viral Infections

HSV1

Ventilator-associated pneumonia (VAP) has always been attributed to bacteria, although on numerous occasions the etiology of VAP remains undetermined. With the advent of better diagnostic tools, recent data indicate that viruses may be implicated in nosocomial infections in non-immunocompromised patients. There are, however, no standardized diagnostic tools. No publication has established a causal relationship between isolation and the infectious episode. In a French prospective study, isolated viruses including rhinovirus, herpes simples, influenza, RSV, enterovirus, parainfluenza, adenovirus, coronavirus and CMV were detected in 25% of the patients [52].

Numerous studies have implicated HSV1 as the most likely virus to cause VAP. The reported frequency varies between 5–64%, with a median of 15–20% [53–57]. Reactivation of a latent virus appears to be the initial mechanism in all patients with HSV1 pneumonia in the ICU. Reactivation is due to instrumentation of the airways and begins by the 3rd–5th day peaking by day 12 [58]. Risk factors for HSV1 include mucocutaneous herpetic lesions, tracheal mucosal lesions, high sequential organ failure assessment (SOFA) and/or APACHE II scores, mechanical ventilation for more than 7 days, old age and prior corticosteroid use [58].

Cytomegalovirus

The seroprevalence of CMV in adults is in the range of 50–90% [59]. As with all herpesviruses, primary CMV infection remains latent lifelong and undergoes episodes of reactivation, and may progress to symptomatic disease. In the last decade, CMV reactivation has been reported in immunocompetent critically ill patients. The incidence is variable, depending on the diagnostic method used (culture or PCR), and ranges from 12–33% [60]. The incidence of active CMV disease was found to be high in a series of 242 immunocompetent patients subjected to ventilation for over 48 hours (16.1%) [61]. CMV should be suspected as the cause of VAP in the presence of persistent infiltrates, a lack of clinical improvement and negative bacterial cultures [62]. Reactivation of CMV occurs between days 14 and 21 of the ICU stay. Reactivation may begin in the lung parenchyma and is usually activated by sepsis. This process can cause a persistent increase in cytokine-mediated inflammatory response. Risk factors for reactivation are blood transfusion, age, previous hospitalization, prior corticosteroid use and burn injury. Several observational studies have shown an association between CMV infection in critically ill patients and poor clinical outcomes [63].

Five drugs – ganciclovir/valganciclovir, cidofovir, foscarnet and fomivirsen – have been approved so far for the treatment of human CMV [64]. Ganciclovir is favored over alternative agents based on its potent activity against CMV and availability of intravenous formulation [65]. Preemptive therapy and prophylaxis appear effective for prevention of symptomatic CMV infection in non-immunocompromised patients. In experimental studies, early prophylactic administration of high-dose ganciclovir was significantly more effective in preventing both CMV reactivation and subsequent pulmonary fibrosis than delayed treatment.

Other Viruses

In a recent study, 19% of ventilated patients with suspected VAP yielded positive serological tests for *Acanthamoeba polyphaga*, a mimivirus. Risk factors consisted of duration of mechanical ventilation, prior bronchoalveolar lavage and absence of enteral nutrition. These patients had mortality rates of about 50% [66].

A host of other viruses may spread between patients by various routes, including community-acquired viruses, as has been seen with measles, during the SARS epidemic, influenza, Avian flu, etc. Nosocomial infections may spread through needlestick injury or exposure to contaminated body fluids, as in HBV, hepatitis C and HIV. All of the above can be associated with a risk of transmission to healthcare workers.

Conclusion

Septic processes remain one of the main causes of morbidity-mortality in ICUs throughout the world. Viruses play a significant role in serious infections warranting admissions to the ICU. The role viruses play in unidentified sepsis may be just the tip of the iceberg. Diagnostic dilemmas and non-availability of appropriate laboratory tests may prevent early and definitive diagnosis of viral sepsis. The limited availability of effective anti-viral agents or vaccines limits therapy. However, certain viruses do respond effectively to appropriate agents (e. g., HSV and VRZ to acyclovir, CCHF to ribavirin, CMV to ganciclovir). ECMO played an important role in improving survival globally in the recent H1N1 epidemic. Advances in HIV therapy provide new hope to the large population of AIDS patients worldwide. A similar hope can be seen for patients with chronic hepatitis B and C infection. In the ICU, healthcare workers need to be cautioned during epidemics of influenza and Ebola virus, ensuring that ICUs follow the necessary protocols to prevent transmission. These microorganisms have been around since even before the era of dinosaurs and have found the means to survival for generations by mutations and alterations in their genetic structure. The question is, can humanity find the means to counter them?

References

1. Gelderblom HR (1996) Structure and Classification of Viruses. In: Baron S (ed) Medical Microbiology. The University of Texas Medical Branch at Galveston, Galveston
2. Belardelli F (1995) Role of interferons and other cytokines in the regulation of the immune response. APMIS 103:161–179
3. Ahmed RGD (1996) Immunological memory and protective immunity: understanding their relation. Science 272:54–60
4. Alcami A (2003) Viral mimicry of cytokines, chemokines and their receptors. Nat Rev Immunol 3:36–50
5. Gomersall CD, Loo S, Joynt GM, Taylor BL (2007) Pandemic preparedness. Curr Opin Crit Care 13:742–747

6. Hampson AW, Mackenzie JS (2006) The influenza viruses. Med J Aust 185:39–43
7. Taylor LH, Latham SM, Woolhouse ME (2001) Risk factors for human disease emergence. Philos Trans R Soc Lond B Biol Sci 356:983–989
8. Chen T, Hudnall SD (2006) Anatomical mapping of human herpesvirus reservoirs of infection. Mod Pathol 19:726–737
9. Lok AS, McMahon BJ, Practice Guidelines Committee AAftSoLD (2004) Chronic hepatitis B: update of recommendations. Hepatology 39:857–861
10. Bentwich Z, Bar-Yehuda S, Nagai K, Wainberg MA, Kalinkovich A, Jehuda-Cohen T (1995) Pending problem of "silent" human immunodeficiency virus infection. Cell Mol Biol 41:345–350
11. Bieniasz PD (2004) Intrinsic immunity: a front-line defense against viral attack. Nat Immunol 5:1109–1115
12. Vivier E, Raulet DH, Moretta A et al (2011) Innate or adaptive immunity? The example of natural killer cells. Science 331:44–49
13. Stetson DB, Medzhitov R (2006) Type I interferons in host defense. Immunity 25:373–381
14. Lee HK, Iwasaki A (2007) Innate control of adaptive immunity: dendritic cells and beyond. Semin Immunol 19:48–55
15. Ishii KJ, Akira S (2006) Innate immune recognition of, and regulation by, DNA. Trends Immunol 27:525–532
16. Fritz JH, Girardin SE, Philpott DJ (2006) Innate immune defense through RNA interference. Sci STKE 2006
17. Bevan MJ (2004) Helping the CD8(+) T-cell response. Nat Rev Immunol 4:595–602
18. Akira S, Takeda K (2004) Toll-like receptor signalling. Nat Rev Immunol 4:499–511
19. Slifka MK, Ahmed R (1996) Long-term humoral immunity against viruses: revisiting the issue of plasma cell longevity. Trends Microbiol 4:394–400
20. Getts DR, Chastain EM, Terry RL, Miller SD (2013) Virus infection, antiviral immunity, and autoimmunity. Immunol Rev 255:197–209
21. Fruh K, Yang Y (1999) Antigen presentation by MHC class I and its regulation by interferon gamma. Curr Opin Immunol 11:76–81
22. Woodland DL, Dutton RW (2003) Heterogeneity of CD4(+) and CD8(+) T cells. Curr Opin Immunol 15:336–342
23. Boonham N, Kreuze J, Winter S et al (2014) Methods in virus diagnostics: from ELISA to next generation sequencing. Virus Res 186:20–31
24. Storch GA (2000) Diagnostic virology. Clin Infect Dis 31:739–751
25. Johnstone J, Majumdar SR, Fox JD, Marrie TJ (2008) Viral infection in adults hospitalized with community-acquired pneumonia: prevalence, pathogens, and presentation. Chest 134:1141–1148
26. Sandrock CE (2008) Severe febrile respiratory illnesses as a cause of mass critical care. Respir Care 53:40–53
27. Beigel JH (2008) Influenza. Crit Care Med 36:2660–2666
28. Davies A, Jones D, Bailey M et al (2009) Extracorporeal membrane oxygenation for 2009 influenza A (H1N1) acute respiratory distress syndrome. JAMA 302:1888–1895
29. Roch A, Lepaul-Ercole R, Grisoli D et al (2010) Extracorporeal membrane oxygenation for severe influenza A (H1N1) acute respiratory distress syndrome: a prospective observational comparative study. Intensive Care Med 36:1899–1905
30. Norfolk SG, Hollingsworth CL, Wolfe CR et al (2010) Rescue therapy in adult and pediatric patients with pH1N1 influenza infection: a tertiary center intensive care unit experience from April to October 2009. Crit Care Med 38:2103–2107
31. Ugarte S, Arancibia F, Soto R (2010) Influenza A pandemics: clinical and organizational aspects: the experience in Chile. Crit Care Med 38:e133–e137
32. Freed DH, Henzler D, White CW et al (2010) Extracorporeal lung support for patients who had severe respiratory failure secondary to influenza A (H1N1) 2009 infection in Canada. Can J Anaesth 57:240–247

33. Liong T, Lee KL, Poon YS et al (2009) The first novel influenza A (H1N1) fatality despite antiviral treatment and extracorporeal membrane oxygenation in Hong Kong. Hong Kong Med J 15:381–384
34. Hall CB (2001) Respiratory syncytial virus and parainfluenza virus. N Engl J Med 344:1917–1928
35. Manocha S, Walley KR, Russell JA (2003) Severe acute respiratory distress syndrome (SARS): a critical care perspective. Crit Care Med 31:2684–2692
36. Kennedy PG (2005) Viral encephalitis. J Neurol 252:268–272
37. Chaudhuri A, Kennedy PG (2002) Diagnosis and treatment of viral encephalitis. Postgrad Med J 78:575–583
38. Steiner I, Budka H, Chaudhuri A et al (2005) Viral encephalitis: a review of diagnostic methods and guidelines for management. Eur J Neurol 12:331–343
39. Kuno G, Chang GJ (2005) Biological transmission of arboviruses: reexamination of and new insights into components, mechanisms, and unique traits as well as their evolutionary trends. Clin Microbiol Rev 18:608–637
40. Staples JE, Breiman RF, Powers AM (2009) Chikungunya fever: an epidemiological review of a re-emerging infectious disease. Clin Infect Dis 49:942–948
41. Campbell GL, Hills SL, Fischer M et al (2011) Estimated global incidence of Japanese encephalitis: a systematic review. Bull World Health Organ 89:766–774 (774A–774E)
42. Tiwari S, Singh RK, Tiwari R, Dhole TN (2012) Japanese encephalitis: a review of the Indian perspective. Braz J Infect Dis 16:564–573
43. Meltzer E (2012) Arboviruses and viral hemorrhagic fevers (VHF). Infect Dis Clin North Am 26:479–496
44. Hoenen T, Groseth A, Falzarano D, Feldmann H (2006) Ebola virus: unravelling pathogenesis to combat a deadly disease. Trends Mol Med 12:206–215
45. Gatherer D (2014) The 2014 Ebola virus disease outbreak in West Africa. J Gen Virol 95:1619–1624
46. Feldmann H, Geisbert TW (2011) Ebola haemorrhagic fever. Lancet 377:849–862
47. Gubler DJ (1998) Dengue and dengue hemorrhagic fever. Clin Microbiol Rev 11:480–496
48. Wilder-Smith A, Schwartz E (2005) Dengue in travelers. N Engl J Med 353:924–932
49. Tripathi NK, Shrivastava A, Dash PK, Jana AM (2011) Detection of dengue virus. Methods Mol Biol 665:51–64
50. Ergonul O (2006) Crimean-Congo haemorrhagic fever. Lancet Infect Dis 6:203–214
51. Vorou R, Pierroutsakos IN, Maltezou HC (2007) Crimean-Congo hemorrhagic fever. Curr Opin Infect Dis 20:495–500
52. Daubin C, Vincent S, Vabret A et al (2005) Nosocomial viral ventilator-associated pneumonia in the intensive care unit: a prospective cohort study. Intensive Care Med 31:1116–1122
53. Bruynseels P, Jorens PG, Demey HE et al (2003) Herpes simplex virus in the respiratory tract of critical care patients: a prospective study. Lancet 362:1536–1541
54. Ong GM, Lowry K, Mahajan S et al (2004) Herpes simplex type 1 shedding is associated with reduced hospital survival in patients receiving assisted ventilation in a tertiary referral intensive care unit. J Med Virol 72:121–125
55. Cook CH, Martin LC, Yenchar JK et al (2003) Occult herpes family viral infections are endemic in critically ill surgical patients. Crit Care Med 31:1923–1929
56. Linssen CF, Jacobs JA, Stelma FF et al (2008) Herpes simplex virus load in bronchoalveolar lavage fluid is related to poor outcome in critically ill patients. Intensive Care Med 34:2202–2209
57. De Vos N, Van Hoovels L, Vankeerberghen A et al (2009) Monitoring of herpes simplex virus in the lower respiratory tract of critically ill patients using real-time PCR: a prospective study. Clin Microbiol Infect 15:358–363
58. Luyt CE, Combes A, Deback C et al (2007) Herpes simplex virus lung infection in patients undergoing prolonged mechanical ventilation. Am J Respir Crit Care Med 175:935–942

59. Chiche L, Forel JM, Papazian L (2011) The role of viruses in nosocomial pneumonia. Curr Opin Infect Dis 24:152–156
60. Limaye AP, Kirby KA, Rubenfeld GD et al (2008) Cytomegalovirus reactivation in critically ill immunocompetent patients. JAMA 300:413–422
61. Chiche L, Forel JM, Roch A et al (2009) Active cytomegalovirus infection is common in mechanically ventilated medical intensive care unit patients. Crit Care Med 37:1850–1857
62. Luyt CE, Brechot N, Chastre J (2014) What role do viruses play in nosocomial pneumonia? Curr Opin Infect Dis 27:194–199
63. Osawa R, Singh N (2009) Cytomegalovirus infection in critically ill patients: a systematic review. Crit Care 13:R68
64. Schreiber A, Harter G, Schubert A, Bunjes D, Mertens T, Michel D (2009) Antiviral treatment of cytomegalovirus infection and resistant strains. Expert Opin Pharmacother 10:191–209
65. Jain M, Duggal S, Chugh TD (2011) Cytomegalovirus infection in non-immunosuppressed critically ill patients. J Infect Dev Ctries 5:571–579
66. Vincent A, La Scola B, Forel JM, Pauly V, Raoult D, Papazian L (2009) Clinical significance of a positive serology for mimivirus in patients presenting a suspicion of ventilator-associated pneumonia. Crit Care Med 37:111–118
67. Storch GA (2000) Diagnostic virology. Clin Infect Dis 31:739–751
68. Ngo NT, Cao XT, Kneen R et al (2001) Acute management of dengue shock syndrome: a randomized double-blind comparison of 4 intravenous fluid regimens in the first hour. Clin Infect Dis 32:204–213
69. World Health Organization (2012) Handbook for Clinical Management of Dengue. http://apps.who.int/iris/bitstream/10665/76887/1/9789241504713_eng.pdf?ua=1. Accessed Nov 2014

Part II
Antimicrobials and Resistance

Light and Shade of New Antibiotics

M. Bassetti, P. Della Siega, and D. Pecori

Introduction

Multidrug-resistant (MDR) bacteria or superbugs represent a challenge for clinicians and a serious and worsening threat to human health both in community and hospital settings [1]. Physicians routinely encounter patients with infections that are not responding to available treatments and when new antibacterials arrive on the market, bacteria quickly develop resistance. The microorganisms that are mainly involved in the resistance process are the so-called ESKAPE pathogens (*Enterococcus faecium, Staphylococcus aureus, Klebsiella pneumoniae, Acinetobacter baumanii, Pseudomonas aeruginosa,* and *enterobacteriaceae*), emphasizing their ability to 'escape' from commonly used antibacterial treatment [2].

Since a standardized definition of MDR, extensively drug-resistant (XDR) and pan-drug-resistant (PDR) pathogens was not available, a group of international experts joined an initiative by the European Center for Disease Prevention and Control (ECDC) and the Centers for Disease Control and Prevention (CDC) in the US to create a new standardized international terminology for describing acquired resistance profiles in bacteria that are often responsible for healthcare-associated infections and that are prone to multidrug resistance [3]. Multidrug resistance was defined as non-susceptibility to at least one agent in three or more antimicrobial categories. Extensive drug resistance was defined as non-susceptibility to at least one agent in all but two or fewer antimicrobial categories. Pan-drug resistance was defined as non-susceptibility to all agents in all antimicrobial categories.

Antibiotic development continues to decline for multifactorial reasons. Drug development, in general, is facing increasing challenges, given the high costs required, currently estimated to be $400–$800 million per approved agent. Furthermore, antibiotics have a lower relative rate of return on investment than do other drugs because they are usually used in short-course therapies. In contrast, chronic dis-

M. Bassetti ✉ · P. Della Siega · D. Pecori
Infectious Diseases Division, Santa Maria Misericordia University Hospital, 33100 Udine, Italy
e-mail: mattba@tin.it

J.-L. Vincent (ed.), *Annual Update in Intensive Care and Emergency Medicine 2015*,
DOI 10.1007/978-3-319-13761-2_5

Table 1 Antibiotics currently in clinical development

Drug class	Drug name	Development phase	Company	Potential activity against Gram-negative pathogens	Potential indications
Cephalosporin	GSK2696266	Phase 1	GlaxoSmithKline (partnered product)		Bacterial infections
Novel cephalosporin + beta-lactamase inhibitor	Ceftolozane + tazobactam	New Drug Application (NDA) submitted (for complicated urinary tract infection and complicated intra-abdominal infection indications)	Cubist pharmaceuticals	Yes	Complicated urinary tract infections, complicated intra-abdominal infections, acute pyelonephritis (kidney infection), hospital-acquired bacterial pneumonia/ventilato-associated pneumonia
	Ceftaroline + avibactam	Phase 2	AstraZeneca/Forest Laboratories	Yes	Complicated urinary tract infections
	Ceftazidime + avibactam (CAZ-AVI)	Phase 3	AstraZeneca/Forest Laboratories	Yes	Complicated urinary tract infections, complicated intra-abdominal infections, acute pyelonephritis (kidney infection), hospital-acquired bacterial pneumonia/ventilator-associated bacterial pneumonia
Monobactam + novel beta-lactamase inhibitor	Aztreonam + avibactam (ATM-AVI)	Phase 1	AstraZeneca/Forest Laboratories	Yes	Bacterial infections

Table 1 (Continuation)

Drug class	Drug name	Development phase	Company	Potential activity against Gram-negative pathogens	Potential indications
Carbapenem + novel betalactamase inhibitor	Carbavance	Phase 1	Rempex Pharmaceuticals/the Medicines Co	Yes	Complicated urinary tract infections, complicated intra-abdominal infections, hospital-acquired bacterial pneumonia/ventilator-associated bacterial pneumonia, febrile neutropenia
	MK-7655 + imipenem/cilastatin	Phase 2	Merck	Yes	Complicated urinary tract infections, acute pyelonephritis, complicated intra-abdominal infections
Aminoglycoside	Plazomicin	Phase 3	Achaogen	Yes	Bloodstream infections and nosocomial pneumonia caused by carbapenem-resistant Enterobacteriaeceae

Table 1 (Continuation)

Drug class	Drug name	Development phase	Company	Potential activity against Gram-negative pathogens	Potential indications
Fluoroquinolone	WCK 771	Phase 1	Wockhardt		Bacterial infections
	WCK 2349 (WCK 771 pro-drug)	Phase 1	Wockhardt		Bacterial infections
	Avarofloxacin	Phase 2	Furiex Pharmaceuticals	Yes	Community-acquired bacterial pneumonia, acute bacterial skin and skin structure infections
	Finafloxacin	Phase 2	MerLion Pharmaceuticals	Yes	Complicated urinary tract infections, acute pyelonephritis (kidney infection), acute intra-abdominal infections, acute bacterial skin and skin structure infections
	Nemonoxacin	Phase 2	TaiGen Biotechnlogy	Yes	Community-acquired bacterial pneumonia, diabetic foot infection, acute bacterial skin and skin structure infections
	Zabofloxacin	Phase 2	Dong Wha Pharmaceutical		Community-acquired bacterial pneumonia
	Delafloxacin	Phase 3	Melinta Pharmaceuticals	Yes	Acute bacterial skin and skin structure infections, community-acquired bacterial pneumonia, uncomplicated gonorrhea

Table 1 (Continuation)

Drug class	Drug name	Development phase	Company	Potential activity against Gram-negative pathogens	Potential indications
Oxazolidinone	Tedizolid	Approved June 20, 2014	Cubist Pharmaceutics		Acute bacterial skin and skin structure infections, hospital acquired bacterial pneumonia/ventilator-acquired bacterial pneumonia
	Cadazolid (Quinolonyl-oxalidinone)	Phase 3	Actelion Pharmaceuticals		*Clostridium difficile*-associated diarrhea
	Radezolid	Phase 2	Melinta Pharmaceutics	Yes	Acute bacterial skin and skin structure infections, community-acquired bacterial pneumonia
	MRX-I	Phase 1	MicuRx Pharmaceuticals		Bacterial infections including community-acquired MRSA and vancomycin-resistant enterococcal infections
	LCB01–0371	Phase 1	LegoChem Biosciences (S. Korea)		Bacterial infections

Table 1 (Continuation)

Drug class		Drug name	Development phase	Company	Potential activity against Gram-negative pathogens	Potential indications
Lipopeptide and glycopeptide		Oritavancin	Approved August 6, 2014	The Medicines Company		Acute bacterial skin and skin structure infections
	Glycopeptide-cephalosporin heterodimer	TD-1607	Phase 1	Theravance, Inc		Serious Gram-positive bacterial infections (acute bacterial skin and skin structure infections, hospital-acquired pneumonia/ventilator-associated pneumonia, bacteremia)
		TD-1792	Phase 2	Theravance, Inc		Acute bacterial skin and skin structure infections, other serious infections caused by Gram-positive bacteria including hospital-acquired pneumonia/ventilator-associated pneumonia and bacteremia
	Lipo-glycopeptide	Dalbavancin	Approved May 23, 2014	Durata Therapeutics		Acute bacterial skin and skin structure infections
		Ramoplanin	Phase 2	Nanotherapeutics		*Clostridium difficile*-associated diarrhea
	Lipopeptide	Surotomycin	Phase 3	Cubist Pharmaceuticals		*Clostridium difficile*-associated diarrhea
Macro-lide	Ketolide	Solithromycin	Phase 3	Cempra Pharmaceuticals	Yes	Community-acquired bacterial pneumonia, uncomplicated urogenital gonorrhea
	LptD inhibitor	POL7080	Phase 2	Polyphor (Roche licensee)	Yes	Ventilator-associated bacterial pneumonia, low respiratory tract infections

Table 1 (Continuation)

Drug class	Drug name	Development phase	Company	Potential activity against Gram-negative pathogens	Potential indications
Tetracycline	Omadacycline	Phase 2	Paratek Pharmaceuticals	Yes	Community-acquired bacterial pneumonia, acute bacterial skin and skin structure infections, complicated urinary tract infections
	Eravacycline	Phase 3	Tetraphase Pharmaceuticals	Yes	Complicated intra-abdominal infections, complicated urinary tract infections, hospital-acquired bacterial pneumonia
Monosulfactam	BAL30072	Phase 1	Basilea Pharmaceutica	Yes	Multidrug-resistant Gram-negative bacterial infections
Fabl inhibitor	Debio 1452	Phase 2	Debiopharm Group		Acute bacterial skin and skin structure infections
	Debio 1450 (Debio 1452 pro-drug)	Phase 1	Debiopharm Group		Bacterial infections
	CG-400549	Phase 2	CrystalGenomics, Inc		Acute bacterial skin and skin structure infections; osteomyelitis
LpxC inhibitor	ACHN-975	Phase 1	Achaogen		Bacterial infections
DNA gyrase inhibitor	AZD0914	Phase 1	AstraZeneca	Yes	Uncomplicated gonorrhea
Methionyl-tRNA synthetase (MetRS) inhibitor	CRS3123	Phase 1	Crestone, Inc		*C. difficile* infection
Peptide deformylase inhibitor	GSK1322322	Phase 2	GlaxoSmithKline		Acute bacterial skin and skin structure infections

Table 1 (Continuation)

Drug class	Drug name	Development phase	Company	Potential activity against Gram-negative pathogens	Potential indications
Type 2 topoisomerase inhibitor	GSK2140944	Phase 2	GlaxoSmithKline		Respiratory tract infections, acute bacterial skin and skin structure infections
Bicyclolide	EDP-788	Phase 1	Enanta Pharmaceuticals		Bacterial infections
Pleuromutilin	Lefamulin (BC-3781)	Phase 2	Nabriva Therapeutics		Acute bacterial skin and skin structure infections, community-acquired bacterial pneumonia
Elongation factor inhibitor	LFF571	Phase 2	Novartis		*C. difficile*-associated diarrhea
Fusidane	Taksta (Fusidic acid)	Phase 2	Cempra Pharmaceutics		Prosthetic joint infections
Defensin-mimetic	Brilacidin	Phase 2	Cellceutix Corp		Acute bacterial skin and skin structure infections
	SMT19969	Phase 2	Summit Corporation Plc.		*C. difficile*-associated diarrhea

eases, including human immunodeficiency virus (HIV) infection and hepatitis, are treated with therapies that suppress symptoms and need to be taken for the life of the patient. Ironically, antibiotics are victims of their own success; they are less desirable to drug companies because they are more successful than other drugs [4].

Numerous agencies and professional societies have highlighted the problem of the lack of new antibiotics, especially for MDR Gram-negative pathogens. Since 2004, repeated calls to reinvigorate pharmaceutical investment in antibiotic research and development have been made by the Infectious Diseases Society of America (IDSA) and several other notable societies [5]. The IDSA have supported a program, called "the 10 × '20 Initiative", aimed at developing 10 new systemic antibacterial drugs within 2020 by discovery of new drug classes or new molecules inside already existing classes of antibiotics [6].

The current assessment of the antibiotic pipeline (last updated, August 2014) shows 45 new antibiotics in development or recently approved (Table 1). Of these, 14 are in Phase 1 clinical trials, 20 in Phase 2, 7 in Phase 3 (one has had new drug applications submitted and three have recently been approved) [7]. Five of the seven antibiotics in Phase 3, as well as one drug submitted for review to the Food and Drug Administration (FDA), have the potential to address infections caused by Gram-negative pathogens, the most pressing unmet need.

In this review we will focus on the light and shade of some of the more interesting new antibiotics, including those recently approved and those in development.

Cephalosporins

Cephalosporins belong to the beta-lactam class of antibiotic and are known for their broad spectrum of activity, proven efficacy and favorable safety profile. Ceftaroline-fosamil was approved in 2010 and has activity against methicillin-resistant *S. aureus* (MRSA) and some Gram-negative bacteria, but not against bacteria producing extended spectrum beta-lactamase (ESBL). To extend the spectrum of activity of this class of antibiotics, a beta-lactamase inhibitor has been associated to new and old cephalosporins.

Ceftolozane/tazobactam

Ceftolozane/tazobactam (formerly known as CXA-201) is a novel oxyimino-aminothia-zolyl anti-pseudomonal cephalosporin associated with a beta-lactamase inhibitor (2 : 1 ratio), marketed and recently submitted by Cubist Pharmaceutics. The spectrum of activity of ceftolozane/tazobactam includes difficult-to-treat Gram-negative pathogens. Specifically, activity against *Escherichia coli* and *K. pneumoniae*, including ESBL strains, has been shown [8, 9]. Furthermore, ceftolozane/tazobactam has demonstrated excellent activity against *P. aeruginosa*, including strains resistant to carbapenems, piperacillin/tazobactam, and other cephalosporins, as well as MDR strains [10]. Spectrum gaps include lack of activity for key resistant Gram-positive pathogens, such as MRSA and vancomycin-resistant *Enterococcus* spp. (VRE).

Ceftolozane/tazobactam is currently in development for treatment of complicated urinary tract infections (UTIs), complicated intra-abdominal infections and hospital-acquired pneumonia (HAP)/ventilator-associated pneumonia (VAP). Phase 2 and 3 trials have shown high efficacy and good tolerability in complicated urinary and intra-abdominal infections compared to standard therapy [11, 12]. New studies are ongoing for the treatment of HAP and VAP.

A number of phase 1 and phase 2 studies have reported that ceftolozane has a good safety and tolerability profile, one that is consistent with that of other cephalosporins [13–15].

Ceftazidime/avibactam

Ceftazidime/avibactam is a novel cephalosporin/beta-lactamase inhibitor (formerly known as CAZ-AVI) in phase 3 of development, promoted by AstraZeneca. Avibactam is a semi-synthetic, non-beta-lactam, beta-lactamase inhibitor (formerly NXL104), developed in combination with ceftazidime, with the intention of inhibiting beta-lactamases with activity against these cephalosporins and, therefore, broadening their spectrum of activity. The addition of avibactam to ceftazidime improves its *in vitro* activity against *Enterobacteriaceae*, including most ceftazidime-resistant isolates [16]. The activity of ceftazidime-avibactam against not-fermenting Gram-negative rods is variable, likely due to the presence of additional mechanisms of resistance (porin alterations, efflux, metallo-beta-lactamases, or OXA beta-lactamases used by *P. aeruginosa* and OXA beta-lactamases used by *Acinetobacter* spp.) [17]. It is not active against *Stenotrophomonas* spp. and has limited activity against Gram-negative anaerobes [18].

Animal studies have shown that ceftazidime-avibactam is effective in ceftazidime-resistant Gram-negative bacteremia, meningitis, pyelonephritis, and pneumonia. Limited clinical trials published to date have reported that ceftazidime-avibactam is as effective as therapy with a carbapenem in complicated UTI and complicated intra-abdominal infection (combined with metronidazole) including infection caused by cephalosporin-resistant Gram-negative isolates [19, 20]. Safety and tolerability of ceftazidime-avibactam in clinical trials has been excellent, with few serious drug-related adverse events reported.

Ceftaroline/avibactam

Ceftaroline/avibactam is a novel cephalosporin/beta-lactamase inhibitor in phase 2 of study, promoted by AstraZeneca. Ceftaroline fosamil is a new cephalosporin with potent activity against Gram-positive organisms, including MRSA and MDR *S. pneumoniae*, approved by the FDA for treatment of bacterial skin and skin structure infection and community-acquired bacterial pneumonia. Ceftaroline is also active against most species of *Enterobacteriaceae* but, like other cephalosporins, has limited activity against isolates producing ESBL, cephalosporinases, or carbapenemases [21]. However, when ceftaroline is combined with avibactam, which inhibits Ambler classes A (e. g., ESBL, *K. pneumoniae* carbapenemase [KPC]) and C (AmpC) enzymes, its spectrum of activity is significantly expanded [22, 23]. Accordingly, it has potent activity against *Enterobacteriaceae* that produce KPC, AmpC and various ESBL and also against MRSA. It has limited activity against *Acinetobacter* spp. and *P. aeruginosa.*

The safety and tolerability of ceftaroline-avibactam have been excellent in clinical trials, with few serious drug-related adverse events reported (gastrointestinal disorders, in particular diarrhea and dry mouth, and nervous system disorders, such as headache, dizziness and tremor) [24].

Carbapenems and Novel Beta-lactamase Inhibitors

Carbapenems have the widest spectrum of antibacterial activity of all the beta-lactams and provide excellent coverage of many Gram-negative and Gram-positive aerobic and anaerobic bacteria. The emergence of carbapenem-hydrolyzing beta-lactamases has threatened the clinical utility of this antibiotic class. The scarcity of new antibiotics against drug-resistant bacteria has led to the development of inhibitors targeting specific resistance mechanisms, which aim to restore the effectiveness of existing agents.

Carbavance (biapenem/RPX7009)

Carbavance is an antibiotic molecule currently in phase 2 of study, promoted by Rempex Pharmaceuticals. RPX7009 is a new boron-based inhibitor of several class A and C beta-lactamases and is being developed in combination with biapenem (RPX2003) but had no effect on the MICs of biapenem for isolates with metallo- (IMP, NDM or VIM) or OXA-48 beta-lactamases; however, most isolates with these enzymes were less resistant to biapenem than to imipenem and, especially, ertapenem [25].

This antibiotic is presently being studied for treating serious Gram-negative infections, such as complicated UTI, acute pyelonephritis, HAP, VAP and bacteremia resistant to currently available carbapenems.

MK-7655

MK-7655 is a novel beta-lactamase diazabicyclooctane inhibitor under clinical investigation as a potential partner for combination with imipenem to overcome class A and C beta-lactamase mediated antibiotic resistance, but it is not active against metallo-carbapenemases. In *in vitro* studies, MK-7655 effectively restored imipenem's activity against imipenem-resistant *Pseudomonas* and *Klebsiella* strains at clinically achievable concentrations [26].

A Phase 2 study is ongoing: the purpose of this study is to determine whether adding 125 mg or 250 mg doses of MK-7655 to imipenem/cilastatin is at least as effective as imipenem/cilastatin alone in adults 18 years or older with complicated intra-abdominal infection.

Aminoglycosides

The aminoglycoside class of antibiotics includes nine antibiotics approved by the FDA and the EMA (gentamicin, tobramycin, amikacin, streptomycin, neomycin, kanamycin, paromomycin, netilmicin, and spectinomycin). They have several important characteristics including rapid bactericidal activity, well-described pharmacokinetics (PK) and excellent solubility and stability. They have been used successfully for the treatment of serious bacterial infections for more than 50 years, in particular infections caused by aerobic Gram-negative bacilli and less common infections caused by *Staphylococcus* spp. and enterococcus spp. (in association with beta-lactams). However, the spread of resistance to currently marketed aminoglycosides has decreased their clinical utility.

Plazomicin

This is a novel semi-synthetic aminoglycoside developed by modifying an existing aminoglycoside, sisomicin, currently in phase 3 of study, promoted by Achaogen. It has bactericidal dose-dependent activity that inhibits bacterial protein synthesis. Plazomicin demonstrated potent *in vitro* activity against members of the *Enterobacteriaceae* family, also against aminoglycoside-not-susceptible *E. coli.* Furthermore, it demonstrated equivalent activity versus ESBL-producing and non-ESBL-producing *E. coli* and *K. pneumoniae* [27] and it is active against clinical *Enterobacteriaceae* possessing most varieties of carbapenem resistance mechanisms. It is active against Gram-negative non-fermenting bacilli; however, it is more active *in vitro* against *P. aeruginosa* and *A. baumannii* isolates with aminoglycoside-modifying enzymes than against those with altered permeability/efflux [28]. Plazomicin demonstrated synergistic activity *in vitro* with daptomycin versus MRSA, vancomycin-intermediate heteroresistant (hVISA), *S. aureus* vancomycin-intermediate (VISA), and vancomycin-resistant (VRSA) and with cefepime, doripenem, imipenem or piperacillin-tazobactam against *P. aeruginosa* [29].

Potential indications for plazomicin are complicated UTI and acute pyelonephritis, including cases with concurrent bacteremia and also the treatment of serious bacterial infections due to MDR *Enterobacteriaceae*, including carbapenem-resistant *Enterobacteriaceae* (CRE) [30].

The advantage compared to approved aminoglycosides is the absence of neprotoxicity and ototoxicity; the most frequently reported adverse events are headache, dizziness (including lightheadedness), somnolence, and blurred vision [31].

Quinolones

The quinolone class of antimicrobial agents has generated considerable interest since its discovery, more than 40 years ago. Clinical utility is diminished due to widespread quinolone resistance, especially in Gram-negative microorganisms. Nevertheless, the quinolone nucleus continues to provide opportunities for future modifications that may produce more valuable compounds.

Delafloxacin (RX-3341, ABT-492)

Delafloxacin is an investigational oral and parenteral fluoroquinolone, which has been demonstrated to be active *in vitro* against quinolone-susceptible and quinolone-resistant Gram-positive pathogens, including streptococci, staphylococci and enterococci, and Gram-negative pathogens, including *P. aeruginosa* and fastidious species. Interestingly, delafloxacin demonstrated potent *in vitro* activity against a set of *S. aureus*, including both MSSA and MRSA [32]. Delafloxacin has been evaluated in three successful Phase 2 trials.

A double-blind study evaluated the intravenous formulation for the treatment of complicated skin and skin structure infections: Delafloxacin was administered at two different doses, 300 mg twice daily and 450 mg twice daily; the comparator was tigecycline [33]. Delafloxacin showed comparable efficacy and an improved tolerance profile compare to tigecycline. The most common adverse events reported in the trial were mild gastrointestinal symptoms, but rates of nausea and vomiting were lower than in patients treated with tigecycline. The oral formulation of delafloxacin has been studied in two trials. In the first, delafloxacin was effective at doses as low as 200 mg once daily in patients with community-acquired pneumonia (CAP). In the second, conducted in patients with acute bacterial exacerbation of chronic bronchitis, delafloxacin, at a once a day dose of 200 mg for 5 days, was as efficacious as levofloxacin, 500 mg once daily for 7 days. Intravenous and oral formulations of delafloxacin are currently being assessed in two Phase 3 studies for the treatment of acute bacterial skin and skin structure infections (ABSSSI) caused by Gram-positive (including MRSA) and Gram-negative bacteria. A Phase 3 clinical study of a single, oral dose of delafloxacin (900 mg) for the treatment of uncomplicated gonorrhea is also ongoing [34].

Oxazolidinones

Oxazolidinones represent a new class of synthetic antibacterial agents active against multiple resistant Gram-positive pathogens, including MRSA, penicillin-resistant streptococci, and VRE. Linezolid, the first and at the moment the only oxazolidinone available, represents an optimal choice in the clinical setting for the treatment of infections caused by Gram-positive organisms. PK properties as well as its good penetration and accumulation in the tissues, including skin, bone, lung, and cerebrospinal fluid, enable it to be used in several types of infections.

Tedizolid Phosphate (TR-701)

Tedizolid, previously known as torezolid phosphate, is an inactive prodrug, which, after oral or intravenous (i.v.) administration, is rapidly converted to the active form (torezolid). Tedizolid is a new oxazolidinone, recently approved by the FDA (June 2014) to treat patients with acute bacterial skin and skin structure infections caused by certain susceptible bacteria, including *S. aureus* (both methicillin-resistant and methicillin-susceptible strains), various *Streptococcus* species, and *Enterococcus faecalis*; furthermore, it shows good antibacterial efficacy against linezolid-resistant strains [35]. Tedizolid has high bioavailability, penetration, and tissue distribution when administered orally or intravenously. *In vitro* studies demonstrate that the activity of tedizolid is greater against *Staphylococcus spp., Streptococcus spp.,* and *Enterococcus spp.*, including strains not susceptible to vancomycin or daptomycin, compared to linezolid. Choi and colleagues showed that tedizolid was four-fold more potent *in vitro* than linezolid against penicillin-resistant *S. pnemoniae* [36]. Pharmacokinetic characteristics of tedizolid allow once-daily administration. Results from a population of healthy volunteers support once daily dosing of 200 mg tedizolid phosphate with both the oral and i.v. formulations, without the need for dose adjustment when switching administration routes [37].

No hematological adverse effects have been reported associated with tedizolid when used up to 3 weeks at the therapeutic dose of 200 mg in Phase 1, 2, or 3 clinical trials. Unlike linezolid, tedizolid does not inhibit monoamine oxidase *in vivo*; therefore interactions with adrenergic, dopaminergic, and serotonergic drugs are not to be expected [38].

Radezolid (RX-1741)

Radezolid is the first biaryloxazolidinone in clinical development. The antimicrobial activity of radezolid was evaluated against respiratory pathogens demonstrating significantly better activity than linezolid against both *S. pneumoniae* and *S. pyogenes*. MIC_{90} values for staphylococci and enterococci ranged from 1 to 4 mcg/ml and from 0.5 to 1 mcg/ml, respectively. Compared with linezolid, radezolid has an expanded spectrum to include fastidious Gram-negative organisms like

Haemophilus influenzae and *Moraxella catarrhalis*, with a MIC_{90} of 1 mcg/ml and 0.5 mcg/ml, respectively [39]. Radezolid was selected for further advancement with two Phase 2 clinical trials completed to date: the first in community-acquired pneumonia and the second in uncomplicated skin and skin structure infections.

Radezolid may represent a future choice for empiric treatment of community-acquired infections because of its activity against the fastidious Gram-negative organisms. It is unclear at this point, based upon published literature, whether radezolid has any appreciable safety advantages over linezolid. To date, Phase 3 trials have not been initiated.

Cadazolid

Cadazolid is a new oxazolidinone currently in clinical development for the treatment of *Clostridium difficile*-associated diarrhea. Cadazolid acts primarily by inhibition of protein synthesis, with weak inhibition of DNA synthesis as a potential second mode of action, and has a low potential for spontaneous resistance development [40]. Cadazolid showed potent *in vitro* bactericidal activity against *C. difficile* with an MIC range of 0.125 to 0.5 µg/ml, including strains resistant to linezolid and fluoroquinolones. In contrast to metronidazole and vancomycin, cadazolid strongly inhibits *de novo* toxin A and B formation in stationary-phase cultures of toxigenic *C. difficile*. [41]. Cadazolid is well tolerated and its systemic exposure is low, thus resulting in high concentrations at the site of action (colon).

Glycopeptides and Lipoglycopeptides

Glycopeptides are large, rigid molecules that inhibit a late stage in bacterial cell wall peptidoglycan synthesis. These antibiotics are effective mainly against Gram-positive cocci. Glycopeptides diffuse well into most body tissues but distribution to lung tissue and the central nervous system is variable and dependent upon disease process. Several derivates of vancomycin are currently being developed, including telavancin, oritavancin and dalbavancin (lipoglycopeptides). Possessing longer half-lives than vancomycin, these newer candidates may demonstrate improvements over vancomycin due to less frequent dosing and activity against vancomycin-resistant bacteria.

Telavancin

Telavancin is a vancomycin-derived lipoglycopeptide approved by the FDA in 2009 for the treatment of complicated skin and skin structure infections. Recently (June 2013), the FDA gave approval for telavancin to treat patients with hospital-acquired and ventilator-associated bacterial pneumonia caused by *S. aureus* when alternative treatments are not suitable.

Telavancin is administered once-daily and characterized by a broad-spectrum of microbiologic activity against Gram-positive bacteria, including vancomycin-resistant staphylococci and enterococci. Large randomized Phase 2 and 3 clinical trials on the efficacy and safety of telavancin in treating complicated skin and skin structure infections reported that telavancin was non-inferior to standard treatment, mostly vancomycin [42].

Two methodologically identical Phase 3 studies demonstrated that telavancin was non-inferior to vancomycin for the treatment of HAP, including VAP, due to *S. aureus* (including methicillin-sensitive *S. aureus* and MRSA). Telavancin showed a similar safety profile to vancomycin, except in patients with moderate-to-severe renal impairment (increased mortality), which warrants caution when using telavancin in this population [43].

Considering the limited therapeutic options for the treatment of nosocomial pneumonia due to MRSA, telavancin may represent a good alternative to standard therapy.

Oritavancin

Oritavancin is a semisynthetic lipoglycopeptide analog of vancomycin with at least three mechanisms of actions: Inhibition of transglycosylation, inhibition of transpeptidation and cell membrane distruption/interaction. Oritavancin was approved by the FDA in August 2014 for treatment of patients with acute bacterial skin and skin structure infections caused by certain susceptible bacteria, including *S. aureus* (methicillin-susceptible and methicillin-resistant strains), various *Streptococcus* species and *E. faecalis*.

Oritavancin has rapid concentration-dependent bactericidal activity. The pharmacodynamics (PD) and PK profiles suggest that oritavancin could be effective given in a single dose. In a recent randomized, double-blind study, a single dose of oritavancin was non-inferior to twice-daily vancomycin administered for 7 to 10 days for the treatment of acute bacterial skin and skin-structure infections caused by Gram-positive pathogens [44]. Oritavancin is not metabolized following intravenous administration. Instead, it is slowly excreted, unchanged, in both urine and the feces (terminal half-life = 393 ± 73.5 h), which means that no dosage adjustment is required for age, or for renal or mild to moderate hepatic dysfunction [45].

In Phase 3 trials, the most commonly reported adverse effects among oritavancin users were headache, nausea, constipation, and phlebitis.

Dalbavancin

Dalbavancin is a new lipoglycopeptide that inhibits cell wall synthesis in Gram-positive bacteria through the formation of a stable complex between its heptapeptide backbone and the D-Ala-D-Ala portion of cell wall precursors. Dalbavancin was approved by the FDA in May 2014 for the treatment of acute bacterial skin and skin structure infections caused by certain susceptible bacteria like *S. aureus* (including methicillin-susceptible and methicillin-resistant strains) and *S. pyogenes*.

Dalbavancin has *in vitro* activity against clinically significant Gram-positive pathogens, including MSSA, MRSA, methicillin-susceptible *S. epidermidis* (MSSE), methicillin-resistant *S. epidermidis* (MRSE) and enterococci, but lacks activity against VanA-type enterococci [46].

Like other glycopeptides, dalbavancin is poorly absorbed when administered orally, thus requiring intravenous administration. The main PK characteristic is the long-half-life: The terminal elimination half-life of dalbavancin ranges from 147 to 258 h, allowing once-weekly dosing. In Phase 3 trials, Discover 1 and Discover 2, patients were treated for two weeks either with intravenous dalbavancin once weekly (1,000 mg on Day 1 followed by 500 mg on Day 8) or with intravenous vancomycin (1,000 mg or 15 mg/kg every 12 h) with the option to switch to oral linezolid after three days. Dalbavancin was non-inferior to the comparator regimen at both an early timepoint and at the end of therapy. The most common treatment-related adverse events in either group were nausea, diarrhea, and pruritus. [47].

Tetracyclines

Tetracyclines are a group of broad-spectrum antibiotics whose general usefulness has been reduced with the onset of bacterial resistance. Despite this, they remain the treatment of choice for some specific indications. Decades after the introduction of doxycycline and minocycline, a team of Wyeth scientists synthesized 7,9-disubstituted tetracycline derivatives, leading to the discovery of tigecycline, the defining member of a new class of tetracyclines known as glycylcyclines, which greatly extend the spectrum of tetracyclines, especially toward tetracycline-resistant microorganisms. Omadacycline and Eravacycline are two novel, promising tetracyclines.

Omadacycline (PTK 0796)

Omadacycline, an aminomethylcycline, is a semisynthetic derivative of minocycline that has *in vitro* potency against Gram-positive and Gram-negative bacteria. It presents activity against MSSA/MRSA, methicillin-sensitive and resistant coagulase-negative staphylococci, *E. faecalis* (including vancomycin-resistant strains), *E. faecium,* penicillin-resistant *S. pneumoniae, K. pneumoniae, Proteus mirabilis/vulgaris, Providencia rettgeri/stuartii, Morganella morganii* and *Bacteroides fragilis*. A randomized, investigator-blind, multicenter Phase 2 trial involving patients with complicated skin and skin structure infections compared the safety and efficacy of omadacycline to those of linezolid. Patients were randomized to receive 100 mg i.v. once a day with an option to transition to 200 mg orally once a day or linezolid at 600 mg i.v. twice daily with an option to transition to

600 mg orally twice daily. Rates of successful clinical response in the intent-to-treat and clinically evaluable populations favored omadacycline. There were no safety concerns [48].

Preliminary results of a Phase 3 trial are consistent with those of the Phase 2 and show comparable efficacy and overall safety/tolerability between omadacycline and linezolid.

Eravacycline (TP-434)

Eravacycline is a novel, fully synthetic fluorocycline belonging to the tetracycline class, with potential for intravenous-to-oral step-down therapy. Eravacycline was evaluated for antimicrobial activity against aerobic and anaerobic Gram-negative and Gram-positive bacteria: The drug showed potent broad-spectrum activity against 90% of the isolates (MIC90) in each panel at concentrations ranging from ≤ 0.008 to 2 µg/ml for all species panels except those of *P. aeruginosa* and *Burkholderia cenocepacia* (MIC90 values of 32 µg/ml for both organisms). The antibacterial activity of eravacycline was minimally affected by expression of resistance mechanisms in clinical isolates. Furthermore, eravacycline was active against MDR bacteria, including those expressing ESBL and carbapenemases [49].

A Phase 2, randomized, double-blind study evaluated efficacy and safety of two dose regimens of eravacycline compared to ertapenem for adult community-acquired complicated intra-abdominal infections. Both dose regimens of eravacycline were as efficacious as the comparator, ertapenem, and were well tolerated. Incidence rates of nausea and vomiting were low in both eravacycline groups [50]. These results support the possible role of eravacycline for the treatment of serious infections, including those caused by drug-resistant Gram-negative pathogens. The results of this study, together with the PK analyses, were key for the analyses of eravacycline dosing in the pivotal Phase 3 study for the treatment of complicated intra-abdominal infections and complicated UTIs and led to the selection of the 1.0 mg/kg twice daily dose.

Conclusion

The development of new antibiotics targeting the growing threat of multidrug resistance is a goal that remains 'alarmingly elusive'. Examples of XDR and PDR bacteria that plague the global healthcare systems include carbapenem-resistant bacteria, such as *Klebsiella*, *Pseudomonas* and *Acinetobacter*, and new classes of antibiotics active against these Gram-negative microorganisms are lacking. Unfortunately, there are also multiple economic barriers to antibiotic development. Low returns on investments and an unpredictable and often unfeasible approval pathway at regulatory agencies have caused many companies to leave the antibiotics market.

There is a number of promising antibiotics in development. Regulatory approvals are crucial over the next five years to return us to a time when reliably effective treatment of bacterial diseases is again a reality, not just a future prospect.

References

1. Pendleton JN, Gorman SP, Gilmore BF (2013) Clinical relevance of the ESKAPE pathogens. Expert Rev Anti Infect Ther 11:297–308
2. Boucher HW, Talbot GH, Bradley JS et al (2009) Bad bugs, no drugs: No ESKAPE! An update from the Infectious Diseases Society of America. Clin Infect Dis 48:1–12
3. Magiorakos AP, Srinivasan A, Carey RB et al (2012) Multidrug-resistant, extensively drug-resistant and pandrug-resistant bacteria: an international expert proposal for interim standard definitions for acquired resistance. Clin Microbiol Infect 18:268–281
4. Spellberg B, Guidos R, Gilbert D et al (2008) Infectious Diseases Society of America; The epidemic of antibiotic-resistant infections: a call to action for the medical community from the Infectious Diseases Society of America. Clin Infect Dis 46:155–164
5. Piddock LJ (2012) The crisis of no new antibiotics–what is the way forward? Lancet Infect Dis 12:249–253
6. Infectious Diseases Society of America (2010) The 10 × '20 Initiative: pursuing a global commitment to develop 10 new antibacterial drugs by 2020. Clin Infect Dis 50:1081–1083
7. The Pew Charitable Trusts (2014) Tracking the Pipeline of Antibiotics in Development. http://www.pewtrusts.org/en/research-and-analysis/issue-briefs/2014/03/12/tracking-the-pipeline-of-antibiotics-in-development. Accessed September 2014
8. Livermore DM, Mushtaq S, Ge Y (2010) Chequerboard titration of cephalosporin CXA-101 (FR264205) and tazobactam versus beta-lactamase-producing Enterobacteriaceae. J Antimicrob Chemother 65:1972–1974
9. Titelman E, Karlsson IM, Ge Y, Giske CG (2011) In vitro activity of CXA-101 plus tazobactam (CXA-201) against CTX-M-14- and CTX-M-15-producing Escherichia coli and Klebsiella pneumoniae. Diagn Microbiol Infect Dis 70:137–141
10. Sader HS, Rhomberg PR, Farrell DJ, Jones RN (2011) Antimicrobial activity of CXA-101, a novel cephalosporin tested in combination with tazobactam against Enterobacteriaceae, Pseudomonas aeruginosa, and Bacteroides fragilis strains having various resistance phenotypes. Antimicrob Agents Chemother 55:2390–2394
11. Umeh O, Cebrik D, Friedland I (2010) A double-blind, randomized, phase 2 study to compare the safety and efficacy of intravenous CXA-101 (CXA) and intravenous ceftazidime (CTZ) in complicated urinary tract infection (cUTI) 50th Interscience Conference on Antimicrobial Agents and Chemotherapy, Boston, MA, September 12–15. (abst)
12. Wagenlehner F, Umeh O, Huntington J et al (2014) Efficacy and safety of ceftolozane/tazobactam versus levofloxacin in the treatment of complicated urinary tract infections (cUTI)/pyelonephritis in hospitalised adults: results from the phase 3 aspect-cUTI trial. 24th European Congress of Clinical Microbiology and Infectious Diseases (ECCMID), May 10–13. Barcelona (abst)
13. Ge Y, Whitehouse MJ, Friedland I, Talbot GH (2010) Pharmacokinetics and safety of CXA-101, a new antipseudomonal cephalosporin, in healthy adult male and female subjects receiving single- and multiple-dose intravenous infusions. Antimicrob Agents Chemother 54:3427–3431
14. Miller B, Hershberger E, Benziger D, Trinh M, Friedland I (2012) Pharmacokinetics and safety of intravenous ceftolozane-tazobactam in healthy adult subjects following single and multiple ascending doses. Antimicrob Agents Chemother 56:3086–3091
15. Lucasti C, Hershberger E, Miller B et al (2014) A multicenter, double-blind, randomized, phase ii trial to assess the safety and efficacy of ceftolozane/tazobactam plus metronidazole compared with meropenem in adult patients with complicated intra-abdominal infections. Antimicrob Agents Chemother 58:5350–5357
16. Zhanel GG, Lawson CD, Adam H et al (2013) Ceftazidime-avibactam: a novel cephalosporin/β-lactamase inhibitor combination. Drugs 73:159–177
17. Mushtaq S, Warner M, Livermore DM (2010) In vitro activity of ceftazidime+NXL104 against Pseudomonas aeruginosa and other non-fermenters. J Antimicrob Chemother 65:2376–2381

18. Citron DM, Tyrrell KL, Merriam V, Goldstein EJ (2011) In vitro activity of ceftazidime-NXL104 against 396 strains of beta-lactamase-producing anaerobes. Antimicrob Agents Chemother 55:3616–3620
19. Lucasti C, Popescu I, Ramesh MK, Lipka J, Sable C (2013) Comparative study of the efficacy and safety of ceftazidime/avibactam plus metronidazole versus meropenem in the treatment of complicated intra-abdominal infections in hospitalized adults: results of a randomized, double-blind, Phase II trial. J Antimicrob Chemother 68:1183–1192
20. Vazquez JA, González Patzán LD, Stricklin D et al (2012) Efficacy and safety of ceftazidime-avibactam versus imipenem-cilastatin in the treatment of complicated urinary tract infections, including acute pyelonephritis, in hospitalized adults: results of a prospective, investigator-blinded, randomized study. Curr Med Res Opin 28:1921–1931
21. Critchley IA, Eckburg PB, Jandourek A, Biek D, Friedland HD, Thye DA (2011) Review of ceftaroline fosamil microbiology: integrated FOCUS studies. J Antimicrob Chemother 66(Suppl 3):iii45–51
22. Stachyra T, Levasseur P, Péchereau MC et al (2009) In vitro activity of the β-lactamase inhibitor NXL104 against KPC-2 carbapenemase and Enterobacteriaceae expressing KPC carbapenemases. J Antimicrob Chemother 64:326–329
23. Mushtaq S, Warner M, Williams G, Critchley I, Livermore DM (2010) Activity of chequerboard combinations of ceftaroline and NXL104 versus beta-lactamase-producing Enterobacteriaceae. J Antimicrob Chemother 65:1428–1432
24. Riccobene TA, Su SF, Rank D (2013) Single- and multiple-dose study to determine the safety, tolerability, and pharmacokinetics of ceftaroline fosamil in combination with avibactam in healthy subjects. Antimicrob Agents Chemother 57:1496–1504
25. Livermore DM, Warner M, Mushtaq S (2013) Activity of MK-7655 combined with imipenem against Enterobacteriaceae and Pseudomonas aeruginosa. J Antimicrob Chemother 68:2286–2290
26. Hirsch EB, Ledesma KR, Chang KT, Schwartz MS, Motyl MR, Tam VH (2012) In vitro activity of MK-7655, a novel β-lactamase inhibitor, in combination with imipenem against carbapenem-resistant Gram-negative bacteria. Antimicrob Agents Chemother 56:3753–3757
27. Walkty A, Adam H, Baxter M et al (2014) In vitro activity of plazomicin against 5,015 gram-negative and gram-positive clinical isolates obtained from patients in canadian hospitals as part of the CANWARD study, 2011–2012. Antimicrob Agents Chemother 58:2554–2563
28. Aggen JB, Armstrong ES, Goldblum AA et al (2010) Synthesis and spectrum of the neoglycoside ACHN-490. Antimicrob Agents Chemother 54:4636–4642
29. Zhanel GG, Lawson CD, Zelenitsky S et al (2012) Comparison of the next-generation aminoglycoside plazomicin to gentamicin, tobramycin and amikacin. Expert Rev Anti Infect Ther 10:459–473
30. Poulikakos P, Falagas ME (2013) Aminoglycoside therapy in infectious diseases. Expert Opin Pharmacother 14:1585–1597
31. Cass RT, Brooks CD, Havrilla NA et al (2011) Pharmacokinetics and safety of single and multiple doses of ACHN-490 injection administered intravenously in healthy subjects. Antimicrob Agents Chemother 55:5874–5880
32. Nilius AM, Shen LL, Hensey-Rudloff D et al (2003) In vitro antibacterial potency and spectrum of ABT-492, a new fluoroquinolone. Antimicrob Agents Chemother 47:3260–3269
33. O'Riordan W, Mehra P, Manos P, Kingsley J, Lawrence L, Cammarata S (2014) A randomized phase 2 study comparing two doses of delafloxacin with tigecycline in adults with complicated stain and stain-structure infections. Int J Infect Dis 30C:67–73
34. Melinta Therapeutics (2014) Delafloxacin. http://www.melinta.com/delafloxacin.php. Accessed September 2014
35. Keel RA, Tessier PR, Crandon JL, Nicolau DP (2012) Comparative efficacies of human simulated exposures of tedizolid and linezolid against Staphylococcus aureus in the murine thigh infection model. Antimicrob Agents and Chemother 56:4403–4407

36. Choi S, Im W, Bartizal K (2012) Activity of Tedizolid Phosphate (TR-701) in murine models of infection with penicillin-resistant and penicillin-sensitive streptococcus pneumoniae. Antimicrob Agents and Chemother 56:4713–4717
37. Flanagan S, Fang E, Muñoz KA, Minassian SL, Prokocimer PG (2014) Single- and multiple-dose pharmacokinetics and absolute bioavailability of tedizolid. Pharmacotherapy 34:891–900
38. Urbina O, Ferrández O, Espona M, Salas E, Ferrández I, Grau S (2013) Potential role of tedizolid phosphate in the treatment of acute bacterial skin infections. Drug Des Devel Ther 7:243–265
39. Lawrence L, Danese P, DeVito J, Franceschi F, Sutcliffe J (2008) In vitro activities of theRx-01 oxazolidinones against hospital and community pathogens. Antimicrob Agents Chemother 52:1653–1662
40. Locher HH, Caspers P, Bruyère T et al (2014) Investigations of the mode of action and resistance development of cadazolid, a new antibiotic for treatment of Clostridium difficile infections. Antimicrob Agents Chemother 58:901–908
41. Locher HH, Seiler P, Chen X et al (2014) In vitro and in vivo antibacterial evaluation of cadazolid, a new antibiotic for treatment of Clostridium difficile infections. Antimicrob Agents Chemother 58:892–900
42. Bassetti M, Mikulska M, Righi E, Nicolini L, Viscoli C (2009) The role of telavancin in the treatment of MRSA infections in hospital. Expert Opin Investig Drugs 18:521–529
43. Barriere SL (2014) The ATTAIN trials: efficacy and safety of telavancin compared with vancomycin for the treatment of hospital-acquired and ventilator-associated bacterial pneumonia. Future Microbiol 9:281–289
44. Corey GR, Kabler H, Mehra P et al (2014) Single-dose oritavancin in the treatment of acute bacterial skin infections. N Engl J Med 370:2180–2190
45. Rubino CM, Van Wart SA, Bhavnani SM, Ambrose PG, McCollam JS, Forrest A (2009) Oritavancin population pharmacokinetics in healthy subjects and patients with complicated skin and skin structure infections or bacteremia. Antimicrob Agents Chemother 53:4422–4428
46. Zhanel GG, Calic D, Schweizer F et al (2010) New lipoglycopeptides: a comparative review of dalbavancin, oritavancin and telavancin. Drugs 70:859–886
47. Boucher HW, Wilcox M, Talbot GH, Puttagunta S, Das AF, Dunne MW (2014) Once-weekly dalbavancin versus daily conventional therapy for skin infection. N Engl J Med 370:2169–79
48. Noel GJ, Draper MP, Hait H, Tanaka SK, Arbeit RD (2012) A randomized, evaluator-blind, phase 2 study comparing the safety and efficacy of omadacycline to those of linezolid for treatment of complicated skin and skin structure infections. Antimicrob Agents Chemother 56:5650–5654
49. Sutcliffe JA, O'Brien W, Fyfe C, Grossman TH (2013) Antibacterial activity of eravacycline (TP-434), a novel fluorocycline, against hospital and community pathogens. Antimicrob Agents Chemother 57:5548–5558
50. Solomkin JS, Ramesh MK, Cesnauskas G et al (2014) Phase 2, randomized, double-blind study of the efficacy and safety of two dose regimens of eravacycline versus ertapenem for adult community-acquired complicated intra-abdominal infections. Antimicrob Agents Chemother 58:1847–1854

Optimizing Antimicrobial Efficacy at Minimal Toxicity: A Novel Indication for Continuous Renal Replacement Therapy?

P. M. Honoré, R. Jacobs, and H. D. Spapen

Introduction

Continuous renal replacement therapy (CRRT) has become a standard adjuvant therapy in the intensive care unit (ICU). Apart from commonly accepted indications, such as acute kidney injury (AKI) of different origins, hemodynamic instability without AKI and fluid overload, CRRT can act as a 'supportive' therapy that allows adequate dosing of antimicrobials whilst limiting some or all of their known toxicities. In particular, CRRT may elegantly reconcile optimal treatment efficacy and safety when high doses of antimicrobial agents have to be administered for an extended time period [1, 2]. In this chapter, we briefly review the literature and share our own experience regarding some antibiotics and antifungals when this 'novel' CRRT approach is realized.

Colistin

In patients with normal kidney function, colistin is predominantly non-renally cleared [3]. Colistin undergoes up to 80% tubular reabsorption. As a consequence, most of the filtered colistin is retained in the body and only an extremely small fraction is excreted unchanged in the urine. Toxicity either depends on drug accumulation by reabsorption or on reaching peak concentrations that are too high. Recent pharmacokinetic (PK) models indicate that a high loading dose is paramount to ensure a rapid bacterial killing effect. Without such a loading dose, steady-state bactericidal colistin concentrations would only be obtained after 24 to 48 h [4]. The AUC:MIC (area under the curve:minimum inhibitory concentration) ratio is the PK parameter that best represents colistin efficacy [1, 2]. To maximize this ratio,

P. M. Honoré ✉ · R. Jacobs · H. D. Spapen
Department of Intensive Care, University Hospital, Vrije Universiteit Brussel, Brussels, Belgium
e-mail: Patrick.Honore@uzbrussel.be

J.-L. Vincent (ed.), *Annual Update in Intensive Care and Emergency Medicine 2015*,
DOI 10.1007/978-3-319-13761-2_6

higher maintenance doses of colistin (i. e., 4.5 million IU twice daily) are warranted in critically ill patients.

Data regarding colistin treatment under conditions of RRT are scarce. Studies assessing colistin elimination during intermittent [5] and continuous [6–8] dialysis do not provide clinically relevant PK information, because the colistin dose was either in a toxic [5] or a low [6–8] range. Colistin handling is dramatically altered during convective CRRT. In fact, the lack of a carrier-mediated mechanism returning colistin from the ultrafiltrate to the blood virtually excludes reabsorption [3]. In practice, a substantially higher maintenance dose (i. e., 4.5 million IU three times daily) must be provided during CRRT [9, 10]. During the procedure, continuous colistin loss by filtration permits accumulation to be avoided whilst bulk membrane adsorption avoids the occurrence of huge peak concentrations [3, 11]. This explains the absence of colistin toxicity during CRRT even when the aforementioned high doses are administered for a prolonged time period.

Continuous venovenous hemofiltration (CVVH) is the most preferred CRRT modality in ICU patients. The current Kidney Disease: Improving Global Outcomes (KDIGO) guidelines recommend a standard dialysis dose of 35 ml/kg/h to guarantee delivery of at least 25 ml/kg/h [14]. High-volume CVVH does not offer any further advantage [15, 16]. CVVH devices equipped with non- or poorly adsorptive membranes are not suitable for colistin clearance. The novel highly-adsorptive AN69 ST (surface treated) membrane allows much higher clearance. Adsorption occurs in part at the (rapidly saturated) membrane surface but predominantly in its (less easily saturated) bulk [10, 12]. Precocious saturation is unlikely and frequent membrane changes (e. g., every 12 to 24 h) are not necessary [10, 12]. This is corroborated by our experience in a small cohort of patients who tolerated colistin doses as high as 4.5 million IU three times daily for more than five consecutive days without adverse effects, toxicity, or need for membrane change [10, 12, 17] (Table 1). Polymethylmetacrylate membranes are able to adsorb similar amounts of colistin into their bulk [10, 17], but colistin elimination with these particular membranes has not been studied. Monitoring of the transmembrane pressure and hemopermeability index permits continuous assessment of the functional capacity of the dialysis membrane. The absence of clotting is an indirect marker

Table 1 Suggested loading and maintenance doses of colistin, aminoglycosides and voriconazole for treatment of highly resistant Gram-negative and fungal infections under CRRT

Drug	Loading dose	Maintenance dose
Colistin	9 MIU	4.5 MIU tid
Amikacin		50–60 mg/kg ± every 24 h, according to MIC and optimal trough level (4–8 μg/ml; TDM)
Gentamicin		20–25 mg/kg ± every 36 h, according to MIC and optimal trough level (5–10 μg/ml; TDM)
Voriconazole	8 mg/kg q12 h	6 mg/kg q12 h

MIU = million international units; tid = three times daily; TDM = therapeutic drug monitoring; MIC: minimum inhibitory concentration.

of the absence of membrane clogging [18]. Citrate is the anticoagulant of choice during CVVH, guaranteeing long-term optimal porosity [19] and – when using the AN69 ST filter – maximal adsorptive capacity of the membrane [20].

Aminoglycosides

Amikacin

Aminoglycosides are concentration-dependent antibiotics and exert optimal bactericidal efficacy at a C_{max}/MIC ratio between 8 and 10 [21]. The formerly recommended 15 mg/kg amikacin dose failed to achieve this PK target in more than 90% of isolates. Inappropriate C_{max} values for amikacin were also observed in burn patients, even when a once-daily dose as high as 25 mg/kg was administered [21]. A similar inadequate dose-response is often present in resuscitated septic shock patients, probably because of an increased distribution volume associated with an enhanced amikacin clearance. Finally, failure to attain PK targets in some patients may also be related to the high MIC of the infecting microorganisms. A Monte Carlo simulation incorporating MIC and PK data indicated that a 25 mg/kg amikacin dose would fail to improve clinical cure at currently accepted C_{max}/MIC standards. For example, a C_{max} of 64 µg/ml for isolates expressing MICs of 8 µg/ml (i. e., susceptible according to the European Committee on Antimicrobial Susceptibility Testing [EUCAST] guidelines) would necessitate a daily amikacin dose exceeding 35 mg/kg to match the larger volume distribution in severe sepsis and septic shock. Moreover, the continuously elevated trough concentrations will precipitate toxicity. Treatment of isolates with intermediate resistance to amikacin (MICs around 16 µg/ml) requires a once-daily amikacin dose of 50 to 60 mg/kg to obtain a cure rate of at least 90%. Patients exposed to such high dosing regimens will all develop AKI [22–24]. Applying CVVH, however, makes administration of such high doses possible. Amikacin is infused over 30 min and, considering that an optimal peak concentration is achieved at 60 min, CVVH with the AN69 ST membrane is initiated 2 h after the start of the amikacin infusion. Amikacin has a sieving coefficient of 0.95 and thus is mainly and rapidly eliminated by convection. As for colistin, membrane adsorption of amikacin occurs predominantly in the bulk of the membrane [19, 25]. Removal through adsorption may eliminate up to 750 mg amikacin per day [25]. Early filter saturation is unlikely and frequent membrane changes are not necessary [10, 12]. The joint convective and adsorptive capacities of CVVH result in swift removal of amikacin from the circulation. The degree of removal is such that a subsequent (high) amikacin dose can already be anticipated within the next 24 h. CVVH is placed in recirculation during the infusion to ensure an optimal peak concentration. To illustrate the feasibility of this concept, a once-daily dose of amikacin as high as 50 mg/kg was recently used to cure refractory *Pseudomonas aeruginosa* infection in two patients receiving continuous veno-venous hemodiafiltration. Trough concentrations between doses could be kept low and toxic effects were not observed [23].

Gentamicin

No data are available regarding the use of a high gentamycin dose (i. e., > 7 mg/kg) during CVVH. However, we recently treated two patients infected by *Pseudomonas* spp. resistant to amikacin and susceptible only to colistin and gentamicin. The MIC for gentamicin was high. Under CVVH, colistin was given as described earlier (9 million IU loading dose, followed by 4.5 million IU three times daily). To optimize therapeutic efficacy, gentamicin was infused at a rate of 20 mg/kg aiming at peak levels 8–10 times above the MIC. For this purpose, CVVH was set in recirculation mode, and restarted 2 h after the infusion. Gentamicin also has a very high sieving coefficient but is adsorbed less by the AN69 ST membrane. Therefore, the dose was repeated every 36 h (instead of every 24 h). CVVH also enabled administration of gentamicin regardless of the presence of higher trough levels. This considerably shortened the time lag between gentamicin peaks whilst avoiding nephrotoxicity. As such, full therapy was continued for 10 days. No signs of renal dysfunction were observed in either patient and one patient was uneventfully discharged from the hospital.

Voriconazole

Sulfobutylether-beta-cyclodextrin (SBECD), an oligosaccharide used to solubilize the intravenous form of voriconazole, is eliminated mainly by renal excretion. High levels of the SBECD vehicle induce vacuolation in epithelial cells of the urinary tract and activate liver and lung macrophages [26, 27]. Despite being rapidly cleared by hemodialysis using high-flux membranes, intermittent elimination of SBECD failed to prevent increasing plasma concentrations after repeated voriconazole doses. In contrast, CVVH adequately protects against SBECD accumulation and also permits administration of higher doses of voriconazole (i. e., 8 mg/kg q12 h loading and 6 mg/kg q12 h as maintenance dose).

Conclusion

CRRT is presented as a 'therapeutic shield' offering potentially life-saving treatment for multidrug-resistant or difficult-to-treat microorganisms in critically ill patients. CRRT not only attenuates or impedes the toxicity of a particular drug but may also optimize antimicrobial PK behavior by allowing administration of high-dose regimens that could otherwise not be tolerated. Among the various CRRT techniques, CVVH using highly adsorptive membranes has been found to be particularly efficient at achieving these goals.

References

1. Honoré PM, Jacobs R, Joannes-Boyau O et al (2014) Continuous renal replacement therapy-related strategies to avoid colistin toxicity: A clinically orientated review. Blood Purif 37:291–295
2. Honore PM, Jacobs R, Joannes-Boyau O et al (2013) Continuous renal replacement therapy allows higher colistin dosing without increasing toxicity. J Transl Intern Med 1:6–8
3. Li J, Nation RL, Turnidge JD et al (2006) Colistin: The re-emerging antibiotic for multidrug-resistant Gram-negative bacterial infections. Lancet Infect Dis 6:589–601
4. Mohamed AF, Karaiskos I, Plachouras D et al (2012) Application of a loading dose of colistin methanesulfonate in critically ill patients: Population pharmacokinetics, protein binding, and prediction of bacterial kill. Antimicrob Agents Chemother 56:4241–4249
5. Marchand S, Frat JP, Petitpas F et al (2010) Removal of colistin during intermittent haemodialysis in two critically ill patients. J Antimicrob Chemother 65:1836–1837
6. Markou N, Fousteri M, Markantonis SL et al (2012) Colistin pharmacokinetics in intensive care unit patients on continuous venovenous haemodiafiltration: Anobservational study. J Antimicrob Chemother 67:2459–2462
7. Cho YS, Yim H, Yang HT et al (2012) Use of parenteral colistin for the treatment of multiresistant Gram-negative organisms in major burn patients in South Korea. Infection 40:27–33
8. Li J, Rayner CR, Nation RL et al (2005) Pharmacokinetics of colistin methanesulfonate and colistin in a critically ill patient receiving continuous venovenous hemodiafiltration. Antimicrob Agents Chemother 49:4814–4815
9. Plachouras D, Karvanen M, Friberg LE et al (2009) Population pharmacokinetic analysis of colistin methanesulfonate and colistin after intravenous administration in critically ill patients with infections caused by gram-negative bacteria. Antimicrob Agents Chemother 53:3430–3436
10. Honore PM, Jacobs R, Lochy S et al (2013) Acute respiratory muscle weakness and apnea in a critically ill patient induced by colistin neurotoxicity: Key potential role of hemoadsorption elimination during continuous venovenous hemofiltration. Int J Nephrol Renovasc Dis 6:107–111
11. Lee J, Han S, Jeon S et al (2013) Population pharmacokinetic analysis of colistin in burn patients. Antimicrob Agents Chemother 57:2141–2146
12. Honore PM, Jacobs R, Joannes-Boyau O et al (2013) Newly designed CRRT membranes for sepsis and SIRS – a pragmatic approach for bedside intensivists summarizing the more recent advances: A systematic structured review. ASAIO J 59:99–106
13. Morimatsu H, Uchino S, Bellomo R, Ronco C (2003) Continuous renal replacement therapy: Does technique influence electrolyte and bicarbonate control? Int J Artif Organs 4:289–296
14. Kellum JA, Lameire N (2013) Diagnosis, evaluation, and management of acute kidney injury: A KDIGO summary (Part 1). Crit Care 17:R204
15. Joannes-Boyau O, Honoré PM, Perez P et al (2013) High-volume versus standard-volume haemofiltration forseptic shock patients with acute kidney injury (IVOIRE study):A multicentre randomized controlled trial. Intensive Care Med 39:1535–1546
16. Zhang P, Yang Y, Lv R et al (2012) Effect of the intensity of continuous renal replacement therapy in patients with sepsis and acute kidney injury: A single-center randomized clinical trial. Nephrol Dial Transplant 27:967–973
17. Spapen HD, Honore PM, Gregoire N et al (2011) Convulsions and apnoea in a patient infected with New Delhi metallo-β-lactamase-1 Escherichia coli treated with colistin. J Infect 63:468–470
18. Honore PM, Joannes-Boyau O, Collin V, Boer W, Gressens B, Janvier G (2008) Practical daily management of extra-renal continuous removal. Reanimation 17:472–478

19. Tian Q, Gomersall CD, Ip M, Joynt GM (2011) Effect of preexposure to aminoglycosides on in vitro adsorption of amikacin by polyacrylonitrile hemofilters. Antimicrob Agents Chemother 55:3641–3642
20. Hofbauer R, Moser D, Frass M et al (1999) Effect of anticoagulation on blood membrane interactions during hemodialysis. Kidney Int 56:1578–1583
21. Conil JM, George B, Breden A et al (2006) Increased amikacin dosage requirements in burn patients receiving a once-daily regimen. Int J Antimicrob Agents 28:226–230
22. Mueller EW, Boucher BA (2009) The use of extended-interval aminoglycoside dosing strategies for the treatment of moderate-to-severe infections encountered in critically ill surgical patients. Surg Infect (Larchmt) 10:563–570
23. Layeux B, Taccone FS, Fagnoul D, Vincent JL, Jacobs F (2010) Amikacin monotherapy for sepsis caused by panresistant Pseudomonas aeruginosa. Antimicrob Agents Chemother 54:4939–4941
24. Drusano GL, Ambrose PG, Bhavnani SM, Bertino JS, Nafziger AN, Louie A (2007) Back to the future: using aminoglycosides again and how to dose them optimally. Clin Infect Dis 45:753–760
25. Tian Q, Gomersall CD, Ip M, Tan PE, Joynt GM, Choi GY (2008) Adsorption of amikacin, a significant mechanism of elimination by hemofiltration. Antimicrob Agents Chemother 52:1009–1013
26. Hafner V, Czock D, Burhenne J et al (2010) Pharmacokinetics of sulfobutylether-beta-cyclodextrin and voriconazole in patients with end-stage renal failure during treatment with two hemodialysis systems and hemodiafiltration. Antimicrob Agents Chemother 54:2596–2602
27. Ghannoum MA, Kuhn DM (2002) Voriconazole-better chances for patients with invasive mycoses. Eur J Med Res 7:242–256

Combatting Resistance in Intensive Care: The Multimodal Approach of the Spanish ICU "*Zero Resistance*" Program

The Scientific Expert Committee for the "Zero Resistance" Project

Introduction

Over the last few decades, a dramatic worldwide increase in infection rates by multidrug-resistant (MDR) pathogens has occurred, which is acknowledged as a public health crisis [1]. Management of infections caused by these pathogens is often difficult due to the scarcity of available active drugs.

The last report of the European Antimicrobial Resistance Surveillance System (EARSS) network, which includes 30 European countries, describes a general European-wide increase in antimicrobial resistance for the Gram-negative pathogens under surveillance (*Escherichia coli*, *Klebsiella pneumoniae* and *Pseudomonas aeruginosa*) [2]. High proportions of antimicrobial-resistant *P. aeruginosa* have been reported by many European countries [3]. In a study performed in 2000 in Spain, 41% of *Acinetobacter baumannii* isolates were resistant to carbapenems [4]. Indeed, the rate of carbapenem resistance has increased dramatically over the last decade, especially in the critical care setting [5]. An ominous emerging threat is the appearance of Gram-negative microorganisms harboring new beta-lactamases that confer high-level resistance to all available classes of beta-lactam antibiotics [6]. Concerning Gram-positive bacteria, methicillin-resistant *Staphylococcus aureus* (MRSA) and *Enterococcus* spp. resistant to vancomycin continue to be the most problematic pathogens. The incidence of MRSA infections seems to have remained stable over recent years, although this pathogen causes severe infections [2, 7].

The issue of increasing incidence of MDR is clearly more complex in intensive care units (ICUs), where selection pressure and emergence of resistance, as well as the risk of patient-to-patient transmission, are highest. The Spanish annual April-to-June ICU National Nosocomial Infection Surveillance Study (Estudio Nacional de Vigilancia de Infección Nosocomial, [ENVIN]) confirms that multi-drug resistance

The Scientific Expert Committee for the "Zero Resistance" Project ✉
Madrid, Spain
e-mail: miguel.sanchez@salud.madrid.org

J.-L. Vincent (ed.), *Annual Update in Intensive Care and Emergency Medicine 2015*,
DOI 10.1007/978-3-319-13761-2_7

is an unresolved problem in Spanish intensive care, with worrisome rates of Gram-negative MDR pathogens [7].

In addition, MDR microorganisms often do not cause true infection, but only colonization, constituting a hidden reservoir for the spread of these pathogens. Importantly, a high proportion of these patients receive antimicrobial treatment.

The prognosis of patients who develop nosocomial infection in the ICU is poor, especially if an MDR pathogen is involved [8]. Mortality rates and economic burden are significantly higher in infections caused by MDR pathogens, than in those caused by susceptible organisms [9]. Moreover, even the acquisition of an MDR pathogen, without concomitant infection, is associated with an increased risk of death, length of hospitalization, and cost [10, 11].

Previous Programs in Spanish ICUs

The Spanish Society of Intensive Care Medicine and Coronary Care Units (SEMICYUC) and the Spanish Society of Intensive Care Nursing (SEEIUC) have recently completed their role as technical lead for two programs aimed at reducing ICU-acquired infections, namely catheter-related bloodstream infections ["Zero Bacteremia"] and ventilator-associated pneumonia (VAP) ["Zero VAP"]. Both projects were developed within a framework of "Zero Tolerance". "Zero Bacteremia" and "Zero VAP" were both promoted by the Spanish Ministry of Health, more than 200 ICUs participated, and the programs consisted of the implementation of evidence-based infection prevention bundles for catheter-related bloodstream infection and VAP. Highly successful results for both initiatives confirmed that these practices could be systematically implemented across Spain, could reduce the rates of these infections and could contribute to diminish antimicrobial use in the participating ICUs [12, 13].

Methodology of "Zero Resistance"

With the experience gained in the two previous projects, a new project named "Zero Resistance" was developed by the SEMICYUC with the support of the Spanish Ministry of Health. This project uses the same structure created for "Zero Bacteremia" and "Zero VAP", which is based on coordination at national, regional and local levels.

A Scientific Expert Committee (SEC) for the development and implementation of this program was appointed as follows: SEMICYUC nominated nine intensivists chosen for their expertise in the field of prevention and management of infections in the critical care setting and SEEIUC designated an intensive care nurse with experience in infection control. A microbiologist, an epidemiologist, an infectious diseases specialist, and two technicians from the Ministry of Health with broad knowledge in the field were also incorporated.

The members of the SEC reviewed the available evidence in PubMed indexed papers, including observational studies, clinical trials, guidelines, systematic reviews

Table 1 Definitions of multidrug-resistant bacteria monitored in the *Zero Resistance* Program

Microorganism	Resistance marker
Gram-positive	
Staphylococcus aureus	methicillin (MRSA)
Enterococcus spp.	vancomycin (VRE)
Gram-negative	
Enterobacteriaceae	3rd generation cephalosporins (particularly ESBL-producing) carbapenems (particularly carbapenemase-producing)
Pseudomonas aeruginosa	$\geq$ 3 antibiotic classes, including carbapenems[a], cephalosporins[b], piperacillin-tazobactam, flouroquinolones, aminoglycosides[d] and colistin
Acinetobacter baumannii	carbapenems

[a] Imipenem, meropenem or doripenem; [b] ceftazidime or cefepime; [c] ciprofloxacin or levofloxacin; gentamicin, tobramycin or amikacin. ESBL: extended spectrum beta-lactamase; MRSA: methicillin-resistant *Staphylococcus aureus;* VRE: vancomycin-resistant enterococcus.

and meta-analyses. The following databases were searched: Medline, Embase, the Cochrane Library, and Centre for Reviews and Dissemination, including the National Health Service Economic Evaluation Database and the Health Technology Assessment database.

The implementation of 'bundles' of effective measures, compared to individual interventions, has been proposed to reduce the incidence of catheter-related bloodstream infections or VAP [14, 15]. With this concept in mind, the SEC developed a bundle of 10 recommendations that was discussed and approved after review and analysis of the existing scientific literature. Admittedly, the evidence supporting some of the chosen recommendations is weak, but all were deemed to reach at least the level of 'expert recommendation'. No grading system was used to support the strength and quality of recommendations. All items include comments intended to facilitate local adaptations.

Criteria for defining MDR pathogens vary from institution to institution and are also not uniform in the published literature, although the most highly resistant strains are readily recognizable. Based on the pathogens considered most problematic in Spanish ICUs, "Zero Resistance" collects information on episodes of infection and colonization of the pathogens listed in Table 1. Finally, because acquiring an infection may be the result of errors in patient-care, all three programs were designed to reduce and prevent these by incorporating an integral patient safety program [16].

Objectives

The main objective of the "Zero Resistance" project is reduction in the cumulative incidence of patients with ICU-acquired MDR infections by 20%. Secondary objectives are to study the epidemiology of MDR infections in Spanish ICUs, to be able to distinguish imported from ICU-acquired cases, to promote and strengthen safety assurance in participating units, and to create a network of ICUs implementing safe, and evidence-based practices. "Zero Resistance" has been active since April 2014.

The Bundle

The primary aim of the bundle recommendations is reduction of the three most influential factors contributing to the development and transmission of MDR, namely: 1) adequate prescription of antibiotics; 2) early detection and prevention of cross-colonization of MDR; and 3) elimination of reservoirs [8].

1. *First recommendation: In each ICU, at least one intensivist will be designated as responsible for the use of antimicrobials. He/She should have extensive experience in infection control and in the treatment of severe infections. This/these physician(s) should routinely assess antimicrobial prescription and advise attending clinicians. Analysis of antimicrobial use should include:*
   a. *Review of the indication for antimicrobials,*
   b. *Evaluation of the appropriateness of the antimicrobial and the correct administration (dosing, intervals and duration),*
   c. *Evaluation of de-escalation of antimicrobial therapy or even antimicrobial cessation.*

   Rationale: Antibiotic prescription in the critical care setting is a complex task that requires profound and extensive knowledge. Moreover, many pathophysiological changes associated with severe acute illness or sepsis, like capillary leak, third spacing, increased volume of distribution, and impaired renal and/or liver function, affect antimicrobial pharmacokinetics/pharmacodynamics [17]. Therefore, it is imperative to identify intensivists with a profound knowledge of infectious diseases in critically ill patients in order to improve prescription quality. This implies choosing optimal empirical antibiotics, appropriate mode of administration, and correct dosage. Administration of antimicrobials to severely ill patients at dosages defined in studies conducted in healthy volunteers often achieves only suboptimal serum concentrations, which are associated with treatment failure and resistance development [17, 18].

   Prompt and adequate antimicrobial therapy reduces morbidity and mortality in severe sepsis and septic shock [19]. However, as soon as microbiological information is available, empiric therapy should be adapted, if appropriate, by either reduction in number and/or narrowing of antimicrobial spectrum. Notwithstanding, many clinicians are reluctant to stop antimicrobials if the patient is improving. In fact, de-escalation of empirical therapy is performed in less than 50% of patients [20]. Recent studies have shown that de-escalation is safe even in critically ill patients with severe sepsis [21] or immunosuppression [22].
2. *Second recommendation: Empirically administer antimicrobials active against MDR pathogens only in cases of severe sepsis or septic shock and high risk of MDR pathogen(s) based on patient risk factors and/or knowledge of local*

ecology. Otherwise, narrow-spectrum or withholding of antimicrobials is recommended until microbiological results become available and targeted therapy with antibiotics active against MDR pathogens (carbapenems, colistin, tigecycline, glycopeptides, daptomycin, linezolid) should be started if needed. In all cases, samples for culture of the potential sources of infection should be obtained before starting antibiotic therapy.

Rationale: Early and adequate antimicrobial therapy is associated with increased survival in patients with severe sepsis and septic shock [19]. However, delaying antimicrobial therapy until microbiological confirmation is available has been shown to be associated with similar outcomes in febrile surgical ICU patients compared to starting antimicrobials immediately after the clinical diagnosis of infection [23]. More recently, a quasi-experimental, before-after observational cohort study concluded that, after adjusting for confounders, aggressive antimicrobial therapy was an independent predictor of mortality. In the aggressive period, antimicrobial treatment was always started in patients suspected of having an infection after appropriate cultures were obtained. In the second period (conservative strategy), antimicrobial treatment was started only after objective findings confirmed the infection [24].

The main limitation of both studies is that they were carried out in surgical patients and data from medical units are lacking. However, it is important to keep in mind that in febrile patients with severe sepsis or septic shock a delay in antimicrobial therapy may be fatal. In addition, the choice of empirical antimicrobial therapy should be based on an updated knowledge of the local ecology. Therefore, it seems prudent to recommend starting empiric antimicrobials active against MDR pathogens immediately only in cases meeting criteria for severe sepsis or septic shock and risk factors for MDR pathogens. Obviously, efforts to reduce the delay of microbiological results (use of rapid diagnostic techniques, direct contact with the microbiologist ...) and close follow-up of the clinical course to rapidly detect signs of alarm are fully endorsed.

3. *Third recommendation: In each Unit, at least one nurse will be designated as leader of this project and responsible for infection control measures aimed at reducing transmission of MDR pathogens.*

   Rationale: Success of quality control programs is particularly dependent on the involvement of all categories of healthcare professionals. Nurses play a critical role in preventing and controlling infectious diseases and measures to prevent patient-to-patient transmission are a significant component of care.

   A multidisciplinary team approach is necessary to develop and implement strategies to prevent infection in the critically ill patient. The participation of nurses is of extraordinary importance for the success of infection control programs in intensive care [25, 26]. In fact, most procedures performed to reduce the risk of nosocomial infection (vascular catheter care, artificial airway care, mouth hygiene, etc.) are part of the nurse's daily tasks.

   Programs that have achieved significant reductions in nosocomial infection rates have designated at least one physician and one nurse in each ICU as team leaders [14]. This model has also been implemented by successful programs designed to reduce nosocomial infection rates in the ICU endorsed by SEMICYUC [11]. The "Zero Resistance" program clearly supports the nomination in every ICU of a nurse leader responsible for infection control to reduce nosocomial infections and transmission of MDR pathogens.

4. *Fourth recommendation: It is recommended to perform an active search for MDR pathogens in all patients on admission to the unit and at least once a week throughout their stay. These samples will be processed to identify MDR pathogens according to the local epidemiology and in collaboration with the Microbiology Service and Infection Control Team of each hospital.*
   Rationale: Guidelines for MDR organisms include recommendations for routine screening cultures and contact precautions for patients after admission to high-risk units, e. g., ICUs [6, 27]. The implementation of contact precautions in patients colonized or infected with MDR is widely accepted. In contrast, the use of routine surveillance cultures in MDR management is still a matter of debate and not widely performed [28]. Initial screening is specially recommended for MRSA, although the same principles and practices apply to Gram-negative MDR organisms, which actually now constitute the main threat.
   Active surveillance programs are time and resource-consuming. The type and number of samples are selected according to local resources and epidemiology and should include at least nasal, rectal and oropharyngeal swabs (bronchial aspirates in intubated patients) [29]. In addition, other samples may be necessary to control potential reservoirs (infections, skin ulcers, etc.)
   Concerning surveillance cultures, two approaches are acceptable: All patients are screened at ICU admission or only those patients with at least one of the risk factors included in the checklist (see Fifth Recommendation).
5. *Fifth recommendation: At admission to the ICU, a 'Checklist' of risk factors (Table 2) must be completed to identify patients at high risk of MDR pathogen carriage. Patients meeting at least one of the risk factors must be cared for under application of contact precautions pending culture results.*
   Rationale: Several risk factors associated with carriage of MDR at admission to the hospital or to the ICU have been identified: Prior antibiotic use, the presence of invasive devices and certain underlying diseases are the most frequently reported [30]. Patients at risk of nosocomial pneumonia caused by MDR pathogens according to American Thoracic Society/Infectious Diseases Society of America (ATS/IDSA) criteria are: Current hospitalization of 5 days or more, prior antibiotic therapy, prior hospitalization, residence in a nursing home or extended-care facility, home infusion therapy within 30 days, chronic dialysis within 30 days, home wound care, family member with an MDR pathogen, and immunosuppression. However, in a prospective evaluation, although these criteria had an excellent negative predictive value (96%), they had a very low positive predictive value (18%) for infection or colonization with an MDR pathogen at ICU admission [31]. In a case-control study, immunosuppression was not independently associated with MDR bacteria in the ICU [32].
   In other studies, risk factors for specific pathogens, like MRSA or *A. baumannii*, have been identified in an attempt to establish control measures that limit spread

Table 2 Checklist of risk factors for carriage of multidrug-resistant (MDR) bacteria

Risk factor		
1. Hospital admission lasting > 5 days, during last 3 months	Yes	NO
2. Institutionalized (prison, healthcare and social centers, geriatric centers, etc.)	Yes	NO
3. Known colonization or infection with MDR pathogens	Yes	NO
4. Antibiotic therapy ≥ 7 days in previous month (particularly 3rd and 4th generation cephalosporins, flouroquinolones and carbapenems)	Yes	NO
5. End-stage renal disease under chronic hemodialysis or ambulatory peritoneal dialysis.	Yes	NO
6. Comorbidities associated with high incidence of colonization or infection with MDR pathogens: Cystic fibrosis, bronchiectasis, chronic skin ulcers, etc.	Yes	NO

[33]. This approach is particularly indicated in ICUs in which a particular microorganism causes the majority of episodes of colonization/infection.

With this information, the SEC generated a Checklist (Table 2) for detection of patients at high risk of carrying MDR pathogens. If one or more of these risk factors is present, screening cultures at ICU admission is mandatory and the patient must be placed in contact isolation until culture results are negative for the target organisms. The prospective validation of this Checklist is one of the pending tasks of this program.

6. *Sixth recommendation: Compliance with preventive measures including those based on transmission mechanisms should be routinely measured.*

   Rationale: Contact precaution and hand hygiene are the mainstay for reducing transmission of microorganisms [34, 35]. Adherence to these practices must be continuously reinforced and monitored [36]. Briefly, contact precautions (by staff and visitors) consist of: Hand hygiene and donning of gown and gloves immediately prior to room entry, and disposal of gown and gloves inside the patient's room, followed by hand hygiene immediately prior to leaving the room. Adherence rates for contact precautions in ICU settings with availability of all facilities were between 75 and 80% in one study [8]. Correct practice includes: (1) Use of a contact precautions sign for every patient colonized/infected by MDR pathogens; (2) availability of contact precautions equipment at patient room entry; (3) barrier disposal containers inside patient room; and (4) monitoring of adherence to the contact precautions protocol by staff/visitors. If there are no closed rooms, precautions must be tightened.

   To achieve the desired results, all staff members should watch compliance with preventive measures. Concerning this issue, the SEC of "Zero Resistance" considers that nurses have a special responsibility in implementing effective prevention. Therefore, the rest of the hospital staff and visitors must follow their recommendations.

7. *Seventh recommendation: All Units should develop a cleaning protocol for rooms of patients with MDR pathogens.*
   Rationale: Many published outbreaks of MDR pathogens detect a common source on environmental surfaces and in moist areas. Studies have documented a widespread deficiency in cleaning practices. Nevertheless, substantial improvements in cleaning and disinfection can be achieved by using standardized protocols in the ICU [37–39]. Cleaning procedures must be adapted to the architectural characteristics of each unit and agreed upon with the cleaning staff and the nosocomial infection control committee. Feedback to all involved personnel is imperative to maintain the benefits. This protocol should include fixed structures (floors and walls) as well as the bed (including main structure, rails and mattress). Cleaning protocols will include daily cleaning and final cleaning at patient discharge. Cleaning protocols for rooms occupied by patients with MDR pathogens must specify methodology, frequency of cleaning and disinfectant products. Because different cleaning products are approved in each hospital, the exact composition or trademark should be specified in the protocol. If deemed necessary, controls will be established to ensure MDR eradication [39].
8. *Eighth recommendation: A file/document specifying the existing equipment in the ICU and its respective cleaning protocols should be available and updated.*
   Rationale: Any clinical or technological equipment could act as a microbiological reservoir for MDR pathogens. Therefore, the first action is to remove all expendable materials, leaving work surfaces as free as possible. Equipment should be filed and information on the following aspects provided: Staff responsible for cleaning, cleaning schedule and cleaning methodology (disinfection, sterilization). Each healthcare worker is responsible for cleaning and disinfection of equipment for personal use (stethoscopes, flashlights . . .) [40].
9. *Ninth recommendation: To include products containing 4% chlorhexidine in daily patient hygiene if colonized or infected with MDR pathogens.*
   Rationale: Several observational studies and single-center trials have concluded that daily chlorhexidine bathing of ICU patients reduces the acquisition of MDR pathogens and the incidence of certain infections [40–43]. A systematic review concluded that chlorhexidine body-washing may be effective in preventing carriage, and possibly bloodstream infections, with Gram-positive MDR pathogens (MRSA and vancomycin-resistant enterococci [VRE]), whereas the evidence that this intervention eradicates carriage or prevents infection with Gram-negative MDR pathogens is weak [44].
   In a recent randomized multicenter trial carried out in 13 ICUs, the effect of different infection control strategies on acquisition of MDR pathogens was assessed. Improved hand hygiene plus unit-wide chlorhexidine body-washing reduced acquisition, particularly of MRSA [45]. Interestingly, in the context of sustained high level compliance of hand hygiene and chlorhexidine bathing, screening and isolation of carriers did not reduce acquisition rates of MDR pathogens. More recently, a multicenter, open, crossover trial documented the clinical benefits of daily bathing with chlorhexidine-impregnated washcloths

in reducing the risks of acquisition of MDR and the development of hospital-acquired bacteremia [46].

Chlorhexidine solutions must contain 0.16 grams of chlorhexidine (digluconate) per liter (dissolve 20 ml of 4% chlorhexidine in 1 liter of warm water). Contraindications for chlorhexidine use and adverse reactions should be taken into account. Because chlorhexidine is a cationic molecule, its activity can be reduced by natural soaps, various inorganic anions, non-ionic surfactants, and hand creams containing anionic emulsifying agents. Daily chlorhexidine bathing is simple to implement and relatively inexpensive and may be an important adjunctive intervention to barrier precautions to reduce acquisition and the subsequent development of infection.

10. *Tenth recommendation: If an outbreak is suspected it is recommended to identify the causative organism with molecular typing methods.*

Rationale: Studies of outbreaks based on the phenotypic characteristics of microorganisms (antigenic properties, metabolic or antibiotic resistance) are limited and do not provide conclusive differences or similarities between them. Therefore, molecular typing methods, to be able to recognize epidemiologically-linked isolates derived from a common precursor microorganism, should be performed. This will also provide understanding of the mechanism of transmission and dissemination and allow strategies to control and eradicate the epidemic to be designed [47, 48].

The "Zero Resistance" Program encourages hospitals without resources for molecular testing to send MDR isolates to a Reference Laboratory (National Center for Microbiology, Institute of Health Carlos III; https://cnm-laboratorios.isciii.es/), where the microbiological test will be performed free of charge.

Implementation of the *"Zero Resistance"* Program

Active implementation of this type of program is clearly necessary in order to achieve the desired results [49]. The Agency for Quality Assurance of the Spanish Ministry of Health will promote implementation in collaboration with the 17 Regional Healthcare Authorities through dissemination, coordination and follow-up. Every autonomous region will create a coordinating team led by an intensivist, responsible for contacting hospital management. The hospital management will notify their local infection and patient quality assurance committees and nominate a local coordinating team consisting of at least an intensivist and an intensive care nurse. The necessary resources for the implementation of the project will be provided.

The "Zero Resistance" program includes a web-based teaching module (http://formacion.sanidadmadrid.org/moodle/?lang=en). It is recommended that the local teams keep track of the number of healthcare workers, physicians, nurses and nurse aides that complete the web-based training modules and report their local educational indices to the regional coordinator. These data are available on the training web page.

Assessment of the Impact of the "Zero Resistance" Project

The impact of "Zero Resistance", as in all quality programs, must be measured using quality indicators that can be broken down into structure, procedure and outcome indicators. Obviously, outcome measures are of greater interest since they reflect all aspects of care and are the ultimate objectives of the intervention. The proposed indicators are explained in detail in the program, but each local team should decide which indicators to monitor depending on the information systems and efforts necessary to obtain these measurements.

ICUs participating in the "Zero Resistance" program are committed to entering data required for calculation of the relevant indices in the web-based "*ENVIN-HELICS*" registry (http://hws.vhebron.net/envin-helics/). "Zero Resistance" data are recorded through a specific adaptation of the "ENVIN-HELICS" web page (http://hws.vhebron.net/resistencia-zero/RZero.asp). Local coordinators record data for individual patients. Summary descriptive statistics are available on-line for every individual unit, which can directly access its data on a daily basis. Local results are displayed together with the corresponding regional and national values.

Conclusion

Bacterial resistance to antibiotics is growing day by day, particularly in hospitals, with a significant impact on mortality and morbidity. The lack of new antibiotics, especially for Gram-negative MDR pathogens, aggravates this serious problem as noted by numerous agencies and professional societies. Antibiotics are often incorrectly prescribed: Inadequate antibiotics or incorrect dosage for a particular infection, administration of antibiotics for non-bacterial infections, and excessively long treatment courses are all frequent.

"Zero Resistance" is a project developed by the SEMICYUC with the technical support of the Spanish Ministry of Health, with the main objective of reducing the cumulative incidence of patients with ICU-acquired MDR by 20%. This project contains a bundle of 10 recommendations aimed at improving prescription of antibiotics, detection and prevention of cross-colonization of MDR pathogens, and elimination of reservoirs. This initiative includes an integral patient safety program and educational modules to facilitate its implementation. Adherence to the project and its results will be evaluated through a series of indicators.

Acknowledgement

Members of the Committee are José Garnacho Montero, for the Working Group of Infectious Diseases and Sepsis (GTEI) of the Spanish Society of Critical Care (SEMICYUC); Francisco Álvarez Lerma, Technical Director of Project "Zero Resistance" and Project "Zero Ventilator-associated Pneumonia"; Paula Ramírez Galleymore (GTEI); Miguel Sánchez García, for the Scientific Committee of SEMI-

CYUC; Mercedes Palomar Martínez, Technical Director of Project "Zero Bacteremia"; Luis Álvarez Rocha (GTEI); Fernando Barcenilla Gaite (GTEI); Joaquín Álvarez Rodríguez, for the Working Group of Planning, Organization and Management of SEMICYUC; Mercedes Catalán González, for "ENVIN" (Spanish National ICU Infection Surveillance Program); Inmaculada Fernández Moreno for the Spanish Society of Critical Care Nursing (SEEIUC); Jesús Rodríguez Baño, Advisor in Infectious Diseases; José Campos Advisor in Microbiology; Jesús Mª Aranaz Andrés, Advisor in Preventive Medicine; Yolanda Agra Varela and Carolina Rodríguez Gay, for the Quality Assurance Agency of the Spanish Ministry of Health.

References

1. Boucher HW, Talbot GH, Bradley JS et al (2009) Bad bugs, no drugs: no ESKAPE! An update from the Infectious Diseases Society of America. Clin Infect Dis 48:1–12
2. Antimicrobial resistance interactive database (EARS-Net). Available at: http://www.ecdc.europa.eu/en/healthtopics/antimicrobial_resistance/database/Pages/database.aspx (Accessed 4 September 2014).
3. Jones RN, Flonta M, Gurler N, Cepparulo M, Mendes RE, Castanheira M (2014) Resistance surveillance program report for selected European nations (2011). Diagn Microbiol Infect Dis 78:429–436
4. Cisneros JM, Rodríguez-Baño J, Fernández-Cuenca F et al (2005) Risk factors for the acquisition of imipenem-resistant Acinetobacter baumannii in Spain. A nationwide study. Clin Microbiol Infect 11:874–879
5. Villar M, Cano ME, Gato E et al (2014) Epidemiologic and clinical impact of Acinetobacter baumannii colonization and infection: A reappraisal. Medicine (Baltimore) 93:202–210
6. Tacconelli E, Cataldo MA, Dancer SJ et al (2014) European Society of Clinical Microbiology. ESCMID guidelines for the management of the infection control measures to reduce transmission of multidrug-resistant Gram-negative bacteria in hospitalized patients. Clin Microbiol Infect 20(Suppl 1):1–55
7. Estudio Nacional De Vigilancia De Infección Nosocomial En Servicios De Medicina Intensiva. Available at: http://hws.vhebron.net/envin-helics/Help/Informe%20ENVIN-UCI%202013.pdf. Accessed Oct 22, 2014
8. Siegel JD, Rhinehart E, Jackson M, Chiarello L (2007) Healthcare Infection Control Practices Advisory Committee. Management of multidrug-resistant organisms in health care settings, 2006. Am J Infect Control 35(10 Suppl 2):S165–S193
9. Neidell MJ, Cohen B, Furuya Y et al (2012) Costs of healthcare- and community-associated infections with antimicrobial-resistant versus antimicrobial-susceptible organisms. Clin Infect Dis 55:807–815
10. García-Garmendia JL, Ortiz-Leyba C, Garnacho-Montero J, Jiménez-Jiménez FJ, Monterrubio-Villar J, Gili-Miner M (1999) Mortality and the increase in length of stay attributable to the acquisition of Acinetobacter in critically ill patients. Crit Care Med 27:1794–1799
11. Zhuo H, Yang K, Lynch SV et al (2008) Increased mortality of ventilated patients with endotracheal Pseudomonas aeruginosa without clinical signs of infection. Crit Care Med 36:2495–2503
12. Palomar M, Álvarez-Lerma F, Riera A et al (2013) Impact of a national multimodal intervention to prevent catheter-related bloodstream infection in the ICU: the Spanish experience. Crit Care Med 41:2364–2372
13. Alvarez Lerma F, Sánchez García M, Lorente L et al (2014) Guidelines for the prevention of ventilator-associated pneumonia and their implementation. The Spanish "Zero-VAP" bundle. Med Intensiva 38:226–236

14. Pronovost P, Needham D, Berenholtz S et al (2006) An intervention to decrease catheter-related bloodstream infections in the ICU. N Engl J Med 355:2725–2732
15. Rello J, Lode H, Cornaglia G, Masterton R, VAP Care Bundle Contributors (2010) A European care bundle for prevention of ventilator-associated pneumonia. Intensive Care Med 36:773–780
16. Burke JP (2003) Infection control – a problem for patient safety. N Engl J Med 348:651–656
17. Pinder M, Bellomo R, Lipman J (2002) Pharmacological principles of antibiotic prescription in the critically ill. Anaesth Intensive Care 30:134–144
18. Thomas JK, Forrest A, Bhavnani SM, Hyatt JM, Cheng A, Ballow CH, Schentag JJ (1998) Pharmacodynamic evaluation of factors associated with the development of bacterial resistance in acutely ill patients during therapy. Antimicrob Agents Chemother 42:521–557
19. Garnacho-Montero J, Garcia-Garmendia JL, Barrero-Almodovar A, Jimenez-Jimenez FJ, Perez-Paredes C, Ortiz-Leyba C (2003) Impact of adequate empirical antibiotic therapy on the outcome of patients admitted to the intensive care unit with sepsis. Crit Care Med 31:2742–2751
20. Heenen S, Jacobs F, Vincent JL (2013) Antibiotic strategies in severe nosocomial sepsis: why do we not deescalate more often? Crit Care Med 40:1404–1409
21. Garnacho-Montero J, Gutiérrez-Pizarraya A, Escoresca-Ortega A et al (2014) De-escalation of empirical therapy is associated with lower mortality in patients with severe sepsis and septic shock. Intensive Care Med 40:32–40
22. Mokart D, Slehofer G, Lambert J et al (2014) De-escalation of antimicrobial treatment in neutropenic patients with severe sepsis: results from an observational study. Intensive Care Med 40:41–49
23. Pelletier SJ, Crabtree TD, Gleason TG et al (1999) Waiting for microbiologic data to direct therapy against nosocomial infections in febrile surgical patients: are outcomes worsened? Arch Surg 134:1300–1307
24. Hranjec T, Rosenberger LH, Swenson B et al (2012) Aggressive versus conservative initiation of antimicrobial treatment in critically ill surgical patients with suspected intensive-care-unit-acquired infection: a quasi-experimental, before and after observational cohort study. Lancet Infect Dis 12:774–780
25. Goeschel CA, Bourgault A, Palleschi M et al (2006) Nursing lessons from the MHA keystone ICU project: developing and implementing an innovative approach to patient safety. Crit Care Nurs Clin North Am 18:481–492
26. Vandijck DM, Labeau SO, Secanell M, Rello J, Blot SI (2009) The role of nurses working in emergency and critical care environments in the prevention of intravascular catheter-related bloodstream infections. Int Emerg Nurs 17:60–68
27. Rodríguez-Baño J, Bischofberger C, Álvarez-Lerma F et al (2008) Vigilancia y control de Staphylococcus aureus resistente a meticilina en hospitales españoles. Documento de consenso GEIH-SEIMC y SEMPSPH. Enferm Infecc Microbiol Clin 26:285–298
28. Sunenshine RH, Liedtke LA, Fridkin SK, Strausbaugh LJ (2005) Infectious Diseases Society of America Emerging Infections Network. Management of inpatients colonized or infected with antimicrobial-resistant bacteria in hospitals in the United States. Infect Control Hosp Epidemiol 26:138–143
29. Martínez Martínez, Eliecer Cano M, Domínguez MA et al (2007) Cultivos de vigilancia epidemiológica de bacterias resistentes a los antimicrobianos de interés nosocomial En: E. Cercenado y R. Cantón. Procedimientos de Microbiología Clínica. Recomendaciones de la Sociedad Española de Enfermedades Infecciosas y Microbiología Clínica (SEIMC). Available at. http://www.seimc.org/documentos/protocolos/microbiologia
30. López-Pueyo MJ, Barcenilla-Gaite F, Amaya-Villar R, Garnacho-Montero J (2011) Multirresistencia antibiótica en unidades de críticos. Med Intensiva 35:41–53
31. Nseir S, Grailles G, Soury-Lavergne A, Minacori F, Alves I, Durocher A (2010) Accuracy of American Thoracic Society/Infectious Diseases Society of America criteria in predicting infection or colonization with multidrug-resistant bacteria at intensive-care unit admission. Clin Microbiol Infect 16:902–908

32. Nseir S, Di Pompeo C, Diarra M et al (2007) Relationship between immunosuppression and intensive care unit-acquired multidrug-resistant bacteria: a case-control study. Crit Care Med 35:1318–1323
33. McKinnell JA, Miller LG, Eells SJ, Cui E, Huang SS (2013) A systematic literature review and meta-analysis of factors associated with methicillin-resistant Staphylococcus aureus colonization at time of hospital or intensive care unit admission. Infect Control Hosp Epidemiol 34:1077–1086
34. Boyce JM, Pittet D (2002) Guideline for Hand Hygiene in Health-Care Settings: recommendations of the Healthcare Infection Control Practices Advisory Committee and the HICPAC/SHEA/APIC/IDSA Hand Hygiene Task Force. Infect Control Hosp Epidemiol 23(12 Suppl):S3–S40
35. Siegel JD, Rhinehart E, Jackson M, Chiarello L (2007) Guideline for isolation precautions: Preventing transmission of infectious agents in health care settings. Am J Infect Control 35(10 Suppl 2):S65–S164
36. Larson EL, Quiros D, Lin SX (2007) Dissemination of the CDC's Hand Hygiene Guideline and impact on infection rates. Am J Infect Control 35:666–675
37. Goodman ER, Platt R, Bass R, Onderdonk AB, Yokoe DS, Huang SS (2008) Impact of an environmental cleaning intervention on the presence of methicillin-resistant Staphylococcus aureus and vancomycin-resistant enterococci on surfaces in intensive care unit rooms. Infect Control Hosp Epidemiol 29:593–599
38. Carling PC, Parry MF, Bruno-Murtha LA, Dick B (2010) Improving environmental hygiene in 27 intensive care units to decrease multidrug-resistant bacterial transmission. Crit Care Med 38:1054–1059
39. Matlow AG (2012) Attitudes and beliefs, not just knowledge, influence the effectiveness of environmental cleaning by environmental service workers. Am J Infect Control 40:260–262
40. Wendt C, Schinke S, Württemberger M, Oberdorfer K, Bock-Hensley O, von Baum H (2007) Value of whole-body washing with chlorhexidine for the eradication of methicillin-resistant Staphylococcus aureus: a randomized, placebo-controlled, double-blind clinical trial. Infect Control Hosp Epidemiol 28:1036–1043
41. Borer A, Gilad J, Porat N et al (2007) Impact of 4% chlorhexidine whole-body washing on multidrug-resistant Acinetobacter baumannii skin colonisation among patients in a medical intensive care unit. J Hosp Infect 67:149–155
42. Popovich KJ, Hota B, Hayes R, Weinstein RA, Hayden MK (2009) Effectiveness of routine patient cleansing with chlorhexidine gluconate for infection prevention in the medical intensive care unit. Infect Control Hosp Epidemiol 30:959–963
43. Climo MW, Sepkowitz KA, Zuccotti G et al (2009) The effect of daily bathing with chlorhexidine on the acquisition of methicillin-resistant Staphylococcus aureus, vancomycin-resistant Enterococcus, and healthcare-associated bloodstream infections: results of a quasi-experimental multicenter trial. Crit Care Med 37:1858–1865
44. Derde LP, Dautzenberg MJ, Bonten MJ (2012) Chlorhexidine body washing to control antimicrobial-resistant bacteria in intensive care units: a systematic review. Intensive Care Med 38:931–939
45. Derde LP, Cooper BS, Goossens H et al (2014) Interventions to reduce colonisation and transmission of antimicrobial-resistant bacteria in intensive care units: an interrupted time series study and cluster randomised trial. Lancet Infect Dis 14:31–39
46. Climo MW, Yokoe DS, Warren DK et al (2013) Effect of daily chlorhexidine bathing on hospital-acquired infection. N Engl J Med 368:533–542
47. Singh A, Goering RV, Simjee S, Foley SL, Zervos MJ (2006) Application of molecular techniques to the study of hospital infection. Clin Microbiol Rev 19:512–530
48. Sabat AJ, Budimir A, Nashev D et al (2013) Overview of molecular typing methods for outbreak detection and epidemiological surveillance. Euro Surveill 18:20380
49. Hawe CS, Ellis KS, Cairns CJ, Longmate A (2009) Reduction of ventilator-associated pneumonia: active versus passive guideline implementation. Intensive Care Med 35:1180–1186

Immune System Dysfunction and Multidrug-resistant Bacteria in Critically Ill Patients: Inflammasones and Future Perspectives

M. Girardis, S. Busani, and S. De Biasi

Introduction

Despite the significant improvements in knowledge, technology and pharmacology obtained in the last few decades, we are not yet ready to provide individualized therapy for critically ill patients with sepsis. Clinicians tend to manage patients according to evidence-based guidelines that are derived from large randomized trials in which single patient characteristics and types of infection are rarely considered. But, as is well known, different types of infection in patients with different characteristics may cause different consequences and may need different treatments.

One of the aspects that remains rather unexplored in clinical practice is the immune response of the patient in the intensive care unit (ICU). On a day-to-day basis in the ICU we are dealing with patients who have a higher susceptibility to nosocomial infections with multidrug-resistant (MDR) bacteria without really understanding the cause. Antibiotic therapy alone in these patients is frequently insufficient, so it is necessary to study an alternative way to make sure that the immune response can actively participate in the elimination of the pathogens [1]. Infection with MDR bacteria frequently occurs in debilitated patients, such as those with shock, surgical complications, prolonged antibiotic therapies and immunosuppressive therapy [2]. The association between MDR infection and immunoparalysis is likely due to a disorder of innate and adaptive immune responses in critically ill patients.

M. Girardis ✉ · S. Busani
Department of Anesthesiology and Intensive Care, Modena University Hospital, Modena, Italy
e-mail: girardis.massimo@unimo.it

S. De Biasi
Department of Surgery, Medicine, Odontoiatrics and Morphological Sciences, University of Modena and Reggio Emilia, Modena, Italy

J.-L. Vincent (ed.), *Annual Update in Intensive Care and Emergency Medicine 2015*,
DOI 10.1007/978-3-319-13761-2_8

Critical Illness and the Host Immune Response

Sepsis

A recent biphasic view highlights the host response in the evolution of the septic process, characterized by a first hyper-inflammatory phase with a storm of cytokines that trigger marked inflammation, and a second step during which an anti-inflammatory immunoparalysis occurs. The balance between these two phases, and the passage from one to the other, likely depends on several factors, including the intrinsic aggressiveness of the pathogen, the baseline immune status of the patient, protracted therapies with debilitating antibiotics and immunosuppressive drugs, and prolonged hospital stay, among others. Concerning the treatment of sepsis, Hotchkiss et al. recently highlighted a possible, different approach [3]. Up to now, the attention of physicians was driven by a sort of race against time in the attempt to neutralize the pathogen, often heedless of the dual pro- and anti-inflammatory responses of the host to the infectious insult. As a result, while the first, pro-inflammatory phase has been investigated by several clinical trials using antagonists of interleukin (IL)-1β and tumor necrosis factor (TNF), Toll-like receptor (TLR) blockers, anticoagulants, etc. [4], the second phase of the host response related to immune-modulation has received much less attention. Meisel et al. [5] carefully investigated the immunosuppressive phase of sepsis in a multicenter trial of granulocyte/macrophage colony-stimulating factor (GM-CSF), and described how therapy with GM-CSF was capable of improving the course of sepsis in patients whose monocytes expressed less than 8,000 molecules of HLA-DR on their surface for 2 days. Not only is native immunity involved in immunoparalysis, adaptive immunity also seems to play a pivotal role. Boomer et al. [6, 7] recently described a profound depletion of B and T lymphocytes and dendritic cells in patients with severe sepsis.

Trauma

Patients with major trauma are characterized by an inflammatory over-boost in which neutrophils are the main performers. Innate immune system activation is caused by the release from the injured tissues of molecules that present so-called damage-associated molecular patterns (DAMPs). This results in four different responses by neutrophils (degranulation, generation of neutrophil extracellular traps [NETs], cytokine production, and chemotaxis) that underlie the pro-inflammatory posttraumatic reaction [8].

Surgery

Surgical stress of the gastrointestinal tract causes a stimulation of innate immunity by the activation of macrophages that secrete cytokines, such as IL-1 and TNF, which are directly related to the degree of surgical stimulus [9].

Hyperglycemia

Stress-induced hyperglycemia in critical illness induces hyper-inflammatory responses and depressed cell functions. Schematically, in monocytes, hyperglycemia enhances cytokine production and regulates adhesion, migration, and transmigration; in macrophages, hyperglycemia promotes proliferation, enhances cytokine production and phagocytosis in response to lipopolysaccharide (LPS) *in vitro,* and impairs the secretion of proinflammatory cytokines, such as TNF-α and IL-6 *ex vivo;* in neutrophils, hyperglycemia inhibits neutrophil function, such as degranulation, and downregulates production of myeloperoxidase [10].

The critically ill patient, therefore, has a state of hyper or under-activation of both native and innate immune systems, which facilitates a variety of possible secondary infections. Therefore, a better understanding of the mechanisms that are triggered in the immunology of critically ill patients may lead to the development of therapies that can counteract the immunoparalysis resulting in a decrease in susceptibility to nosocomial infections, in particular those sustained by MDR germs. Among such mechanisms, those related to the triggering and modulation of acute and chronic inflammation are acquiring a pivotal role.

Inflammasomes

Inflammasomes are key signaling platforms that detect pathogenic microorganisms and sterile stressors, and that activate the highly pro-inflammatory cytokines, IL-1β and IL-18 [11]. Inflammasomes are essential protein complexes (nucleotide-binding-and-oligomerization domain [NOD]-like receptors [NLR]) that direct the innate immune system's responses to pathogenic stimuli, such as pattern recognition receptors (PRR), components of the innate immune system that recognize danger signals, such as invading bacteria, and initiate the immune response. Inflammasomes process proinflammatory cytokines, and induce their maturation in several types of cell, including those of the myeloid series, such as macrophages and dendritic cells, leading to a potent inflammatory response.

Inflammasomes are formed by three main components: a cytosolic pattern-recognition receptor (NLR), the enzyme caspase 1 and an adaptor protein (ASC) that facilitates the interaction between NLR and caspases 1 [12]. Formation of the complex leads to pro-caspase-1 self-cleavage and generates active caspase-1, which processes pro-IL-1β and pro-IL-18 to mature IL-1β and IL-18, respectively, triggering inflammation and inducing a type of cell death defined "pyroptosis" [13]. Members of the NLR family, including NLRP1, NLRP3 and NLRC4, and the cytosolic AIM2 are critical components of inflammasomes and link microbial and endogenous danger signals to the activation of caspase 1. In response to microbial infection, activation of the inflammasomes contributes to host protection by inducing immune responses that limit microbial invasion (Fig. 1) [14].

NLR are defined by a tripartite structure comprising the following: an amino-terminal caspase-recruiting domain (CARD), pyrin domain, and acidic transacti-

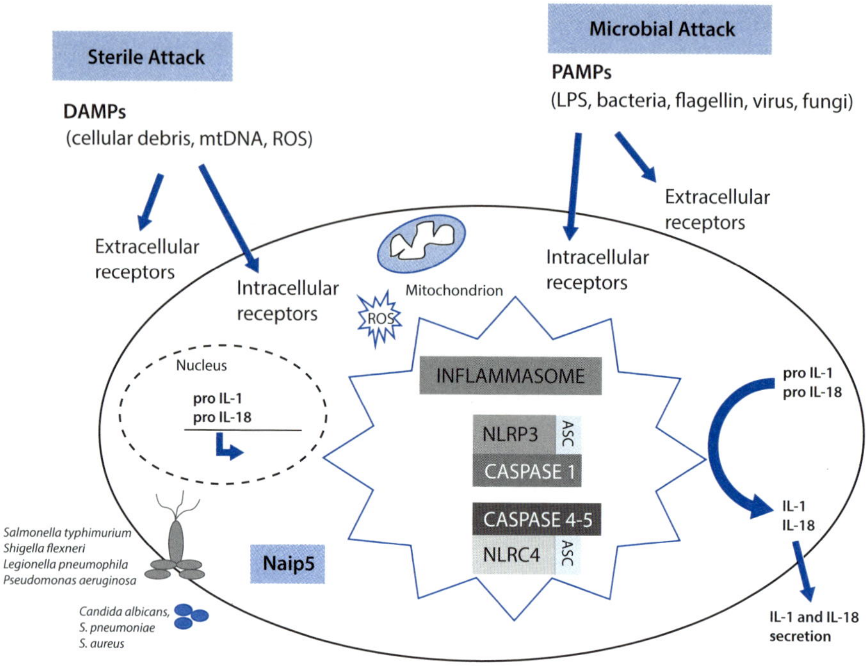

Fig. 1 Inflammasome activation by microbes and danger signals. Several NOD-like receptors (NLRs) can form multiprotein complex inflammasomes. Activation of the inflammasome consists in the auto-activation of the cysteine protease caspase-1 that processes pro-IL-1b and pro-IL-18 into mature IL-1b and IL-18. Activation of the NLRC4 inflammasome following infection of macrophages with *S. typhimurium*, *P. aeruginosa*, *S. flexneri*, or *L. pneumophila* requires a functional type III or type IV secretion system. Bacterial-derived cytosolic flagellin augments caspase-1 activation following infection with *L. pneumophila*, *S. typhimurium*, and *P. aeruginosa* possibly through a Naip5-dependent pathway. A wide variety of stimuli, including bacterial pore-forming toxins, ATP, DNA, bacterial RNA, and crystals, activate the NLRP3 inflammasome. NLRP3-activating pathogen-associated molecular patterns (PAMP) and danger-associated molecular patterns (DAMPs) also induce the generation of mitochondrial-derived reactive oxygen species (ROS) that, in turn, can activate the inflammasome and maintain the inflammatory process

vating domain, which mediate downstream protein-protein interaction; a central NOD that mediates self-oligomerization; and carboxy-terminal leucine-rich repeats (LRRs) that are thought to sense different microbial and endogenous damage stimuli [14, 15].

Several stimuli, including ATP and bacterial toxins, activate the canonical NLR family, pyrin domain containing 3 (NLRP3) inflammasome. In contrast, many Gram-negative bacteria, including *Legionella pneumophila*, *Pseudomonas aeruginosa*, and enteric pathogens *Salmonella enterica serovar typhimurium* and *Shigella flexneri*, induce activation of a non-canonical inflammasome that depends on activation of a pro-capase 11 (human orthologs are pro-caspase 4 and pro-caspase 5) via the NLRC4 inflammasome (Fig. 1) [14, 16].

The inflammasome assembled by NLRC4 responds to bacterial flagellin and a conserved type III secretion system (TTSS) rod component. NAIP5, a BIR-domain NLR protein, is a universal component of the flagellin–NLRC4 pathway. NAIP5 directly and specifically interacts with flagellin, which determins the inflammasome-stimulation activities of different bacterial flagellins. NAIP5 engagement by flagellin promoted a physical NAIP5–NLRC4 association, rendering full reconstitution of a flagellin-responsive NLRC4 inflammasome in non-macrophage cells. The related NAIP2 functioned analogously to NAIP5, serving as a specific inflammasome receptor for TTSS rod proteins [17]. Moreover, innate immune recognition of bacterial ligands by NAIPs determines inflammasome specificity, identifying NAIPs as immune sensor proteins and providing biochemical evidence for a simple receptor–ligand model for activation of the NAIP–NLRC4 inflammasomes [18].

Inflammasomes and Immune-depression/Immunoparalysis

Hyperactivation of the immune system that leads to chronic inflammation and consequent exhaustion of the components of the innate and adaptive immunity exists in autoimmune diseases. In such disorders, a hyperactive innate immune response is characterized by an exaggerated release of proinflammatory cytokines, such as IL-1β, IL-18 and TNF-α. To date, several auto-inflammatory disorders have been strongly linked with mutations of NLRs, which form subunits of the inflammasome complex. Autoimmune diseases exist in which overactivating mutations in the NLRP3 inflammasome are related to an increased production and release of IL-1β, causing familial cold auto-inflammatory syndrome, Muckle–Wells syndrome and chronic infantile neurological, cutaneous, and articular syndrome. Moreover, the NLRP3 inflammasome has also been linked with polygenic disorders [19, 20].

Polymorphisms in the NALP3/NLRP3 gene have also been associated with increased susceptibility to infectious agents, such as human immunodeficiency virus (HIV)-1 [21] and *Candida albicans* [22], reinforcing the idea that a deregulation in inflammasome and in IL-1β secretion could lead to an impaired immune response. In particular, in human monocytes, HIV-1 infection induces IL-1β production via TLR8 protein-dependent and NLRP3 inflammasome mechanisms [23]. Moreover, HIV-1 induces NALP3-inflammasome expression and IL-1β secretion in dendritic cells from healthy individuals but not from HIV-positive patients. In other words, HIV-1 does not activate inflammasome and cytokine production in HIV-dendritic cells [24].

Furthermore, the NLRP3 inflammasome is involved in the regulation of acute graft-versus-host disease in which intestinal commensal bacteria contribute to NLRP3 inflammasome–mediated IL-1β production [25].

Inflammasomes and Sepsis

The immune response to sepsis can be considered as a PRR-mediated dysregulation of the immune system following pathogen invasion in which a careful balance between inflammatory and anti-inflammatory responses is vital [4]. The most frequently isolated pathogens, rich in PRR (pathogen-associated molecular patterns [PAMP] and DAMP), in patients with sepsis include the Gram-positive bacteria *Streptococcus pneumoniae* and *Staphylococus aureus* and the Gram-negative *Escherichia coli*, *Klebsiella* spp., and *P. aeruginosa*. In addition, fungal sepsis, mainly caused by Candida species, is on the increase, at least in part due to an increase in immunocompromised patients. Pathogens associated with sepsis express an imposing arsenal of virulence factors, each of which contributes to the severity of the infectious insult [26].

LPS, a surface component of Gram-negative bacteria, activates innate immune signaling by binding to TLR4. This pathway has been strongly implicated in the pathogenesis of sepsis. High concentrations of LPS provide priming signals that induce the expression of NLRP3 and activation of pro-caspase 11, a 'non-canonical' inflammasome [11, 27].

Inflammasome Blockers as Therapy for Sepsis

PAMPs are recognized by naturally occurring antibodies that can also act as innate immune receptors. Severe sepsis is associated with a decrease in circulating immunoglobulins levels [28]. There is little direct evidence of the effects of intravenous immunoglobulin on caspase signaling in sepsis, thus inhibition of these pathways may be potentially beneficial [29]. However, cytokine neutralization is an important component of anti-inflammatory intravenous immunoglobulin activity as well as complement activation, which has impaired scavenger properties in sepsis patients [28]. The roles of immunoglobulins in sepsis are varied and many of these are still to be determined, but pathogen clearance, toxin scavenging and anti-apoptotic effects have been already defined [30].

Considering the two inflammasome-dependent responses, pyroptosis and cytokine release, blockade of inflammasome activity could not only be achieved at the level of final effector pathways (i. e., caspase 1 and cytokines), but all the different steps involved in inflammasome assembly and activation should be taken into account [31]. To target inflammasome-activating plasma membrane receptors, drug-like P2X7R blockers are being tested in several chronic inflammatory diseases, such as osteoarthritis, rheumatoid arthritis, chronic obstructive pulmonary disease (COPD) [31].

To target the products of inflammasome activity, monotherapy blocking IL-1β activity in autoinflammatory syndromes results in a rapid and sustained reduction in disease severity, including reversal of inflammation-mediated loss of sight, hearing and organ function. So far, three IL-1β-targeted agents have been approved: The IL-1β receptor antagonist, anakinra, the soluble decoy receptor, rilonacept, and the neutralizing monoclonal anti-IL1β antibody, canakinumab. In addition, a monoclonal antibody directed against the IL-1 receptor and a neutralizing anti-IL1 antibody are in clinical trials [32]. Moreover, two protease inhibitors, ritonavir and disulfiram, were shown to inhibit caspase-1 activation [31].

Conclusion

The study of therapies that stimulate the immune system in patients with severe infections by MDR microorganisms remains one of the unexplored frontiers of our profession. Since the discovery of new antibiotics to combat MDR microorganisms is proceeding extremely slowly, it is necessary to focus resources and tools to the search for drugs that can hinder immune dysfunction in these patients. The activation of inflammasomes and NLRs may be one of the keystones of this still rather obscure process. Similar to the improvements needed for therapies that regulate the host response, we also need to set up trials to identify biomarkers in patients whose immune system is dysfunctional, in order to individualize immunological therapy for each patient.

References

1. Venet F, Lukaszewicz AC, Payen D, Hotchkiss R, Monneret G (2013) Monitoring the immune response in sepsis: a rational approach to administration of immunoadjuvant therapies. Curr Opin Immunol 25:477–483
2. Pop-Vicas A, Opal SM (2014) The clinical impact of multidrug-resistant gram-negative bacilli in the management of septic shock. Virulence 5:206–212
3. Hotchkiss RS, Monneret G, Payen D (2013) Immunosuppression in sepsis: a novel understanding of the disorder and a new therapeutic approach. Lancet Infect Dis 13:260–268
4. Boomer JS, Green JM, Hotchkiss RS (2014) The changing immune system in sepsis: is individualized immuno-modulatory therapy the answer? Virulence 5:45–56
5. Meisel C, Schefold JC, Pschowski R et al (2009) Granulocyte-macrophage colony-stimulating factor to reverse sepsis-associated immunosuppression: a double-blind, randomized, placebo-controlled multicenter trial. Am J Respir Crit Care Med 180:640–648
6. Boomer JS, To K, Chang KC et al (2011) Immunosuppression in patients who die of sepsis and multiple organ failure. JAMA 306:2594–2605
7. Boomer JS, Shuherk-Shaffer J, Hotchkiss RS, Green JM (2012) A prospective analysis of lymphocyte phenotype and function over the course of acute sepsis. Crit Care 16:R112
8. Hazeldine J, Hampson P, Lord JM (2014) The impact of trauma on neutrophil function. Injury 45:1824–1833
9. Karanika S, Karantanos T, Theodoropoulos GE (2013) Immune response after laparoscopic colectomy for cancer: a review. Gastroenterol Rep (Oxf) 1:85–94
10. Xiu F, Stanojcic M, Diao L, Jeschke MG (2014) Stress hyperglycemia, insulin treatment, and innate immune cells. Int J Endocrinol 2014:486403
11. Latz E, Xiao TS, Stutz A (2013) Activation and regulation of the inflammasomes. Nat Rev Immunol 13:397–411
12. Walsh JG, Muruve DA, Power C (2014) Inflammasomes in the CNS. Nat Rev Neurosci 15:84–97

13. Kepp O, Galluzzi L, Zitvogel L, Kroemer G (2010) Pyroptosis – a cell death modality of its kind? Eur J Immunol 40:627–630
14. Franchi L, Munoz-Planillo R, Nunez G (2012) Sensing and reacting to microbes through the inflammasomes. Nat Immunol 13:325–332
15. Franchi L, Kamada N, Nakamura Y et al (2012) NLRC4-driven production of IL-1beta discriminates between pathogenic and commensal bacteria and promotes host intestinal defense. Nat Immunol 13:449–456
16. Broz P, Monack DM (2013) Noncanonical inflammasomes: caspase-11 activation and effector mechanisms. PLoS Pathog 9:e1003144
17. Zhao Y, Yang J, Shi J et al (2011) The NLRC4 inflammasome receptors for bacterial flagellin and type III secretion apparatus. Nature 477:596–600
18. Kofoed EM, Vance RE (2011) Innate immune recognition of bacterial ligands by NAIPs determines inflammasome specificity. Nature 477:592–595
19. Shaw PJ, McDermott MF, Kanneganti TD (2011) Inflammasomes and autoimmunity. Trends Mol Med 17:57–64
20. Choi AJ, Ryter SW (2014) Inflammasomes: molecular regulation and implications for metabolic and cognitive diseases. Mol Cells 37:441–448
21. Pontillo A, Brandao LA, Guimaraes RL, Segat L, Athanasakis E, Crovella S (2010) A 3′UTR SNP in NLRP3 gene is associated with susceptibility to HIV-1 infection. J Acquir Immune Defic Syndr 54:236–240
22. Lev-Sagie A, Prus D, Linhares IM, Lavy Y, Ledger WJ, Witkin SS (2009) Polymorphism in a gene coding for the inflammasome component NALP3 and recurrent vulvovaginal candidiasis in women with vulvar vestibulitis syndrome. Am J Obstet Gynecol 200:303e1–303e6
23. Guo H, Gao J, Taxman DJ, Ting JP, Su L (2014) HIV-1 Infection Induces Interleukin-1beta Production via TLR8 Protein-dependent and NLRP3 Inflammasome Mechanisms in Human Monocytes. J Biol Chem 289:21716–21726
24. Pontillo A, Silva LT, Oshiro TM, Finazzo C, Crovella S, Duarte AJ (2012) HIV-1 induces NALP3-inflammasome expression and interleukin-1beta secretion in dendritic cells from healthy individuals but not from HIV-positive patients. AIDS 26:11–18
25. Jankovic D, Ganesan J, Bscheider M et al (2013) The Nlrp3 inflammasome regulates acute graft-versus-host disease. J Exp Med 210:1899–1910
26. Wiersinga WJ, Leopold SJ, Cranendonk DR, van der Poll T (2014) Host innate immune responses to sepsis. Virulence 5:36–44
27. Papatriantafyllou M (2013) When LPS sneaks into the cell. Nat Rev Immunol 13:772–773
28. Shankar-Hari M, Spencer J, Sewell WA, Rowan KM, Singer M (2012) Bench-to-bedside review: Immunoglobulin therapy for sepsis – biological plausibility from a critical care perspective. Crit Care 16:206
29. Arredondo J, Chernyavsky AI, Karaouni A, Grando SA (2005) Novel mechanisms of target cell death and survival and of therapeutic action of IVIg in Pemphigus. Am J Pathol 167:1531–1544
30. Ehrenstein MR, Notley CA (2010) The importance of natural IgM: scavenger, protector and regulator. Nat Rev Immunol 10:778–786
31. Adinolfi E, Raffaghello L, Giuliani AL et al (2012) Expression of P2X7 receptor increases in vivo tumor growth. Cancer Res 72:2957–2969
32. Dinarello CA, Simon A, van der Meer JW (2012) Treating inflammation by blocking interleukin-1 in a broad spectrum of diseases. Nat Rev Drug Discov 11:633–652

Part III
Sepsis

Tachycardia in Septic Shock: Pathophysiological Implications and Pharmacological Treatment

A. Morelli, A. D'Egidio, and M. Passariello

Introduction

Heart rate is measured in every critically ill patient and high values often reflect the severity of underlying disease. Nevertheless, in clinical practice the pathophysiological implications of an increase in heart rate are often undervalued. The importance of elevated heart rate and its role in determining or contributing to cardiovascular diseases began to be recognized at the end of the 1970s. Nowadays, it is clear that tachycardia represents an independent risk factor for mortality and morbidity in several clinical conditions, including coronary artery disease, myocardial infarction, and congestive heart failure [1–7]. Furthermore, it has also been demonstrated that with respect to other cardiovascular factors, a high heart rate is the best predictor of mortality in different categories of patients [6]. Results of numerous large epidemiological trials confirm that an elevated heart rate not only represents a clinical sign of altered cardiac function but also contributes to cardiac dysfunction. Although the role of an elevated heart rate is well established and has clearly been linked to outcome in cardiology patients, the topic has gained less attention in septic patients. To date only a few small clinical studies have evaluated the relationship between increased heart rate and mortality in patients suffering from septic shock. However, the results of such studies strongly suggest that elevated heart rate is a risk factor for increased mortality, even in septic shock patients [8–10]. A reduction in heart rate could, therefore, improve outcomes for septic shock patients by lowering cardiac workload and improving diastolic coronary perfusion of the septic heart. Recently, the results from a monocenter trial that investigated the hemodynamic effects of reducing heart rate with the β-blocker esmolol in septic shock patients attracted the interest of critical care physicians [10]. The aim of this article is to

A. Morelli ✉ · A. D'Egidio · M. Passariello
Department of Cardiovascular, Respiratory, Nephrological, Anesthesiological and Geriatric Sciences, University of Rome "La Sapienza", Rome, Italy
e-mail: andrea.morelli@uniroma1.it

J.-L. Vincent (ed.), *Annual Update in Intensive Care and Emergency Medicine 2015*,
DOI 10.1007/978-3-319-13761-2_9

provide an overview of the pathophysiology of sepsis-induced tachycardia and its implications in the clinical management of affected patients.

Tachycardia in Septic Shock: Prognostic Implications

Only a few clinical studies have specifically focused on the relationship between increased heart rate and mortality in septic shock patients. Azimi and Vincent [8] reported that despite achieving hemodynamic stability, septic shock patients with a persistently high heart rate (102 ± 6 bpm) and greater ongoing norepinephrine requirements after 24 hours subsequently died, yet lactate levels were only marginally elevated. In survivors, the heart rate decreased to 87 ± 4 bpm after stabilization and lactate levels were comparable [8]. In another study of 48 septic shock patients, statistically significant predictors of survival included heart rate < 106 bpm on ICU admission or < 95 bpm at 24 hours, or an incremental fall in heart rate > 18 bpm within this 24 hour period [9]. Our research group performed a randomized controlled trial investigating the hemodynamic effects of esmolol-titrated reduction in heart rate below a predefined threshold of 95 bpm in septic shock patients in whom tachycardia persisted after conventional hemodynamic stabilization [10]. In agreement with these previous studies [8, 9], in the control group in which patients remained tachycardic after adequate volume resuscitation, we observed a mortality rate of 80% [10]. More recently, these findings were confirmed by a retrospective analysis of records of consecutive septic shock patients in eight European (the Netherlands, UK, France and Italy) intensive care units (ICUs), in which mortality was higher in patients with heart rate ≥ 95 bpm and increasing catecholamine dose requirements. In this subgroup of septic shock patients, the mortality rate peaked at 88% (presented at 27th ESICM Annual Congress 2014, Barcelona). These studies [8–12] demonstrate that a relatively low heart rate or a decrease in heart rate at 24 hours predicts survival, reflecting successful hemodynamic optimization. A lack of decrease or an increase in heart rate from 0 to 24 h indicates a poor prognosis. Employing this prognostic factor, a very high risk subgroup of septic shock patients can be identified early in their course.

Tachycardia in Septic Shock: Is it Just Compensatory?

In the early phase of septic shock, overwhelming inflammation leads to vasodilation and capillary leakage, which alter cardiac output by preload reduction [13–15]. The results of such alterations are severe hypovolemia and arterial hypotension, which trigger massive sympathetic activation in a physiologic attempt to maintain vital organ perfusion. This activation is typically associated with tachycardia and vasoconstriction to compensate for systemic vasodilatation [15]. The tachycardia observed in sepsis is, therefore, classically considered as the main compensatory mechanism to maintain cardiac output despite a reduction in preload. Based on this pathophysiological assumption, current sepsis guidelines recommend resuscitation with intravascular fluid administration as the first approach to counteract hypotension [16]. In fact, the majority of septic patients respond to volume administration with a reduction in tachycardia thanks to the fact that baro- and chemo-receptor activities are still preserved. Anemia, pain and agitation may also contribute to elevated heart rate but these contributing factors can be easily recognized and promptly treated at the bedside [5, 10–12, 17]. However, even after excluding hypovolemia, septic patients often have an elevated heart rate. This tachycardia is typically resistant to aggressive fluid resuscitation due to an altered chronotropic response. The underlying mechanism of such chronotropic dysfunction is an impairment of the sympathetic nervous system with disturbances in neurally mediated organ interactions. It is now well recognized that some septic shock patients may suffer from a protracted and overshooting stimulation of the sympathetic nervous system, which exceeds in time and scope the beneficial short-term compensatory effect, leading to several adverse effects, such as an elevated heart rate [5, 10–12, 17, 18]. In this context, it should be remembered that 75–80% of myocardial adrenergic receptors are β_1 and adrenergic stress is predominantly mediated by β receptors. Therefore, the heart has to be considered as a main target of sympathetic overstimulation [17]. This abnormal stimulation is further sustained by high levels of circulating catecholamines produced at the level of gut, lymphocyte, macrophages and neutrophils [18]. The autonomic dysfunction in these patients is extremely complex and also involves an imbalance of the two parasympathetic and sympathetic components. It has been demonstrated that patients with septic shock and an elevated heart rate also show reduced heart rate variability, indicating a strong attenuation of the vagal tone [19]. Why such an impairment of the autonomic nervous system occurs in some patients and not in others is not clear, but it is widely accepted that autonomic function is reduced in relation to the severity of sepsis [10, 19]. Among factors that can alter the autonomic nervous system, mediators and toxins play a pivotal role by interfering with the nerve connections at several stages: Afferent, central, or efferent [20]. Nevertheless, despite increased sympathetic outflow, there is an attenuation of the adrenergic response at the level of target organs. This impaired adrenergic response is mediated by cytokines and nitric oxide (NO), which cause down-regulation of α- and β-adrenergic receptors and depression of post-receptor signaling pathways [18]. The adrenergic response is further blunted by neuronal apoptosis in the cardiovascular autonomic centers and by catecholamine inactivation by reactive oxygen species (ROS) [18]. Down-regulation of α- and β-adrenergic receptors is, therefore, among the main underlying mechanisms of septic cardiovascular dysfunction but also accounts for the need of additional exogenous catecholamines to maintain organ perfusion. Incremental doses of exogenous catecholamines, such as dobutamine or norepinephrine, may, therefore, be required to achieve therapeutic goals. However, in the presence of an elevated endogenous sympathetic outflow, such as in septic shock, incremental doses of exogenous catecholamines further increase heart rate and the risk of tachyarrhythmia [12].

A pathologic increase in heart rate may also be the result of inputs from peripheral sympathetic afferent fibers that are activated by metabolic signals in peripheral tissues [18, 21]. These signals can be activated by tissue ischemia and inflammation that typically occur during septic shock [21]. Finally, the direct effect of cytokines and NO on the pacemaker cardiomyocytes constitutes an additional cellular mechanism that alters heart rate [22–24]. NO has been shown to modulate several cardiac ionic currents and may stimulate the sinoatrial pacemaker current. This stimulation may further contribute to sinus tachycardia in septic shock [23, 24]. Taken together, all these findings suggest that, in septic shock, tachycardia that does not respond to adequate volume resuscitation, indicates an altered chronotropic response rather than hypovolemia or demand for supranormal oxygen delivery and thus can be considered as an early manifestation of septic myocardial dysfunction.

Tachycardia and Septic Myocardial Dysfunction

In the failing heart, an increase in oxygen demand is crucial in developing ischemia. Heart rate is a major determinant of myocardial oxygen consumption, metabolic demand and importantly cardiac workload. In a state of oxygen delivery/oxygen consumption mismatch such as in septic shock, an increase in heart rate may, therefore, further deteriorate myocardial performance and lower the ischemic threshold of the septic heart [21]. In such a condition of decreased cardiac efficiency, the increase in peripheral resistance (especially in the small vessels) with vasoconstrictor agents to maintain mean arterial pressure (MAP) is an important contributor to increasing cardiac workload. This assumption is supported by an echocardiographic evaluation performed in a series of septic shock patients [25]. Among the 67 patients investigated, in 14 patients with previously non-hypokinetic hearts, global left ventricular hypokinesia occurred after 24 hours or 48 hours of continuous norepinephrine infusion. The unfavorable interplay between elevated heart rate and an increase in peripheral resistance in septic myocardial dysfunction can be better understood by looking at the physiology of ventriculo-arterial coupling. Matching between the ventricle and arterial load is crucial to provide adequate blood flow to the peripheral tissues. A sufficient cardiac output is the net result of different combinations of myocardial contractility (stroke volume) and afterload (systemic vascular resistance) and the cardiovascular system chooses any combination of these to optimize coupling between the ventricle and the arterial system [26, 27]. The maximum efficiency of the cardiovascular system with lower energy costs is obtained when the whole pulsating energy produced by the left heart is transmitted downstream to the peripheral districts [26, 27]. In this case, the left ventricle provides an adequate stroke volume with the lowest possible energetic consumption [26]. Recently, Guarracino et al demonstrated that patients suffering from septic myocardial dysfunction may show some degree of ventriculo-arterial uncoupling, due to an imbalance between the increased arterial elastance induced by pharmacological vasoconstriction and the decreased ventricular elastance caused by the reduction in myocardial contractility [27]. In the light of this, the findings of Vieillard-Baron et al. [25] suggest that in the septic heart increasing left ventricular afterload with norepinephrine impaired ventriculo-arterial coupling leading to myocardial failure. Furthermore, frequency potentiation of contractile function is a major mechanism of the increase in myocardial performance thanks to an improvement in ventricular-arterial coupling. In this case, stroke volume increases in parallel with heart rate due to a perfect matching between cardiac function and venous return [28]. In the failing heart, such as the septic heart, this positive force-frequency relation is impaired with ventricular-arterial coupling, which becomes negatively affected by elevated heart rate [26, 27, 29, 30]. When this occurs, an increase in heart rate is not associated with an increase in stroke volume; in fact stroke volume likely decreases due to a reduction in sarcoplasmic reticulum calcium uptake capacity [29, 30]. Therefore, in septic myocardial dysfunction, tachycardia and pharmacological increase in vascular resistance contribute to ventricular-arterial uncoupling. The efficiency and cardiac energetics of such a hemodynamic profile are unfavorable especially if prolonged in time as typically occurs in septic shock. Such a condition further aggravates septic myocardial failure [26, 27].

Furthermore, an elevated heart rate influences the diastolic duration, contributing to a reduction in myocardial perfusion and loss of cardiac efficiency. An increase in heart rate reduces the global time of the cardiac cycle leading to a proportional decrease in the coronary perfusion duration and the time for filling the ventricle. Under normal conditions, in the left coronary circulation, maximum coronary blood flow occurs during diastole, whereas the right coronary circulation has a systolic flow dominance. A decrease in diastolic duration results in a reduction in left coronary perfusion, whereas hypotension causes a flow decrease in both coronary arteries [21]. In septic myocardial dysfunction, an increase in heart rate may lead to an oxygen supply/oxygen demand mismatch due to an increase in oxygen consumption with a concomitant decrease in oxygen delivery caused by the reduction of coronary perfusion duration [31]. This becomes crucial in septic patients with fixed coronary artery disease.

Tachycardia also impacts on intraventricular diastolic pressure due to sepsis-related impairment of frequency-dependent acceleration of relaxation [29, 30]. In this condition, the decrease in intraventricular diastolic pressure after aortic valve closure is slowed down, leading to a higher intraventricular diastolic pressure for longer than normal. Such a prolonged higher intraventricular diastolic pressure increases myocardial wall stress and may cause a mechanical compression of the subendocardial layer, which negatively affects subendocardial perfusion [31, 32]. These pathophysiological alterations may precipitate diastolic dysfunction in septic patients who suffer from preexisting alterations of ventricular relaxation (coronary artery disease, arterial hypertension, aortic stenosis, diabetes mellitus). Patients with septic shock, therefore, frequently suffer from both systolic and diastolic dysfunction, rendering hemodynamic management extremely difficult. It is important to highlight that tachycardia *per se* and pharmacological hemodynamic support inducing tachycardia (catecholamines) may contribute to worsen preexisting diastolic dysfunction. Notably, patients with systolic dysfunction have better survival and myocardial dysfunction recovers if patients survive the septic course [18]. Conversely, diastolic dysfunction does not improve and is associated with high mortality [33]. Due to a growing elderly and cardiac morbid patient population treated in modern ICUs, the number of septic patients in whom tachycardia may negatively affect outcome is likely to increase in the near future [34].

Treating Non-compensatory Tachycardia in Sepsis: How Low Should We Go?

Since tachycardia is associated with a higher mortality in septic shock, a reduction in heart rate should be considered as one of the therapeutic targets to improve patient outcome. However, this does not necessarily imply that lowering heart rate improves survival; an elevated heart rate may simply be a biomarker rather than a cause of a poor outcome. Reducing heart rate in septic shock is difficult, because the correct timeframe for intervention and the optimal heart rate range are currently undefined. More importantly, the degree of reduction needs to be individualized according to the patient's overall hemodynamic condition, and any pre-existing co-morbidities. Before controlling heart rate it becomes crucial to distinguish between the compensatory (anemia, low stroke volume due to low preload or low contractility) or non-compensatory (maladaptive sympathetic overstimulation, pain, agitation) nature of tachycardia. As discussed previously, in the very early phase of septic shock (prior to fluid resuscitation), tachycardia constitutes the main mechanism that compensates for the decrease in stroke volume. At this stage, reducing heart rate may blunt this adaptive physiologic response, leading to a dramatic fall in cardiac output. Conversely, if the elevated heart rate does not represent a compensatory mechanism, it can be cautiously reduced without affecting systemic hemodynamics and organ perfusion [10, 34–36]. In this context, combined utilization of echocardiography and cardiovascular monitoring instruments may help to define the meaning of the elevated heart rate.

Based on the pathophysiology of the cardiac cycle, several beneficial effects can be achieved by lowering heart rate (Figs. 1 and 2). A decrease in heart rate leads to a decrease in myocardial oxygen consumption and cardiac workload with a parallel increase in coronary blood flow. In the presence of an adequate preload, a reduction in heart rate allows better ventricular filling during diastole resulting in a maintained or even increased stroke volume due to increased end-diastolic volume [10, 21, 34–36]. If we consider that end-diastolic volume is in the numerator and denominator of the ejection fraction calculation, as a consequence of heart rate reduction, the fraction increases without changes in myocardial contractility [21]. Furthermore, for a given cardiac output, a hemodynamic profile characterized by a decrease in heart rate together with a concomitant increase in stroke volume can be interpreted as an economy of cardiac work and oxygen consumption [36]. On the other hand, it is important to highlight that reducing heart rate may have negative consequences on systemic hemodynamics. Lowering heart rate may dramatically decrease stroke volume in the presence of hypovolemia or limitation to venous return [21]. In addition, although changes in stroke volume may compensate for the decrease in heart rate to maintain cardiac output, the capacity to do so is limited by the passive filling characteristics of the ventricles [21]. A reduction in heart rate may, therefore, lead to a decreased cardiac output if end-diastolic volume cannot increase. Furthermore, an increase in diastolic duration may result in increased ventricular diastolic volume and pressure (both right and left) with an increased wall

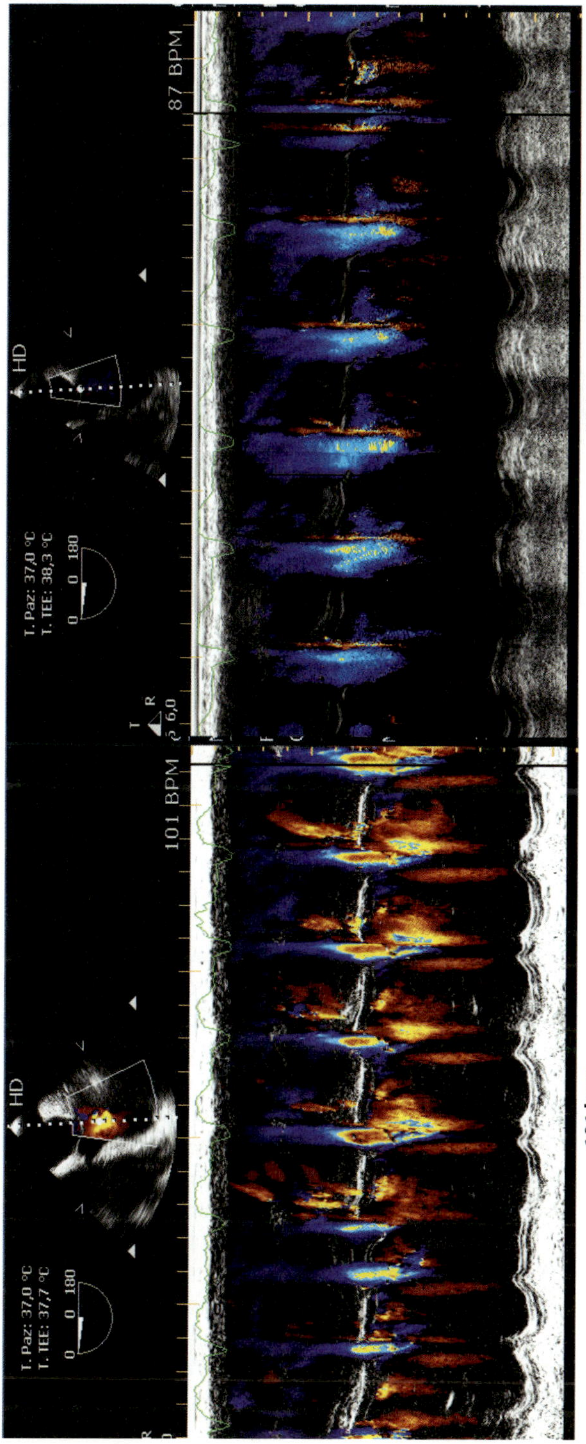

Fig. 1 Echocardiographic evaluation of ventricular filling. The figure shows the improvement in left ventricular filling after heart rate reduction with esmolol. bpm: beats per minute

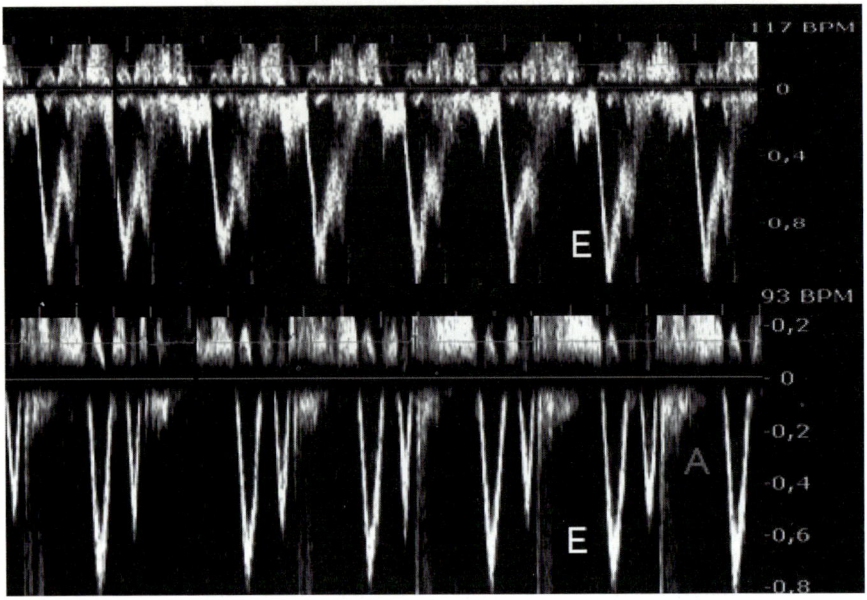

Fig. 2 Echocardiographic evaluation of diastolic function. The figure shows the improvement in diastolic function after heart rate reduction from 117 to 93 beats per minute with esmolol

stress and thus increased myocardial oxygen demand [21]. It is, therefore, clear that the clinical response of lowering heart rate depends on the nature of tachycardia, the degree of heart rate reduction, the adequacy of preload and the characteristics of myocardium. Once a non-compensatory tachycardia has been ascertained, the major problem is to determine whether a predefined heart rate threshold or a percentage of reduction exists that maintains hemodynamic stability. In a retrospective analysis of critically ill patients with a high risk of cardiac complications [6], a heart rate > 95 bpm was associated with a greater occurrence of major cardiac events including non-fatal myocardial infarction, non-fatal cardiac arrest and cardiac death (48.7% vs. 13.3%), and new onset atrial fibrillation (41.0% vs. 6.7%). Kumar et al reported that in patients with septic shock, a heart rate threshold of 95 bpm could be considered as an optimal predictive cut-off value to differentiate between survivors and non-survivors [37]. A reduction in heart rate by 20% from baseline in tachycardic patients with sepsis did not adversely affect tissue perfusion [38]. A good safety profile was reported in septic shock patients given oral metoprolol to achieve a heart rate < 95 bpm [36]. Balik et al. showed that reducing the heart rate by 30 bpm did not worsen systemic hemodynamics for rates above 110 bpm [34]. In line with these findings, our research group recently demonstrated that a heart rate range between 80–94 bpm was a sufficient compromise between improving cardiac performance and preserving systemic hemodynamics [10, 35]. Taken together these findings suggest that adopting a predefined heart rate range between 80–94 bpm or a heart rate reduction of 20–30% does not negatively affect systemic hemodynamics and organ perfusion in rates above 110 bpm [10, 34–38]. Although the predefined heart rate thresholds and percentages of heart rate reduction previously mentioned [10, 34–38] were chosen arbitrarily rather than being individualized according to the specific myocardial characteristics of each patient, in clinical practice they offer a readily achievable target without the need for a skilled echocardiographer. However, larger prospective, controlled studies are needed to confirm the efficacy and safety of such thresholds. At present, an initial echocardiography before heart rate reduction, combined with continuous monitoring or with repeated echocardiographic exams should be performed to find an adequate heart rate threshold for each patient.

How to Treat Non-compensatory Tachycardia: Pharmacological Options

Based on the underlying mechanisms of non-compensatory tachycardia in septic shock, β-blockers and ivabradine, a blocker of HCN channels, appear to be the most appropriate drugs for treating non-compensatory tachycardia.

Since a high sympathetic stress is involved in the chronotropic dysfunction observed in septic shock, β-blockers theoretically are the treatment of choice, because they can enable heart rate control and limit the adverse events related to sympathetic overstimulation. Evidence suggests that to obtain effective and safe β-adrenergic blockade, slow titration of the dose against hemodynamic endpoints has to be preferred to the administration of fixed doses [10, 34, 35]. When adopting this approach in the septic patient, it is important to consider the pharmacokinetics of β-blockers and the route of administration. In this regard, an ultra-short acting compound is preferred because it can be titrated and tailored to every patient. For the route of administration, it should be remembered that septic shock patients often have impaired gastrointestinal perfusion, which may compromise oral absorption of β-blockers, leading to unpredictable clinical effects. Among all the available β-blockers, esmolol can be considered the best option (Table 1). Because of its half-life of approximately 2 min [39], it allows titration against a predefined heart rate target and, crucially, a rapid resolution of any potential adverse effect on drug discontinuation [10, 35, 39]. Due to its high β_1-receptor selectivity, esmolol can be safely used in patients with chronic obstructive pulmonary disease (COPD). Further advantages of esmolol are related to its metabolism, which occurs via hydrolysis of the ester group in the red blood cells and is independent of renal or hepatic function. Therefore, no special precautions are necessary when administering esmolol to patients with liver or kidney dysfunction, which are frequent in septic shock. Although kidney dysfunction does not affect the pharmacokinetics of esmolol, it may contribute to the accumulation of its acid metabolite, since this is excreted by the kidney. However, due to the weak β-receptor antagonist activity of this metabolite, no significant adverse effects are expected as a result of an increase in its concentration in plasma [39].

Table 1 Intravenous selective β_1-adrenergic antagonists

Class	Drug	Onset of action	Half-life	Duration of action	Site of action (receptors)	Metabolism
Short-acting	esmolol	2 min	9 min	10 to 20 min	β_1	Red blood cell
Long-acting	metoprolol	20 min	3 to 7 h	5 to 8 h	β_1	Hepatic
Long-acting	atenolol	5 min	6 to 7 h	12 h	β_1	Renal

Considering the strong rationale of β-blockers for controlling heart rate, it is surprising that only a few human studies with several limitations are available in the current literature. This suggests that such a strategy in septic shock has never gained wide acceptance. In fact, although the first human study appeared at the end of the 1960s [40], it was not until 30 years later that Gore and Wolfe decreased heart rate by using esmolol in six septic patients [38]. It is noteworthy that in this study all the investigated patients had an MAP exceeding 70 mmHg without vasopressor support. In this hemodynamic condition, a reduction of heart rate by 20% from baseline did not adversely affect hepatic or peripheral blood flow [38]. More recently, Balik et al. showed that in 10 septic shock patients, a decrease in heart rate from a mean of 142 ± 11 bpm to 112 ± 9 bpm by titrating esmolol infusion for 24 hours, did not negatively affect hemodynamics or myocardial performance assessed by echocardiography [34]. Our research group performed an observational pilot study to investigate the effects of reducing heart rate to < 95 bpm with esmolol in patients with septic shock and persistent tachycardia (> 95 bpm) despite fluid resuscitation, with a specific focus on systemic hemodynamics and microcirculation. After 24 hours' therapy, stroke volume and microvascular blood flow were maintained while norepinephrine dosage was reduced with no negative effect on lactate concentration or mixed venous oxygen saturation (SvO_2). This pilot study supports the hypothesis that a reduction in heart rate with esmolol may safely preserve myocardial function in septic shock by decreasing cardiac workload without compromising the microcirculation. By applying the same protocol with titrated esmolol to maintain heart rate between 84 and 95 bpm, we performed an open, randomized, prospective controlled trial assessing the impact of esmolol on systemic hemodynamics and organ function in septic shock. In this controlled study, heart rate control by esmolol was continued until ICU discharge or death. Compared with the control group, stroke index and left ventricular stroke work index were higher, whereas the doses of norepinephrine, the need for fluids and lactate concentrations were lower in the esmolol group [10]. Interestingly, we found an unexpected significant difference in 28-day mortality between the two groups: 49.4% in the esmolol group vs. 80.5% in the control group [10]. In accordance with previous studies [8, 9, 37], such high mortality rates confirm that a high-dose norepinephrine requirement and tachycardia persisting at 24 hours after initiation of vasopressors identify a particularly severe subset of patients. It is, therefore, important to clarify that this subset of patients has higher mortality rates compared to septic patients with lower heart rates and lower vasopressor requirements at 24 hours. To strengthen this hypothesis, we recently completed a retrospective analysis of records of 430 consecutive septic patients admitted to our ICU between March 2008 and October 2009. Among them, 118 patients were tachycardic (> 95 bpm) and receiving a high dose of norepinephrine (0.74 ± 0.3 µg/kg/min) 24 hour after the ICU admission. Interestingly, the 28-day mortality in this subgroup of patients was 88%. We then performed a retrospective analysis of records of 541 consecutive septic patients admitted to our ICU from April 2012 to October 2013: 172 patients had tachycardia (> 95 bpm) and were receiving high doses of norepinephrine (0.85 ± 0.6 µg/kg/min) 24 hours after the ICU admission. These patients received titrated esmolol according to our institutional policy to maintain heart rate between 80 and 95 bpm until ICU discharge [10, 35]. In line with our previous study [10], the 28-day mortality in this subgroup of patients was 48.5% (unpublished data). In addition to decreasing the heart rate, esmolol can potentially decrease cardiac contractility. Nevertheless, Balik et al. demonstrated no changes in left ventricular ejection fraction (LVEF) after reducing heart rate with esmolol [34]. Similar results were found by our research group who reported that, in 44 septic shock patients, a decrease in heart rate (115 ± 10 to 91 ± 7 bpm) following esmolol administration was associated with an improvement in tricuspid annular plane solid excursion (15 ± 3 to 20 ± 3 mm) and an unchanged LVEF (46 ± 10 to 48 ± 10%) [41]. A likely explanation for these findings is that the administration of β-blockers may reduce the downregulation of β_1-adrenergic receptors and thus restore the β_1-adreneregic receptor density and responsiveness as demonstrated in experimental sepsis [42]. Finally, the beneficial effects of β-blockade could extend beyond the reduction in heart rate, including modulation of coagulation, metabolism and inflammation, all of which are important functions frequently altered in septic shock [15]. Accordingly, long-term prescription of any type of β-blocker may confer a survival advantage for patients who subsequently develop severe sepsis [43].

Bacterial toxins and cytokines interfere with pacemaker cardiomyocytes. In these cells, the pacemaker current is mainly mediated by HCN channel (hyperpolarization-activated cyclic nucleotide gated channel) activity (I_f current). The I_f current could also be stimulated by myocardial overproduction of NO, as in septic shock [22–24]. All these mechanisms contribute to tachycardia and support the use of ivabradine for controlling heart rate in septic patients. Ivabradine is a pure heart rate-lowering drug that acts specifically on the sinoatrial node by selectively inhibiting the HCN channel of cardiac pacemaker cells by entering and binding to a site in the channel pore from the intracellular side without affecting the other cardiac ionic currents [44]. Interestingly, whereas ivabradine decreases heart rate by prolonging diastole, β-blockers prolong not only diastole but potentially also systole due to their negative impact on inotropism. As a consequence, for the same decrease in heart rate, ivabradine produces a greater duration of diastolic time than β-blockers [44, 45]. Very recently, De Santis et al. administered fixed doses of oral ivabradin (starting dose 10 mg followed by a maintenance dose of 5 mg every 12 h) for 18 h in three septic shock patients with multiple organ dysfunction syndrome. Heart rate (mean difference −27.6) and cardiac index decreased following ivabradine administration, whereas end-diastolic volume index, stroke volume index, MAP and SvO_2 increased. Pulmonary capillary wedge pressure and right atrial pressure did not change over time; arterial lactate concentrations decreased and norepinephrine requirements were reduced [44]. Notably, such hemodynamic effects were similar to those previously observed after heart rate reduction with esmolol [10, 35], suggesting that the reduction in heart rate *per se* is probably the main factor in determining these results. As for esmolol, these very preliminary findings suggest that a heart rate reduction with ivabradine could improve outcome of septic shock patients by lowering myocardial oxygen demand, improving diastolic coronary perfusion and acting on the negative force-frequency relationship of the failing septic heart [44]. The results of the ongoing MODI(f)Y (reducing elevated heart rate in patients with multiple organ dysfunction syndrome by the I_f inhibitor ivabradine) trial are needed to confirm these preliminary findings [46]. Nevertheless, the oral administration and the pharmacokinetic profile of ivabradine, which do not allow an accurate titration of effect and dose, is an important limitation of its use when compared with ultra-short acting compounds, such as esmolol.

Conclusion

Tachycardia persisting at 24 hours after volume resuscitation and commencement of vasopressors identifies early a particularly severe subset of septic shock patients. These high-risk patients would likely benefit most from heart rate control. However, before controlling heart rate it is crucial to ascertain the non-compensatory (maladaptive sympathetic overstimulation) nature of tachycardia. Based on the underlying mechanisms of non-compensatory tachycardia in septic shock, at the present esmolol and ivabradine appear to be the most appropriate drugs for treating tachycardia. Despite the strong rationale and the beneficial hemodynamic effects associated with heart rate reduction in septic patients, several aspects need to be elucidated in larger trials. The effectiveness and safety of these agents, the degree of heart rate reduction, and the appropriate target population, should be better defined before widely adopting this therapeutic strategy.

References

1. Copie X, Hnatkova K, Staunton A, Fei L, Camm AJ, Malik M (1996) Predictive power of increased heart rate versus depressed left ventricular ejection fraction and heart rate variability for risk stratification after myocardial infarction. Results of a two-year follow-up study. J Am Coll Cardiol 27:270–276
2. Dyer AR, Persky V, Stamler J et al (1980) Heart rate is a prognostic factor for coronary heart disease and mortality: findings in three Chicago epidemiologic studies. Am J Epidemiol 112:736–749
3. Diaz A, Bourassa MG, Guertin MC, Tardif JC (2005) Long-term prognostic value of resting heart rate in patients with suspected or proven coronary artery disease. Eur Heart J 26:967–974

4. Disegni E, Goldbourt U, Reicher-Reiss H et al (1995) The predictive value of admission heart rate on mortality in patients with acute myocardial infarction. SPRINT study group. Secondary Prevention, Reinfarction, Israeli Nifedipine Trial. J Clin Epidemol 48:1197–1205
5. Sander O, Welters ID, Foëx P, Sear JW (2005) Impact of prolonged elevated heart rate on incidence of major cardiac events in critically ill patients with a high risk of cardiac complications. Crit Care Med 33:81–88
6. Singh BN (2003) Increased heart rate as a risk factor for cardiovascular disease. Eur Heart J Suppl 5(Suppl G):G3–G9
7. Kannel WB, Kannel C, Paffenberger RS Jr, Cupples LA (1987) Heart rate and cardiovascular mortality: the Framingham study. Am Heart J 113:1489–1494
8. Azimi G, Vincent JL (1986) Ultimate survival from septic shock. Resuscitation 14:245–253
9. Parker MM, Shelhamer JH, Natanson C, Alling DW, Parrillo JE (1987) Serial cardiovascular variables in survivors and nonsurvivors of human septic shock: heart rate as an early predictor of prognosis. Crit Care Med 15:923–929
10. Morelli A, Ertmer C, Westphal M et al (2013) Effect of heart rate control with esmolol on hemodynamic and clinical outcomes in patients with septic shock: a randomized clinical trial. JAMA 310:1683–1691
11. Leibovici L, Gafter-Gvili A, Paul M et al (2007) Relative tachycardia in patients with sepsis: an independent risk factor for mortality. QJM 100:629–634
12. Schmittinger CA, Torgersen C, Luckner G, Schröder DC, Lorenz I, Dünser MW (2012) Adverse cardiac events during catecholamine vasopressor therapy: a prospective observational study. Intensive Care Med 38:950–958
13. Bhagat K, Hingorani AD, Palacios M, Charles IG, Vallance P (1999) Cytokine-induced venodilatation in humans in vivo: eNOS masquerading as iNOS. Cardiovasc Res 41:754–764
14. Marx G, Vangerow B, Burczyk C et al (2000) Evaluation of noninvasive determinants for capillary leakage syndrome in septic shock patients. Intensive Care Med 26:1252–1258
15. Parillo JE (1993) Pathogenetic mechanisms of septic shock. N Engl J Med 328:1471–1477
16. Dellinger RP, Levy MM, Rhodes A (2013) Surviving sepsis campaign: international guidelines for management of severe sepsis and septic shock: 2012. Crit Care Med 41:580–637
17. Dünser MW, Hasibeder WR (2009) Sympathetic overstimulation during critical illness: adverse effects of adrenergic stress. J Intensive Care Med 24:293–316
18. Rudiger A, Singer M (2013) The heart in sepsis. Curr Vasc Pharmacol 11:187–195
19. Schmidt H, Muller-Werdan U, Hoffmann T et al (2005) Autonomic dysfunction predicts mortality in patients with multiple organ dysfunction syndrome of different age groups. Crit Care Med 33:1994–2002
20. Sharshar T, Gray F, de la Lorin Grandmaison G et al (2003) Apoptosis of neurons in cardiovascular autonomic centres triggered by inducible nitric oxide synthase after death from septic shock. Lancet 362:1799–1805
21. Magder SA (2012) The ups and downs of heart rate. Crit Care Med 40:239–245
22. Werdan K, Schmidt H, Ebelt H et al (2009) Impaired regulation of cardiac function in sepsis, SIRS, and MODS. Can J Physiol Pharmacol 87:266–274
23. Musialek P, Lei M, Brown HF, Paterson DJ, Casadei B (1997) Nitric oxide can increase heart rate by stimulating the hyperpolarization-activated inward current, I(f). Circ Res 81:60–68
24. Aoki Y, Hatakeyama N, Yamamoto S et al (2012) Role of ion channels in sepsis-induced atrial tachyarrhythmias in guinea pigs. Br J Pharmacol 166:390–400
25. Vieillard-Baron A, Caille V, Charron C, Belliard G, Page B, Jardin F (2008) Actual incidence of global left ventricular hypokinesia in adult septic shock. Crit Care Med 36:1701–1706
26. Guarracino F, Baldassarri R, Pinsky MR (2013) Ventriculo-arterial decoupling in acutely altered hemodynamic states. Crit Care 17:213
27. Guarracino F, Ferro B, Morelli A, Bertini P, Baldassarri R, Pinsky MR (2014) Ventriculoarterial decoupling in human septic shock. Crit Care 18:R80
28. Notarius CF, Levy RD, Tully A et al (1998) Cardiac vs. non-cardiac limits to exercise following heart transplantation. Am Heart J 135:339–348

29. Joulin O, Marechaux S, Hassoun S, Montaigne D, Lancel S, Neviere R (2009) Cardiac force–frequency relationship and frequency-dependent acceleration of relaxation are impaired in LPS-treated rats. Crit Care 13:R14
30. Masutani S, Cheng HJ, Tachibana H, Little WC, Cheng CP (2011) Levosimendan restores the positive force-frequency relation in heart failure. Am J Physiol Heart Circ Physiol 301:H488–H496
31. Kern MJ (2000) Coronary physiology revisited: practical insights from the cardiac catheterization laboratory. Circulation 101:1344–1351
32. Grosse P, Clementy J (1995) Coronary reserve in experimental myocardial hypertrophy. Eur Heart J 16(Suppl 1):22–25
33. Marik PE (2006) Management of the critically ill geriatric patient. Crit Care Med 34:176–182
34. Balik M, Rulisek J, Leden P et al (2012) Concomitant use of beta-1 adrenoreceptor blocker and norepinephrine in patients with septic shock. Wien Klin Wochenschr 124:552–556
35. Morelli A, Donati A, Ertmer C et al (2013) Microvascular effects of heart rate control with esmolol in patients with septic shock: a pilot study. Crit Care Med 41:2162–2168
36. Schmittinger CA, Dünser MW, Haller M et al (2008) Combined milrinone and enteral metoprolol therapy in patients with septic myocardial depression. Crit Care 12:R99
37. Kumar A, Schupp E, Bunnell E, Ali A, Milcarek B, Parrillo JE (2008) Cardiovascular response to dobutamine stress predicts outcome in severe sepsis and septic shock. Crit Care 12:R35
38. Gore DC, Wolfe RR (2006) Hemodynamic and metabolic effects of selective beta1 adrenergic blockade during sepsis. Surgery 139:686–694
39. Volz-Zang C, Eckrich B, Jahn P, Schneidrowski B, Schulte B, Palm D (1994) Esmolol, an ultrashort acting selective beta 1-adrenoreceptor antagonist: pharmacodynamic and pharmacokinetic properties. Eur J Clin Pharmacol 46:399–404
40. Berk JL, Hagen JF, Beyer WH, Gerber MJ, Dochat GR (1969) The treatment of endotoxin shock by beta adrenergic blockade. Ann Surg 169:74–81
41. Morelli A, D'Egidio A, Orecchioni A, Marraffa E, Romano S (2014) Heart rate reduction with Esmolol in septic shock: effects on myocardial performance. Crit Care 18(Suppl 1):P162
42. Suzuki T, Morisaki H, Serita R et al (2005) Infusion of the beta-adrenergic blocker esmolol attenuates myocardial dysfunction in septic rats. Crit Care Med 33:2294–2301
43. Macchia A, Romero M, Comignani et al (2012) Previous prescription of β-blockers is associated with reduced mortality among patients hospitalized in intensive care units for sepsis. Crit Care Med 40:2768–2772
44. De Santis V, Frati G, Greco E, Tritapepe L (2014) Ivabradine: a preliminary observation for a new terapeutic role in patients with multiple organ dysfunction syndrome. Clin Res Cardiol 103:831–834
45. Fox KM, Ferrari R (2011) Heart rate: a forgotten link in coronary artery disease? Nat Rev Cardiol :369–379
46. Nuding S, Ebelt H, Hoke RS et al (2011) Reducing elevated heart rate in patients with multiple organ dysfunction syndrome by the If (funny channel current) inhibitor ivabradine. MODIfY Trial. Clin Res Cardiol 100:915–23

Angiotensin II in Septic Shock

T. D. Corrêa, J. Takala, and S. M. Jakob

Introduction

Systemic vasodilatation and arterial hypotension are landmarks of septic shock. Whenever fluid resuscitation fails to restore arterial blood pressure and tissue perfusion, vasopressors agents are necessary [1]. Norepinephrine, a strong α-adrenergic agonist, is the standard vasopressor to treat septic shock-induced hypotension [1]. Adrenergic vasopressors have been associated with several detrimental effects, including organ dysfunction and increased mortality [2, 3]. Therefore, alternative agents have been proposed, yet with disappointing results so far [4].

The renin-angiotensin system (RAS) provides an important physiologic mechanism to prevent systemic hypotension under hypovolemic conditions, such as unresuscitated septic shock [5]. In addition to its classical hemodynamic function of regulating arterial blood pressure, angiotensin II plays a key role in several biological processes, including cell growth, apoptosis, inflammatory response, and coagulation. It may also affect mitochondrial function [6, 7].

This review briefly discusses the main physiological functions of the RAS, and presents recent evidence suggesting a role for exogenous angiotensin II administration as a vasopressor in septic shock.

The Renin-angiotensin System

Since the discovery of renin by Robert Tigerstedt and Per Gunnar Bergman in 1898, a lot of progress has been made towards better understanding of the role of the RAS

T. D. Corrêa
Intensive Care Unit, Hospital Israelita Albert Einstein, São Paulo, Brazil

J. Takala · S. M. Jakob ✉
Inselspital, Department of Intensive Care Medicine, Bern University Hospital, Bern, Switzerland
University of Bern, Bern, Switzerland
e-mail: stephan.jakob@insel.ch

J.-L. Vincent (ed.), *Annual Update in Intensive Care and Emergency Medicine 2015*,
DOI 10.1007/978-3-319-13761-2_10

in body homeostasis and in disease. The classical circulating RAS includes angiotensinogen (the precursor of angiotensin), the enzymes renin and angiotensin converting enzyme (ACE), which produces the bioactive angiotensin II, and its receptors, AT-1 and AT-2. Aldosterone is often considered together with the circulating RAS, then referred to as the RAAS (renin-angiotensin-aldosterone system). The major components of the classical 'circulating' RAS were described at the beginning of the 1970s. In the subsequent decades, knowledge about angiotensin receptors and the complex interaction between the RAS and other neuroendocrine pathways has increased [5]. One of the most remarkable advances has been the discovery of a tissue (or local) RAS, and more recently, the discovery of an intracellular RAS [8].

The local RAS contains all the components of the circulating RAS and exerts different functions in different organs. The local RAS has been identified in heart, brain, kidney, pancreas, and lymphatic and adipose tissues. It can operate independently, as in the brain, or in close connection with the circulating RAS, as in the kidneys and the heart [5]. While the circulating RAS is mainly responsible for blood pressure control and fluid and electrolyte homeostasis, the local RAS is predominantly related to inflammatory processes, modulating vascular permeability, apoptosis, cellular growth, migration and differentiation [6].

Agiontensin II Production

Juxtaglomerular cells of the renal afferent arteriole are responsible for renin synthesis. Renin, a proteolytic enzyme, is stored as an inactive form, called pro-renin. Extracellular fluid volume depletion and/or decreased arterial blood pressure trigger several enzymatic reactions resulting in the release of active renin into surrounding tissues and the systemic circulation. However, renin has no hemodynamic effects (Fig. 1) [8].

Angiotensin I, a decapeptide with weak biological activity, is produced from angiotensinogen, an α_2-globulin produced primarily in the liver and, to a lesser extent, in the kidneys and other organs. Angiotensin is rapidly converted to angiotensin II by an ACE and, to a lesser extent, by other chymases stored in secretory granules of mast cells. Angiotensin II, an octapeptide, has strong vasopressor activity [8].

ACE is present mainly in lung capillaries, although it can also be found in the plasma and vascular beds of other organs, such as the kidneys, brain, heart and skeletal muscle. The action of angiotensin II is terminated by its rapid degradation into angiotensin 2–8 heptapeptide (angiotensin III) and ultimately into angiotensin 3–8 heptapeptide (angiotensin IV) by aminopeptidases A and M, respectively [8]. ACE-2 is a carboxypeptidase responsible for the production of angiotensin 1–9 from angiotensin I and angiotensin 1–7 from angiotensin II [9, 10]. Angiotensin 1–7 is a heptapeptide, which produces vasodilatation mediated by its interaction with the prostaglandin-bradykinin-nitric oxide system [10].

The balance between ACE and ACE-2 may play an important role in cardiovascular pathophysiology by modulating and controlling angiotensin II blood concen-

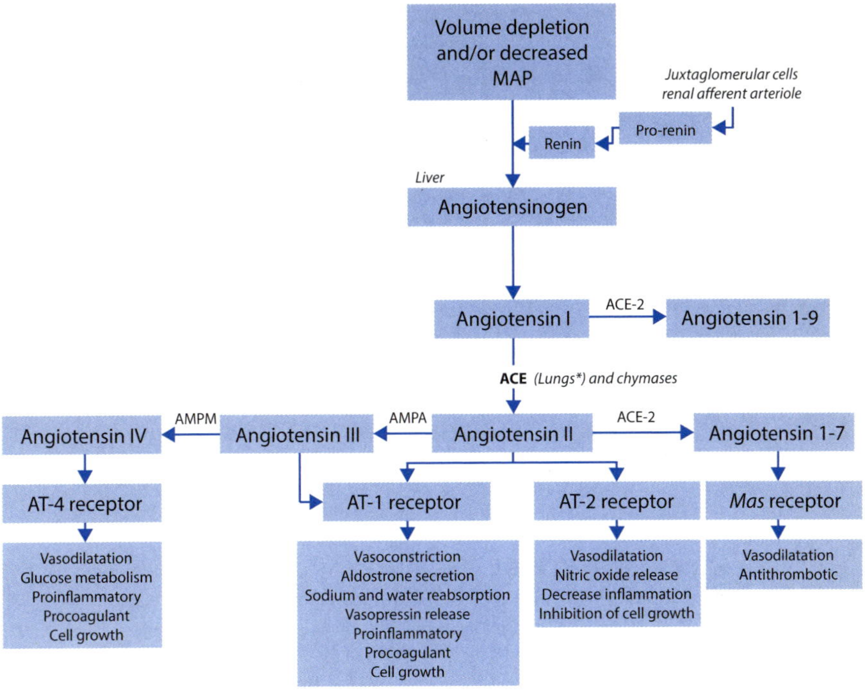

Fig. 1 Overview of the renin-angiotensin system. MAP: mean arterial blood pressure; AT: angiotensin; ACE: angiotensin-converting enzyme; AMPA: aminopeptidase A; AMPM: aminopeptidase M; *: ACE is present mainly in lung capillaries, although it can also be found in the plasma and vascular beds of other organs, such as the kidneys, brain, heart and skeletal muscle

trations. The RAS is primary regulated by a negative feedback effect of angiotensin II on renin production by the juxtaglomerular cells of the renal afferent arteriole [5].

Angiotensin II Receptors

The physiological effects of angiotensin II result from its binding to specific G protein-coupled receptors. So far, four angiotensin receptors have been described: AT-1, AT-2, AT-4 and *Mas* [11]. Additionally, two isoforms of AT-1 receptors (AT-1a and AT-1b) have been identified in rodents [12, 13]. It has been postulated that human cells express only AT-1a receptors, located in the kidneys, vascular smooth muscle, heart, brain, adrenals, pituitary gland, liver and several other organs and tissues [11].

The major physiological activities of angiotensin II are mediated by AT-1 receptors. Thereby, angiotensin II acts to control arterial blood pressure, aldosterone release by the adrenal zona glomerulosa, sodium and water reabsorption in the proximal tubular cells, and vasopressin secretion (Fig. 1) [14]. When chronically

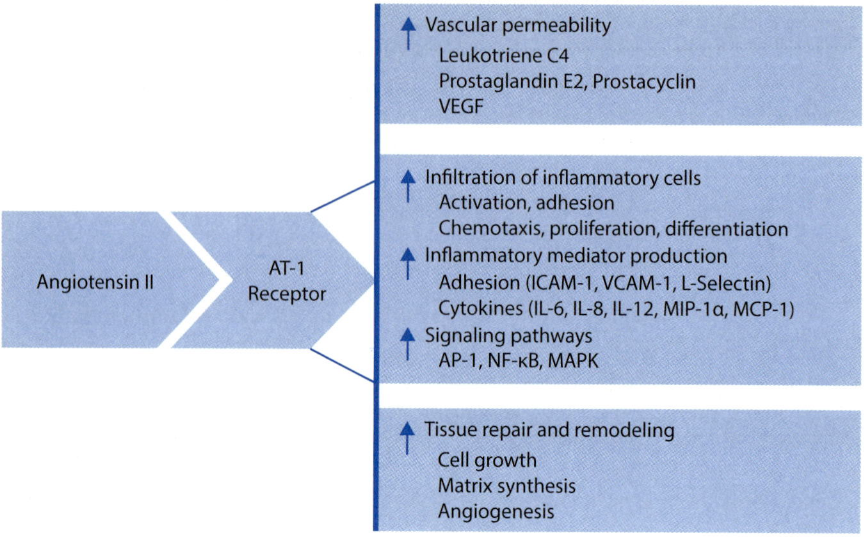

Fig. 2 Key potential mechanism attributed to angiotensin II's action via AT-1 receptors. AT-1: angiotensin receptor 1; VEGF: vascular endothelial growth factor; ICAM-1: intercellular adhesion molecule-1; VCAM-1: vascular cell adhesion molecule-1; IL: interleukin; MIP-1α: macrophage inflammatory protein-1α; MCP-1: monocyte chemotactic protein-1; AP-1: activating protein-1; NF-κB: nuclear factor-kappa B; MAPK: mitogen-activated protein kinase

stimulated, AT-1 receptors have been shown to mediate cardiac hypertrophy and induce cardiac remodeling [15].

The function of AT-2 receptors in adults has not been completely determined and some authors suggest that their stimulation might counteract the AT-1 effects on blood pressure regulation, inflammation and cell growth [11]. Indeed, angiotensin II binding to AT-2 receptors results in vasodilatation and decreased systemic vascular resistance (Fig. 1) [5].

A large number of experimental studies have shown that angiotensin II mediates countless key elements of inflammatory processes [6] (Fig. 2). By binding to AT-1 receptors, angiotensin II enhances the expression of proinflammatory mediators, increases vascular permeability by inducing vascular endothelial growth factor (VEGF), and stimulates the expression of endothelial adhesion molecules (P-selectin and E-selectin), intercellular adhesion molecule-1 (ICAM-1) and vascular cell adhesion molecule-1 (VCAM-1) (Fig. 2) [6]. Angiotensin II also promotes reactive oxygen species (ROS) production, cell growth, apoptosis, angiogenesis, endothelial dysfunction, cell migration and differentiation, leukocyte rolling, adhesion and migration, extracellular matrix remodeling. Finally, it can play a role in multiple intracellular signaling pathways leading to organ and mitochondrial injury [16].

The Renin-angiotensin System in Sepsis

Activation of the RAS during sepsis is a well know phenomenon, observed in experimental [17] and clinical studies [18–20]. However, so far, most of our knowledge about the RAS system during septic shock has come from a few experimental studies performed with healthy rodents [17, 21–26], sheep [27, 28] or pigs [7]. The role of exogenous angiotensin II administration or its inhibition in sepsis is poorly understood [29].

Unresuscitated septic shock is characterized by marked hypovolemia, extracellular fluid volume depletion, decreased cardiac output, low arterial blood pressure and decreased systemic vascular resistance [30]. Septic shock triggers a complex neurohumoral response, releasing several vasoactive substances in the circulation [31]. Four main mechanisms are involved in effective circulating volume and arterial blood pressure restoration in septic shock [32]. These mechanisms are sympathetic nervous system activation, the release of arginine vasopressin by the posterior pituitary gland, inhibition of atrial and cerebral natriuretic peptide secretion from the atria of the heart, and the increase in renin secretion by the juxtaglomerular cells, resulting in elevated angiotensin II plasma levels and an increased secretion of aldosterone from the adrenal cortex [32].

During sepsis, the activity of plasma renin, angiotensin I and angiotensin II are increased [19]. Despite the high angiotensin II plasma levels, pronounced hypotension, associated with a reduced vasopressor effect of angiotensin II, has been reported [17]. Moreover, RAS activation contributes to oxidative stress and endothelial dysfunction [24], which has been associated with development of kidney [33] and pulmonary [25, 26] injury and with the severity of organ dysfunction [19].

Data from experimental animal models have suggested that sepsis can induce a systemic downregulation of both AT-1 [21] and AT-2 receptors [22]. Proinflammatory cytokines, e.g., interleukin (IL)-1β, tumor necrosis factor (TNF)-α, interferon (IFN)γ and nitric oxide (NO), released during Gram-positive and Gram-negative sepsis, downregulate AT-1 receptor expression. This leads to systemic hypotension and low aldosterone secretion despite increased plasma renin activity and angiotensin-II levels [21, 22]. Very recently, it has been demonstrated that sepsis down-regulates the expression of an AT-1 receptor-associated protein (Arap1), which contributes to the development of hypotension secondary to reduced vascular sensitivity to angiotensin II [23]. Downregulation of adrenal AT-2 receptors may impair catecholamine release by the adrenal medulla and, thereby, play a critical role in the pathogenesis of sepsis-induced hypotension [22]. Mediators of the RAS have also been associated with microvascular dysfunction in patients with severe sepsis and septic shock [19].

Infusion of Angiotensin II in Septic Shock

Some early observations suggested that angiotensin II may be used as an alternative vasopressor in cases of norepinephrine unresponsive septic shock [34–36]. The main concern about exogenous administration of angiotensin II in septic shock is related to its strong vasoconstrictor effect, which may impair regional blood flow and aggravate tissue perfusion. Angiotensin II binding to AT-1 receptors causes dose-dependent vasoconstriction of both afferent and efferent glomerular arterioles. Indeed, the most pronounced effect of angiotensin II occurs on efferent arterioles [37], resulting in reduced renal blood flow and increased glomerular filtration pressure [27].

Wan et al. demonstrated in a hyperdynamic sepsis model in conscious sheep that a six-hour infusion of angiotensin II was effective in restoring arterial blood pressure and increased urinary output and creatinine clearance, despite a marked decrease in renal blood flow [27]. In this study, mesenteric, coronary and iliac artery blood flow were also affected but to a lesser degree [27]. In a similar model in anesthetized sheep, the same group reported an equal decrease in renal blood flow in controls and angiotensin II treated animals, but renal conductance was lower in angiotensin II-treated animals [28].

We recently evaluated in pigs the long term effects of exogenous angiotensin II administration on systemic and regional hemodynamics, tissue perfusion, inflammatory response, coagulation and mitochondrial function [7]. In this study, 16 pigs were randomized to receive either norepinephrine or angiotensin II for 48 hours after a 12-hour period of untreated sepsis. An additional group was pre-treated with enalapril (20 mg/d orally) for one week prior to the experiment, and then with intravenous enalapril (0.02 mg/kg/h) until the end of the study. We found that angiotensin II was as effective as norepinephrine to restore arterial blood pressure, and cardiac output increased similarly as in animals resuscitated with norepinephrine. Renal plasma flow, incidence of acute kidney injury, inflammation and coagulation patterns did not differ between the two groups [7]. However, enalapril-treated animals did not achieve the blood pressure targets despite receiving high norepinephrine doses (approximately 2.0 mcg/kg/min), and they had a higher incidence of acute kidney injury at the end of the study [7].

Our data demonstrate that the effects of angiotensin II on regional perfusion are different in vasodilatatory states compared to normal conditions: in healthy pigs, angiotensin II infusion resulted in net reduction of renal blood flow, while portal blood flow decreased in parallel with cardiac output, and fractional blood flow increased dose-dependently in carotid, hepatic and femoral arteries [38]. As in sepsis, angiotensin II infusion had no effects on diuresis or creatinine clearance [38]. The discrepant findings on renal perfusion can be explained by sepsis-induced hyporeactivity of the renal arteries [39]. It seems, therefore, that organ perfusion is not at risk in experimental septic shock treated with angiotensin II.

Currently, a few studies are recruiting septic patients for evaluation of the effects of angiotensin II as a vasopressor (Clinicaltrials.gov: NCT00711789 and NCT01393782).

Angiotensin II and Mitochondrial Function

In sepsis, mitochondrial dysfunction occurs, but its relevance in the development of organ failure is unclear [40]. Angiotensin II itself can stimulate mitochondrial ROS production in endothelial cells [41] and alter cardiac mitochondrial electron transport chains [15].

Evidence has indicated a direct interaction between angiotensin II and mitochondrial components [42–45]. In a study using 125 I-labeled angiotensin II in rats, angiotensin II was detected in the mitochondria and nuclei of the heart, brain and smooth muscle cells [42, 43]. In rat adrenal zona glomerulosa, renin, angiotensinogen and ACE were detected within intramitochondrial dense bodies [44], and renin has been detected in the cytosol of cardiomyocyte cell lines [45]. However, we recently demonstrated that high-affinity angiotensin II binding sites are actually located in the mitochondria-associated membrane fraction of rat liver cells, but not in purified mitochondria [46]. Moreover, we found that angiotensin II had no effect on the function of isolated mitochondria at physiologically relevant concentrations [46]. It, therefore, seems unlikely that the effects of angiotensin II on cellular energy metabolism are mediated through its direct binding to mitochondrial targets.

In septic pigs, a 48-hour angiotensin II infusion did not affect kidney, heart or liver mitochondrial respiration in comparison to norepinephrine-treated animals [7]. Although other mitochondrial functions, such as ROS production or enzymatic activity, were not assessed in this study, it seems unlikely that angiotensin II diminishes oxygen consumption in sepsis.

Conclusion

The RAS plays a key role in fluid and electrolyte homeostasis, arterial blood pressure and blood flow regulation. A better understanding of its complex interactions with other neuroendocrine regulating systems is crucial for the development of new therapeutic options to treat septic shock. Angiotensin II is a powerful vasopressor in experimental septic shock, and has proved to be safe in the tested settings. Administration of angiotensin II as an alternative to norepinephrine should be further evaluated in clinical trials.

References

1. Dellinger RP, Levy MM, Rhodes A et al (2012) Surviving sepsis campaign: international guidelines for management of severe sepsis and septic shock. Crit Care Med 41:580–637
2. Dunser MW, Ruokonen E, Pettila V et al (2009) Association of arterial blood pressure and vasopressor load with septic shock mortality: a post hoc analysis of a multicenter trial. Crit Care 13:R181
3. De Backer D, Aldecoa C, Njimi H, Vincent JL (2012) Dopamine versus norepinephrine in the treatment of septic shock: a meta-analysis. Crit Care Med 40:725–730

4. Russell JA, Walley KR, Singer J et al (2008) Vasopressin versus norepinephrine infusion in patients with septic shock. N Engl J Med 358:877–887
5. Fyhrquist F, Saijonmaa O (2008) Renin-angiotensin system revisited. J Intern Med 264:224–236
6. Suzuki Y, Ruiz-Ortega M, Lorenzo O, Ruperez M, Esteban V, Egido J (2003) Inflammation and angiotensin II. Int J Biochem Cell Biol 35:881–900
7. Correa TD, Jeger V, Pereira AJ, Takala J, Djafarzadeh S, Jakob SM (2014) Angiotensin II in septic shock: effects on tissue perfusion, organ function, and mitochondrial respiration in a porcine model of fecal peritonitis. Crit Care Med 42:e550–e559
8. Paul M, Poyan MA, Kreutz R (2006) Physiology of local renin-angiotensin systems. Physiol Rev 86:747–803
9. Donoghue M, Hsieh F, Baronas E et al (2000) A novel angiotensin-converting enzyme-related carboxypeptidase (ACE2) converts angiotensin I to angiotensin 1–9. Circ Res 2000 87:E1–E9
10. Santos RA, Ferreira AJ (2007) Angiotensin-(1–7) and the renin-angiotensin system. Curr Opin Nephrol Hypertens 16:122–128
11. Zhuo JL, Li XC (2011) New insights and perspectives on intrarenal renin-angiotensin system: focus on intracrine/intracellular angiotensin II. Peptides 32:1551–1565
12. Sasamura H, Hein L, Krieger JE, Pratt RE, Kobilka BK, Dzau VJ (1992) Cloning, characterization, and expression of two angiotensin receptor (AT-1) isoforms from the mouse genome. Biochem Biophys Res Commun 185:253–259
13. Iwai N, Inagami T (1992) Identification of two subtypes in the rat type I angiotensin II receptor. FEBS Lett 298:257–260
14. Lavoie JL, Sigmund CD (2003) Minireview: overview of the renin-angiotensin system – an endocrine and paracrine system. Endocrinology 144:2179–2183
15. Larkin JE, Frank BC, Gaspard RM, Duka I, Gavras H, Quackenbush J (2004) Cardiac transcriptional response to acute and chronic angiotensin II treatments. Physiol Genomics 18:152–166
16. Benigni A, Cassis P, Remuzzi G (2010) Angiotensin II revisited: new roles in inflammation, immunology and aging. EMBO Mol Med 2:247–257
17. Schaller MD, Waeber B, Nussberger J, Brunner HR (1985) Angiotensin II, vasopressin, and sympathetic activity in conscious rats with endotoxemia. Am J Physiol 249:H1086–H1092
18. Tamion F, Le Cam-Duchez V, Menard JF, Girault C, Coquerel A, Bonmarchand G (2004) Erythropoietin and renin as biological markers in critically ill patients. Crit Care :R328–R335
19. Doerschug KC, Delsing AS, Schmidt GA, Ashare A (2010) Renin-angiotensin system activation correlates with microvascular dysfunction in a prospective cohort study of clinical sepsis. Crit Care 14:R24
20. Hilgenfeldt U, Kienapfel G, Kellermann W, Schott R, Schmidt M (1987) Renin-angiotensin system in sepsis. Clin Exp Hypertens A 9:1493–1504
21. Bucher M, Ittner KP, Hobbhahn J, Taeger K, Kurtz A (2001) Downregulation of angiotensin II type 1 receptors during sepsis. Hypertension 38:177–182
22. Bucher M, Hobbhahn J, Kurtz A (2001) Nitric oxide-dependent down-regulation of angiotensin II type 2 receptors during experimental sepsis. Crit Care Med 29:1750–1755
23. Mederle K, Schweda F, Kattler V et al (2013) The angiotensin II AT1 receptor-associated protein Arap1 is involved in sepsis-induced hypotension. Crit Care 17:R130
24. Lund DD, Brooks RM, Faraci FM, Heistad DD (2007) Role of angiotensin II in endothelial dysfunction induced by lipopolysaccharide in mice. Am J Physiol Heart Circ Physiol 293:H3726–H3731
25. Imai Y, Kuba K, Rao S et al (2005) Angiotensin-converting enzyme 2 protects from severe acute lung failure. Nature 436:112–116
26. Klein N, Gembardt F, Supe S et al (2013) Angiotensin-(1–7) protects from experimental acute lung injury. Crit Care Med 41:e334–e343
27. Wan L, Langenberg C, Bellomo R, May CN (2009) Angiotensin II in experimental hyperdynamic sepsis. Crit Care 13:R190

28. May CN, Ishikawa K, Wan L et al (2012) Renal bioenergetics during early gram-negative mammalian sepsis and angiotensin II infusion. Intensive Care Med 38:886–893
29. Salgado DR, Rocco JR, Silva E, Vincent JL (2010) Modulation of the renin-angiotensin-aldosterone system in sepsis: a new therapeutic approach? Expert Opin Ther Targets 14:11–20
30. Correa TD, Vuda M, Blaser AR et al (2012) Effect of treatment delay on disease severity and need for resuscitation in porcine fecal peritonitis. Crit Care Med 40:2841–2849
31. Cuesta JM, Singer M (2012) The stress response and critical illness: a review. Crit Care Med 40:3283–3289
32. Rolih CA, Ober KP (1995) The endocrine response to critical illness. Med Clin North Am 79:211–224
33. du Cheyron D, Lesage A, Daubin C, Ramakers M, Charbonneau P (2003) Hyperreninemic hypoaldosteronism: a possible etiological factor of septic shock-induced acute renal failure. Intensive Care Med 29:1703–1709
34. Thomas VL, Nielsen MS (1991) Administration of angiotensin II in refractory septic shock. Crit Care Med 19:1084–1086
35. Wray GM, Coakley JH (1995) Severe septic shock unresponsive to noradrenaline. Lancet 346:1604
36. Yunge M, Petros A (2000) Angiotensin for septic shock unresponsive to noradrenaline. Arch Dis Child 82:388–389
37. Denton KM, Anderson WP, Sinniah R (2000) Effects of angiotensin II on regional afferent and efferent arteriole dimensions and the glomerular pole. Am J Physiol Regul Integr Comp Physiol 279:R629–R638
38. Pereira AJ, Jeger V, Fahrner R et al (2014) Interference of angiotensin II and enalapril with hepatic blood flow regulation. Am J Physiol Gastrointest Liver Physiol 307:G655–663
39. Yu HP, Hsu JC, Yen CH, Ma YH, Lau YT (2008) Hyporeactivity of renal artery to angiotensin II in septic rats. Chin J Physiol 51:301–307
40. Jeger V, Djafarzadeh S, Jakob SM, Takala J (2013) Mitochondrial function in sepsis. Eur J Clin Invest 43:532–542
41. Kimura S, Zhang GX, Nishiyama A et al (2005) Mitochondria-derived reactive oxygen species and vascular MAP kinases: comparison of angiotensin II and diazoxide. Hypertension 45:438–444
42. Robertson AL Jr., Khairallah PA (1971) Angiotensin II: rapid localization in nuclei of smooth and cardiac muscle. Science 172:1138–1139
43. Sirett NE, McLean AS, Bray JJ, Hubbard JI (1977) Distribution of angiotensin II receptors in rat brain. Brain Res 122:299–312
44. Peters J, Kranzlin B, Schaeffer S et al (1996) Presence of renin within intramitochondrial dense bodies of the rat adrenal cortex. Am J Physiol 271:E439–E450
45. Wanka H, Kessler N, Ellmer J et al (2009) Cytosolic renin is targeted to mitochondria and induces apoptosis in H9c2 rat cardiomyoblasts. J Cell Mol Med 13:2926–2937
46. Astin R, Bentham R, Djafarzadeh S et al (2013) No evidence for a local renin-angiotensin system in liver mitochondria. Sci Rep 3:2467

β-Blockers in Critically Ill Patients: From Physiology to Clinical Evidence

S. Coppola, S. Froio, and D. Chiumello

Introduction

β-blockers are commonly used in the treatment of cardiovascular diseases and to reduce the risk of re-infarction and the related mortality after myocardial infarction [1]. In fact, they almost universally reduce myocardial oxygen consumption and hence the degree of cardiac ischemia. Two randomized controlled trials (RCT) demonstrated that the perioperative use of β-blockers could reduce the incidence of cardiac complications responsible for significant morbidity and mortality after cardiac surgery [2, 3]. However, these results were not confirmed in three subsequent RCTs and in a large cohort study [4–7]. Similarly, the Perioperative Ischemic Evaluation Study (POISE) found that individuals receiving metoprolol succinate 30 days before surgery had a reduced risk of postoperative myocardial infarction compared to the control group but an increased risk of stroke and death associated with an increased incidence of hypotension, bradycardia and bleeding [8]. Over the years, these surprising results led to different changes in practice guidelines; specifically, the recent 2014 American College of Cardiology/American Heart Association (ACC/AHA) guidelines recommend that perioperative β-blockers should be started only in patients considered to be at intermediate or high risk for myocardial ischemia [9].

The physiopathological concept that β-blockers can decrease tissue oxygen consumption has led several authors to investigate the role of β-blockers in critical illness, which is characterized by increased resting energy expenditure due to sympathetic activation and a hypermetabolic state. Critically ill patients admitted to an intensive care unit (ICU) are affected by different degrees of systemic inflammatory response syndrome and cardiovascular comorbidities. In this context, Christensen et al. performed the first study to investigate the association between preadmission

S. Coppola · S. Froio · D. Chiumello ✉
Dipartimento di Anestesia, Rianimazione (Intensiva e Subintensiva) e Terapia del Dolore
Fondazione IRCCS Ca' Granda - Ospedale Maggiore Policlinico, Milan University, Milan, Italy
e-mail: chiumello@libero.it

J.-L. Vincent (ed.), *Annual Update in Intensive Care and Emergency Medicine 2015*,
DOI 10.1007/978-3-319-13761-2_11

Table 1 Clinical studies investigating the role of β-blocker exposure in critically ill patients. Selection of clinical studies from the last 10 years. Studies are grouped according to specific categories of critical illness: General admission to ICU, septic shock, acute respiratory failure, trauma and traumatic brain injury

	Author	Study design	N°	β-blocker	Groups	Main Outcomes	Limitations
ICU	Christensen, 2011 [10]	Observational	8087	Metoprolol (63.4%), others (36.5%) Preadmission oral use	β-blockers: 1556 No β-blockers: 6531	β-blocker group: lower 30-day mortality	No data on in-hospital β-blocker use No data on severity scores Study design
Septic Shock	Gore, 2006 [20]	Interventional clinical study	6	Intravenous esmolol 3 hours of infusion 6–22 mg/min to achieve 20% ↓ HR	Septic, mechanically ventilated patients: 6	↓ 20% HR ↓ Cardiac index O_2 consumption not altered	No control group Small population
	Schmittinger, 2008 [22]	Retrospective	40	Enteral metoprolol Within 48 hours after the onset of shock or ICU admission	Septic shock and cardiac depression in patients with chronic β-blocker therapy: 40	↓ HR (target 65–95 bpm); ↑ SVI ↓ NE, AVP and milrinone dosages ↓ lactate, creatinine	No control group Study design
	Macchia, 2012 [23]	Retrospective	9465	Preadmission oral use	β-blockers: 1061 No β-blockers: 8404	β-blocker group: lower 28-day mortality	Study design No data on severity scores Lack of information on β-blockers
	Morelli, 2013 [13]	RCT	154	Intravenous esmolol ICU treated to maintain HR 80–94 bpm 25–2000 mg/h	β-blocker: 77 Usual care: 77	β-blocker group: ↓ HR (80–94 bpm) ↑ SVI ↓ NE ↓ fluids ↓ 28-day mortality	Single center Arbitrary selection of HR threshold

Table 1 (Continuation)

	Author	Study design	N°	β-blocker	Groups	Main Outcomes	Limitations
Acute Respiratory Failure	Noveanu, 2010 [29]	Retrospective	314	Preadmission oral use Metoprolol (36%), carvedilol (18%), bisoprolol (16%), nebivolo (22%), atenolol (4%), sotalol (3%), celiproplol (2%)	In-hospital non-survivors: 51 In-hospital survivors: 263	More β-blocker use in survivors ↑ mortality if discontinuation of β-blockers	Study design Post-hoc analyses
	Kargin, 2014 [35]	Retrospective	188	Intravenous bolus metoprolol + enteral maintenance; enteral bisoprolol or carvedilol ICU treatment	β-blockers: 74 Other HRLD: 114	Similar mortality	Study design No data on spirometry
Trauma	Arbabi, 2007 [47]	Retrospective	4117	In hospital treatment	β-blocker: 303 No β-blocker: 3814	Similar mortality rate	Study design No data on HR No data on severity scores Lack of information on β-blockers
	Cotton, 2007 [46]	Retrospective	420	β-blocker therapy for 2 or more consecutive days in hospital Metoprolol, propranolol, labetalol, atenolol, esmolol, sotalol	β-blocker: 174 No β-blocker: 246	β-blocker: reduction in mortality despite more severe injury, older patients, lower predicted survival	Study design Lack of information on β-blockers Different β-blockers No data on neurological outcomes

Table 1 (Continuation)

	Author	Study design	N°	β-blocker	Groups	Main Outcomes	Limitations
TBI	Riordan, 2007 [48]	Retro-spective	446	Esmolol (e.v.), propranolol (e.v. or enteral), labetalol (e.v.), metoprolol (e.v. or enteral)	β-blocker: 138 No β-blocker: 308	Reduced mortality in β-block group despite older and more severely injured patients	Study design Different β-blockers
	Inaba, 2008 [42]	Retro-spective	1156	In-hospital treatment	β-blocker: 203 No β-blocker: 953	Reduced mortality in β-block group despite older and more severely injured patients	Study design Lack of information on β-blockers
	Schroeppel, 2010 [49]	Retro-spective	2601	In-hospital treatment Atenolo, carvedilol, esmolol, labetalol, metoprolol, nadolol, propranolol, sotalol	β-blocker: 506 No β-blocker: 2095	Similar mortality between groups despite older and more severely injured β-blocker patients	Study design Different β-blockers

ICU: intensive care unit; HR: heart rate; BP: blood pressure; TBI: traumatic brain injury; HRLD: heart rate-limiting drug; SVI: stroke volume index; NE: norepinephrine; AVP: arginine-vasopressin; RCT: randomized control trial; bpm: beat per minute; e.v.: endovenous.

β-blocker use and 30-day mortality among ICU patients and found reduced mortality in β-blocker users [10]. Over the last 10 years, there has been a growing interest in this topic (Table 1). The aim of this clinical review is to review the literature regarding the use of β-blockers in critically ill patients affected by sepsis, acute respiratory failure and traumatic brain injury (TBI).

Beta-blockers: Basic Concepts

β-blockers act on β-adrenergic receptors interfering with the ability of catecholamines or sympathomimetics to induce β-adrenergic responses. The clinical effects of β-adrenergic agonism or antagonism depend on the subtypes of receptor and on their locations. β_1-adrenergic receptors are located in the heart, on cardiomyocytes, sino atrial node and atrioventricular node, in the kidney, on adipocytes and on the platelets, causing an increase in heart rate, contractility, speed of atrioventricular conduction, renin secretion, lipolysis and aggregation of platelets, respectively. They can also be found presynaptically where their activation causes an increase in norepinephrine release.

β_2-adrenergic receptors are located on smooth muscle fibers of bronchioles, arteries, arterioles and of visceral organs, and on liver cells. Their activation results in bronchodilation, vasodilatation, glycogenolysis in the liver and tremor in skeletal muscle [11].

β-adrenoceptor antagonists with a specific affinity for β_1-receptors are defined as cardioselective (atenolol, bisoprolol, esmolol, metoprolol), those acting on β_1- and β_2-receptors are defined as non-selective (propranolol, pindolol, timolol and nadolol). This receptor selectivity is dose-dependent and is lost when large doses of antagonist are administered.

The clinical effects and comparative characteristics of β-adrenergic receptor antagonists are summarized in Fig. 1. The principal properties exploited in clinical practice are negative inotropism and chronotropism to reduce heart rate, blood pressure and myocardial work. Of course, the decrease in heart rate also ensures an improvement in diastolic perfusion time and consequently in myocardial perfusion [12].

β-blocker molecules differ from each other because of their elimination half-time. The long action of some β-adrenergic blockers represents an obvious limit for their application in critically ill patients. By contrast, the pharmacological characteristics of esmolol, an ultrashort acting β-selective drug, allow titration of the dosage to specific hemodynamic endpoints, thus minimizing the incidence of adverse events, which has recently led to investigation of its application in septic shock [13].

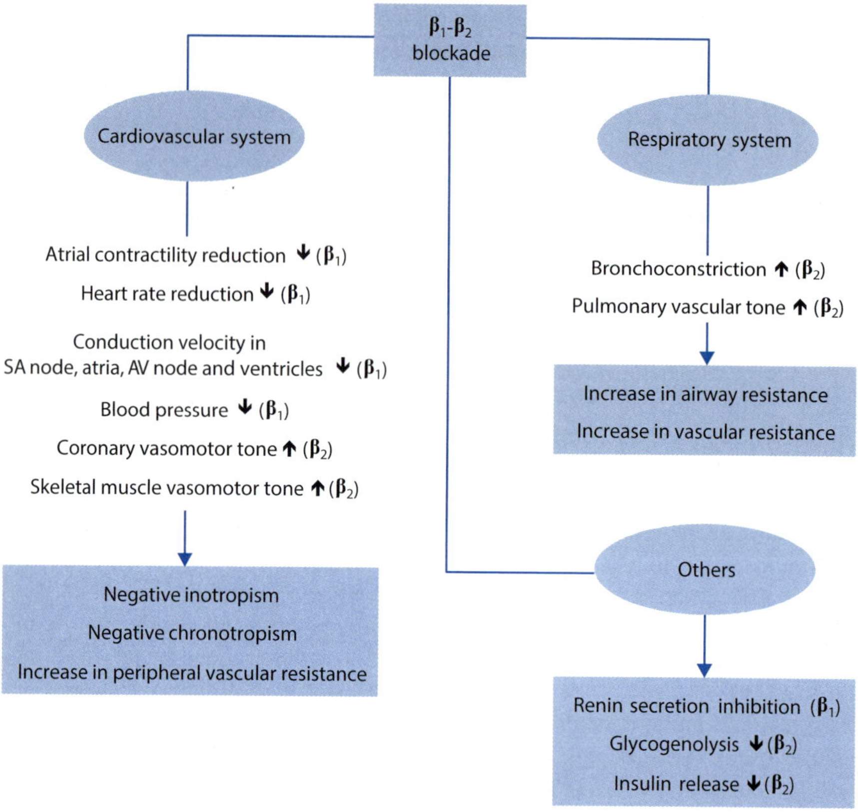

	Receptors	Clearance	Half-time	Route
Propranolol	$\beta_1-\beta_2$	Hepatic	2-3 hours	Oral/Intravenous
Pindolol	$\beta_1-\beta_2$	Hepatic-Renal	3-4 hours	Oral/Intravenous
Timolol	$\beta_1-\beta_2$	Hepatic	3-4 hours	Oral/Intravenous
Nadolol	$\beta_1-\beta_2$	Renal	20-24 hours	Oral
Atenolol	β_1	Renal	6-7 hours	Oral/Intravenous
Bisoprolol	β_1	Renal	9-12 hours	Oral
Metoprolol	β_1	Hepatic	3-4 hours	Oral/Intravenous
Landilol	β_1	Plasma Hydrolysis	3-4 minutes	Intravenous
Esmolol	β_1	Plasma Hydrolysis	10 minutes	Intravenous

Fig. 1 Clinical effects and comparative characteristics of β-adrenergic receptor antagonists. SA: sinoatrial; AV: atrioventricular

Sepsis and Septic Shock

Physiologic Rationale

Despite recent advances in the management of septic shock [14], mortality and morbidity remain unacceptably high and sepsis treatment is an active area of research. Recent data suggest that β-blockers can provide beneficial effects in the setting of sepsis. As is well-known, sepsis is the systemic inflammatory response to infection, characterized by a multitude of pathophysiological changes in terms of cardiovascular alterations, metabolic derangements and immunomodulation. The mechanism underlying these modifications is the production of mediators, such as epinephrine, which is the adrenergic response of our organism to an external aggression. This intense adrenergic stimulation results in cardiac (increased contractility, heart rate and myocardial energy demand) and extra cardiac (catabolic state, hyperglycemia, hypercoagulability, release modulation of systemic inflammatory cytokines) effects [15, 16].

Although these physiological responses allow the human body to react against injury, the sympathetic activation can become deleterious when excessive and its clinical effects persist. In fact, when sepsis progresses or tachycardia persists after fluid resuscitation and pain/agitation control, cardiac energy demand can overcome supply with the risk of cardiac dysfunction and multiorgan failure [17].

The heart is the main victim of the adrenergic stimulation because adrenergic stress is mainly mediated by β-receptors and 80% of myocardial adrenergic receptors are β_1 subtype [13]. In early sepsis, the adrenergic response increases cardiac contractility and heart rate to meet metabolic demands, but then cardiac depression with impaired left ventricular ejection fraction (LVEF), apical ballooning, myocardial stunning, apoptosis and necrosis occurs in up to 60% of patients with septic shock and contributes to increased mortality [18]. It has been hypothesized that the sepsis-induced cardiac depression is due to catecholamine-induced cardiomyocyte toxic effects following excessive sympathetic activation. However, it could be, at least partially, an adaptive and protective mechanism from an overwhelming stress response, whereby the heart tries to attenuate the adrenergic response by downregulation of β-adrenergic receptors and depression of post-receptor signaling.

In this context, increasing cardiac output above supernormal values by dobutamine administration showed no benefit [19], while the use of β-blockers to modulate this pathway has been suggested to have a protective role [17]. The physiologic rationale behind the clinical application of β-blockers in septic shock is not limited to the modulation of the cardiac effects of excessive sympathetic stimulation but also to the modulation of the extracardiac effects. In fact, the overwhelming adrenergic response during sepsis induces an overall catabolic state, an impairment of glucose metabolism and a derangement of the physiologic inflammatory state.

Literature Findings

Preclinical studies on the use of β-blockers in different models of sepsis have provided conflicting results. Nevertheless, Berk et al. in 1970, testing the administration of propranolol infusion in 5 septic patients with refractory shock, and Gore and Wolfe in 2006 testing a 3-hour esmolol infusion in 6 normotensive septic patients, reported no detrimental cardiac effects [20, 21]. Subsequently, Schmittinger et al., in a retrospective study enrolling 40 septic shock patients who were given enteral metoprolol to achieve a target heart rate of less than 95 beats/min, reported increased stroke volume and blood pressure with stable cardiac index and lactate, although no data on outcome were presented [22].

Recently, Macchia et al. analyzed a database of Italian ICU patients hospitalized for sepsis and found a 28-day survival advantage in patients who were taking β-blockers at the time of admission and who subsequently developed sepsis [23]. The recent study conducted by Morelli et al. is the first RCT on this topic [13]. These authors reported that a continuous esmolol infusion titrated to maintain heart rate between 80 and 94 beats/min in septic shock patients with a heart rate of 95/min or higher and requiring norepinephrine to maintain mean arterial pressure (MAP) of 65 mmHg, initiated 24 hours after hemodynamic optimization, was associated with a significant reduction in norepinephrine and fluid requirements and with a decrease in 28-day mortality compared to standard care. Although Morelli et al. recognize that the right timeframe for intervention and the optimal heart rate threshold should be individualized according to a patient's hemodynamic status and pre-existing comorbidities, their findings suggest that lowering heart rate improves cardiac efficiency without any detrimental effects in tissue perfusion [13]. However, some concern has been expressed regarding the interpretation of these results. In fact, the 80% mortality rate in the control group is unusually high compared to mortality rates reported in similar populations [24]; patients received large amounts of fluids during the first 96 hours although this strategy is recommended for the first 6 hours of resuscitation [14]; and the baseline cardiovascular parameters were slightly worst in the control group [24].

Moreover, as Morelli et al. hypothesized, the non-cardiac effects of esmolol in modulating the adverse effects of catecholamines on the catabolic state, glucose metabolism, the coagulation system and cytokine production could have contributed to the observed improvement in mortality.

Indeed, it has been suggested that β-blockers can counteract the hypermetabolism of the hyperdynamic phase of sepsis to prevent the catabolic phase of the decompensated period of sepsis [11, 15]. In particular, propranolol has been shown to decrease plasma glucose concentrations during stress, inhibiting the decrease in insulin-mediated glucose uptake and normalizing gluconeogenesis [25]. This mechanism does not seem to be influenced by selective β_1-antagonism [20], suggesting that non-selective β-blockade can be beneficial for glucose modulation in sepsis [11].

Moreover, it is well known that β-adrenergic receptors are involved in the cytokine production and the modulation of the cellular immune system [26, 27]. However, results from sepsis models on the immunomodulatory role of β-blockade are conflicting and immunological effects in critically ill patients have not yet been investigated. In summary, from the literature in septic shock patients, the use of esmolol can reduce heart rate without adverse events; more research is necessary to investigate the effect of this approach on outcome and to reveal the clinical significance of extra-cardiac effects.

Acute Respiratory Failure

Physiologic Rationale

Acute respiratory failure is one of the major complications that can occur in patients already admitted in the ICU [28]. Among patients admitted to the ICU for acute respiratory failure, patients with acute exacerbation of chronic obstructive pulmonary disease (COPD) are often treated with oral β-blockers [29].

COPD patients generally have cardiovascular comorbidities, for example a history of coronary artery disease, chronic heart failure, arterial hypertension, atrial fibrillation and diabetes mellitus. In these patients with a high risk of cardiac events, chronic respiratory therapy with β_2-agonists seems to increase the incidence of cardiovascular morbidity [30]. However, the use of β-blockers has been demonstrated safe and beneficial for outcome in patients with COPD and co-existing coronary artery disease because the potential benefits may outweigh the risks [31, 32]. Despite this evidence in COPD patients, the use of β-blockers in patients with acute respiratory failure is controversial. It has been reported that both selective and non-selective β-blockers increase airway hyper-responsiveness [33].

On this basis, there is a growing interest in the clinical role of β-adrenergic antagonism in COPD patients with acute respiratory failure. Moreover, the acute respiratory distress syndrome (ARDS), independent of etiology, is a critical illness and is, therefore, accompanied by sympathetic overstimulation resulting in a hyperdynamic circulation that also affects the pulmonary vasculature. In this clinical context, the potential role of β-antagonists represents an interesting field of research.

Literature Findings

The effect of β-blockers in critically ill patients with acute respiratory failure has been investigated recently, without any definitive results. In 2010, Noveanu et al. retrospectively explored the impact of oral β-blocker therapy at ICU admission or before hospital discharge on in-hospital and 1-year mortality in unselected ICU patients with acute respiratory failure [29]. Patients taking oral β-blockers at the time of admission had lower in-hospital and 1-year mortality rates than other patients. This study showed for the first time a positive effect on outcome of oral β-blocker therapy in ICU patients affected by acute respiratory failure and that discontinuation of established therapy during hospitalization was associated with higher mortality rates independent of the cardiac or non-cardiac etiology of the respiratory failure. Nevertheless, the retrospective nature of this study limits the relevance of the observed results [34].

More recently, Kargin et al. performed a retrospective case-control study to compare the outcome of COPD patients admitted to the ICU for acute respiratory failure who received β-blockers (metoprolol, bisoprolol or carvedilol) *versus* non β-blocker drugs (diltiazem and/or digoxin and/or amiodarone) for heart rate control during the ICU stay [35]. Similar ICU, hospital and 30-day mortality rates and lengths of ICU stay were found between groups [35]. The rate of application of non-invasive ventilation was higher in patients treated with β-blockers, and the need for invasive mechanical ventilation was not significantly different between groups, suggesting that β-blockers did not lead to a worsening of respiratory conditions and that they can be used to limit heart rate in COPD patients with acute respiratory failure in the ICU. Unfortunately, spirometric data were not recorded [35]. However, previously, a meta-analysis had already demonstrated that selective β-adrenoceptor antagonists in COPD patients did not induce any significant changes in forced expiratory volume in 1 second (FEV_1) or in respiratory symptoms and did not significantly affect the FEV_1 treatment response to β_2-agonists [32]. Despite the limited evidence, β-blockers thus seem safe in patients with acute respiratory failure.

In experimental models, cardioselective β_1-blockers were found to be lung-protective. Hagiwara et al. tested the effect of landilol in a rat model of lipopolysaccharide (LPS)-induced sepsis. Wet-to-dry ratio, parenchymal congestion, edema, hemorrhage and inflammatory cells were significantly reduced in animals treated with the β_1-blocker [36]. More recently, an increase in the PaO_2/FiO_2 ratio was observed 3 hours after administration of esmolol in a pig model of endotoxin shock, suggesting that the β_1-blocker did not have any negative effects [37]. In these preclinical settings, the administration of β_1-blockers seems to reduce pulmonary vascular flow and, thereby, the endothelial damage in the injured lung.

The clinical effect of β_1-blocker therapy in ARDS patients in terms of mitigation of pulmonary blood flow without a decrease in systemic hemodynamics should be further investigated. Because of the lack of evidence, RCTs testing β-adrenoreceptor antagonists in acute respiratory failure are needed to confirm the potential benefits of β-blocker therapy [34, 35].

Acute Brain Injury

Physiologic Rationale

Acute brain injury, both traumatic and non-traumatic, is frequently associated with severe autonomic dysfunction. The underlying causes of death among patients with severe brain injury are the result not only of the primary head injury, but also of the development of non-neurologic organ dysfunction that appears to be due to sympathetic hyperactivity [38]. In fact, the interplay between the neuroendocrine system and the injured brain has been studied for decades.

The reduction in normal heart rate variability as well as the disruption in the autonomic control of heart rate was observed to correlate with the degree of the neurologic injury in patients with severe brain damage [39]. A catecholamine surge, as measured by plasma and urinary catecholamine levels, has been clearly demonstrated after TBI [38]. These abnormal levels correlated with the admission Glasgow Coma Scale (GCS) score, and with outcome, in particular with the GCS at 1 week, survival, length of stay and ventilator-dependent days. A similar hyperadrenergic state has been identified in patients with non-traumatic subarachnoid hemorrhage [40]. The clinical manifestations of these hyperadrenergic responses present with tachycardia, hypertension, mydriasis, diaphoresis, arrhythmias, ventricular wall abnormalities, myocardial ischemia and neurogenic pulmonary edema. Of note, the development of stress cardiomyopathy and of neurogenic pulmonary edema have been demonstrated to contribute to poor outcome independently of the severity of the initial brain injury [41].

Although the pathophysiology of stress cardiomyopathy (also called apical ballooning syndrome or Takotsubo syndrome) is still not completely understood, sympathetic overstimulation seems to have an important role in the development of the left ventricular dysfunction [34]. In this context, β-blockade exposure to modulate the effects of the catecholaminergic storm activated by acute brain injury after trauma or subarachnoid hemorrhage could be beneficial. Locally β-blockade may attenuate the vasoconstriction of parenchymal vessels and reduce the risk of secondary brain injury, improving perfusion and oxygenation [42]. Systemically, it can have a cardioprotective role in terms of rhythm disturbances, myocardial necrosis and left ventricular function.

Literature Findings

Based on these physiological considerations, several authors have evaluated the potential benefit of β-blockers as a therapeutic option to attenuate the cerebral adverse effects and the systemic sequelae of the sympathetic activation after TBI. Unfortunately, although there are numerous preclinical studies on the use of β-blockers to mitigate inflammatory response and cardiac effects after acute brain insult, the results are conflicting. A relatively recent systematic review on the effects of β-blockers in controlled trials in TBI animal models suggested improved neurological outcome and lessened cerebral edema but with a poor methodological quality of the included studies [43].

Two small early RCTs found decreased intensity and duration of the hyperadrenergic state in patients with brain disease treated with propranolol but no data on mortality were provided [44, 45]. More recently, two retrospective studies demonstrated that the use of β-blockers was associated with reduced mortality in TBI patients with GCS ≤ 13 [46, 47]. In the most severe form of TBI, β-blocker exposure was associated with improved survival [48]. Similarly, Inaba et al. demonstrated that β-blocker exposure was an independent protective factor against death in 203 patients with isolated TBI compared to 903 patients who did not receive β-blockers. Moreover, a subgroup of elderly patients (>55 years old) with severe head injury who received β-blockers had a mortality of 28%, compared with 60% if they did not [42]. Similar findings were observed in a large retrospective study of 2601 blunt TBI patients [49].

Despite these results, the exact mechanism of the positive effects of β-blockers on the outcome of brain injured patients remains unclear. The current state of evidence suggests that the use of β-blockers in acute brain injury seems to have a valid rationale, although several unsolved problems regarding clinical application remain, such as whether to use selective or non-selective β-blockers, duration of treatment and dose.

Conclusion

Many questions about using β-blockers in critically ill patients are unanswered:

- *When should β-blocker treatment be started*? During septic shock, recent clinical data suggest starting a β-blocker 24 hours after hemodynamic optimization [13]. During acute respiratory failure some clinical and experimental studies seem to suggest starting a β-blocker before signs of fulminant sepsis occur, whereas after brain injury β-blocker treatment should be started as soon as possible.
- *Which β-blocker should be used?* Currently, esmolol is the only β-blocker that has been tested in a randomized controlled study. There is not enough evidence to propose the use of a specific agent in each specific critical condition.
- *How should the β-blocker be administered?* Probably, as studies on perioperative patients have demonstrated, a fixed dose is not a good choice; physiological titration to heart rate or oxygen delivery in relation to oxygen demand seems more advisable.
- *Finally, which patients may benefit from this therapy?* Individualized treatment based on presence of comorbidities and the degree of sympathetic activation may provide better results in terms of outcome.

In conclusion, further clinical research is needed to find a balance between β-blockade and β-stimulation in acutely ill patients.

References

1. Sanfilippo F, Santonocito C, Foex P (2014) Use of beta-blockers in non-cardiac surgery: an open debate. Minerva Anestesiol 80:482–494
2. Mangano DT, Layug EL, Wallace A, Tateo I (1996) Effect of atenolol on mortality and cardiovascular morbidity after noncardiac surgery. Multicenter Study of Perioperative Ischemia Research Group. N Engl J Med 335:1713–1720
3. Poldermans D, Boersma E, Bax JJ et al (1999) The effect of bisoprolol on perioperative mortality and myocardial infarction in high-risk patients undergoing vascular surgery. Dutch Echocardiographic Cardiac Risk Evaluation Applying Stress Echocardiography Study Group. N Engl J Med 341:1789–1794
4. Brady AR, Gibbs JS, Greenhalgh RM, Powell JT, Sydes MR (2005) Perioperative beta-blockade (POBBLE) for patients undergoing infrarenal vascular surgery: results of a randomized double-blind controlled trial. J Vasc Surg 41:602–609
5. Juul AB, Wetterslev J, Gluud C et al (2006) Effect of perioperative beta blockade in patients with diabetes undergoing major non-cardiac surgery: randomised placebo controlled, blinded multicentre trial. BMJ 332:1482
6. Lindenauer PK, Pekow P, Wang K, Mamidi DK, Gutierrez B, Benjamin EM (2005) Perioperative beta-blocker therapy and mortality after major noncardiac surgery. N Engl J Med 353:349–361
7. Yang H, Raymer K, Butler R, Parlow J, Roberts R (2006) The effects of perioperative beta-blockade: results of the Metoprolol after Vascular Surgery (MaVS) study, a randomized controlled trial. Am Heart J 152:983–990
8. Devereaux PJ, Yang H, Yusuf S et al (2008) Effects of extended-release metoprolol succinate in patients undergoing non-cardiac surgery (POISE trial): a randomised controlled trial. Lancet 371:1839–1847

9. Fleisher LA, Fleischmann KE, Auerbach AD et al (2014) 2014 ACC/AHA Guideline on Perioperative Cardiovascular Evaluation and Management of Patients Undergoing Noncardiac Surgery: A Report of the American College of Cardiology/American Heart Association Task Force on Practice Guidelines. J Am Coll Cardiol 64:e77–e137
10. Christensen S, Johansen MB, Tonnesen E et al (2011) Preadmission beta-blocker use and 30-day mortality among patients in intensive care: a cohort study. Crit Care 15:R87
11. Novotny NM, Lahm T, Markel TA et al (2009) beta-Blockers in sepsis: reexamining the evidence. Shock 31:113–119
12. Stoelting RK, Hilller SC (2006) Alpha and beta-adrenergic receptor antagonists. In: Pharmacology & Physiology in Anesthetic Practice, 4th edn. Lippincott, Williams & Wilkins, Philadelphia, pp 321–337
13. Morelli A, Ertmer C, Westphal M et al (2013) Effect of heart rate control with esmolol on hemodynamic and clinical outcomes in patients with septic shock: a randomized clinical trial. JAMA 310:1683–1691
14. Dellinger RP, Levy MM, Carlet JM et al (2008) Surviving Sepsis Campaign: international guidelines for management of severe sepsis and septic shock: 2008. Crit Care Med 36:296–327
15. Ginsberg F (2012) beta-blockers: more good news? Crit Care Med 40:2901–2902
16. Hamzaoui O, Teboul JL (2015) The role of beta-blockers in septic patients. Minerva Anestesiol (in press)
17. Rudiger A (2010) Beta-block the septic heart. Crit Care Med 38:608–S612
18. Vieillard-Baron A, Caille V, Charron C, Belliard G, Page B, Jardin F (2008) Actual incidence of global left ventricular hypokinesia in adult septic shock. Crit Care Med 36:1701–1706
19. Gattinoni L, Brazzi L, Pelosi P et al (1995) A trial of goal-oriented hemodynamic therapy in critically ill patients. SvO2 Collaborative Group. N Engl J Med 333:1025–1032
20. Gore DC, Wolfe RR (2006) Hemodynamic and metabolic effects of selective beta1 adrenergic blockade during sepsis. Surgery 139:686–694
21. Berk JL, Hagen JF, Dunn JM (1970) The role of beta adrenergic blockade in the treatment of septic shock. Surg Gynecol Obstet 130:1025–1034
22. Schmittinger CA, Dunser MW, Haller M et al (2008) Combined milrinone and enteral metoprolol therapy in patients with septic myocardial depression. Crit Care 12:R99
23. Macchia A, Romero M, Comignani PD et al (2012) Previous prescription of beta-blockers is associated with reduced mortality among patients hospitalized in intensive care units for sepsis. Crit Care Med 40:2768–2772
24. Orbegozo CD, Njimi H, Dell'Anna AM, Taccone FS (2014) Esmolol for septic shock: more than just heart rate control? Minerva Anestesiol 80:254–258
25. Shaw JH, Holdaway CM, Humberstone DA (1998) Metabolic intervention in surgical patients: the effect of alpha- or beta-blockade on glucose and protein metabolism in surgical patients receiving total parenteral nutrition. Surgery 103:520–525
26. Dinarello CA, Abraham E (2002) Does blocking cytokines in sepsis work? Am J Respir Crit Care Med 166:1156–1157
27. Oberbeck R, van Griensven M, Nickel E, Tschernig T, Wittwer T, Pape HC (2002) Influence of beta-adrenoceptor antagonists on hemorrhage-induced cellular immune suppression. Shock 18:331–335
28. Ware LB, Matthay MA (2000) The acute respiratory distress syndrome. N Engl J Med 342:1334–1349
29. Noveanu M, Breidthardt T, Reichlin T et al (2010) Effect of oral beta-blocker on short and long-term mortality in patients with acute respiratory failure: results from the BASEL-II-ICU study. Crit Care 14:R198
30. Au DH, Curtis JR, Every NR, McDonell MB, Fihn SD (2002) Association between inhaled beta-agonists and the risk of unstable angina and myocardial infarction. Chest 121:846–851
31. Albouaini K, Andron M, Alahmar A, Egred M (2007) Beta-blockers use in patients with chronic obstructive pulmonary disease and concomitant cardiovascular conditions. Int J Chron Obstruct Pulmon Dis 2:535–540

32. Salpeter SR, Ormiston TM, Salpeter EE, Poole PJ, Cates CJ (2003) Cardioselective beta-blockers for chronic obstructive pulmonary disease: a meta-analysis. Respir Med 97:1094–1101
33. van der Woude HJ, Zaagsma J, Postma DS, Winter TH, van Huist M, Aalbers R (2005) Detrimental effects of beta-blockers in COPD: a concern for nonselective beta-blockers. Chest 127:818–824
34. van der Jagt M, van der Miranda DR (2012) Beta-blockers in intensive care medicine: potential benefit in acute brain injury and acute respiratory distress syndrome. Recent Pat Cardiovasc Drug Discov 7:141–151
35. Kargin F, Takir HB, Salturk C et al (2014) The safety of beta-blocker use in chronic obstructive pulmonary disease patients with respiratory failure in the intensive care unit. Multidiscip Respir Med 9:8
36. Hagiwara S, Iwasaka H, Maeda H, Noguchi T (2009) Landiolol, an ultrashort-acting beta1-adrenoceptor antagonist, has protective effects in an LPS-induced systemic inflammation model. Shock 31:515–520
37. Aboab J, Sebille V, Jourdain M et al (2011) Effects of esmolol on systemic and pulmonary hemodynamics and on oxygenation in pigs with hypodynamic endotoxin shock. Intensive Care Med 37:1344–1351
38. Woolf PD, Hamill RW, Lee LA, Cox C, McDonald JV (1987) The predictive value of catecholamines in assessing outcome in traumatic brain injury. J Neurosurg 66:875–882
39. Goldstein B, Toweill D, Lai S, Sonnenthal K, Kimberly B (1998) Uncoupling of the autonomic and cardiovascular systems in acute brain injury. Am J Physiol 275:R1287–R1292
40. Hortnagl H, Hammerle AF, Hackl JM, Brucke T, Rumpl E, Hortnagl H (1980) The activity of the sympathetic nervous system following severe head injury. Intensive Care Med 6:169–170
41. Bruder N, Rabinstein A (2011) Cardiovascular and pulmonary complications of aneurysmal subarachnoid hemorrhage. Neurocrit Care 15:257–269
42. Inaba K, Teixeira PG, David JS et al (2008) Beta-blockers in isolated blunt head injury. J Am Coll Surg 206:432–438
43. Ker K, Perel P, Blackhall K (2009) Beta-2 receptor antagonists for traumatic brain injury: a systematic review of controlled trials in animal models. CNS Neurosci Ther 15:52–64
44. Greendyke RM, Kanter DR, Schuster DB, Verstreate S, Wootton J (1986) Propranolol treatment of assaultive patients with organic brain disease. A double-blind crossover, placebo-controlled study. J Nerv Ment Dis 174:290–294
45. Feibel JH, Baldwin CA, Joynt RJ (1981) Catecholamine-associated refractory hypertension following acute intracranial hemorrhage: control with propranolol. Ann Neurol :340–343
46. Cotton BA, Snodgrass KB, Fleming SB et al (2007) Beta-blocker exposure is associated with improved survival after severe traumatic brain injury. J Trauma 62:26–33
47. Arbabi S, Campion EM, Hemmila MR et al (2007) Beta-blocker use is associated with improved outcomes in adult trauma patients. J Trauma 62:56–61
48. Riordan WP Jr., Cotton BA, Norris PR, Waitman LR, Jenkins JM, Morris JA Jr (2007) Beta-blocker exposure in patients with severe traumatic brain injury (TBI) and cardiac uncoupling. J Trauma 63:503–510
49. Schroeppel TJ, Fischer PE, Zarzaur BL et al (2010) Beta-adrenergic blockade and traumatic brain injury: protective? J Trauma 69:776–782

Part IV
Oxygenation and Respiratory Failure

Prehospital Endotracheal Intubation: Elemental or Detrimental?

P. E. Pepe, L. P. Roppolo, and R. L. Fowler

Introduction

Modern out-of-hospital emergency medical services (EMS) systems, as we have come to recognize them today, were established in the 1960s and 1970s when a cadre of intrepid physicians ventured into the streets and later published their successful experiences with lifesaving approaches to managing acute coronary syndromes, trauma care, and cardiopulmonary arrest on-scene [1–3].

Although physician-staffed ambulance services had been in place in many venues worldwide for more than a century, the late 20th century evolution of prehospital care was highlighted by documentation of life-saving outcomes in those first modern EMS programs and their use of invasive 'advanced life support' (ALS) procedures including prehospital endotracheal intubation (ETI) and intravascular (i.v.) cannulation for drug administration [1–3]. These life-saving reports helped to propel the widespread adoption of EMS systems and the concomitant introduction of specially-trained (non-physician) emergency medical technicians called 'paramedics' [1–5]. Eventually nursing personnel also ventured into the realm of on-scene emergency response, particularly in the arena of air medical services.

This evolution in out-of-hospital care was especially remarkable in that the formal training of these non-physician personnel included those advanced care interventions such as ETI and i.v. drug administration, interventions traditionally provided in the in-hospital setting by expert physician specialists [1–9]. Paramedic skill portfolios ranged from basic spinal immobilization and extremity splinting to the more advanced skills of electrocardiographic (EKG) interpretation, defibrillation attempts, ETI, i.v. catheter placement and even pericardiocentesis and tracheotomies in some communities [10].

P. E. Pepe ✉ · L. P. Roppolo · R. L. Fowler
Department of Emergency Medicine, University of Texas Southwestern Medical Center, Dallas, USA
The Parkland Health and Hospital System, Dallas County, USA
e-mail: Paul.Pepe@UTSW.edu

J.-L. Vincent (ed.), *Annual Update in Intensive Care and Emergency Medicine 2015*,
DOI 10.1007/978-3-319-13761-2_12

The skill of ETI had become the definitive airway control for most critically ill and injured patients, be they in the operating room, in the early phases of an intensive care unit (ICU) hospitalization, or in the out-of-hospital setting [2–9, 11]. The presumed presence of significant physiological derangements (e. g., hypoxemia, hypercarbia, hypoperfusion) in cardiopulmonary arrest, head injury and hemorrhagic states made ETI an intuitive procedure to perform as soon as feasible in the critically ill and injured [4, 5, 9, 11].

In addition, there were other clinical care imperatives (e. g., airway protection, ventilatory control, end-tidal carbon monoxide monitoring, drug administration and airway suctioning) that drove a strong philosophy that EMS personnel should provide a definitive airway as soon as possible in the out-of-hospital setting for cardiopulmonary arrest, severe trauma and other life-threatening emergencies [2–9, 11]. Nevertheless, although these invasive skills were now being provided by paramedics and nurses, for the most part they were still being delegated under the direction of accountable physician supervisor experts in out-of-hospital care [12]. Early studies conducted in EMS systems with intensive, expert physician supervision, comprehensive training programs and on-scene supervision of EMS personnel reported extremely high rates of successful ETI for both children and adults [2–8, 13–15].

In most of these studies, success was defined not only by accurate anatomic placement of the endotracheal tube (ETT), but also by absence of significant complications [3–7]. Moreover, prehospital ETI was soon correlated with positive outcomes particularly in the most dire of circumstances [7, 8, 15].

For the most part, prehospital ETI has usually been performed in cardiopulmonary arrest cases and in the most severely injured trauma patients with significant physiological impairment (unconscious) and, generally, no gag reflex [5]. As a result, the procedure can be relatively easy to perform by highly-experienced care providers. However, using unqualified univariate analysis, ETI is typically performed in those patients with a high-risk of associated morbidity and mortality and thus can be simplistically *correlated* with a poor outcome [16–20]. Paradoxically, in some selected EMS systems, ETI has actually been correlated positively with survival, particularly in cases of post-traumatic circulatory arrest [7, 8]. In turn, this paradoxical finding infers a likely value of ETI in these worst-case scenarios [7, 8, 21].

However, despite intuitive biases and impressive inferential studies indicating the positive effects of prehospital ETI in certain settings, another evolving body of studies and experiences has unveiled a detrimental effect of prehospital ETI or, at least, no significant advantage to providing the procedure [17, 20, 22–29]. Most notably, a controlled clinical trial conducted in the 1990s in a pediatric population generated significant concern about prehospital ETI in that vulnerable population and subsequent studies in adult head injury patients amplified that concern [25, 26]. In the pediatric ETI trial, 830 children (age 12 years or younger) were studied over a three-year period [26]. Although not statistically significant, survivors with positive neurological outcomes were slightly more frequent (92 of 104; 23%) in those managed with bag-valve-mask (BVM) devices (23%), versus 85 of 416 (20%) receiving

ETI [26]. In a subsequent case-control study of severely head-injured patients receiving ETI that was facilitated by rapid sequence induction (RSI), outcomes were worse for patients receiving the procedure versus those with similar injuries not receiving it [25]. Also, in deference to other studies indicating a survival advantage to ETI in post-traumatic circulatory arrest [7, 8], the on-going univariate association of ETI with mortality in recent studies, though predictable, has fueled the debate that ETI should no longer be used in the out-of-hospital setting [16–18, 23].

Adding to this debate has been the concern over interruptions in well-performed chest compressions during cardiopulmonary resuscitation (CPR), the key factor in restoring return of spontaneous circulation and eventual survival following cardiac resuscitation. It is argued that pausing to intubate could, therefore, be detrimental under these circumstances [30, 31]. In turn, ETI has lost priority standing in many venues.

Along with its lowered prioritization in cardiac arrest management, it has been argued that, overall, there is no strong evidenced-based support for ETI in terms of survival advantage. So despite the logical value of performing it in critically ill and injured patients, many have argued that a true value cannot be demonstrated, particularly in children [20, 23, 26, 31].

Regardless of this evolving sentiment to avoid prehospital ETI altogether and even consider it as a deleterious procedure, that 'evidence-based' position may indeed be overly simplistic. In the ensuing discussion, it will be delineated how several under-recognized confounding variables have a major impact on the performance of this skill and even related outcomes. These variables include non-intuitive factors, such as how the EMS providers are deployed or how they have been trained to ventilate [32–44]. These concepts and how they relate to the success of prehospital ETI for the critically ill and injured will be addressed in the rest of this article. It is hoped that by being provided these perspectives, one can better delineate the circumstances in which ETI should be utilized and those in which it should truly be discouraged.

Factors That Affect Successful Prehospital ETI

Unique Training Challenges

As previously stated, the original EMS programs that first published success with paramedic-staffed responses generally reported extremely high rates of success with prehospital ETI placement [2–10, 15]. Also, as stated, others have not demonstrated similar successes [17, 20, 25, 26, 28]. In retrospect, when examining the differences in systems that have or have not had successes in ETI, it appears that several factors are actually strong determinants of paramedic and nursing proficiency in the skill of ETI. These determinants include: 1) the quality, orientation and types of experiences in the initial training; 2) the frequency of performance; and 3) on-scene oversight and supervision of ETI performance [3–6, 12, 13, 29, 32–36].

Proper training for the prehospital environment clearly needs to be somewhat unique. In contrast to the typical operating room training experience, the skill of ETI performed in the emergency care setting, and particularly in the out-of-hospital environment, is wrought with unique challenges [5]. These challenges range from vomit-flooded airways and ground-level patient positions to ambient lighting and oro-pharyngeal injuries. With full stomachs, relaxed esophageal sphincters and inadvertent gastric insufflation from BVM or mouth-to-mouth ventilation, it is commonplace to approach an airway welled-up with vomit in a circumstance with often less-than-adequate (or delayed) suctioning. In turn, this often requires the ability to intubate almost instantly without adjuncts.

Unlike the controlled in-hospital environment, in a sunny, bright outdoors setting, the ambient light causes glare and pupillary constriction for the rescuers. This circumstance requires that the practitioners are taught and understand the 'tricks of the trade', such as placing a coat or blanket over one's head (and the head of the patient) in order to create a makeshift darkened room akin to an old-time photographer's camera hood. In contrast, even in the dark of night, heavy rain or

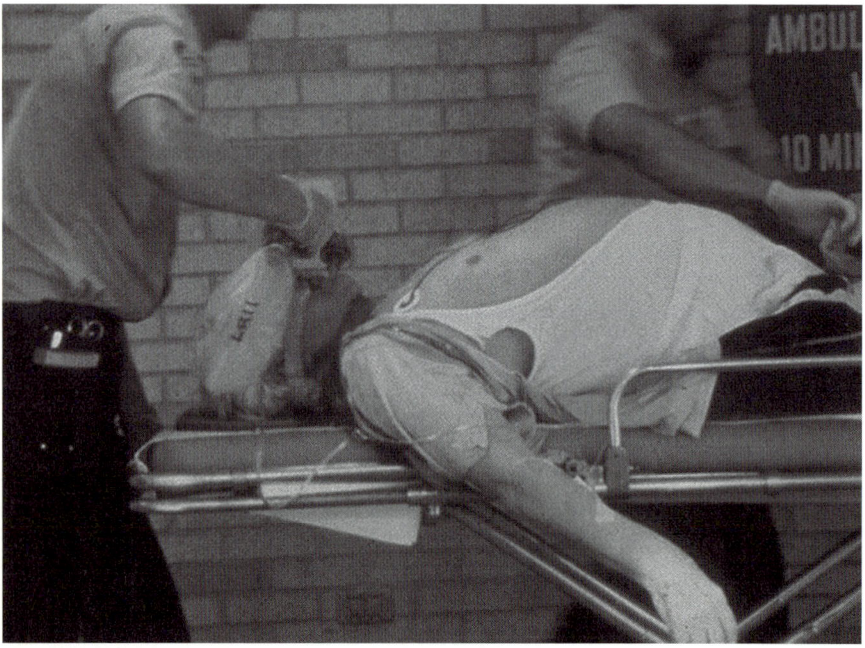

Fig. 1 Endotracheal intubation in the out-of-hospital setting. In the early years of out-of-hospital emergency medical services (EMS) systems, advanced life support personnel were not only trained in the nuances of how to avoid overzealous ventilation and properly place an endotracheal tube in very challenging circumstances, but they were also well-supervised on-scene by expert physicians who themselves were highly-experienced and exceptionally familiar with those challenges as well as methods to overcome them (photo by Dr. Paul Pepe)

awkward confined spaces may pose their own barriers to easily visualizing vocal cords. Therefore, many of the classical techniques used by other practitioners in more traditional settings would not be as effective in the fast-paced, poorly controlled and mobile prehospital settings where resources and support are limited (Fig. 1).

In turn, a key to successful EMS intubation in the out-of-hospital setting is the street-wise experience of expert highly-experienced medical trainers and EMS medical directors who not only understand these principles, but also are themselves facile in such techniques in the out-of-hospital setting [5, 6, 12].

Frequent Skill Usage and System Staffing Configurations

Even if initial training techniques are expert and well-taught, both in the classroom and on-scene, frequency of performance is a critical factor. For example, studies have shown the success rates for ETI can be related to the deployment strategy of the EMS system [2, 3, 32, 33]. In EMS systems using tiered ambulance deployments in which paramedics (ALS providers) are spared for the most critical calls, many fewer paramedics are needed on the roster and the individual experience of each paramedic, including frequency of ETI performance, can be enhanced dramatically [2, 32]. Accordingly, this approach has been correlated with improved success rates in terms of ETI performance [2, 32].

This need to enable frequent experience is critical in EMS. While ETI skills may deteriorate a little with a hiatus from practice, collective experience [2, 32] has demonstrated that most prehospital personnel who have performed ETI a hundred times or more in the out-of-hospital setting may still be able to perform the technique quite well despite the hiatus. However, the key issue is getting to that threshold of experience and this prerequisite goal requires high exposure and frequent performance. Unfortunately, that level of performance is not always achieved in most EMS systems today. As an example, for a five-year 'veteran' paramedic to have achieved a successful ETI over 100 times, it would mean successful performance of that procedure at least 20 times a year for five years. Most paramedic units are usually staffed by two paramedics, so if ETI experience were to be shared with a paramedic partner, the implication is that this particular team would need to face 40 ETI situations a year on their particular ambulance and shift. In fact, accounting for sick time, vacation time and other factors, it typically takes 5 to 6 fulltime equivalent paramedics to staff one of those two positions and thus 10–12 different paramedics will be needed just for that one ambulance around the clock. Therefore, that particular response unit would need to face approximately 200 to 250 ETI cases a year for each ALS provider to get 20 opportunities to intubate.

Considering that cardiac arrest, respiratory distress and major trauma cases requiring ETI constitute only 2–3% of all EMS on-scene emergency responses [32], the ambulance in question would need to experience nearly 10,000 EMS incidents a year overall. In most EMS system configurations, this level of volume would be a logistical-temporal impossibility for a single ambulance. Unless alternate deployment strategies were to be utilized, frequent exposure to ETI cases would be clearly limited.

Indeed, alternative deployments are key. Specifically, in some communities, paramedics (or other types of ALS personnel, such as doctors or nurses) are spared from the majority of EMS responses. Instead of ALS providers, basic emergency medical technicians (EMTs) trained to do the non-invasive procedures such as spinal immobilization and splinting are used for most of the responses [2, 3, 32, 33]. Under such circumstances, overall staffing could, therefore, involve a much smaller cadre of paramedics. This would permit more frequent exposure to critical illness and injury for the individual paramedics (ALS providers). The same concept would apply to nurses or apprentice physicians who staff ambulances and air medical units, particularly in some European countries [2, 32, 33]. The fact that air medical units are typically triaged only to the most critical cases means that those ALS providers staffing the helicopters are part of a deployment strategy that enhances skill use. Using this so-called 'tiered' approach, individual paramedics (ALS personnel), nurses or doctors each get more chances to perform an ETI.

While there is great variation from one city to another, on average a city with a population of 1 million in the U.S. (for example) might be expected to have 100,000 EMS response incidents annually [45]. This volume of cases might predict two or three thousand potential circumstances for ETI each year. To optimize individual paramedic exposure, it would be best to limit the number of paramedic (ALS) ambulances to a maximum of 10 ambulances (250 ETI exposures per ambulance per year × 10 ambulances covers 2 to 3 thousand cases). In this circumstance, a cadre of 100 to 120 paramedics might be required for the 10 paramedic-staffed units.

In a contrast, in a system experiencing 100,000 EMS responses a year and using all-paramedic staffing, 35 to 40 ambulances would typically be required minimally and thus 400 to 500 paramedics would be needed [32, 33]. This all-ALS provider approach decreases individual exposure to ETI attempts at least 4 to 5-fold. To make matters worse, in some cities, additional paramedics are also placed on first-responder vehicles such as responding fire engines [26, 28]. In turn, this further compounds the infrequency of exposure for individuals. Moreover, some ambulances are situated in lower call volume areas than others, creating even less exposure to ETI opportunities [36].

Fortunately, the great majority (85 to 95%) of EMS incidents do not require an ALS provider (e. g., authorized physician, nurse, paramedic) and can be managed by basic EMTs [32]. In turn, using well-established and well-documented dispatch triage protocols, paramedics (ALS providers) can be spared and basic EMTs (basic life support [BLS] providers) are deployed directly to manage the cases [32]. In other situations, after an initial paramedic (ALS) response is made, the basic EMT ambulance can be called in to transport the less critical patients thus freeing up paramedics (ALS providers) for the more critical cases.

Not only does this type of system configuration permit the need for fewer ALS personnel, but it also improves response intervals because paramedics are not tied up transporting patients and are thus more available. Ironically, by having fewer paramedics, paramedic response can be improved [32].

Beyond on-scene procedures and moving the patient from the scene, the time to transport, provide hospital transition, create a record and then return to the primary response territory is the greatest deterrent to the availability of ambulance crews and thus a factor in compromised response times. Not surprisingly then, the original EMS systems reporting excellent paramedic track records with ETI were largely this type of tiered response system with staffing configurations that utilized basic EMTs for the majority of responses and spared the much smaller cadre of relatively busy paramedics for the more critical calls, therefore creating more opportunities for ETI skills usage [2, 3, 32, 44].

Furthermore, the paramedics in these systems rapidly achieved experience seeing many dozens of cases per year and they eventually became reliably facile. In turn, as they became exceptionally facile, they deferred ETI attempts to new trainees. As a result, in these sophisticated EMS systems, the lesser-experienced medics rapidly developed their own skills even faster. Veterans also maintained their skills by teaching, supervising and getting to attempt and perform the more difficult intubations when the more novice personnel could not place the tube.

Unfortunately, today in the U.S. and other countries, the majority of EMS systems actually utilize all-paramedic (all-ALS) staffing on their ambulances. In addition, many first-responder crews often supplement ambulance response with additional paramedics (ALS providers) staffing the first response vehicles as well [26, 28, 33]. Therefore, it is no surprise that paramedics may not perform ETI as well as their forerunners 40 years ago.

Despite the described impact of using an all-paramedic system, one remedy might be to create a de facto 'tier' in those all-ALS systems by creating a team of supervisors, field training officers, or expert physician responders who routinely respond to critical calls. Depending upon the geography, vertical (high-rise) challenges, and traffic, it would be wise to create a small number of senior personnel who can respond across a designated territory (or even into a fellow senior officer's territory for back-up) as a modified approach to ensure high level skills performance. Just as there may be 10 or so battalion fire chiefs in a city of a million residents spread out over a large geographical territory, staffing and responding a similar number of senior EMS personnel into high level cases could be another alternative and one that is now being adopted by many progressive EMS systems.

Expert on-Scene Supervision

Finally, even with appropriate, tailored initial training and tiered response systems with a high frequency of performance for individual paramedics, if the on-scene medics in training are not properly supervised, they may still develop bad habits in a vacuum. It is critical to reinforce what constitutes a proper technique (e. g., sniffing position in those at low risk of neck injury) and to provide renewed coaching in the actual patient care setting, especially in terms of confirmation of tube placement and proper ventilatory techniques. In most EMS systems that provide high rates of ETI success, in-field medical directors, highly-experienced EMS supervisors and well-coached veteran paramedics are the norm [2, 6, 12].

Why Successful ETI Attempts Can Even Be Detrimental

Detrimental Effects of Ventilatory Techniques Following Intubation

Even if paramedics or other prehospital care providers are expertly trained, highly-skilled, highly-experienced and highly-supervised performers of intubation for both adults and children, their ventilatory techniques may still adversely affect outcome [25, 37–39]. The types of patients most likely to need ETI are those with cardiac arrest, chronic lung disease and severe post-traumatic shock conditions. Yet these patients are also the most vulnerable to the detrimental cardiovascular effects of the positive pressure breaths that are being delivered through the ETT [39].

Despite the basic physiological principle that ventilation should match perfusion (blood flow), over the years, in many venues, EMS personnel have been trained traditionally to aggressively ventilate patients, usually with the ill-advised rationale that such an approach was the way to ensure oxygenation and offset metabolic acidosis [37, 38]. Even with more judicious training, however, emergency workers can still have the tendency to over-zealously ventilate such patients in the heat of the emergency [38]. Ironically, while such patients in deep shock actually require infrequent breaths and a lesser minute ventilation, once the ETT is placed, they may now receive excessive levels of assisted breathing, not only because of some unsound rote training, but also because of adrenaline-modulated behaviors [38].

Accordingly, it is now speculated that low national survival rates for out-of-hospital cardiac arrest and the negative outcomes of several prehospital clinical trials may have been, in part, the result of uncontrolled ventilatory rates using positive pressure breaths [39]. For example, in the study of severe traumatic brain injury (TBI) in which RSI-facilitated ETI was associated with worse outcomes, a key correlation with mortality was the finding "hyperventilation", defined as an arterial $PCO_2 < 24$ mmHg [25]. While one might suspect that these negative outcomes may, therefore, be caused by effects of respiratory alkalosis, such as myocardial depression, cerebral vasoconstriction and a left shift in the hemoglobin dissociation curve, it is most likely that the low arterial PCO_2 is simply a surrogate variable for overzealous positive pressure ventilation [37–39].

As Aufderheide and colleagues have shown, despite aggressive, targeted re-training on respiratory rates and delivery techniques, paramedics still overzealously ventilate and prolong the duration of positive pressure breaths in the adrenaline-charged environment of a critical emergency [38]. It is likely that this scenario is exaggerated in children, considering that paramedics and other emergency care providers are trained to think that pediatric arrests are mostly the result of hypoxemia and that proscribed respiratory rates are generally higher than those proscribed for adults [19, 26, 39]. Also, emotions run even higher in childhood critical emergencies, theoretically compounding any predisposition to overzealously ventilate. Therefore, clinical trials that indicated worse outcomes with ETI may have been confounded by unrecognized detrimental ventilatory techniques [37–39].

So, paradoxically, in systems where many paramedics are deployed to *all* prehospital emergency cases with the rationale of improving response times for ALS procedures (and thus improved survival chances), worse outcomes might actually be expected, especially with successful ETI. In the EMS system in which the clinical trial of pediatric intubation was conducted [26], more than 2000 paramedics were trained to perform what resulted in being less than 150 annual pediatric intubations across the system during the study period.

Experience-wise, this type of system configuration issue makes it difficult for the individual paramedic to get much exposure, even to adult intubations. Clearly, pediatric intubation situations would be uncommon, or even unlikely over his or her entire career. This is a set-up for misplaced tubes or significantly delayed ETI. It also means too frequent and too lengthy pauses in chest compressions if the crews are not facile at placing the tube. Overall, this scenario provides a clear set-up for under-skilled attempts at ETI altogether [2, 32]. Coupled with high anxiety when dealing with kids, an EMS system that follows typical protocols for ventilation and/or does not control for overzealous ventilation, may likely experience even poorer outcomes.

Under these circumstances, one can make a strong argument against using ETI or attempting ETI, especially in children and other vulnerable groups such as spontaneously-breathing head injured patients. Nevertheless, it must be kept in mind that there are communities that can safely enjoy high success rates for ETI and associated good outcomes for patients, even using certain RSI techniques [3, 7, 8, 21, 46]. But, again, these EMS systems are typified by street-wise training, tiered paramedic ambulance response systems, and patient care protocols involving controlled ventilatory techniques for critical cases. Places like Houston and Seattle in the 1980s were delivering only one positive pressure breath every ten seconds to their patients with circulatory arrest and outcomes were exceptional when compared to other sites [3, 7, 8, 21].

Most importantly, these sites also involved intensive on-scene expert medical oversight [2, 12, 46]. Therefore, ETI should not be discouraged in such appropriate settings. On the other hand, as other researchers have implied, ETI and/or RSI should be discouraged in those EMS systems that are unable to adapt to those appropriate characteristics that facilitate ETI and its proper use.

Conclusion

While ETI remains the gold standard for definitive airway management in the emergency care setting, it may be inappropriate in the prehospital setting in the absence of paramedic-sparing deployment systems, controlled ventilatory techniques and intensive medical oversight that provides street-wise training as well as expert, on-scene supervision of the EMS personnel providing the ETI. While ETI may very well be life-saving, particularly in cases of severe trauma with circulatory arrest, ETI may also be detrimental in certain EMS systems. Successful placement and use of an ETI is more likely to occur in EMS systems that provide:

1) 'street-wise' training that is provided by experts in out-of-hospital patient care who themselves are well-experienced in on-scene emergency ETI;
2) tiered EMS deployment systems that spare a small cadre of highly-skilled (and relatively busy) paramedics from the majority of EMS incidents (focusing them on the more critical cases, thus resulting in a very high frequency of ETI performance by each individual in the system); and
3) intensive, street-wise and expert out-of-hospital medical oversight.

But, even when paramedics (and other ALS providers) are facile at ETI in the unique environmental conditions and challenges of the out-of-hospital setting, inappropriate and overzealous ventilation can still result in detrimental outcomes. In summary, systems unable to adopt the appropriate configurations, protocols, training, monitoring, and all other characteristics that optimize ETI may, therefore, need to be discouraged from performing ETI or they need to develop alternative mechanisms to better ensure routine success with placement of the tube and its appropriate use.

References

1. Pantridge JF, Geddes JS (1967) A mobile intensive care unit in the management of myocardial infarction. Lancet 290:271–273
2. Cobb LA, Alvarez H, Copass MK (1976) A rapid response system for out-of-hospital cardiac emergencies. Med Clin North Am 60:283–293
3. McManus WF, Tresch DD, Darin JC (1977) An effective prehospital emergency system. J Trauma 17:304–310
4. Jacobs LM, Berrizbeitia LD, Bennett B, Madigan C (1983) Endotracheal intubation in the prehospital phase of emergency medical care. JAMA 250:2175–2177
5. Pepe PE, Copass MK, Joyce TH (1985) Prehospital endotracheal intubation: rationale for training emergency medical personnel. Ann Emerg Med 14:1085–1092
6. Stewart RD, Paris P, Winter PM et al (1984) Field endotracheal intubation by paramedical personnel: success rates and complications. Chest 85:341–345
7. Copass MK, Oreskovich MR, Blaedogroen MR, Carrico CJ (1984) Prehospital cardiopulmonary resuscitation of the critically injured patient. Am J Surg 148:20–24
8. Durham LA, Richardson RJ, Wall MH, Pepe PE, Mattox KL (1992) Emergency center thoracotomy: impact of prehospital resuscitation. J Trauma 32:775–779
9. Miller JD, Sweet RC, Narayan R, Becker DP (1978) Early insults to the injured brain. JAMA 240:439–442
10. Page JO (1979) The paramedics: an illustrated history of paramedics in their first decade in the U.S.A. Backdraft Publications, Morristown, New Jersey, USA, pp 1–179
11. American College of Surgeons Committee on Trauma (1997) Advanced trauma life support program for physicians, 6th edn. American College of Surgeons, Chicago, pp 21–124 (Chapters 1–3)
12. Pepe PE, Copass MK, Fowler RL, Racht EM (2009) Medical direction of emergency medical services systems. In: Cone DC, Fowler R, O'Connor RE (eds) Textbook of the National Association of EMS Physicians. Kendall Hunt Publications, Dubuque, Iowa, USA, pp 22–52
13. Warner KJ, Carlbom D, Cooke CR, Bulger EM, Copass MK, Sharar SR (2010) Paramedic training for proficient prehospital endotracheal intubation. Prehospital Emerg Care 14:103–108
14. Sirbaugh PE, Pepe PE, Shook JE et al (1999) A prospective, population-based study of the demographics, epidemiology, management and outcome of out-of-hospital pediatric cardiopulmonary arrest. Ann Emerg Med 33:174–184

15. Winchell RJ, Hoyt DB (1997) Endotracheal intubation in the field improves survival in patients with severe head injury. Arch Surg 132:592–597
16. Eckstein M, Chan L, Schneir A, Palmer R (2000) The effect of prehospital advanced life support on outcomes of major trauma patients. J Trauma 48:643–648
17. Hasegawa K, Hiraide A, Chang Y, Brown DF (2013) Association of prehospital advanced airway management with neurologic outcome and survival in patients with out-of-hospital cardiac arrest. JAMA 309:257–66
18. Holmberg M, Holmberg S, Herlitz J (2002) Low chance of survival among patients requiring adrenaline (epinephrine) or intubation after out-of-hospital cardiac arrest in Sweden. Resuscitation 54:37–45
19. Atkins DL, Everson-Stewart S, Sears GK, Daya M, Osmond MH, Warden CR (2009) Epidemiology and outcomes from out-of-hospital cardiac arrest in children: the Resuscitation Outcomes Consortium Epistry-Cardiac Arrest. Circulation 119:1484–1491 (for the Resuscitation Outcomes Consortium)
20. Hanif MA, Kaji AH, Niemann JT (2010) Advanced airway management does not improve outcome of out-of-hospital cardiac arrest. Acad Emerg Med 17:926–931
21. Key CB, Pepe PE, Sirbaugh PE, Shook JE, Kimball KT (1996) Does endotracheal intubation affect outcome in out-of-hospital pediatric cardiac arrest? Acad Emerg Med 3:404–405
22. Wang HE, Yealy DM (2006) Out-of-hospital endotracheal intubation: where are we? Ann Emerg Med 47:532–541
23. Strote J, Roth R, Cone DC, Wang HE (2009) Prehospital endotracheal intubation: the controversy continues. Am J Emerg Med 27:1142–1147
24. Lossius HM, Sollid SJM, Rehn M, Lockey DJ (2011) Revisiting the value of pre-hospital tracheal intubation: an all-time systematic literature review extracting the Utstein airway core variables. Crit Care 15:R26
25. Davis DP, Hoyt DB, Ochs M et al (2003) The effect of paramedic rapid sequence intubation on outcome in patients with severe traumatic brain injury. J Trauma 54:444–453
26. Gausche M, Lewis RJ, Stratton S et al (2000) Effect of out-of-hospital pediatric endotracheal intubation on survival and neurological outcome. JAMA 283:783–790
27. Pepe PE, Eckstein M (1998) Reappraising the prehospital care of the patient with major trauma. Emerg Med Clin N Am 16:1–15
28. Katz SH, Falk JL (2001) Misplaced endotracheal tubes by paramedics in an urban emergency medical services systems. Ann Emerg Med 37:32–37
29. Wang HE, Kupas DF, Paris PM et al (2003) Preliminary experience with a prospective, multicentered evaluation of out-of-hospital endotracheal intubation. Resuscitation 58:49–58
30. Christenson J, Andrusiek D, Everson-Stewart S, Kudenchuk P, Hostler D, Powell J (2009) Chest compression fraction determines survival in patients with out-of-hospital ventricular fibrillation. Circulation 120:1241–1247
31. Bobrow BJ, Clark LL, Ewy G et al (2008) Minimally interrupted cardiac resuscitation. JAMA 299:1158–1165
32. Curka PA, Pepe PE, Ginger VF, Ivy MV, Sherrard RC, Zachariah BS (1993) Emergency medical services priority dispatch. Ann Emerg Med 22:1688–1695
33. Stout J, Pepe PE, Mosesso VN (2000) All-advanced life support versus tiered-response ambulance systems. Prehospital Emerg Care 4:1–6
34. Pepe PE, Zachariah BS, Chandra N (1993) Invasive airway techniques in resuscitation. Ann Emerg Med 22(Part II):393–403
35. Silvestri S, Ralls G, Krauss B et al (2005) The effectiveness of out-of-hospital use of continuous end-tidal carbon dioxide monitoring on the rate of unrecognized misplaced intubation within a regional emergency medical service system. Ann Emerg Med 45:497–503
36. Burton JH, Baumann MR, Maoz T et al (2003) Endotracheal intubation in a rural state: Procedure utilization and impact of skills maintenance guidelines. Prehospital Emerg Care 7:352–356
37. Pepe PE, Lurie KG, Wigginton JG, Raedler C, Idris AH (2004) Detrimental hemodynamic effects of assisted ventilation in hemorrhagic states. Crit Care Med 32(Suppl):414–420

38. Aufderheide TP, Sigurdsson G, Pirrallo RG et al (2004) Hyperventilation-induced hypotension during cardiopulmonary resuscitation. Circulation 109:1960–1965
39. Roppolo LP, Wigginton JG, Pepe PE (2004) Emergency ventilatory management as a detrimental factor in resuscitation practices and clinical research efforts. In: Vincent JL (ed) 2004 Intensive Care and Emergency Medicine. Springer-Verlag, Berlin, pp 139–151
40. Bernhard M, Becker TK, Böttiger BW (2013) Prehospital airway management for out-of-hospital cardiac arrest. JAMA 309:1888
41. Wang HE, Balasubrami GK, Lave JR et al (2009) Paramedic endotracheal intubation experience improves patient survival. Prehosp Emerg Care 19:90–91
42. Helm M, Hossfeld B, Schafer S, Hoitz J, Lampl L (2005) Factors influencing emergency intubation in the pre-hospital setting – a multicentre study in the German helicopter emergency medical service. Br J Anaesthesia 96:67–71
43. Jensen JL, Cheung KW, Tallon JM, Travers AH (2010) Comparison of tracheal intubation and alternative airway techniques performed in the prehospital setting by paramedics: a systematic review. Can J Emerg Med 12:135–40
44. Wang HE, Szydlo D, Stouffer JA, Lin S, Carlson JN, Vaillancourt C (2012) Endotracheal intubation versus supraglottic airway insertion in out-of-hospital cardiac arrest. Resuscitation 83:1061–1066
45. Pepe PE, Mattox KL, Fischer RP, Matsumoto CM (1990) Geographical patterns of urban trauma according to mechanism and severity of injury. J Trauma 30:1125–1132
46. Persse DE, Key CB, Bradley RN et al (2003) Cardiac arrest survival as a function of ambulance deployment strategy in a large urban medical services system. Resuscitation 59:97–104

Hyperoxia in Intensive Care and Emergency Medicine: Dr. Jekyll or Mr. Hyde? An Update

S. Hafner, P. Radermacher, and P. Asfar

Introduction

Since the discovery of molecular oxygen (O_2) at the end of the 18th century, its 'friend and foe' character has been recognized. On the one hand, O_2 is vital for survival of mammalian cells since it allows for a sustained, high synthesis rate of adenosine triphosphate (ATP) in the respiratory chain because of its unique properties as a final electron acceptor [1]. On the other hand, this chemical property also renders it one of the strongest oxidizing agents that can damage any biological molecule [1], a phenomenon which led to the paradigm of 'oxygen toxicity'. Oxygen toxicity is the result of enhanced formation of reactive oxygen species (ROS), the rate of formation being directly related to the O_2 partial pressure [2]. The ambiguous role of O_2 as a crucial molecule for ATP synthesis in the respiratory chain is also valid in the context of ROS formation. Approximately 1–3% of mitochondrial O_2 consumption leads to ROS production; in other words, the more ATP is produced, the more ROS are released [2]! Moreover, ROS share the Janus-headed character of O_2: While their toxic potential is well-established, they are also vital, both for host defense and as signaling molecules [3].

By definition, circulatory shock "... represents an imbalance between O_2 supply and requirements ..." [4], and intuitively, increasing the inspired O_2 fraction (FiO_2) is a logical therapeutic measure. In fact, this concept is nearly as old as the knowledge of the possible toxic side effects of breathing O_2, and the recommendation that "... the administration of oxygen should be started immediately to increase O_2 delivery ..." [4] represents part of the 'V' (ventilate) component of the

S. Hafner · P. Radermacher ✉
Klinik für Anästhesiologie, Universitätsklinikum Ulm, Ulm, Germany
e-mail: peter.radermacher@uni-ulm.de

P. Asfar
Département de Réanimation Médicale et de Médecine Hyperbare, Centre Hospitalier Universitaire, 49933 Angers, France
Laboratoire de Biologie Neurovasculaire et Mitochondriale Intégrée, Université Angers, Angers, France

J.-L. Vincent (ed.), *Annual Update in Intensive Care and Emergency Medicine 2015*,
DOI 10.1007/978-3-319-13761-2_13

Table 1 Beneficial and deleterious effects of hyperoxia during circulatory shock and/or in medical emergencies

Beneficial effects	Deleterious effects
Improved blood O_2-content due to increased O_2 partial pressure	Impaired gas exchange due to aggravated pulmonary right-to-left shunt resulting from adsorption atelectasis and inhibition of hypoxic pulmonary vasoconstriction
Improved pericapillary oxygenation due to increased O_2 diffusion gradient	Impaired microcirculatory perfusion due to reduced local NO availability
Accelerated re-oxygenation after low-flow conditions and/or ischemia	Aggravated ischemia/reperfusion-injury due to enhanced oxidative stress
Vasoconstrictor-related hemodynamic stabilization during hypotensive vasodilatory shock	Vasoconstrictor-related impairment of microcirculatory perfusion
Attenuation of inflammation due to accelerated HIF-1α degradation	Diffuse alveolitis and lung permeability edema due to ROS and RNS formation and activation of signal transduction
Improved host defense and antimicrobial activity due to ROS formation	Aggravated oxidative and nitrosative stress due to increased ROS formation and NO consumption
Restoration of mitochondrial O_2 availability and thereby enhanced rate of ATP synthesis	ROS-induced uncoupling of the mitochondrial respiratory chain
Improved yield of the respiratory chain due to overall reduction of O_2 consumption together with shift to preferential carbohydrate utilization	Aggravation of cytopathic hypoxia due to reduced activity of the mitochondrial respiratory chain

NO: nitric oxide; ROS: reactive oxygen species; HIF: hypoxia inducible factor; RNS: reactive nitrogen species

"VIP" (ventilate – infuse – pump) rule for shock resuscitation [5]. Accordingly, supplemental O_2 was an integral part of all resuscitation protocols in the recently published Protocol-based Care for Early Septic Shock (ProCESS) trial [6]. Nevertheless, the administration of high-dose O_2 is a matter of ongoing, controversial debate [7, 8]. Table 1 summarizes the key 'pro and con' arguments concerning the use of O_2 therapy during shock states.

Given the possible deleterious side effects of hyperoxia, current guidelines recommend using the lowest FiO_2 possible, but available data from prospective, controlled, randomized trials on the use of therapeutic hyperoxia are surprisingly scarce. Therefore, the present chapter reviews the (patho-)physiological effects of ventilation with high FiO_2 (0.8–1.0), with a special focus on the most recent clinical data on use of therapeutic hyperoxia in the management of circulatory shock and/or in medical emergencies.

Window of Opportunity

It is textbook knowledge that the effect on total blood O_2 content of changing from air to pure O_2 breathing will be moderate when cardiopulmonary function is normal: Hemoglobin O_2 saturation is already near-complete at arterial PO_2 (PaO_2) levels of 90–100 mmHg, and, consequently, increasing the FiO_2 from 0.21 to 1.0, will only increase the amount of physically dissolved O_2 (at best by a factor of 5) with hardly any change in hemoglobin-bound O_2. Nevertheless, pure O_2 breathing markedly increases the margin of safety during anesthesia induction and/or securing the airway: The 'safe time of apnea' (i. e., the time until transcutaneous O_2 saturation decreased < 90%) was doubled when the FiO_2 was increased from 60 to 100% [9]. From the above-mentioned estimate, it is self-evident that the effect of hyperoxia on blood O_2 content will be more pronounced the lower the hemoglobin content. Consequently, it is not surprising that pure O_2 ventilation was particularly protective in models of critical hemodilution (for review see [10]), the most prominent example being the "Live without blood" experiment in 1960 [11]: In pigs, 45 minutes of mechanical ventilation with an $FiO_2 = 1.0$ prevented the otherwise profound electrocardiographic (EKG) alterations of hemodilution to a hematocrit < 1–2%, and after re-transfusion animals had no apparent sequelae. Nevertheless, although commonly routine practice, no clinical studies on the effect of mechanical ventilation with $FiO_2 = 1.0$ during hemorrhagic shock have been published, most likely because of ethical constraints. The available pre-clinical data are equivocal inasmuch as both deleterious and beneficial effects were reported [10]. Recent data in murine combined traumatic brain injury (TBI) and hemorrhagic shock reproduce this ambiguity: Immediate post-shock pure O_2 breathing decreased brain tissue anti-oxidant content, but improved neuronal survival [12].

Pulmonary Effects

Since central nervous O_2 toxicity, i. e., convulsions, is only present during pure O_2 breathing under supra-atmospheric pressures, under ICU conditions the term 'oxygen toxicity' refers to pulmonary effects during normobaric hyperoxia. It has been well-established for more than a century that pulmonary O_2 toxicity may cause severe pulmonary inflammation, ultimately leading to hemorrhagic pulmonary edema. In experimental animals, this requires long-term exposure and/or injurious ventilation, whereas lung-protective ventilation with high positive end-expiratory pressure (PEEP) levels and low tidal volumes over shorter periods had no deleterious effect at all. In humans, the exposure period needed to provoke clinical and histological signs of tracheitis and/or alveolitis varied between 6–25 hours [10], while the only data available from mechanically ventilated patients originate from hyperoxic mechanical ventilation over 14 hours to 30 days [13]. Although these latter reports do not mention ventilator settings, the publication year (1972) makes it unlikely that patients were ventilated with low tidal volumes and higher PEEP levels according to current guidelines. Thus, no 'threshold time' inducing O_2 toxicity-related pulmonary inflammation is known in mechanically ventilated patients.

Any long-term pulmonary O_2 toxicity must be discriminated from the induction of adsorption atelectasis occurring already within a few minutes after pure O_2

breathing, e. g., during induction of anesthesia [9]. This effect is the result of instability of still open but poorly ventilated lung regions in relation to perfusion, so-called low ventilation/perfusion-ratio (V_A/Q) regions, when the inert carrier gas, N_2, is washed out: Whereas normobaric pure O_2 breathing doubled intra-pulmonary right-to-left shunt, hyperbaric air breathing at the same inspiratory O_2 partial pressure, i. e., at 4.9 atmospheres of ambient pressure, had no effect on gas exchange [10]. In mechanically ventilated patients, hyperoxia-induced adsorption atelectasis can be prevented by using higher PEEP levels: Increasing PEEP from 5 to 14 cm H_2O completely blunted the decrease in the PaO_2/FiO_2 ratio from 200 to 150 mmHg that was induced by increasing the FiO_2 from 0.6 to 1.0 [14].

Vascular Effects

It has been known for a century that hyperoxia decreases cardiac output, mainly due to a fall in heart rate resulting from increased parasympathetic tone, and due to an increase in systemic vascular resistance [15]. Stamler et al. elegantly demonstrated that the latter is caused by reduced local release of nitric oxide (NO) from cysteine-binding in the hemoglobin-molecule (*S*-nitrosothiol) resulting from the hyperoxia-induced increase in venous PO_2 [16]. The degree of the hyperoxia-induced vasoconstriction varies among different vascular beds, and is particularly pronounced in the cerebral and coronary circulation. So far, it remains a matter of debate whether this hyperoxia-induced vasoconstriction is beneficial or deleterious: Clearly, it could be argued that tissue O_2 delivery may be impaired in patients with sepsis [17] or cardiovascular disease [15]. It must be noted, however, that most of the studies on hyperoxia-induced systemic or regional vasoconstriction were performed under stable hemodynamic conditions without an imbalance between O_2 supply and demand, in particular not during circulatory shock. In addition, any hyperoxia-related increase in vasomotor tone would have the potential of reducing vasopressor demands required to counteract shock-induced hypotension. Moreover, the vasoconstrictor effect of pure O_2 ventilation coincided with reduced whole body [18] and myocardial [19] O_2, suggesting an improved balance between O_2 supply and demand rather than impaired O_2 utilization: There was no deleterious effect on any marker of systemic energy balance, and myocardial lactate extraction was even enhanced. Finally, experimental data suggest that pure O_2 ventilation may even redistribute cardiac output in favor of the hepatosplanchnic system and the kidney [10] and, thereby, improve organ function. These experimental studies also suggest that therapeutic hyperoxia shifted energy metabolism to preferential utilization of carbohydrates, which is well-known to increase the yield of the mitochondrial respiratory chain, i. e., the molar ratio of O_2 consumption and ATP formation [20]. So far, scarce data are available on the effects of ventilation with $FiO_2 = 1.0$ on systemic or regional hemodynamics, metabolism, and organ function in patients with circulatory shock, but the prospective, controlled, randomized Hyperoxia and Hypertonic Saline in Septic Shock (HYPER2S, clinical trials.gov Identifier NCT01722422) trial (see Table 2) should help address this issue.

Table 2 Ongoing or recently completed/terminated clinical trials on the effects of hyperoxia in intensive care and emergency medicine

Study acronym	Trial registration number	Patients	Intervention	Primary outcome measures	Planned enrolment
OXY-GEN-ICU	NCT 01319643	ICU treatment for ≥ 3 days	FiO_2 titrated to SpO_2 94–98/PaO_2 70–100 mmHg *vs.* SpO_2 >97%/PaO_2 100–150 mmHg	Mortality at 30 days	660
HYPER 2S	NCT 01722422	Septic shock	FiO_2 titrated to SpO_2 88–95% *vs.* $FiO_2 = 1.0$ over the first 24 hours	Mortality at 28 days	Terminated at n = 441
AVOID	NCT 01272713	Acute myocardial infarction	Air (unless $SpO_2 < 94\%$) *vs.* 8 l/min O_2 during pre-hospital phase, thereafter according to hospital protocol	Infarct size, time course of CK-MB and cTnI	490
DETO 2X-AMI	NCT 01787110	Acute coronary syndrome	Air (unless $SpO_2 < 90\%$) *vs.* 6 l/min O_2 over 6–12 hours	Mortality at 1 year	6600
BRAIN-OXY	NCT 01201291	TBI, GCS ≤ 8	FiO_2 0.4 *vs.* 0.7	GOS/GOSE at 6 months	Not specified; terminated (slow recruitment)
REOX	NCT 01881243	Cardiac arrest	Observational study; association between hyperoxia and outcome	Blood isofuranes/-prostanes	133

ICU: intensive care unit; FiO_2: fraction of inspired O_2 concentration; SpO_2: transcutaneous hemoglobin O_2 saturation; PaO_2 arterial O_2 partial pressure; CK-MB: myocardial creatine kinase; cTnI: cardiac troponin I; TBI: traumatic brain injury; GCS: Glasgow Coma Score; GOS: Glasgow Outcome Score; GOSE: Extended Glasgow Outcome Score.

Acute Coronary Syndrome

Since the 1940s, supplemental O_2 breathing has been a cornerstone of the management of the acute coronary syndrome. This approach has recently been questioned [21] because of the above-mentioned hyperoxia-induced coronary vasoconstriction, which was confirmed in patients undergoing cardiac catheterization for coronary artery disease. It must be noted, however, that these data originate from patients with stable vascular disease and not with acute myocardial infarction. Nevertheless, the latest guidelines of the European Resuscitation Council on the initial management of acute coronary syndromes recommend that an "O_2 saturation of 94–98%, or 88–92% if the patient is at risk of hypercapnic respiratory failure" should be achieved, in other words, "supplementary O_2 should be given only to those patients with hypoxemia, breathlessness or pulmonary congestion" [22]. The evidence for these guidelines is surprisingly scarce: Over the last four decades (!) four clinical trials enrolling a total of only 447 patients have been published on the effects of O_2 therapy in patients with myocardial infarction [23–26], and the available results are far from allowing a definitive conclusion. Rawles and Kenmure [23] reported no difference in the incidence of arrhythmias and use of analgesics after 6 l/min O_2 over 24 hours when compared to air breathing; however, there was a tendency (3.9 vs. 11.3%, $p=0.08$) towards increased mortality in the O_2-group. Recently, Ranchord et al. found "no evidence of benefit or harm" from high-concentration (6 l/min O_2 over 6 hours) vs. titrated O_2 therapy (to achieve O_2 saturations of 93–96%) in initially uncomplicated ST-elevation myocardial infarction [24]. In contrast, Madias et al. had earlier shown reduced ischemic injury as assessed by pre-cordial ST-mapping during 48–80 minutes of breathing 15 l/min O_2; however, this study included only 17 patients, without a control group [25]. Finally, Ukholkina et al. demonstrated that an FiO_2 of 0.3–0.4 until three hours after interventional myocardial revascularization reduced the number of early post-intervention arrhythmias and lowered the peak values of the activity of the myocardial creatine kinase, ultimately resulting in a smaller relative area of ischemic damage; however, 37% of the patients had baseline O_2 saturations <94% and, for reasons unexplained, time to revascularization was longer in the O_2-group [26]. Therefore, as highlighted in recent reviews [21], there is an urgent need for large clinical trials to determine whether or not O_2 therapy should be used for the management of acute coronary syndromes. The Air Verses Oxygen In myocarDial Infarction (AVOID, NCT01272713) and DETermination of the Role of OXygen in Suspected Acute Myocardial Infarction (DETO2X-AMI, NCT01787110) studies (see Table 2) are designed to answer this question.

Despite this uncertainty, it should be noted that the concept of a prolonged window of opportunity seems to be valid in coronary artery disease at least for O_2 breathing as a preventive measure: Breathing 15 l/min O_2 prevented the recurrence of pacing-angina [27] and prolonged the time until occurrence of exercise-induced angina [28].

Traumatic Brain Injury and Stroke

Theoretically, the above-mentioned hyperoxia-induced vasoconstriction could be referred to as particularly interesting in the context of brain injury, inasmuch it would allow reduction of intracranial blood volume and thereby decreased intracranial pressure (ICP). This effect on ICP was clearly demonstrated in patients with TBI during *hyperbaric* oxygenation (HBO; 60 minutes of mechanical ventilation with pure O_2 at 1.5 atmospheres of ambient pressure) [29]. Moreover, combining HBO with subsequent *normobaric* hyperoxia was even associated with improved long-term outcome: At six months, mortality was reduced (3 out of 20 vs. 9 out of 22 patients, $p = 0.048$) and overall outcome more favorable as assessed using the sliding dichotomized Glasgow Outcome Score (14 out of 19 vs. 8 out of 21 patients, $p = 0.024$) [30]. In contrast, normobaric hyperoxia alone yielded equivocal results with respect to tissue oxygenation and metabolism as assessed by microdialysis, possibly at least in part as a result of the lack of effect on brain tissue PO_2 in hypoperfused regions [31]. Despite recent findings of a potential benefit of hyperoxia in the perilesional penumbra using magnetic resonance imaging (MRI) [32], the role of hyperoxia in TBI remains a matter of debate because of the controversial outcome data currently available [33]. In a retrospective analysis of 1,116 patients, a univariate analysis showed a significant association between hyperoxemia ($PaO_2 > 100$ mmHg) and a decreased risk of six-month mortality. However, a multivariate logistic regression model to adjust for markers of illness severity no longer showed any significant relationship [34]. In two other retrospective studies on a total of 1,759 patients, multivariate analyses demonstrated that more pronounced hyperoxemia ($PaO_2 > 200$ or > 300 mmHg, respectively) was independently associated with higher in-hospital mortality [35, 36]. Unfortunately, the Impact of Inspired Oxygen Fraction on Outcome in Patients With Traumatic Brain Injury (BRAINOXY, NCT01201291) study, which was designed to answer this question, was terminated due to slow recruitment.

Despite the compelling experimental evidence and some encouraging pilot studies in patients, there is substantial evidence that hyperoxia is deleterious in patients with stroke and/or intracranial bleeding, i. e., in ischemic brain injury. In a prospective, single-center observational study in 252 patients, Jeon et al. showed that hyperoxemia (defined as a $PaO_2 > 173$ mmHg) was associated with delayed cerebral ischemia and, consequently, poor outcome [37]. More recently, a retrospective analysis of 2,894 mechanically ventilated patients with ischemic stroke, subarachnoid or intracerebral hemorrhage, showed that profound hyperoxemia ($PaO_2 > 300$ mmHg) was associated with a significantly higher in-hospital mortality at day 28 [38]. The 'Normobaric Oxygen Therapy in Acute Ischemic Stroke Trial' (NCT00414726), which was to study the effects of high-flow O_2 (30–45 l/min for eight hours via facemask) was terminated prematurely after enrolment of 85 of 240 patients, because of an imbalance in deaths favoring the control arm (hyperoxia: 17 out of 43 patients, room air: 7 out of 42 patients, $p = 0.03$). The question of whether hyperoxia is definitely deleterious, however, remains unanswered because the deaths were not attributed to treatment by the blinded external medical monitor.

Even low-flow O_2 therapy (2 l/min either continuously over 72 hours or overnight only) to compensate for mild, in particular nocturnal, hypoxemia (Stroke Oxygen Study, SO2S) did not improve outcome after ischemic stroke: Despite promising pilot data in 289 patients at one week and six months [39, 40], the complete study (ISRCTN register ID number ISRCTN52416964) in 8,003 patients did not show any difference in morbidity (disability at day 90 as assessed by the modified Rankin Scale) or mortality (Roffe, unpublished data).

Cardiac Arrest

The specific effects of hyperoxia on the cerebral circulation, together with its potential to aggravate ischemia/reperfusion-injury, have prompted investigations into the association between hyperoxia and outcome after cardiac arrest. So far only retrospective analyses are available and, again, the results are equivocal: A multicenter cohort study in 6,326 patients showed that hyperoxemia ($PaO_2 > 300$ mmHg) was associated with higher mortality than normoxemia and even hypoxemia ($PaO_2 < 60$ mmHg) [41]. Moreover, a secondary analysis of 4,459 patients from this study demonstrated a linear relationship between PaO_2 increments and increased risk of mortality, a PaO_2 of 100 mmHg being associated with a 24% higher odds ratio for unfavorable outcome [42]. In contrast, another retrospective analysis of mortality as a function of PaO_2 deciles in 12,108 patients found that the odds ratio adjusted for illness severity did not suggest a robust association between hyperoxemia ($PaO_2 > 309$ mmHg) and mortality [43]. Other authors analyzing smaller databases confirmed this latter finding [44]. Finally, studies focusing on the impact of $PaCO_2$ did not reveal any deleterious effect of hyperoxemia *per se* on neurological outcome. It could be argued that different temperature management in the various countries was responsible for these discrepancies, but a single-center, retrospective analysis of 170 patients treated with therapeutic hypothermia showed that non-survivors and patients with poor neurological outcome presented with significantly higher maximum PaO_2 values (median 254 vs. 198 mmHg) during the first 24 hours after cardiac arrest [45]. Consequently, a recent meta-analysis concluded that hyperoxemia ($PaO_2 > 300$ mmHg) "... appears to be correlated with increased in-hospital mortality ...", which, however, "... should be interpreted cautiously because of the significant heterogeneity ... of studies analyzed" [46]. Overall, all these studies demonstrate the urgent need for data from prospective, randomized controlled trials, and the ongoing Reoxygenation After Cardiac Arrest (REOX, NCT01881243) trial should at least help to answer this demand.

Perioperative Hyperoxia

Clearly, the use of intraoperative (and, in a broader sense, perioperative) hyperoxia to prevent surgical site infection does not refer to the treatment of circulatory shock and medical emergencies, but several of the pathophysiological effects of hyperoxemia are also relevant in this context. Since the recognition of "oxygen as an antibiotic" [47] in the 1980s, several studies have been conducted enrolling more than 5,000 patients. Recent meta-analyses of these studies concluded that high FiO_2 values (0.8 vs. 0.3 as the standard approach) decreased the risk of surgical site infection after elective and emergency surgery, without a major risk of postoperative atelectasis [48]. The protection against infection was particularly pronounced in colorectal surgery, possibly due to an improved patency of anastomoses [49]; however, it was no longer present in obese patients. The molecular mechanism of any hyperoxia-related reduction in surgical site infection is still not entirely clear:

Some authors reported that hyperoxic ventilation restored the local inflammatory response to normal, rather than causing deleterious hyper-inflammation, and thereby augmented the antimicrobial potential of alveolar macrophages. In contrast, other studies found that *ex vivo* exposure to hyperoxia enhanced ROS formation and even reduced secretion of tumor necrosis factor (TNF)-α in endotoxin-stimulated leukocytes. It should be noted that, despite the above-mentioned possible short-term benefit, high intraoperative FiO_2 was associated with greater long-term (> two years) post-operative mortality in cancer patients [50], which coincided with shorter cancer-free intervals [51].

What is the Optimal PaO_2 for ICU Survival?

Again, a definitive answer is pending: de Jonge et al. demonstrated a U-shaped relationship of in-hospital mortality and arterial PO_2 in 36,307 patients during the first 24 hours of ICU stay, the nadir average mortality being at PaO_2 values of 15–20 kPa (110–150 mmHg), whereas mortality sharply increased at $PaO_2 < 9$ (67 mmHg) and > 30 (225 mmHg) kPa [52]. A more recent study of unadjusted odds ratios for PaO_2 deciles in 152,680 patients confirmed the impact of hypoxemia, while even hyperoxemia > 40 kPa (300 mmHg) had no impact on outcome [53]. The results of the Normal Oxygenation Maintenance in Intensive Care Unit (OXYGEN-ICU, NCT01319643) trial (see Table 2) will certainly contribute to answering this question.

Conclusion

Hyperoxia (i. e., ventilation with an $FiO_2 = 1.0$) is a cornerstone in the acute management of circulatory shock, a concept which is based on compelling experimental evidence that compensating the imbalance between O_2 supply and requirements (i. e., the oxygen debt) is crucial for survival. On the other hand, oxygen toxicity from the increased formation of ROS limits its use, because it may provoke serious deleterious adverse effects, especially in conditions of ischemia/reperfusion. These effects are particularly pronounced during long-term administration, i. e., beyond 12–24 hours. Moreover, numerous retrospective studies also suggest that even hyperoxemia of shorter duration is associated with increased mortality and morbidity in various important medical emergencies. The clinical evidence from prospective studies is, however, surprisingly scarce. Therefore, there is a need for the results from large scale, randomized, controlled clinical trials on the use of hyperoxia, which are to be expected within the next two to three years. Until these data are available, "conservative" O_2 therapy [54] may be the treatment of choice to avoid both hypoxemia and excess hyperoxic exposure.

Acknowledgements

Supported by the Deutsche Forschungsgemeinschaft (KFO 200, DFG RA 396/9-2) and the Bundesministerium der Verteidigung (Vertragsforschungsvorhaben E/U2AD/CF523/DF556).

References

1. Leverve XM (2008) To cope with oxygen: a long and still tumultuous story for life. Crit Care Med 36:637–638
2. Turrens JF (2003) Mitochondrial formation of reactive oxygen species. J Physiol 552:335–344
3. Magder S (2006) Reactive oxygen species: toxic molecules or spark of life? Crit Care 10:208
4. Vincent JL, De Backer D (2013) Circulatory shock. N Engl J Med 369:1726–1734
5. Weil MH, Shubin H (1969) The "VIP" approach to the bedside management of shock. JAMA 207:337–340
6. The ProCESS Investigators (2014) A randomized trial of protocol-based care for early septic shock. N Engl J Med 370:1683–1693
7. Bitterman H (2009) Bench-to-bedside review: Oxygen as a drug. Crit Care 13:205
8. Cornet AD, Kooter AJ, Peters MJL, Smulders YM (2013) The potential harm of oxygen therapy in medical emergencies. Crit Care 17:313
9. Edmark L, Kostova-Aherdan K, Enlund M, Hedenstierna G (2003) Optimal oxygen concentration during induction of general anesthesia. Anesthesiology 98:28–33
10. Calzia E, Asfar P, Hauser B et al (2010) Hyperoxia may be beneficial. Crit Care Med 38 (suppl):S559–S568
11. Boerema I, Meyne NG, Brummelkamp WK et al (1960) [Life without blood]. Ned Tijdschr Geneeskd 104:949–954
12. Blasiole B, Bayir H, Vagni VA et al (2013) Effect of hyperoxia on resuscitation of experimental combined traumatic brain injury and hemorrhagic shock in mice. Anesthesiology 118:649–663
13. Kapanci Y, Tosco R, Eggermann J, Gould VE (1972) Oxygen pneumonitis in man. Chest 62:162–169
14. Aboab J, Jonson B, Kouatchet A, Taille S, Niklason L, Brochard L (2006) Effect of inspired oxygen fraction on alveolar derecruitment in acute respiratory distress syndrome. Intensive Care Med 32:1979–1986
15. Mak S, Azevedo ER, Liu PP, Newton GE (2001) Effect of hyperoxia on left ventricular function and filling pressures in patients with and without congestive heart failure. Chest 120:467–473
16. Stamler JS, Jia L, Eu JP et al (1997) Blood flow regulation by S-nitrosohemoglobin in the physiological oxygen gradient. Science 276:2034–2037
17. Rossi P, Tauzin L, Weiss M, Rostain JC, Sainty JM, Bousuges A (2007) Could hyperoxic ventilation impair oxygen delivery in septic patients? Clin Physiol Funct Imaging 27:180–184
18. Reinhart K, Bloos F, König F, Bredle D, Hannemann L (1991) Reversible decrease of oxygen consumption by hyperoxia. Chest 99:690–694
19. Ganz W, Donoso R, Marcus H, Swan HJC (1972) Coronary hemodynamics and myocardial oxygen metabolism during oxygen breathing in patients with and without coronary artery disease. Circulation 45:763–768
20. Leverve XM (2007) Mitochondrial function and substrate availability. Crit Care Med 35 (Suppl):S454–S460
21. Shuvy M, Atar D, Steg PG et al (2013) Oxygen therapy in acute coronary syndrome: are the benefits worth the risk? Eur Heart J 34:1630–1635

22. Arntz HR, Bossaert LL, Danchin N, Nikolaou NI (2010) European Resuscitation Council Guidelines for Resuscitation 2010 Section 5. Initial management of acute coronary syndromes. Resuscitation 81:1353–1363
23. Rawles JM, Kenmure ACF (1976) Controlled trial of oxygen in uncomplicated myocardial infarction. BMJ 1:1121–1123
24. Ranchord AM, Argyle R, Beynoon R et al (2012) High-concentration versus titrated oxygen therapy in ST-elevation myocardial infarction: A pilot randomized controlled trial. Am Heart J 163:168–175
25. Madias JE, Madias NE, Hood WB (1976) Precordial ST-segment mapping. 2. Effects of oxygen inhalation in patients with acute myocardial infarction. Circulation 53:411–417
26. Ukholkina GB, Kostyanov IY, Kuchkina NV, Gofman YB (2005) Oxygen therapy in combination with endovascular reperfusion during the first hours of acute myocardial infarction: clinical and laboratory findings. Int J Intervent Cardioangiol 9:45–51
27. Horvat M, Yoshida S, Prakash R, Marcus HS, Swan HJC, Ganz W (1972) Effect of oxygen breathing on pacing-induced angina pectoris and other manifestations of coronary insufficiency. Circulation 45:837–844
28. Ranchord AM, Perrin K, Weatherall M, Beasley R, Simmonds M (2012) A randomised controlled trial of the effect of high concentration oxygen on myocardial ischemia during exercise. Int J Cardiol 160:201–205
29. Rockswold SB, Rockswold GL, Zaun DA et al (2010) A prospective, randomized clinical trial to compare the effect of hyperbaric to normobaric hyperoxia on cerebral metabolism, intracranial pressure, and oxygen toxicity in severe traumatic brain injury. J Neurosurg 112:1080–1094
30. Rockswold SB, Rockswold GL, Zaun DA, Liu J (2013) A prospective, randomized Phase II clinical trial to evaluate the effect of combined hyperbaric and normobaric hyperoxia on cerebral metabolism, intracranial pressure, oxygen toxicity, and clinical outcome in severe traumatic brain injury. J Neurosurg 118:1317–1328
31. Hlatky R, Valadka AB, Gopinath SP, Robertson CS (2007) Brain tissue oxygen tension response to induced hyperoxia in hypoperfused brain. J Neurosurg 108:53–58
32. Veenith TV, Carter EL, Grossac J et al (2014) Use of diffusion tensor imaging to assess the impact of normobaric hyperoxia within at-risk pericontusional tissue after traumatic brain injury. J Cereb Blood Flow Metab 34:1622–1627
33. Narotam P (2013) Eubaric hpyeroxia. Controversies in the management of acute traumatic brain injury. Crit Care 17:197
34. Raj R, Bendel S, Reinikainen M et al (2013) Hyperoxia and long-term outcome after traumatic brain injury. Crit Care 17:R177
35. Brenner M, Stein D, Hu P, Kufera J, Wooford M, Scalea T (2012) Association between early hyperoxia and worse outcomes after traumatic brain injury. Arch Surg 147:1042–1046
36. Rincon F, Kang J, Vibbert M, Urtecho J, Athar MK, Jallo J (2014) Significance of arterial hyperoxia and relationship with case fatality in traumatic brain injury; a multicentre cohort study. J Neurol Neurosurg Psychiatry 85:799–805
37. Jeon SB, Choi HA, Badjata N et al (2014) Hyperoxia may be related to delayed cerebral ischemia and poor outcome after subarachnoid haemorrhage. J Neurol Neurosurg Psychiatry 85:1301–1307
38. Rincon F, Kang J, Maltenfort M et al (2014) Association between hyperoxia and mortality after stroke: a multicenter cohort study. Crit Care Med 42:387–396
39. Roffe C1, Ali K, Warusevitane A et al (2011) The SOS pilot study: a RCT of routine oxygen supplementation early after acute stroke – effect on recovery of neurological function at one week. PloS One 6:e19113
40. Ali K, Warusevitane A, Lally F et al (2013) The stroke oxygen pilot study: a randomized controlled trial of the effects of routine oxygen supplementation early after acute stroke – effect on key outcomes at six months. PloS One 8:e59274

41. Kilgannon JH, Jones AE, Shapiro NI et al (2010) Association between arterial hyperoxia following resuscitation from cardiac arrest and in-hospital mortality. JAMA 303:2165–2171
42. Kilgannon JH, Jones AE, Parrillo JE et al (2011) Relationship between supranormal oxygen tension and outcome after resuscitation from cardiac arrest. Circulation 123:2717–2722
43. Bellomo R, Bailey M, Eastwood GM et al (2011) Arterial hyperoxia and in-hospital mortality after resuscitation from cardiac arrest. Crit Care 15:R90
44. Vaahersalo J, Bendel S, Reinikainen M et al (2014) Arterial blood gas tensions after resuscitation from out-of-hospital cardiac arrest: associations with long-term neurologic outcome. Crit Care Med 42:1463–1470
45. Janz DR, Hollenbeck RD, Pollock JS, McPherson JA, Rice TW (2012) Hyperoxia is associated with increased mortality in patients treated with mild therapeutic hypothermia after sudden cardiac arrest. Crit Care Med 40:3135–3139
46. Wang CH, Chang WT, Huang CH et al (2014) The effect of hyperoxia on survival following adult cardiac arrest: A systematic review and meta-analysis of observational studies. Resuscitation 85:1142–1148
47. Knighton DR, Halliday B, Hunt TK (1984) Oxygen as an antibiotic. The effect of inspired oxygen on infection. Arch Surg 119:199–204
48. Hovaguimian F, Lysakowski C, Elia N, Tramèr MR (2013) Effect of intraoperative high inspired oxygen fraction on surgical site infection, postoperative nausea and vomiting, and pulmonary function: systematic review and meta-analysis of randomized controlled trials. Anesthesiology 119:303–316
49. Schietroma M, Cecilia EM, Sista F, Carlei F, Pessia B, Amicucci G (2014) High-concentration supplemental perioperative oxygen and surgical site infection following elective colorectal surgery for rectal cancer: a prospective, randomized, double-blind, controlled, single-site trial. Am J Surg 208:719–726
50. Meyhoff CS, Jorgensen LN, Wetterslev J, Christensen KB, Rasmussen LS, PROXI Trial group (2012) Increased long-term mortality after high perioperative inspiratory oxygen fraction during abdominal surgery: Follo-up of a randomized clinical trial. Anesth Analg 115:849–854
51. Meyhoff CS, Jorgensen LN, Wetterslev J, Siersma VD, Rasmussen LS, PROXI Trial group (2014) Risk of new or recurrent cancer after a high perioperative inspiratory oxygen fraction during abdominal surgery. Brit J Anaesth 113 (Suppl 1):i74–i81
52. de Jonge E, Peelen L, Keijzers PJ et al (2008) Association between administered oxygen, arterial partial oxygen pressure and mortality in mechanically ventilated intenisve care unit patients. Crit Care 12:R156
53. Eastwood G, Bellomo R, Bailey M et al (2012) Arterial oxygen tension and mortality in mechanically ventilated patients. Intensive Care Med 38:91–98
54. Suzuki S, Eastwood GM, Glassford NJ et al (2014) Conservative oxygen therapy in mechanically ventilated patients: a pilot before-and-after trial. Crit Care Med 42:1414–1422

Extracorporeal Gas Exchange for Acute Respiratory Failure in Adult Patients: A Systematic Review

M. Schmidt, C. Hodgson, and A. Combes

Introduction

Mechanical ventilation remains the cornerstone of respiratory support for patients with acute respiratory failure. However, high pressure and volume associated with tidal ventilation are known to aggravate lung injury in this setting [1]. Furthermore, profound gas-exchange abnormalities threatening patients' lives can occur in the most severe forms of the disease despite recourse to conventional salvage therapies [2, 3]. Extracorporeal gas exchange devices, i. e., venovenous extracorporeal membrane oxygenation (ECMO) and extracorporeal carbon dioxide removal ($ECCO_2R$), were developed more than 40 years ago [4, 5] to rescue these dying patients. Whereas venovenous ECMO provides complete extracorporeal blood oxygenation and decarboxylation using high blood flows (4–6 l/min) and large (20–30 Fr) cannulas [6–9], efficient extracorporeal CO_2 removal (with minimal blood oxygenation) can be achieved with $ECCO_2R$ devices using limited extracorporeal blood flow (0.4–1 l/min) and thin double lumen venous catheters (14–18 Fr) [10, 11], because CO_2 clearance is more effective than oxygenation due to the greater solubility and more rapid diffusion of CO_2 [12]. Extracorporeal gas exchange devices also permit 'ultraprotective' mechanical ventilation with further reduction of volume and pressure, which may ultimately enhance lung protection and improve clinical outcomes for patients with acute respiratory distress syndrome (ARDS). However, results of trials evaluating extracorporeal gas exchange for respiratory failure performed in the 1970s, 80s and 90s were often disappointing [13, 14]. In recent years, major technological advances have occurred and the latest gen-

M. Schmidt · A. Combes ✉
Medical-Surgical Intensive Care Unit, iCAN, Institute of Cardiometabolism and Nutrition, Hôpital de la Pitié–Salpêtrière, Assistance Publique–Hôpitaux de Paris, Université Pierre et Marie Curie, Paris, France
e-mail: alain.combes@psl.aphp.fr

C. Hodgson
The Australian & New Zealand Intensive Care Research Centre and the Intensive Care Department, Alfred Hospital, Melbourne, Australia

J.-L. Vincent (ed.), *Annual Update in Intensive Care and Emergency Medicine 2015*,
DOI 10.1007/978-3-319-13761-2_14

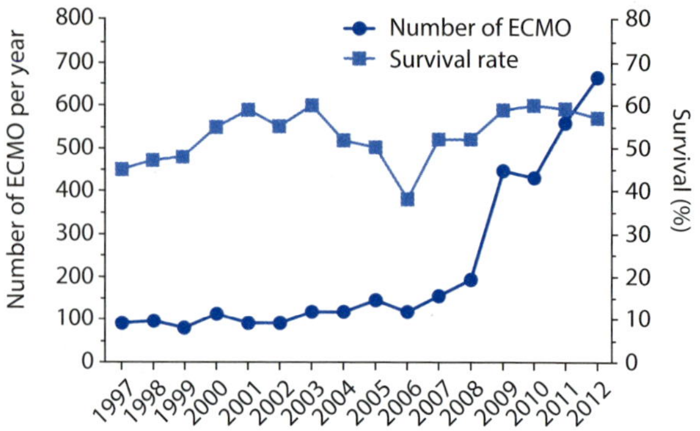

Fig. 1 Number of annual adult respiratory cases treated by ECMO and relative survival rates over 15 years (adapted from [73])

eration extracorporeal gas exchange devices, with polymethylpentene hollow-fiber membrane lungs and Mendler-designed centrifugal pumps offer lower resistance to blood flow, have smaller priming volumes, higher effective gas exchange properties and are coated with more biocompatible materials.

The successful use of ECMO for the most severe ARDS cases associated with the recent influenza A(H1N1) pandemic, in whom conventional ventilation was not successful [15–17], and positive results of the randomized Conventional ventilatory support versus Extracorporeal membrane oxygenation for Severe Adult Respiratory failure (CESAR) trial [18] have been associated with a steep increase in the number of VV-ECMO procedures performed in very recent years (Fig. 1). In addition, a proof-of-concept study suggested that the very low tidal volume ventilation (3.5–5 ml/kg of predicted body weight) permitted by $ECCO_2R$ can improve pulmonary protection and decrease pulmonary inflammation in ARDS patients [19] and a recent randomized trial suggested that this strategy may be associated with better outcomes for moderate to severe ARDS patients [11].

The aim of this systematic review was to analyze studies reporting indications, associated complications and short- and long-term outcomes of extracorporeal gas exchange in adult patients with acute respiratory failure. It may ultimately help critical care physicians and researchers select better candidates for extracorporeal gas exchange and to design future observational and randomized clinical trials to evaluate these techniques.

Methods

To achieve a high standard of reporting, we adopted Preferred Reporting Items for Systematic Reviews and Meta-Analyses (PRISMA) guidelines [20, 21].

Search Strategy

The detailed search strategy (identification, screening, eligibility and inclusion process) used to identify relevant studies is summarized in Fig. 2. We used a detailed PubMed/MEDLINE, EMBASE and CINAHL query to identify randomized controlled trials (RCTs), controlled observational studies (retrospective and prospec-

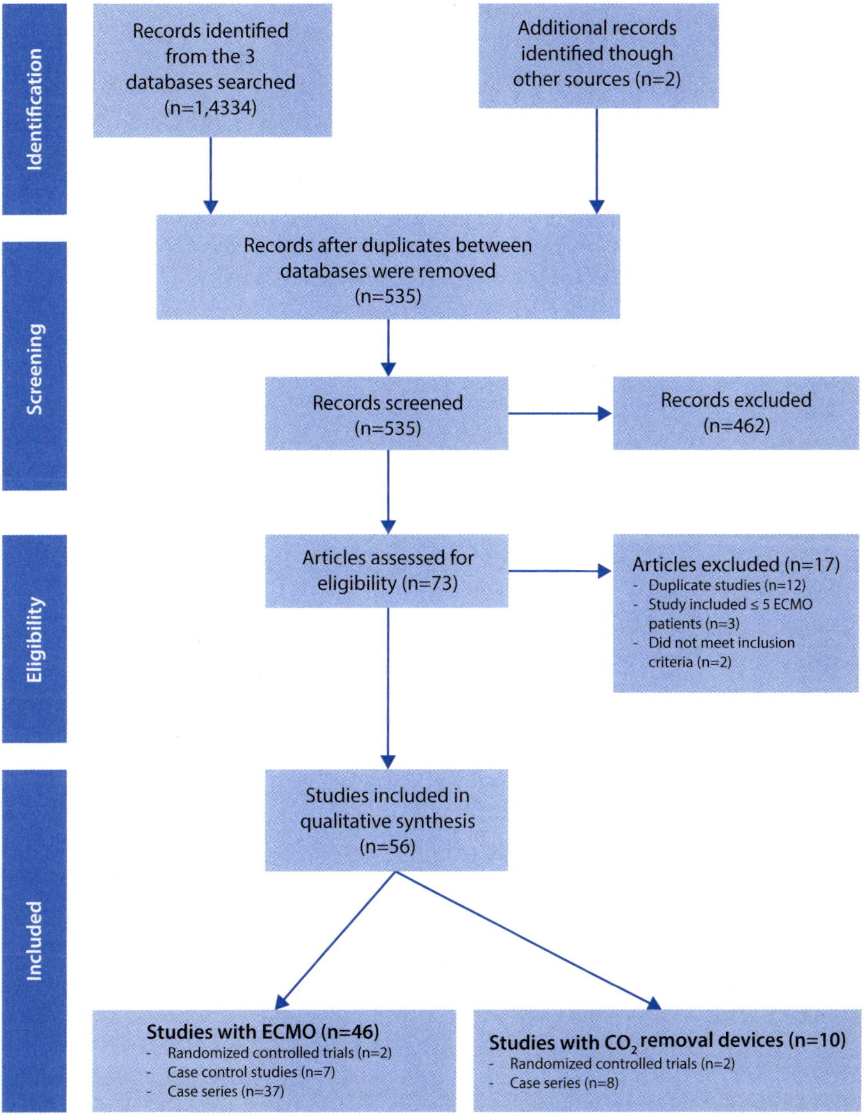

Fig. 2 Summary of evidence search and selection: PRISMA flow Chart

tive) and case series with >5 patients who received extracorporeal gas exchange. Additionally, reference lists from relevant reviews, observational studies and clinical trials were hand-searched. Neonatal and pediatric studies (patients <18 years of age) were excluded. Language of publication was limited to English and no restriction on the time was set on the primary literature searches. The query was last updated in June 2014.

Study Selection

Two independent researchers (MS and AC) conducted a two-step literature search. Studies were included according to the following criteria: 1) original study published in a peer-reviewed journal; and 2) analyzed/reported the use of extracorporeal gas exchange (i. e., ECMO or pumpless extracorporeal lung assist or extracorporeal CO_2 removal) and its specific outcomes for acute respiratory failure in adult patients. Any discrepancies between the two reviewers who examined the titles and abstracts of all relevant citations were resolved by discussion.

Data Extraction, Quality Assessment and Analysis

The two reviewers (MS and AC) independently read the entire texts of the retrieved reports and rated study quality using well-established criteria [21, 22]. RCT quality was graded using a nine-point scale combining elements from Jadad's [21] and Chalmers' [23, 24] scales, whereas the quality of case-controlled studies was appraised using the Newcastle-Ottawa scale [25]. In addition, both reviewers extracted the following data: First author, year of publication, country, study design, number of patients, demographic data, pre-ECMO ventilation and blood gas data and outcomes. Because of very high heterogeneity between studies, related to different generation ECMO and $ECCO_2R$ devices used in the last 40 years, different patient populations evaluated, and the scarcity of randomized or quasi-randomized trials (most of which were flawed by major methodological limitations) performed with the latest generation extracorporeal gas exchange techniques, we did not perform meta-analyses of randomized or quasi-randomized trials and choose to report and discuss only crude study results.

Results

Number of Studies Selected

The initial search yielded 535 articles, of which 462 were excluded through title and abstract review, leaving 73 articles potentially meeting our inclusion criteria. After a complete analysis of these, 17 articles were excluded. Of the remaining 56 studies that were evaluated, 4 were RCTs, 7 case-control studies, and 45 case series (Fig. 2 and Tables 1–6). With the exception of two studies [13, 18], all ECMO cohorts had an observational design. Sixteen studies reported on the outcomes of ARDS cases associated with the recent influenza A(H1N1) pandemic (Tables 4 and 5). Ten studies (2 randomized) reporting on $ECCO_2R$ devices in ARDS patients were retained for the review (Table 6). Overall study validity was adequate, with an average score of 8.1/9.0 on the Newcastle-Ottawa scale appraising the quality of case-control studies.

ECMO and ARDS: Studies of Historical Interest

In 1968, Kolobow et al. developed the first membrane oxygenator for long-term extracorporeal oxygenation [5]. Three years later, Donald Hill and colleagues described the first use of an ECMO device for acute respiratory failure in humans [4]. They reported on a 24-year-old polytrauma patient, who survived after 75 hours of veno-arterial ECMO. In cohort studies published up to the mid-2000s, the oldest ECMO technology combining roller pump, silicone membrane oxygenator and blood reservoir was used. Survival was 50% in a cohort of 1,473 patients (1986 to 2006, mean age 34 years, 78% had VV-ECMO) from the Extracorporeal Life Support Organization (ELSO) registry [26]. In that report, survival was comparable across study periods, although age and severity of disease were significantly higher for the most recent patients. Similarly, Hemmila et al. from Michigan University reported a survival of 52% in 255 adult patients treated with ECMO between 1989 and 2003 [27]. Other case-control studies reported similar survival rates for patients treated with ECMO [28, 29]. Interestingly, in a cohort of 150 patients with ARDS (mean age 42 years, mean SAPS II 45), of whom 32 received ECMO as a rescue therapy, ECMO support was not independently associated with a higher mortality [30].

ECMO and ARDS: Results of Randomized Controlled Trials

Over the last 30 years, only two RCTs of ECMO for ARDS patients have been conducted [13, 18]. The National Institutes of Health (NIH) performed the first multicenter trial in the 1970s, enrolling 90 patients with severe ARDS refractory to conventional ventilation [13], of whom 42 received ECMO. Survival was extremely low (< 10%) and not different between groups. However, that study suffered from major methodological limitations. For example, the mode of ECMO support was only veno-arterial and when no improvement was observed after 5 days, ECMO was removed, which precluded the possibility of late clinical improvement. Because the ECMO group did not receive lung-protective ventilation, severe complications related to barotrauma occurred and since ECMO circuitry was not heparin-coated at that time, a very high percentage of patients had severe hemorrhagic complications due to excessive anticoagulation.

The most recent trial (CESAR), which was conducted in the UK from 2001 to 2006, evaluated a strategy of transfer to a single center (Glenfield, Leicester)

Table 1 Large, recent studies of ECMO for acute respiratory failure: Key patient features

First author [ref]	Design	Prospective	Setting	Quality assessment[§]	Follow up	ECMO patients	Years	Age	Pneumonia, %	Mobile ECMO team, %	SOFA score
Peek, ECMO Arm, CESAR trial [18]	RCT	Y	Multi	RCT6	6 months	68	2001–2006	40 ± 13	62	0	–
Schmidt [50]	Case series	Y	Multi	–	Hospital discharge	2,355	2000–2012	41 (28–54)	34	–	–
Brogan [26]	Case series	N	Multi	–	Hospital discharge	1,473	1986–2006	35 (22–53)	26	–	–
Enger [51]	Case series	Y	Single	–	Hospital discharge	284	2008–2013	46 (43–48) †	49	47	11 (11–12)
Hemmila [27]	Case series	N	Single	–	Hospital discharge	280	1989–2003	38 ± 13	31	37	–
Schmid [32]	Case series	N	Single	–	ICU discharge	176	2007–2010	48 ± 17	58	34	12 ± 4
Schmidt [33]	Case series	N	Multi	–	6 months	140	2008–2012	44 (30–56)	71 [£]	68	12 (10–15)
Lindskov [31]	Case series	Y	Single	–	ICU discharge	124	1977–2011	42 (16–67)	64	85	–
Roch [49]	Case series	N	Single	–	Hospital discharge	85	2009–2013	47 ± 15	86	100	9 (7–11)

Table 1 (Continuation)

First author [ref]	Design	Pros-pective	Setting	Quality assessment[§]	Follow up	ECMO patients	Years	Age	Pneu-monia, %	Mobile ECMO team,%	SOFA score
Rega [74]	Case series	N	Single	–	90 days	70	1997–2005	43 ± 18	41	–	–
Mols [28]	Case-control	Y	Single	7	Hospital discharge	62	1991–1999	35 ± 11	58	0	7 (6–9)
Muller [35]	Case series	Y	Single	–	ICU discharge	60	2006–2008	53 (21–78)	42	17	14 (11–16)
Lewandowski [29]	Case-control	Y	Single	9	ICU discharge	49	1989–1995	31 ± 14	37	–	–
Forrest [34]	Case series	N	Multi	–	Hospital discharge	38	2007–2010	34 (26–42)	89 [#]	100	8 (5–10)
Frenckner [75]	Case series	N	Single	–	ICU discharge	38	1995–2002	38 (17–61)	60	32	
Michaels [46]	Case series	N	Single	–	ICU discharge	36	2009–2012	40 ± 6	58 [$]	69	–
Beiderlinden [30]	Case-control	Y	Single	9	Hospital discharge	32	1998–2003	42 ± 13	53	–	14 ± 3

ICU, intensive care unit; Multi, multicenter; N, no; RCT, randomized control trial; SOFA; Sequential Organ Failure Assessment; Y, yes.
Data are given as mean ± SD or median (interquartile range). £ 26% were H1N1 pneumonia; # 42% were H1N1 pneumonia; $ 44% were H1N1 pneumonia.
§ Randomized controlled trial quality was graded using a nine-point scale combining elements from Jadad's [21] and Chalmers' scales [23, 24] whereas the validity of case-controlled studies was appraised with the Newcastle-Ottawa scale [25]; † in the survivors.

Table 2 Large, recent studies of ECMO for acute respiratory failure: Key pre-ECMO data and outcomes

First author [ref]	PaO_2/FiO_2	pH	Plateau pressure	PEEP	LIS	Delay MV – ECMO, hours	Rescue therapies, %	Duration of ECMO, days	Hemorrhage, %	Intracerebral hemorrhage, %	Mortality, n (%)
Peek, ECMO Arm, CESAR trial [18]	76 ± 29	7.1 ± 0.1	–	14 ± 9	3.5 ± 0.6	36 (17–104)	–	10 (5–23)	–	0	33 (37%)
Schmidt [50]	59 (48–75)	7.25 (7.15–7.35)	36 (31–43) *	13 (10–16)	–	57 (19–151)	30	7 (4–13)	–	–	1,017 (43%)
Brogan [26]	57 (45–71)	7.27 (7.18–7.36)	40 (35–48) *	13 (10–16)	–	52 (20–160)	–	23 ± 20	30	4	732 (50%)
Enger [51]	69 (65–74) †	7.22 (7.22–7.25) †	35 (34–36) *†	16 (16–17) †	3.5 (3.4–3.5) †	120 (96–168) †	–	10 (9–11) †	–	–	117 (41%)
Hemmila [27]	55 ± 16	7.31 ± 0.12	44 ± 11*	13 ± 5	–	96 ± 72	–	9 ± 8	–	3	123 (48%)
Schmid [32]	77 ± 47	7.2 ± 0.2	35 ± 6 *	18 ± 6	3.4 ± 0.5	144 ± 240	–	12 ± 9	–	–	78 (44%)
Schmidt [33]	53 (43–60)	7.22 (7.15–7.32)	32 (30–35)	10 (8–12)	–	120 (24–264)	94	15 (8–30)	46	3	50 (36%)
Lindskov [31]	48 (37–60)	7.26 ± 0.15	37 (35–41)	–	–	–	–	9 (1–23)	–	9	36 (29%)
Roch [49]	60 (50–70)	7.1 ± 0.2	32 (29–35)	–	3.5 (3.3–3.7)	48 (24– 194)	85	9 (7–13)	29	2	48 (56%)
Rega [74]	56 ± 18	7.22 ± 0.18	44 ± 11*	13 ± 3	–	108 ± 178	–	7 ± 5	20	–	40 (57%)

Table 2 (Continuation)

First author [ref]	PaO_2/FiO_2	pH	Plateau pressure	PEEP	LIS	Delay MV – ECMO, hours	Rescue thera-pies, %	Duration of ECMO, days	Hemor-rhage, %	Intracere-bral he-morrhage, %	Mortality, n (%)
Mols [28]	96 ± 51	7.30 (7.22–7.40)	–	–	3.2 ± 0.4	–	–	12 ± 7	7	2	28 (45%)
Muller [35]	64 (48–86)	7.20 (7.13–7.30)	36 (32–40)*	16 (13–20)	3.6 (3.3–3.8)	1.0 (1.0–4.8)	–	9 (5–13)	30	–	33 (55%)
Lewandowski [29]	–	7.32 ± 0.10	39 ± 7*	12 ± 3	3.4 ± 0.2	312 ± 216	–	23 ± 17	–	–	22 (45%)
Forrest [34]	57 (47–65)	7.20 (7.13–7.3)	–	16 (12–18)	3.7 (3.5–3.7)	48 (24–48)	34	10 (7–17)	37	3	5 (13%)
Frenckner [75]	47 (31–65)	–	41 (29–54)*	13 (0–20)	3.5 (3.0–4.0)	120 (24–672)	100	17 (2–57)	16	8	13 (34%)
Michaels [46]	52 ± 3	–	–	–	–	68 ± 9	–	7 ± 1	–	6	15 (40%)
Beiderlinden [30]	63 ± 28	7.1 ± 0.2	–	19 ± 3	3.8 ± 0.3	132 ± 168	–	10 (7–15)	–	–	15 (47%)

LIS, lung injury score; MV, mechanical ventilation; PEEP, positive end-expiratory pressure;
Data are given as mean ± SD or median (interquartile range). * Peak pressure; † in the survivors.

Table 3 Studies of ECMO for ARDS published before 1997 or including < 30 patients

First author [ref]	Design	Pros-pective	Setting	Follow up	Quality of the study	ECMO patients	Years	Age, years	Pre ECMO PaO_2/FiO_2, mmHg	Length of ECMO, days	Mortality, n (%)
Zapol [13]	RCT	Y	Multi	ICU discharge	RCT4	42	1979	12 to 65	< 83	< 5 days	39 (92%)
Macha [76]	Case series	N	Single	Hospital discharge	–	33	1990–1995	36 ± 2	59 ± 5	6 ± 1	13 (39%)
Cordell-Smith [77]	Case series	N	Single	ICU discharge	–	28	1992–2000	27 *	62 *	6 *	8 (29%)
Haneya [78]	Case series	Y	Single	ICU discharge	–	22	2010–2011	47 (36–61)	60 (46–75)	13 (8–19)	7 (32%)
Hodgson [66]	Case series	N	Single	8 months	–	21 £	2009–2011	36 ± 12	69 (50–105)	11 (4–16)	3 (14%)
Huang [79]	Case series	N	Single	ICU discharge	–	16	2003–2005	32 ± 22	54 ± 8	7 ± 4	6 (37%)
Isgrò [80]	Case series	Y	Single	Hospital discharge	–	12	2004–2009	35 ± 19	60 ± 11	–	6 (54%)
Oshima [81]	Case series	N	Single	ICU discharge	–	11	2003–2008	52 ± 24	90 ± 10	10 ± 9	5 (45%)
Bermudez [82]	Case series	N	Single	ICU discharge	–	11	2009–2010	34 (25–54)	45 (28–248)	3 (0–11)	5 (45%)
Goulon [83]	Case series	N	Single	8 months	–	11	1973–1976	29 (22–37)	39 ± 12	3 (1–4)	9 (82%)
Park [84]	Case series	N	Multi	60 days	–	10	2011	47 (14–71)	50 (36–56)	5 (3–32)	6 (60%)
Park [85]	Case series	N	Single	ICU discharge	–	9	2008–2011	56 (51–64)	57 ± 8	12 ± 6	10 (55%)
Huang [79]	Case series	N	Single	11 (8–51) months	–	9	2004–2007	35 ± 10	49 (31–64)	6 (3–19)	7 (78%)
Rossaint [86]	Case series	N	Single	Hospital discharge	–	8	1993–1995	35 (24–49)	43 ± 4	8 ± 9	2 (25%)

ICU: intensive care unit; Multi: multicenter; N: no; RCT: randomized controlled trial; Y: yes.
Data are given as mean ± SD or median (interquartile range). * Mean; £ 55% were H1N1 pneumonia.

that had ECMO capability while the patients randomized to the control group were treated conventionally at designated treatment centers [18]. The primary endpoint combining mortality or severe disability 6 months after randomization was lower for the 90 patients randomized to the ECMO group (37% vs. 53%, $p = 0.03$). However, the results of that trial should be analyzed carefully. First, 22 patients randomized to the ECMO arm did not receive ECMO (died before or during transport, improved with conventional management at the referral center or had a contraindication to heparin). Second, no standardized protocol for lung-protective mechanical ventilation existed in the control group and the time spent receiving 'protective' mechanical ventilation was significantly higher in the ECMO arm. Third, more patients received corticosteroids in the ECMO group.

ECMO and ARDS: Retrospective Series Using the Latest Technology

In the most recent series, patients benefited from the latest ECMO technology, which includes a centrifugal pump, a polymethylpentene membrane oxygenator and tubing with biocompatible surface treatment. Mortality rates range from 36 to 56% in the studies performed in the last 15 years and reporting outcomes of > 30 ECMO patients (Tables 1 and 2). Interestingly, ECMO was provided through a mobile ECMO rescue team in some of these studies. For example, in a series of 124 patients treated at a Danish center between 1997 and 2011 [31], survival was 71% and 85% of these patients received ECMO via a mobile unit before being transferred to the referral hospital. Similarly, in the Regensburg cohort, 59/176 received ECMO at another hospital by a mobile unit [32]. In a multicenter French cohort of 140 patients treated between 2008 and 2012, 68% patients were retrieved via a mobile ECMO team and their prognosis was comparable to those who received VV-ECMO support in their initial hospital [33].

ECMO support may also cause frequent, severe and potentially life-threatening complications (Table 2), such as bleeding, infections, intravascular hemolysis, thrombocytopenia or consumption coagulopathy [26, 33–36].

Results of ECMO for Pandemic Influenza A (H1N1)-Associated ARDS

Mortality rates ranged from 14 to 64% in the 16 studies from 11 countries reporting on the experience of ECMO for influenza A(H1N1)-associated ARDS (Tables 4 and 5) [15–17, 33, 37–48]. The Australia and New Zealand collaborative group (ANZICS) was the first to report its experience [15]. Despite extreme disease severity at the time of ECMO initiation (median PaO_2/FiO_2 ratio 56 mmHg, median positive end-expiratory pressure [PEEP] 18 cmH_2O and median lung injury score [LIS] of 3.8), only 25% of the 68 ECMO patients died. A British collaborative cohort series [16] depicted the outcome of 80 patients transferred into ECMO referral centers in the United Kingdom of whom 69 received ECMO. Mortality in this cohort was 27.5%. A propensity-matched analysis comparing survival of patients referred for consideration of ECMO to other ARDS patients showed better outcomes for referred patients. By contrast, mortality of propensity-matched patients treated conventionally was comparable to that of ECMO patients in French ICUs of the REVA network. However, only 50% of ECMO patients were successfully matched with control ARDS patients, while unmatched ECMO patients were younger, suffered more severe respiratory failure and had considerably lower mortality [17]. Interestingly, a higher plateau pressure under ECMO was independently associated with mortality, indicating for the first time that an ultraprotective ventilation strategy with reduction of plateau pressure to around 25 cmH_2O following ECMO installation might improve outcomes. Lastly, mortality was 29% in a cohort of 49 proven influenza A(H1N1) patients from the 14 ECMO centers of the ECMO-NET Italian collaborative group [48]. In this series, patients ventilated for less than 7 days before ECMO initiation had a significantly higher survival.

Mortality Risk Factors and Outcome Prediction for ECMO Candidates

Factors associated with poor outcomes after ECMO for acute respiratory failure include older age [26, 27, 30, 32, 33, 49, 50], a greater number of days of mechanical ventilation before ECMO establishment [26, 27, 30, 33, 50], a higher number of organ failures [26, 27, 30, 32, 33, 49, 50], low pre-ECMO respiratory system compliance [50], and immunosuppression [33, 50, 51]. Predictive survival models have been recently developed that might help clinicians select appropriate candidates for ECMO [33, 49–52]. For example, the Respiratory Extracorporeal Membrane Oxygenation Survival (RESP) score [50], constructed on data extracted from a large multicenter international population ($n = 2,355$), computes 12 simple pre-ECMO parameters, to provide a relevant and validated tool predicting survival after ECMO for acute respiratory failure. Cumulative predicted hospital survival rates were 92, 76, 57, 33 and 18% for five RESP-score risk classes, I (≥ 6), II (3 to 5), III (-1 to 2), IV (-5 to -2) and V (≤ -6), respectively.

Volume-outcome Effect and ECMO Activity Organization

Recent analyses of large pediatric databases have suggested a significant relationship between the volume of patients treated by center and ECMO patient prognosis [53–55]. ECMO case-series published after the pandemic influenza A(H1N1) might also allow a comparative analysis of worldwide results obtained for a very homogeneous disease (Tables 4 and 5). These data suggest that the best results were obtained for patients managed in expert centers treating a sufficient number of patients and in countries where ECMO activity was organized and regulated, as was the case in the United Kingdom [56], Italy [57] and in Australia and New Zealand [58]. A recent position paper [59] by an international group of physicians with expertise in ECMO for severe respiratory failure advocated for regional and interregional organization of ECMO activity through networks of hospitals around an

Table 4 Large studies of ECMO for H1N1-induced ARDS

	Pham [17]	Noah [16]	Davies [15]	Patroniti [48]	Schmidt [33]	Michaels [46]	Takeda [43]	Holzgraefe [40]
Patients, n	123$	69£	68	49	36	15	14	13
Number of centers	33	4	15	14	3	1	12	1
Study design	Case control	Case control	Case control	Case series	Case series	Case series	Case series	Case series
Newcastle-Ottawa scale	9	8	8	7	–	–	–	–
Age, years	42 (32–53)	34 (28–46)	36 (27–45)	39 (32–46)	39 (28–53)	34 ± 4	54 (43–60)	31 (25–50)
BMI, kg/m^2	30.5 ± 8.0	–	29 (23–36)	27 (24–35)	29 (25–36)	–	–	35 (31–42)
Pregnant or postpartum, n (%)	18 (15)	10 (17)	10 (16)	4 (8)	7 (19)	1(7)	1 (7)	3 (23)
SOFA	9.5 ± 4.0	9 (7–10)		7 (6–9)	11 (9–14)	–	16 (12–19)	–
Interval MV-ECMO, d	2 (1–5)	4 (2–7)	2 (1–5)	2 (1–5)	2 (0–5)	3.5 ± 0.8	5.0 (0.8–8.5)	1 (0–7)

Table 4 (Continuation)

	Pham [17]	Noah [16]	Davies [15]	Patroniti [48]	Schmidt [33]	Michaels [46]	Takeda [43]	Holzgraefe [40]
Pre-ECMO parameters								
pH	7.26 ± 0.12	–	7.20 (7.10–7.30)	7.30 (7.22–7.40)	7.22 (7.15–7.32)	–	–	7.30 (7.30–7.40)
PaO_2/FiO_2, mmHg	59 (51–71)	55 (46–63)	56 (48–63)	63 (56–79)	50 (41–55)	62 ± 6	50 (40–55)	52 (38–60)
Plateau pressure, mmHg	32 (29–35)	–	36 (33–38)	33 (30–35)	32 (30–35)	–	30 (29–35)	37 (31–38)
Lung injury score	3.5 (3.0–4.0)	3.5 (3.5–3.7)	3.8 (3.5–4.0)	3.8 (3.3–3.8)	–	–	–	3.6 (3.3–4.0)
Any rescue therapy	91 (74)	–	–	–	35 (97)	–	4 (29)	–
Nitric oxide, %	72	19	32	15	89	–	7	–
Prone position, %	45	34	20	28	67	–	21	–
Duration of ECMO, days	11 (8–22)	9 (6–12)	10 (7–15)	10 (7–17)	20 (9–38)	9 ± 1	9 (4–11)	16 (9–30)
Mortality, n (%)	44 (36)	22 (28)	17 (25)	14 (29)	6 (17)	6 (40)	9 (64)	2 (15)

BMI: body mass index; SOFA: sequential organ failure assessment; MV: mechanical ventilation
Data are given as mean ± SD or median (interquartile range)
$ Winter 2009–2010: 73 patients, winter 2010–2011: 50 patients
£ 80 patients were transferred to Leicester for consideration to receive ECMO and 69 received the device.

Table 5 Studies of ECMO for H1N1-associated ARDS reporting on $\leq$ 10 patients

	Roncon [42]	D'Ancona [38]	Roch [41]	Hou [45]	Bonastre [47]	Turner [44]	Chan [37]	Freed [39]
Country	Portugal	Italy	France	China	Spain	USA	Hong Kong	Canada
Patients, n	10	10	9	9	9	7	7	6
Study design	Case series	Case series	Case series	Case series	Case series	Case series	Case series	Case series
Number of centers	1	1	1	1	5	1	3	4
Age, years	40 (36–47)	36 (23–55)	49 (26–57)	31 ± 11	36 (28–42)	24 (16–25)	42 (39–50)	33 ± 7
BMI, kg/m^2	–	26 (21–48)	30 (25–80)	–	–	27 (26–29)	26 (26–27)	33 ± 7
Pregnant or postpartum	1(10)	0 (0)	1 (11)	4 (44)	–	1 (14)	0 (0)	–
SOFA	–	–	9 (8–10)	–	–	–	–	–
Interval MV-ECMO, d	6.5 (2.2–12.2)	–	0.5 (0.25–4.0)	6 (2–10)	5 (2–7)	6.0 (1.5–12.5)	–	5.0 (2.5–8.3)

Table 5 (Continuation)

	Roncon [42]	D'Ancona [38]	Roch [41]	Hou [45]	Bonastre [47]	Turner [44]	Chan [37]	Freed [39]
Pre-ECMO parameter								
pH	7.33 (7.28–7.38)	–	7.17 (7.04–7.25)	–		–	7.30 (7.19–7.36)	7.31 ± 0.05
PaO_2/FiO_2, mmHg	69 (56–84)	–	52 (50–60)	53 (45–64)	66 (64–102)	57 (51–62)	56 (53–71)	58 ± 17
Plateau pressure, mmHg	35 (32–36)	–	31 (30–35)	–	–	–	33 (30–35) *	44 ± 42 *
Lung injury score	3.5 (3.3–3.8)	–	3.6 (3.3–3.7)	3.6 (3.25–3.75)	–	–	3.8 (3.8–3.9)	–
Any rescue therapy, %	70	100	–	–	–	100	14	100
Nitric oxide, %	60	–	67	–		100	0	67
Prone position, %	10	–	22	–		0	14	33
Duration of ECMO, days	22 (14–32)	–	9 (4–14)	18 (3–90)	6 (5–22)	13 (8–37)	6 (6–10)	15 (14–15)
Mortality, n (%)	4 (40)	5 (50)	5 (56)	4 (44)	5 (56)	2 (28)	1 (14)	2 (33)

BMI: Body mass index; SOFA: Sequential Organ Failure Assessment; MV: mechanical ventilation; Data are given as mean ± SD or median (interquartile range). * Peak pressure.

ECMO referral center with a mobile ECMO unit [34, 60, 61] to retrieve the most severe ARDS patients. This group also suggested that at least 20 ECMO cases should be performed per year at each referral center [59]. Furthermore, high volume and expert referral centers may provide better prevention and management of the severe complications that can occur during long ECMO runs (Table 2).

Long Term Outcomes After ECMO

Durations of intensive care and hospital stays of ECMO patients are long and frequently exceed one month [26, 33]. Thus, evaluation of the impact of such complex therapy on long-term pulmonary function, quality of life and psychological status appears crucial in the decision process to use ECMO in ARDS patients. To date, long-term prognosis after ECMO for ARDS has rarely been evaluated. Linden et al. reported long-term outcomes of 21 ARDS survivors rescued with ECMO [62]. In this study, most of the patients had limited fibrosis lesions on CT scan. Respiratory function tests were within normal limits. However, patients reported deterioration in pulmonary symptoms measured by the St George Respiratory Questionnaire, although these symptoms were comparable to those reported in other series of ARDS patients treated conventionally. Similarly, patients in the ECMO arm of the CESAR trial [18] exhibited comparable or better health-related quality of life scores (measured by the SF-36 questionnaire) than those reported by patients with ARDS treated with conventional management [63, 64]. Exertional dyspnea was reported by 50% and 40% of 12 influenza A(H1N1) ECMO patients and 25 controls, respectively [65]. Anxiety and depressive symptoms were reported by 50% and 28% of ECMO patients, respectively, whereas 41% were at risk of post-traumatic stress disorder (PTSD) [65]. By contrast, results of the Melbourne group were poorer, with only 26% of long-term survivors having returned to their previous work at eight-month-follow-up [66]. Similar to previous studies, mean SF-36 scores in the ECMO population were lower than these previously described with ARDS survivors in the domains of general health, mental health, vitality and social function. Lastly, the largest study published to date was reported by Schmidt et al. [33] on a population of 84 6-month survivors. In that series, 36% of the patients reported exertional dyspnea, whereas 30% were still receiving pulmonary treatments after a median 17-month follow-up. Health-related quality of life evaluation in 80% of the 6-month survivors revealed satisfactory mental health but persistent physical and emotional-related difficulties, with anxiety, depression or PTSD symptoms reported by 34, 25 and 16%, respectively.

Results of Extracorporeal CO_2 Removal Techniques for ARDS Patients

To date, studies on $ECCO_2R$ in ARDS patients are scarce and mostly small retrospective case series (Table 6). Gattinoni et al. reported in 1986 the first cohort of 43 patients with severe ARDS treated with veno-venous, low flow (200–

Table 6 Studies reporting on $ECCO_2R$ for ARDS

	Gattinoni [67]	Morris [14]	Bein [11]	Flörchinger [69]	Brunet [87]	Muellenbach [88]	Nierhaus [89]	Cho [90]	Conrad [91]	Iglesias [68]
Country	Italy	USA	Germany	Germany	France	Germany	Germany	Korea	USA	Spain
Design	Case series	RCT	RCT	Case series	Case series	Case series	Case series	Case series	Case series	Case series
Prospective	Y	Y	Y	Y	Y	N	N	Y	Y	Y
Setting	Single	Mulit	Multi	Single	Single	Single	Single	Single	Multi	Single
Quality assessment §	–	RCT5	RCT6	–	–	–	–	–	–	–
Type of CO_2 removal device, AV/VV	VV	VV	AV	AV	VV	AV	AV	AV	AV	AV
Patients received $ECCO_2R$, n	43	21	40	159	23	22	13	11	8	7
Years	1980–1985	1987–1991	2007–2010	1996–2007	1989–1991	2002–2006	–	2010	1997–1999	2005–2006
Age, years			50 ± 12	44 ± 17	29 ± 10	38 ± 15	52 ± 19	58 ± 15	44 ± 8	53.7 ± 16.0
SOFA score			–	159	15 ± 5	–	–	8.8 ± 1.8	–	–

Table 6 (Continuation)

	Gattinoni [67]	Morris [14]	Bein [11]	Flörchinger [69]	Brunet [87]	Muellenbach [88]	Nierhaus [89]	Cho [90]	Conrad [91]	Iglesias [68]
Pre-CO_2 removal										
PO_2/FiO_2, mmHg	67		152 ± 37	72 ± 37	84 ± 30	61 (47–85)$	100 ± 29	110 ± 36.6	–	90
PCo_2, mmHg	49 ± 11		57 ± 12	65 ± 24	56 ± 20	65 (54–72) $	80 ± 23	84 ± 23	90.8 ± 7.5	70
Plateau pressure, cmH_2O	–		29 ± 5	37 ± 6 *	51 ± 9 *	40 (36–46)*$	34 ± 3*	30.1 ± 7.1	–	22.0 ± 7.4
Lung injury score	–		2.8 ± 0.7	–	3.4 ± 0.4	3.5 (3–3.7)	–	–	–	2.9 ± 0.3
Delay MV – extracorporeal CO_2 removal, days	–		< 7	7 ± 13	9.2 ± 7.7	1 (0.5–1.9)	9.4 ± 10.2	8.6 ± 12.6	–	4 ± 2
Post-cannulation PCo_2 (24 h), mmHg	–		–	35 ± 7	41 ± 7	39 (36–42) $	54 ± 19	40.7 ± 10.2	51.8 ± 3.1	45
Length of CO_2 removal device, days	8 ± 5		7.4 ± 4.0	8 ± 6	13 (1–55)	5.3 (3.2–8.2)	12 ± 22	8.6 ± 9.4	–	4.3 ± 2.5

Table 6 (Continuation)

	Gattinoni [67]	Morris [14]	Bein [11]	Flörchinger [69]	Brunet [87]	Muellen-bach [88]	Nierhaus [89]	Cho [90]	Conrad [91]	Iglesias [68]
Serious complica-tion, n (%)	3 (7)		3 (7)	25 (16)	5 (22)	5 (23)	2 (15)	3 (27)	0 (0)	1 (14
Ischemia lower limb	–		1 (2)	13 (8)	–	3 (14)	0	0	0	0
Compartment syndrome	–		–	4 (2.5)	–	1 (4)	0	0	0	0
Cannula thrombosis	–		–	8 (5)	–	–	0	0	0	1
Mortality, n (%)	22 (51)	7 (33)	7 (17)	104 (65)	12 (52)	6 (27)	7 (54)	9 (82)	4 (50)	1 (14)

AV: arteriovenous; VV: veno-venous; Multi: multicenter; MV: mechanical ventilation; N: no; RCT: randomized controlled trial; SOFA: Sequential Organ Failure Assessment; Y: yes; *Peak pressure; §RCT quality was graded using a nine-point scale combining elements from Jadad's [21] and Chalmers' scales [23, 24] whereas the validity of case-controlled studies was appraised with the Newcastle-Ottawa scale [25]. Data are given as mean ± SD or median (interquartile range).

300 ml/min) $ECCO_2R$, which needed a boot volume of almost two liters of blood [67]. In this series, $ECCO_2R$ duration was 5 days, daily blood losses were large (> 1,800 ml/24 hours) and survival was 49%. A randomized study using the same technology was carried out in the early 1990s by Morris et al. [14]. It was stopped for futility after the enrolment of only 40 patients and mortality was 67% in the 21 patients randomized to $ECCO_2R$. In the 2000s, case series, which used the pumpless arteriovenous shunt (extracorporeal interventional lung assist, iLA, Novalung®, Heilbronn, Germany) were published. Iglesias et al. [68] reported the outcome of seven patients with ARDS after pneumonectomy. The $ECCO_2R$ device was left in place for four days, CO_2 removal was 255 ml/min allowing significant reduction in tidal volume and 6/7 patients survived (Table 6). In a larger German cohort of 156 patients, a higher mortality was reported (65%). Of note, 16% of the patients experienced serious complications in that cohort, particularly leg ischemia related to femoral arterial cannulation and need for higher dose catecholamines (Table 6) [69].

The concept of ultraprotective mechanical ventilation was tested in a proof-of concept trial, with CO_2 removal performed by a modified veno-venous hemofiltration platform. In 10 patients with plateau pressure of 28–30 cmH_2O at baseline, $ECCO_2R$ allowed a reduction of tidal volume (from 6 to 4 ml/kg) and of plateau pressure (from 29 to 25 cmH_2O), while maintaining $PaCO_2$ around 50 mmHg [19]. This protective ventilation strategy was also associated with a significant reduction in pro-inflammatory cytokine levels in bronchoalveolar (BAL) fluid. This ultraprotective ventilation strategy was recently evaluated in the Xtravent trial [11], which randomized 79 patients to conventional mechanical ventilation using the ARDSNet strategy [70] or to tidal volume reduction to 3 ml/kg permitted by CO_2 removal with the Novalung AV pumpless $ECCO_2R$ device. The numbers of ventilator-free days at day 60 were not different between groups. However, a post-hoc subgroup analysis revealed that patients with lower PaO_2/FiO_2 ($\leq$ 150 mmHg) at randomization had significantly more ventilator-free days at days 28 and 60 and were more rapidly weaned from mechanical ventilation.

Conclusion and Perspectives

We report the results of 56 studies (including 4 RCTs) evaluating extracorporeal gas exchange techniques (ECMO or $ECCO_2$-R) to treat moderate to severe acute respiratory failure in adult patients. Major heterogeneity in study populations, disease severity, type of device used and time at which studies were performed creates insuperable hurdles to design relevant meta-analyses. Results of the most recent randomized CESAR trial, which was conducted in the UK from 2001 to 2006, suggested that a strategy of transfer to an ECMO referral center for consideration to receive ECMO was associated with better outcomes. However, that trial was highly criticized for methodological limitations. Additionally, non-randomized case-series of ECMO, including propensity-matched case-control studies, are prone to important selection biases weakening interpretation of their results. Although early implementation of VV-ECMO in severe ARDS patients might allow significant reduction in ventilator-induced lung injury (VILI) and may rescue patients dying of refractory hypoxemia, more evidence is urgently needed to evaluate the actual impact of the technique on patient-centered outcomes compared to optimization of conventional treatments, including prone positioning [2]. This is the main objective of the ongoing international multicenter randomized Extracorporeal Membrane Oxygenation for Severe Acute Respiratory Distress Syndrome (EOLIA) trial (ClinicalTrials.gov Identifier: NCT01470703), which will test the efficacy of early VV-ECMO in patients with severe ARDS with tight control of mechanical ventilation in the control group, initiation of ECMO prior to transportation to ECMO centers, and the use of ECMO in every patient randomly assigned to receive it [71].

Pathophysiological, experimental and clinical data suggest that an 'ultraprotective' mechanical ventilation strategy reducing tidal volume to 3–4 ml/kg predicted body weight and plateau pressure to $<25\,cmH_2O$ may further reduce VILI and ARDS-associated morbidity and mortality in less severe ARDS patients. Hypercapnia induced by tidal volume reduction in this setting might be efficiently controlled by the latest generation low-flow, venovenous $ECCO_2R$ devices, which are more efficient, more biocompatible and associated with fewer hemorrhagic complications because they require less anticoagulation than devices evaluated in the 1980s and 90s, which did not achieve significant mortality reduction. However, the uncritical and large adoption of this strategy is premature and problematic without rigorous evaluation of associated risks and benefits. This will be the objective of the large randomized Strategy of Ultra Protective lung ventilation with Extracorporeal CO_2 Removal for New-Onset moderate to severe ARDS (SUPERNOVA) trial, which will test the benefits of early tidal volume and plateau pressure reduction allowed by the latest generation $ECCO_2R$ device in patients with moderate forms of ARDS [72].

Lastly, future studies of extracorporeal gas exchange should also include detailed evaluation of physical and psychosocial rehabilitation that could lead to improved long-term health-related quality of life in this population of patients.

Acknowledgement

Matthieu Schmidt was supported by the French Intensive Care Society (SRLF), the "Fonds de dotation Recherche en Santé Respiratoire, 2012", the "Collège des Enseignants de Réanimation Médicale" and the "Département du Développement professionnel continu médical – Assistance publique-Hôpitaux de Paris".

References

1. Dreyfuss D, Soler P, Basset G, Saumon G (1988) High inflation pressure pulmonary edema. Respective effects of high airway pressure, high tidal volume, and positive end-expiratory pressure. Am Rev Respir Dis 137:1159–1164
2. Guerin C, Reignier J, Richard JC et al (2013) Prone positioning in severe acute respiratory distress syndrome. N Engl J Med 368:2159–2168
3. Papazian L, Forel JM, Gacouin A et al (2010) Neuromuscular blockers in early acute respiratory distress syndrome. N Engl J Med 363:1107–1116
4. Hill JD, O'Brien TG, Murray JJ et al (1972) Prolonged extracorporeal oxygenation for acute post-traumatic respiratory failure (shock-lung syndrome). Use of the Bramson membrane lung. N Engl J Med 286:629–634
5. Kolobow T, Zapol W, Pierce JE, Keeley AF, Replogle RL, Haller A (1968) Partial extracorporeal gas exchange in alert newborn lambs with a membrane artificial lung perfused via an A-V shunt for periods up to 96 hours. Trans Am Soc Artif Intern Organs 14:328–334
6. Combes A, Brechot N, Luyt CE, Schmidt M (2012) What is the niche for extracorporeal membrane oxygenation in severe acute respiratory distress syndrome? Curr Opin Crit Care 18:527–532
7. Brodie D, Bacchetta M (2012) Extracorporeal membrane oxygenation for ARDS in adults. N Engl J Med 365:1905–1914
8. Combes A, Bacchetta M, Brodie D, Muller T, Pellegrino V (2012) Extracorporeal membrane oxygenation for respiratory failure in adults. Curr Opin Crit Care 18:99–104
9. MacLaren G, Combes A, Bartlett RH (2012) Contemporary extracorporeal membrane oxygenation for adult respiratory failure: life support in the new era. Intensive Care Med 38:210–220
10. Cove ME, Maclaren G, Federspiel WJ, Kellum JA (2012) Bench to bedside review: Extracorporeal carbon dioxide removal, past present and future. Crit Care 16:232
11. Bein T, Weber-Carstens S, Goldmann A et al (2013) Lower tidal volume strategy (approximately 3 ml/kg) combined with extracorporeal CO2 removal versus 'conventional' protective ventilation (6 ml/kg) in severe ARDS: the prospective randomized Xtravent-study. Intensive Care Med 39:847–856
12. Schmidt M, Tachon G, Devilliers C et al (2013) Blood oxygenation and decarboxylation determinants during venovenous ECMO for respiratory failure in adults. Intensive Care Med 39:838–846
13. Zapol WM, Snider MT, Hill JD et al (1979) Extracorporeal membrane oxygenation in severe acute respiratory failure. A randomized prospective study. JAMA 242:2193–2196
14. Morris AH, Wallace CJ, Menlove RL et al (1994) Randomized clinical trial of pressure-controlled inverse ratio ventilation and extracorporeal CO2 removal for adult respiratory distress syndrome. Am J Respir Crit Care Med 149:295–305
15. Davies A, Jones D, Bailey M et al (2009) Extracorporeal Membrane Oxygenation for 2009 Influenza A(H1N1) Acute Respiratory Distress Syndrome. JAMA 302:1888–1895
16. Noah MA, Peek GJ, Finney SJ et al (2011) Referral to an extracorporeal membrane oxygenation center and mortality among patients with severe 2009 influenza A(H1N1). JAMA 306:1659–1668
17. Pham T, Combes A, Roze H et al (2013) Extracorporeal membrane oxygenation for pandemic influenza A(H1N1)-induced acute respiratory distress syndrome: A cohort study and propensity-matched analysis. Am J Respir Crit Care Med 187:276–285
18. Peek GJ, Mugford M, Tiruvoipati R et al (2009) Efficacy and economic assessment of conventional ventilatory support versus extracorporeal membrane oxygenation for severe adult respiratory failure (CESAR): a multicentre randomised controlled trial. Lancet 374:1351–1363
19. Terragni PP, Del Sorbo L, Mascia L et al (2009) Tidal volume lower than 6 ml/kg enhances lung protection: role of extracorporeal carbon dioxide removal. Anesthesiology 111:826–835

20. Moher D, Liberati A, Tetzlaff J, Altman DG (2009) Preferred reporting items for systematic reviews and meta-analyses: the PRISMA statement. Ann Intern Med 151:264–269 (W264)
21. Jadad AR, Moore RA, Carroll D et al (1996) Assessing the quality of reports of randomized clinical trials: is blinding necessary? Control Clin Trials 17:1–12
22. Wells GA, Shea B, O'Connell D et al The Newcastle-Ottawa Scale (NOS) for assessing the quality of nonrandomised studies in meta-analyses. http://www.ohri.ca/programs/clinical_epidemiology/oxford.asp
23. Chalmers TC, Smith H Jr, Blackburn B et al (1981) A method for assessing the quality of a randomized control trial. Control Clin Trials 2:31–49
24. Mitchell MD, Mikkelsen ME, Umscheid CA, Lee I, Fuchs BD, Halpern SD (2010) A systematic review to inform institutional decisions about the use of extracorporeal membrane oxygenation during the H1N1 influenza pandemic. Crit Care Med 38:1398–1404
25. Stang A (2010) Critical evaluation of the Newcastle-Ottawa scale for the assessment of the quality of nonrandomized studies in meta-analyses. Eur J Epidemiol 25:603–605
26. Brogan TV, Thiagarajan RR, Rycus PT, Bartlett RH, Bratton SL (2009) Extracorporeal membrane oxygenation in adults with severe respiratory failure: a multi-center database. Intensive Care Med 35:2105–2114
27. Hemmila MR, Rowe SA, Boules TN et al (2004) Extracorporeal life support for severe acute respiratory distress syndrome in adults. Ann Surg 240:595–605
28. Mols G, Loop T, Geiger K, Farthmann E, Benzing A (2000) Extracorporeal membrane oxygenation: a ten-year experience. Am J Surg 180:144–154
29. Lewandowski K, Rossaint R, Pappert D et al (1997) High survival rate in 122 ARDS patients managed according to a clinical algorithm including extracorporeal membrane oxygenation. Intensive Care Med 23:819–835
30. Beiderlinden M, Eikermann M, Boes T, Breitfeld C, Peters J (2006) Treatment of severe acute respiratory distress syndrome: role of extracorporeal gas exchange. Intensive Care Med 32:1627–1631
31. Lindskov C, Jensen RH, Sprogoe P et al (2013) Extracorporeal membrane oxygenation in adult patients with severe acute respiratory failure. Acta Anaesthesiol Scand 57:303–311
32. Schmid C, Philipp A, Hilker M et al (2012) Venovenous extracorporeal membrane oxygenation for acute lung failure in adults. J Heart Lung Transplant 31:9–15
33. Schmidt M, Zogheib E, Roze H et al (2013) The PRESERVE mortality risk score and analysis of long-term outcomes after extracorporeal membrane oxygenation for severe acute respiratory distress syndrome. Intensive Care Med 39:1704–1713
34. Forrest P, Ratchford J, Burns B et al (2011) Retrieval of critically ill adults using extracorporeal membrane oxygenation: an Australian experience. Intensive Care Med 37:824–830
35. Muller T, Philipp A, Luchner A et al (2009) A new miniaturized system for extracorporeal membrane oxygenation in adult respiratory failure. Crit Care 13:R205
36. Schmidt M, Brechot N, Hariri S et al (2012) Nosocomial infections in adult cardiogenic shock patients supported by venoarterial extracorporeal membrane oxygenation. Clin Infect Dis 55:1633–1641
37. Chan KK, Lee KL, Lam PK, Law KI, Joynt GM, Yan WW (2010) Hong Kong's experience on the use of extracorporeal membrane oxygenation for the treatment of influenza A (H1N1). Hong Kong Med J 16:447–454
38. D'Ancona G, Capitanio G, Chiaramonte G et al (2011) Extracorporeal membrane oxygenator rescue and airborne transportation of patients with influenza A (H1N1) acute respiratory distress syndrome in a Mediterranean underserved area. Interact Cardiovasc Thorac Surg 12:935–937
39. Freed DH, Henzler D, White CW et al (2010) Extracorporeal lung support for patients who had severe respiratory failure secondary to influenza A (H1N1) 2009 infection in Canada. Can J Anaesth 57:240–247
40. Holzgraefe B, Broome M, Kalzen H, Konrad D, Palmer K, Frenckner B (2010) Extracorporeal membrane oxygenation for pandemic H1N1 2009 respiratory failure. Minerva Anestesiol 76:1043–1051

41. Roch A, Lepaul-Ercole R, Grisoli D et al (2010) Extracorporeal membrane oxygenation for severe influenza A (H1N1) acute respiratory distress syndrome: a prospective observational comparative study. Intensive Care Med 36:1899–1905
42. Roncon-Albuquerque R Jr., Basilio C, Figueiredo P et al (2012) Portable miniaturized extracorporeal membrane oxygenation systems for H1N1-related severe acute respiratory distress syndrome: A case series. J Crit Care 27:454–463
43. Takeda S, Kotani T, Nakagawa S et al (2012) Extracorporeal membrane oxygenation for 2009 influenza A(H1N1) severe respiratory failure in Japan. J Anesth 26:650–657
44. Turner DA, Rehder KJ, Peterson-Carmichael SL et al (2011) Extracorporeal membrane oxygenation for severe refractory respiratory failure secondary to 2009 H1N1 influenza A. Respir Care 56:941–946
45. Hou X, Guo L, Zhan Q et al (2012) Extracorporeal membrane oxygenation for critically ill patients with 2009 influenza A (H1N1)-related acute respiratory distress syndrome: preliminary experience from a single center. Artif Organs 36:780–786
46. Michaels AJ, Hill JG, Bliss D et al (2013) Pandemic flu and the sudden demand for ECMO resources: a mature trauma program can provide surge capacity in acute critical care crises. J Trauma Acute Care Surg 74:1493–1497
47. Bonastre J, Suberviola B, Pozo JC et al (2012) Extracorporeal lung support in patients with severe respiratory failure secondary to the 2010–2011 winter seasonal outbreak of influenza A (H1N1) in Spain. Med Intensiva 36:193–199
48. Patroniti N, Zangrillo A, Pappalardo F et al (2011) The Italian ECMO network experience during the 2009 influenza A(H1N1) pandemic: preparation for severe respiratory emergency outbreaks. Intensive Care Med 37:1447–1457
49. Roch A, Hraiech S, Masson E et al (2014) Outcome of acute respiratory distress syndrome patients treated with extracorporeal membrane oxygenation and brought to a referral center. Intensive Care Med 40:74–83
50. Schmidt M, Bailey M, Sheldrake J et al (2014) Predicting survival after extracorporeal membrane oxygenation for severe acute respiratory failure. The Respiratory Extracorporeal Membrane Oxygenation Survival Prediction (RESP) Score. Am J Respir Crit Care Med 189:1374–1382
51. Enger T, Philipp A, Videm V et al (2014) Prediction of mortality in adult patients with severe acute lung failure receiving veno-venous extracorporeal membrane oxygenation: a prospective observational study. Crit Care 18:R67
52. Pappalardo F, Pieri M, Greco T et al (2013) Predicting mortality risk in patients undergoing venovenous ECMO for ARDS due to influenza A (H1N1) pneumonia: the ECMOnet score. Intensive Care Med 39:275–281
53. Campbell BT, Braun TM, Schumacher RE, Bartlett RH, Hirschl RB (2003) Impact of ECMO on neonatal mortality in Michigan (1980–1999). J Pediatr Surg 38:290–295
54. Jen HC, Shew SB (2010) Hospital readmissions and survival after nonneonatal pediatric ECMO. Pediatrics 125:1217–1223
55. Karamlou T, Vafaeezadeh M, Parrish AM et al (2013) Increased extracorporeal membrane oxygenation center case volume is associated with improved extracorporeal membrane oxygenation survival among pediatric patients. J Thorac Cardiovasc Surg 145:470–475
56. Extracorporeal membrane oxygenation for severe acute respiratory failure in adults: NHS NICE GUIDANCE Available at: http://www.nice.org.uk/guidance/IPG391 Accessed December 2014
57. ECMOnet. Available at: http://www.ecmonet.org/. Accessed March 14th 2014
58. NSW Critical Care Tertiary Referral Networks and Transfer of Care (ADULTS). Available at: http://www0.health.nsw.gov.au/policies/pd/2010/pdf/PD2010_021.pdf Accessed December 14, 2014
59. Combes A, Brodie D, Bartlett R et al (2014) Position paper for the organization of extracorporeal membrane oxygenation programs for acute respiratory failure in adult patients. Am J Respir Crit Care Med 190:488–496

60. Beurtheret S, Mordant P, Paoletti X et al (2013) Emergency circulatory support in refractory cardiogenic shock patients in remote institutions: a pilot study (the cardiac-RESCUE program). Eur Heart J 34:112–120
61. Linden V, Palmer K, Reinhard J et al (2000) High survival in adult patients with acute respiratory distress syndrome treated by extracorporeal membrane oxygenation, minimal sedation, and pressure supported ventilation. Intensive Care Med 26:1630–1637
62. Linden VB, Lidegran MK, Frisen G, Dahlgren P, Frenckner BP, Larsen F (2009) ECMO in ARDS: a long-term follow-up study regarding pulmonary morphology and function and health-related quality of life. Acta Anaesthesiol Scand 53:489–495
63. Herridge MS, Cheung AM, Tansey CM et al (2003) One-year outcomes in survivors of the acute respiratory distress syndrome. N Engl J Med 348:683–693
64. Schelling G, Stoll C, Haller M et al (1998) Health-related quality of life and posttraumatic stress disorder in survivors of the acute respiratory distress syndrome. Crit Care Med 26:651–659
65. Luyt CE, Combes A, Becquemin MH et al (2012) Long-term outcomes of pandemic 2009 influenza A(H1N1)-associated severe ARDS. Chest 142:583–592
66. Hodgson CL, Hayes K, Everard T et al (2012) Long-term quality of life in patients with acute respiratory distress syndrome requiring extracorporeal membrane oxygenation for refractory hypoxaemia. Crit Care 16:R202
67. Gattinoni L, Pesenti A, Mascheroni D et al (1986) Low-frequency positive-pressure ventilation with extracorporeal CO2 removal in severe acute respiratory failure. JAMA 256:881–886
68. Iglesias M, Martinez E, Badia JR, Macchiarini P (2008) Extrapulmonary ventilation for unresponsive severe acute respiratory distress syndrome after pulmonary resection. Ann Thorac Surg 85:237–244
69. Florchinger B, Philipp A, Klose A et al (2008) Pumpless extracorporeal lung assist: a 10-year institutional experience. Ann Thorac Surg 86:410–417 (discussion 417)
70. The Acute Respiratory Distress Syndrome Network (2000) Ventilation with lower tidal volumes as compared with traditional tidal volumes for acute lung injury and the acute respiratory distress syndrome. N Engl J Med 342:1301–1308
71. EOLIA trial. Available at: http://www.clinicaltrials.gov/ct2/show/NCT01470703?term=eolia&rank=1. Accessed December 2014
72. SUPERNOVA trial of ECCO2-R for moderate ARDS. Available at: http://www.esicm.org/research/trials-group/supernova. Accessed December 2014
73. Paden ML, Conrad SA, Rycus PT, Thiagarajan RR (2013) Extracorporeal Life Support Organization Registry Report 2012. ASAIO J 59:202–210
74. Rega FR, Evrard V, Bollen H et al (2007) pH 48 h after onset of extracorporeal membrane oxygenation is an independent predictor of survival in patients with respiratory failure. Artif Organs 31:384–389
75. Frenckner B, Palmer P, Linden V (2002) Extracorporeal respiratory support and minimally invasive ventilation in severe ARDS. Minerva Anestesiol 68:381–386
76. Macha M, Griffith BP, Keenan R et al (1996) ECMO support for adult patients with acute respiratory failure. ASAIO J 42:M841–844
77. Cordell-Smith JA, Roberts N, Peek GJ, Firmin RK (2006) Traumatic lung injury treated by extracorporeal membrane oxygenation (ECMO). Injury 37:29–32
78. Haneya A, Philipp A, Foltan M et al (2012) First experience with the new portable extracorporeal membrane oxygenation system Cardiohelp for severe respiratory failure in adults. Perfusion 27:150–155
79. Huang YK, Liu KS, Lu MS, Wu MY, Tsai FC, Lin PJ (2009) Extracorporeal life support in post-traumatic respiratory distress patients. Resuscitation 80:535–539
80. Isgro S, Patroniti N, Bombino M et al (2011) Extracorporeal membrane oxygenation for interhospital transfer of severe acute respiratory distress syndrome patients: 5-year experience. Int J Artif Organs 34:1052–1060

81. Oshima K, Kunimoto F, Hinohara H et al (2010) Evaluation of prognosis in patients with respiratory failure requiring venovenous extracorporeal membrane oxygenation (ECMO). Ann Thorac Cardiovasc Surg 16:156–162
82. Bermudez CA, Rocha RV, Sappington PL, Toyoda Y, Murray HN, Boujoukos AJ (2010) Initial experience with single cannulation for venovenous extracorporeal oxygenation in adults. Ann Thorac Surg 90:991–995
83. Goulon M, Raphael JC, Gajdos P, Barois A, Babinet P, Margent P (1978) Membrane oxygenators for acute respiratory insufficiency. Clinical use in 11 patients. Intensive Care Med 4:173–179
84. Park M, Azevedo LC, Mendes PV et al (2012) First-year experience of a Brazilian tertiary medical center in supporting severely ill patients using extracorporeal membrane oxygenation. Clinics (Sao Paulo, Brazil) 67:1157–1163
85. Park YH, Hwang S, Park HW et al (2012) Effect of pulmonary support using extracorporeal membrane oxygenation for adult liver transplant recipients with respiratory failure. Transplant Proc 44:757–761
86. Rossaint R, Pappert D, Gerlach H, Lewandowski K, Keh D, Falke K (1997) Extracorporeal membrane oxygenation for transport of hypoxaemic patients with severe ARDS. Br J Anaesth 78:241–246
87. Brunet F, Belghith M, Mira JP et al (1993) Extracorporeal carbon dioxide removal and low-frequency positive-pressure ventilation. Improvement in arterial oxygenation with reduction of risk of pulmonary barotrauma in patients with adult respiratory distress syndrome. Chest 104:889–898
88. Muellenbach RM, Kredel M, Wunder C et al (2008) Arteriovenous extracorporeal lung assist as integral part of a multimodal treatment concept: a retrospective analysis of 22 patients with ARDS refractory to standard care. Eur J Anaesthesiol 25:897–904
89. Nierhaus A, Frings D, Braune S et al (2011) Interventional lung assist enables lung protective mechanical ventilation in acute respiratory distress syndrome. Minerva Anestesiol 77:797–801
90. Cho WH, Lee K, Huh JW, Lim CM, Koh Y, Hong SB (2012) Physiologic effect and safety of the pumpless extracorporeal interventional lung assist system in patients with acute respiratory failure – a pilot study. Artif Organs 36:434–438
91. Conrad SA, Zwischenberger JB, Grier LR, Alpard SK, Bidani A (2001) Total extracorporeal arteriovenous carbon dioxide removal in acute respiratory failure: a phase I clinical study. Intensive Care Med 27:1340–1351

Update on the Role of Extracorporeal CO_2 Removal as an Adjunct to Mechanical Ventilation in ARDS

P. Morimont, A. Batchinsky, and B. Lambermont

Introduction

Despite new promising therapeutic interventions including protective ventilation, prone positioning, use of neuromuscular blockers and conservative fluid balance, acute respiratory distress syndrome (ARDS) remains a devastating disease [1, 2]. Mortality rates for ARDS have decreased over time but still remain around 40%, in large part a result of the hemodynamic complications of this syndrome [3]. ARDS has various etiologies and early diagnosis and intervention are key to improving outcomes [4]. Dominant features of ARDS include injury to the alveolar-capillary membrane, which results in severe hypoxemia, decrease in pulmonary compliance, and increase in pulmonary vascular resistance [5, 6]. At present, positive-pressure mechanical ventilation is the mainstay of symptomatic treatment for ARDS [1], but may further increase pulmonary hypertension and right ventricular (RV) afterload, leading to acute *cor pulmonale* and RV failure [6]. Moreover, mechanical ventilation induces additional lung injuries due to overdistention, repeated stretch to the alveoli, atelectotrauma, and increased inflammatory mediator levels [7]. The ARDSNet study reported a reduction in mortality with a ventilation strategy involving limitation of mean tidal volume to 6 ml/kg, as compared with a more traditional tidal volume of 12 ml/kg [1]. However, utilization of lower tidal volumes leads to permissive hypercapnia and most clinicians seldom use very low tidal volumes in practice. Indeed, the need to substantially reduce tidal volume to improve outcome in ARDS patients remains questionable because of the deleterious effects of hypercapnia [8]. In addition, lung injury persists even when tidal volumes are small

P. Morimont ✉ · B. Lambermont
Medical and Coronary Intensive Care Unit, Department of Internal Medicine, University Hospital of Liege, Liege, Belgium
e-mail: ph.morimont@chu.ulg.ac.be

A. Batchinsky
U.S. Army Institute of Surgical Research, Battlefield Health and Trauma Research Institute, Fort Sam Houston, San Antonio, USA

J.-L. Vincent (ed.), *Annual Update in Intensive Care and Emergency Medicine 2015*,
DOI 10.1007/978-3-319-13761-2_15

[9] and further reduction in tidal volume beyond those recommended by ARDSNet may have outcome benefits [10], although not all agree [11]. Thus, modern care for ARDS requires a decision to maximally reduce ventilator settings to ensure lung protection and reduce exacerbation of lung injury while facing the metabolic consequences of this intervention. How can we enhance lung protection in ARDS while not causing metabolic disturbances?

As the discussion about optimization of mechanical ventilation in ARDS patients continues, a new promising adjunct is low-flow partial lung support or extracorporeal CO_2 removal (ECCO$_2$R). This approach takes advantage of a concept proposed many years ago [12] which, carried out with modern technology, has been shown to effectively remove metabolically produced CO_2 while permitting significant reductions in minute ventilation in preclinical [13, 14] and clinical settings [15]. Specifically, combination therapy using reduction in tidal volumes to around 4 ml/kg and concomitant use of ECCO$_2$R has been shown to effectively manage permissive hypercapnia in ARDS [15]. Thus ECCO$_2$R could be an effective strategy in ARDS management and a viable option to combat the deleterious effects of low-tidal volume ventilation, such as permissive hypercapnia.

The purpose of this manuscript is to elaborate on potential applications of ECCO$_2$R as an adjunct to mechanical ventilation for the treatment of ARDS. We discuss the effects of hypercapnia in ARDS and the emerging evidence for the utility of ECCO$_2$R during hypercapnia; as well as the potential role of ECCO$_2$R in optimizing RV-pulmonary artery coupling and RV function in lung failure.

Hypercapnic Acidosis: More Deleterious than Beneficial?

Cellular and Metabolic Effects

Depending on its degree and duration, permissive hypercapnia has a series of potential adverse effects related to systemic and cerebral vasodilatation, cardiovascular depression, arrhythmia, and increase in gastric hydrogen ion secretion [16]. Until recently, however, cellular and metabolic effects of hypercapnia in ARDS have not been clearly defined. Some investigators have hypothesized that hypercapnia *per se* might improve outcome in ARDS and have proposed the concept of 'therapeutic' hypercapnia [17]. The logic of this approach is that since inflammation contributes to respiratory failure and ARDS and respiratory acidosis has been shown to inhibit several inflammatory mediators [18], it seems reasonable that hypercapnia may be protective in ARDS. In support of this concept, hypercapnia has been demonstrated to attenuate acute lung injury induced by free radicals, pulmonary and systemic ischemia-reperfusion, pulmonary endotoxin, and excessive lung stretch [19]. These effects seem to be due in part to the anti-inflammatory effects of hypercapnia, including attenuation of neutrophil function, reduction in free radicals, decreased oxidant-induced tissue damage, and reduction in the levels of pro-inflammatory cytokines, such as tumor necrosis factor (TNF)-α, interleukin (IL)-1 and IL-8 [20]. However, some of these beneficial effects were likely caused by systemic acidosis rather than hypercapnia *per se*, because buffering of respiratory acidosis worsened experimental lung injury [21]. Recent studies confirm that CO_2 can also act as a signaling molecule via pH-independent mechanisms, leading to deleterious effects in the lung. These effects include inhibition of cell membrane repair, impairment of alveolar fluid clearance, and suppression of innate immunity and host defense [19]. Briva et al. [22] showed that elevated CO_2 levels impaired Na,K-ATPase function independently of extra- and intra-cellular acidosis. Taken together, the above reports do not suggest convincingly that hypercapnia could be beneficial and means to mitigate excessive CO_2 accumulation in the blood are likely to be useful tools in the arsenal of medical providers.

Hypercapnia, Pulmonary Hemodynamics and Right Ventricular Function

Hypercapnic acidosis enhances pulmonary vasoconstriction [23]. Several clinical studies demonstrated that hypercapnic acidosis causes an increase in mean pulmonary arterial pressure in ARDS [6]. Acute pulmonary hypertension increases RV afterload [24, 25], which individually and collectively with microvascular obstruction, the effects of positive-pressure ventilation, and hypercapnic acidosis exacerbate RV failure in ARDS [6]. Acute *cor pulmonale* in ARDS patients is associated with high mortality rates [6]. Impaired RV function in early stage ARDS may be under-diagnosed and yet it might be the harbinger of a downward spiral in the patient's condition [6]. We previously established that pulmonary vascular resistance and RV ejection fraction (RVEF) are poor indicators of RV-arterial performance [24]. RV-arterial coupling is beneficial for cardiovascular performance and can be assessed by the ratio of two elastances: Ees/Ea, where Ees is the RV elastance characterizing the RV system and Ea is the arterial elastance characterizing the pulmonary vascular system. When Ees/Ea is > 1, the system is coupled. However, when Ees/Ea is < 1, the cardio-pulmonary system is uncoupled [24]. Thus, the Ees/Ea ratio reflects the mechano-energetic aspects of RV-vascular coupling. It can be demonstrated that efficiency of energy transfer from the RV to the pulmonary circulatory system is optimal when Ees/Ea = 2 whereas mechanical RV work is maximal when Ees/Ea = 1 [26]. In ARDS patients, increased RV afterload is responsible for increased Ea while Ees may decrease because of hypercapnic acidosis, hypoxia, and often associated sepsis, leading to uncoupling between the right ventricle and the pulmonary circulation, and finally precipitating RV failure (Fig. 1) [27]. Therapies should ideally be oriented to restore the coupling between the heart and pulmonary vasculature by avoiding any increase in pulmonary vascular tone as well as depression in RV contractility [27, 28]. Alternatively, safe adjuncts to current ARDS management approaches should be considered as we learn more about the pros and cons of hypercapnia in ARDS.

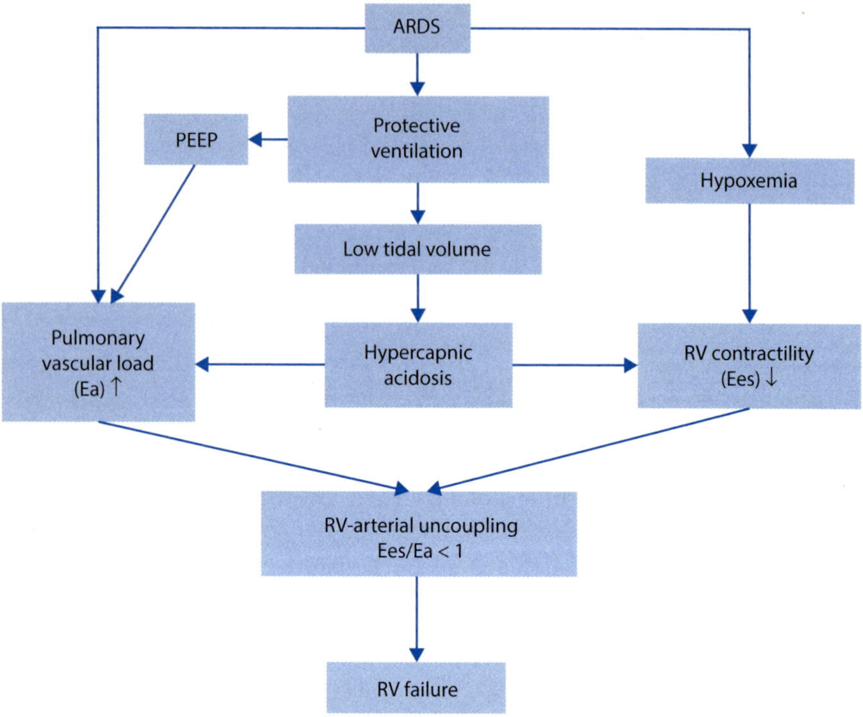

Fig. 1 Schematic representation of the key role played by hypercapnic acidosis in right ventricular (RV) failure in patients with acute respiratory distress syndrome (ARDS). PEEP: positive end-expiratory pressure

New Extracorporeal Devices for CO_2 Removal

The premise of intervening with the ventilatory function of the lung stems from early work by Kolobow, Gattinoni and Pesenti, which showed that partial-to-total CO_2 removal and so 'ventilation' is possible by means of extracorporeal circulation of the blood through a gas exchange membrane [12, 29, 30]. Of all the available forms of extracorporeal gas exchange, partial lung support, also known as $ECCO_2R$ or respiratory dialysis, is the most promising, because it offers unique advantages while carrying a low potential for complications [31, 32]. In this context, the recent successes of full extracorporeal membrane oxygenation (ECMO) are also relevant as lung support with full ECMO can replace total lung function to include oxygenation and ventilation. Although full ECMO can also be used for 'ventilation' or as an $ECCO_2R$ approach, it comes at a higher logistical and economic burden [33] when compared to use of special $ECCO_2R$ devices which, in contrast to ECMO, are logistically simpler and do not require dedicated personnel, reducing the cost of care. Although the question about whether various lung support technologies have the potential to avoid mechanical ventilation altogether in select patients remains to be determined [34], partial lung support via $ECCO_2R$ at flows of 300–500 ml/min has already been shown to provide replacement of about 50% or more of the ventilatory function of the lung [13] and poses a viable therapeutic adjunct to mechanical ventilation. $ECCO_2R$ significantly reduces mechanical ventilator settings while successfully combating hypercapnia and acidosis in humans with ARDS [13, 15]. When compared to oxygenation, removal of CO_2 from blood can be accomplished at lower blood flows [35]. As a result, less invasive veno-venous devices have been specifically designed for CO_2 removal with high gas exchange efficiency at relatively low blood flow rates (300–1,500 ml/min). Theoretically, flow rates as low as 0.5 l/min should be enough to eliminate all the CO_2 that the body produces, because a liter of blood with a $PaCO_2$ of 5 kPa contains around 500 ml of CO_2 or on average two times more CO_2 than the body produces per minute. However, the exact level of CO_2 removed will depend on several factors – mainly blood flow through the circuitry and the CO_2 level before the membrane [36].

There is an increasing number of modern $ECCO_2R$ devices on the market. These devices use 13–17 F veno-venous dual lumen catheters which can be placed percutaneously using the Seldinger technique. The $ECCO_2R$ circuitry is heparin-coated, which reduces heparinization requirements. These $ECCO_2R$ devices use advanced low impact mechanical pumps to propel the blood and efficient hollow-fiber gas exchangers or membrane lungs. The micropores in the membrane lungs create microscopic blood-gas interfaces allowing efficient gas exchange on a counter-current principle with sweep gas blown through the blood-polymer interface. As micropores also cause plasma leak, non-microporous poly-4-methyl-1-pentene has been recently established as a standard material for gas exchangers, providing better gas exchange, better bio compatibility and less plasma leak compared to older silicone or polypropylene materials [37]. Fibers in the membrane lungs are arranged into a complex mat allowing optimal blood flow and improving gas transfer efficiency by enhancing diffusion. Membranes are also coated with covalently bound heparin to enhance biocompatibility and reduce thrombogenicity. Modern membrane lungs achieve adequate gas exchange with surface areas of 0.67 to 3 m^2. Rotary pumps used in modern $ECCO_2R$ devices are either centrifugal or diagonal flow pumps designed to minimize blood trauma. To eliminate the need for a drive shaft or bearings and to reduce heating, most advanced centrifugal pump impellors are completely suspended in an electromagnetic field which reduces shear stress. The pump and membrane lung are either separate components or incorporated into a single console. Most importantly, the design and components of the modern veno-venous (VV)-$ECCO_2R$ systems reduce the degree of anticoagulation required and minimize the damaging effects of blood coming into contact with foreign surfaces. There are currently four commercially available VV-$ECCO_2R$ systems, all approved for use in Europe but none with Food and Drug Administration (FDA) approval status for use in the USA.

1. The Pump-Assisted Lung Protection (PALP) (Maquet, Rastatt, Germany) system is a low-flow system based on Maquet's CARDIOHELP® console, which is a portable heart–lung support system. PALP is not an ECMO device and has been designed to serve as a partial lung support device with primary effect

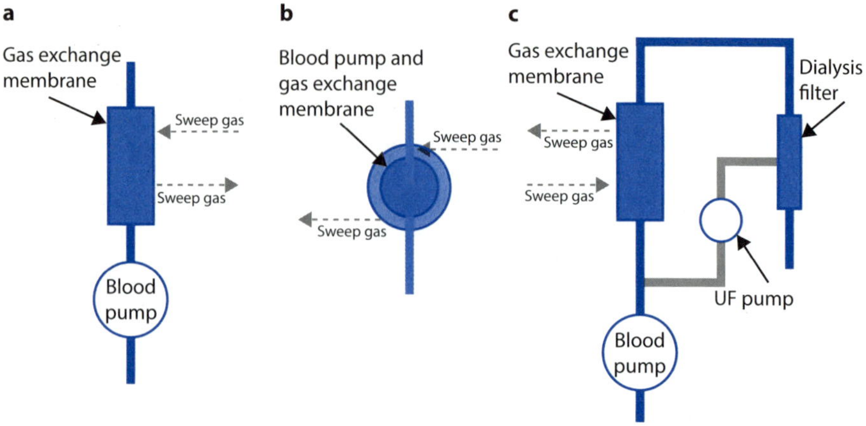

Fig. 2 Schematic representation of the three commercially available types of CO_2 removal devices. UF: ultrafiltrate

on the side of CO_2 removal (Fig. 2a). However, the PALP can be seamlessly bridged into full ECMO by simply switching out the membrane for a full ECMO oxygenator while using the same operational console which can travel with the patient. The latter is a unique feature of the Maquet system and constitutes a mobile partial lung support to total lung support solution.

2. The iLA Activve® (Novalung, Germany) is based on the same principle (Fig. 2a), but uses a small portable diagonal pump and operational console and has the capacity to run at low or high flow rates (0.5–4.5 l/min). It covers the full range of respiratory support from highly effective CO_2 elimination at lower flows to complete oxygenation and ventilation support. This capability is similar to the Maquet system in the sense that the footprint of therapy can be increased from partial to full lung support.
3. The Hemolung® system (Alung Technologies, Pittsburgh, USA) has a small $0.67\,m^2$ surface area and is the only system specifically designed for CO_2 removal and targeting CO_2 retention syndromes, such as chronic obstructive pulmonary disease (COPD). The Hemolung integrates blood pump and gas exchange membrane into a single unit (Fig. 2b). Blood flows centrally into a rotating core, is radially pumped through a stationary annular fiber bundle, and returns to the patient via an outlet port. The system has not been designed for oxygenation and is generally recommended for COPD patients as a primary indication.
4. The Decap® system (Hemodec, Salerno, Italy) uses a membrane lung connected in series with a hemodialysis filter and roller pump (Fig. 2c). Ultrafiltrate from the filter is returned to the blood stream prior to the membrane lung inflow, allowing additional CO_2 removal. Consequently, smaller membrane lungs can be used (0.3 to $1.35\,m^2$) with lower flow rates (< 500 ml/min). This configuration is useful for patients requiring both pulmonary and renal support and is a unique feature of the Decap.

Rationale for the Use of $ECCO_2R$ in ARDS

Experimental Evidence

Recent experimental studies have demonstrated that new generations of VV-$ECCO_2R$ devices are highly efficient at CO_2 removal. A 50% reduction in minute ventilation was obtained in healthy mechanically ventilated swine while maintaining normocarbia using the Hemolung system [13]. In this study, a 15-F dual-lumen catheter was inserted in the external jugular vein and connected to the Hemolung system. Minute ventilation was reduced from 5.6 l/min at baseline to 2.6 l/min 2 h after device insertion and was kept low until the end of the study, while normocarbia ($PaCO_2$ 35–45 mm Hg) was maintained. CO_2 removal by Hemolung remained steady over 72 h, averaging 72 ± 1.2 ml/min at blood flows of 447 ± 5 ml/min. After insertion, O_2 consumption did not change; CO_2 production by the lung decreased by 50% and stayed at that level ($p < 0.001$). Plasma-free hemoglobin did not change during the course of the study signifying the safety of the device with respect to hemolysis [13]. In this study, $ECCO_2R$ using the Hemolung permitted significant CO_2 removal in a safe and feasible manner while requiring only a partial increase in activated clotting time titrated by continuous heparin infusion.

The hemodynamic effects of CO_2 removal seem to be beneficial by decreasing pulmonary hypertension and improving RV-arterial coupling in an experimental model of ARDS. In a recent study, we sought to determine whether low-flow CO_2 removal therapy used at an early stage of ARDS could have beneficial hemodynamic effects on the pulmonary circulation. This study was performed in an experimental model of ARDS in pigs. ARDS was obtained by repeated bronchoalveolar lavage (BAL, 0.09% saline solution). Protective ventilation at low tidal volume was then established according to the ARDSNet study. Drainage (12 F) and re-

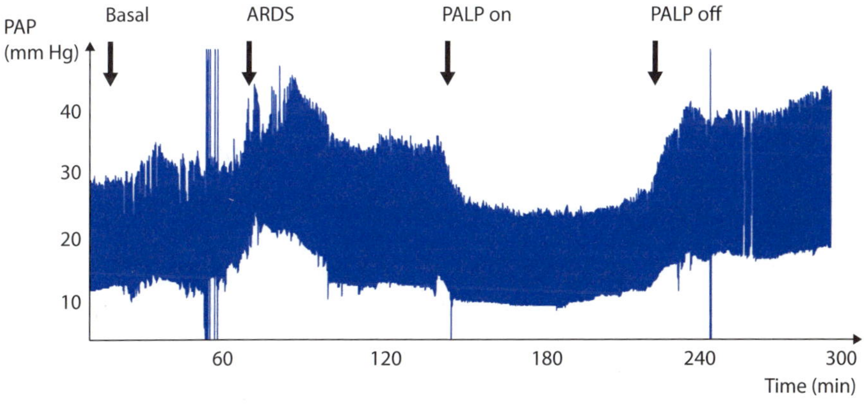

Fig. 3 Effects of PALP ('Pump Assisted Lung Protection', Maquet, Germany) therapy on systolic pulmonary artery pressure (PAP) in an experimental model of acute respiratory distress syndrome (ARDS)

infusion (10 F) cannulae were inserted into the inferior and the superior vena cava, respectively. These cannulae were connected to the PALP system for CO_2 removal. ARDS induced severe hypercapnic acidosis with significantly increased pulmonary artery pressure (PAP). After the PALP was started, acidosis was rapidly corrected and normocarbia was maintained despite protective ventilation. PAP significantly decreased and a significant drop in Ea was observed during PALP therapy (Fig. 3). Mean blood flow through the PALP was 0.645 l/min and sweep gas flow was 8 l/min. RV-arterial coupling assessed by the ratio of Ees on Ea was improved [38].

Other promising approaches for efficient CO_2 removal are still in development [39, 40]. Novel methods to maximize CO_2 removal, such as regional blood acidification which increases the bioavailability of CO_2 by unbinding it from the bicarbonate ion in circulating blood, are also under investigation [40].

Clinical Evidence

There is accumulating evidence that VV-$ECCO_2R$ can effectively reduce $PaCO_2$ in patients with ARDS and that VV-$ECCO_2R$ facilitates a lung-protective ventilation strategy by allowing a reduction in tidal volume and inspiratory airway pressures [32, 41]. Terragni et al. used VV-$ECCO_2R$ to facilitate 'ultraprotective' ventilation [15]. They recruited 32 patients with early (<72 h) ARDS and ventilated them according to the ARDSNet protocol for 72 h, at which point the tidal volume was reduced from 6 to 4 ml/kg in all patients (n = 10) who had a plateau pressure of between 28 and 30 cmH_2O, thus facilitating further reductions in plateau pressures. VV-$ECCO_2R$ using the Decap device successfully treated the hypercapnic acidosis in all cases and allowed the plateau pressure to be lowered to 25 cmH_2O (4 ml/kg tidal volume and higher levels of positive end-expiratory pressure [PEEP]) while mitigating the resultant changes in pH and $PaCO_2$. The study also demonstrated a reduction in bronchoalveolar inflammatory cytokines (IL-6, IL-8, IL-1b, IL-1 receptor antagonist [IL-Ira]) in the Decap group. There were no harmful effects related to the ultra-protective ventilation strategy or the VV-$ECCO_2R$. Although this study was uncontrolled and small, it suggests that there may be benefit to an ultra-protective ventilation strategy facilitated by VV-$ECCO_2R$ within 72 hours of diagnosing ARDS. A similar approach was taken by another group using the NovaLung device in arterio-venous configuration. In the prospective randomized Xtravent-study, Bein et al. [42] demonstrated that use of very low tidal volumes (3 ml/kg PBW) combined with extracorporeal elimination of CO_2 was feasible without major side effects and might be beneficial in the treatment of patients with severe ARDS. Although that study did not show a mortality benefit, ventilator-free days assessed at 28 and 60 days were significantly higher in the $ECCO_2R$ group. Adjunct use of $ECCO_2R$ and mechanical ventilation facilitated liberation of patients from excessive sedation and increased levels of spontaneous breathing. Thus, integration of spontaneous breathing into the management of patients with ARDS might be easier and more comfortable with extracorporeal CO_2-removal, and a reduced demand for sedative and analgesic medication could be advantageous [42]. Forster et al. [43] demonstrated, in a small series of 10 patients, that low-flow CO_2 removal integrated into a renal-replacement circuit could reduce acidosis and decrease vasopressor requirements. The gas exchanger was integrated into the continuous hemodialysis system after the dialysis filter. The authors used a 13.5-F double-lumen catheter placed in the jugular vein. Similarly, we reported a case of refractory hypercapnia in a severely burned adult treated with a simplified VV-$ECCO_2R$ technique [44]. We integrated a pediatric oxygenator into a continuous veno-venous hemofiltration circuit. This technique, used for at least 96 h, was feasible and efficiently removed up to 32% of CO_2. Future studies are required to determine whether 'ultraprotective' ventilation with adjunct use of $ECCO_2R$ will improve survival in patients suffering from moderate to severe ARDS. At this time, the effect of $ECCO_2R$ on survival in patients with ARDS is accumulating but is not yet conclusive [15, 42, 45].

There are clinical trials planned for several of the new $ECCO_2R$ devices. The rationale for adjunct use of $ECCO_2R$ will depend on the clinical situation in each individual patient. However, with the new Berlin definition of ARDS, the therapeutic window for $ECCO_2R$ in ARDS may be expanded [46]. Because the intensity of therapeutic intervention increases proportionally to the level of hypoxemia, adjunct use of $ECCO_2R$ will likely be considered at earlier stages of ARDS, for example when the PaO_2/FiO_2 ratio is < 200. At that time, $ECCO_2R$ could be initiated in combination with tidal volume reduction in order to achieve ultraprotective ventilation. This approach will need to be tested in prospective randomized fashion but the preliminary evidence suggests that, at least in some patients with slow ARDS progression, this early intervention may be of use. A few areas of concern remain for both $ECCO_2R$ and ECMO alike, including cannula thrombosis, need to exchange membranes due to thrombosis and pump malfunction [45]. Intense research is oriented toward solution of these problems and major improvements in anticoagulation protocols and updates to clinical practice guidelines are expected as the results of this research become available. In our opinion, alternative anticoagulation approaches, such as the work by Cardenas et al. utilizing regional citrate anticoagulation, could provide a promising solution to future $ECCO_2R$ approaches, especially in line with the tendency for developing modular therapeutic solutions permitting concomitant lung and renal interventions [39, 47]. Other novel approaches are emerging with respect to heparin-free antibody-based interventions to the coagulation cascade as a means to induce thromboprotection during extracorporeal circulation [48]. Specific anticoagulation requirements for low-flow systems must be studied systematically and will be the cornerstone of further acceptance of $ECCO_2R$ as well as full ECMO into daily practice, especially in patients with ARDS due to multiple trauma and burns, in whom heparinization is not desired.

Conclusion

ARDS remains a life-threatening condition with long-term consequences in survivors. Protective ventilation reduces alveolar stress and strain and clearly improves mortality. However, these beneficial effects are tempered by the fact that low tidal volume ventilation induces hypercapnic acidosis responsible for deleterious effects. Uncoupling between impaired RV function and increased pulmonary vascular tone enhanced by hypercapnic acidosis and positive pressure ventilation is a starting point in the downward spiral of ARDS patients. New generation $ECCO_2R$ therapy can be seen as a low impact and safe 'respiratory dialysis' allowing control of hypercapnia and acidosis. $ECCO_2R$ should be considered as a therapeutic adjunct in moderate to severe ARDS, combined with further decrease in tidal volume. Recent major technological improvements in devices make them simpler, safer, less invasive and more efficient, requiring lower blood flow rates and smaller access cannulas with reduced anticoagulation requirements. However, while the efficiency of modern $ECCO_2R$ devices has been clearly demonstrated in experimental and clinical settings, current evidence on their impact on survival in ARDS is just accumulating and more data will be needed before these techniques can be incorporated into routine use.

References

1. The Acute Respiratory Distress Syndrome Network (2000) Ventilation with lower tidal volumes as compared with traditional tidal volumes for acute lung injury and the acute respiratory distress syndrome. The Acute Respiratory Distress Syndrome Network. N Engl J Med 342:1301–1308
2. Zambon M, Vincent JL (2008) Mortality rates for patients with acute lung injury/ARDS have decreased over time. Chest 133:1120–1127
3. Squara P, Dhainaut JF, Artigas A, Carlet J (1998) Hemodynamic profile in severe ARDS: results of the European Collaborative ARDS Study. Intensive Care Med 24:1018–1028
4. Gajic O, Dabbagh O, Park PK et al (2011) Early identification of patients at risk of acute lung injury: evaluation of lung injury prediction score in a multicenter cohort study. Am J Respir Crit Care Med 183:462–470
5. Cancio LC, Batchinsky AI, Dubick MA et al (2007) Inhalation injury: pathophysiology and clinical care proceedings of a symposium conducted at the Trauma Institute of San Antonio, San Antonio, TX, USA on 28 March 2006. Burns 33:681–692
6. Lheritier G, Legras A, Caille A et al (2013) Prevalence and prognostic value of acute cor pulmonale and patent foramen ovale in ventilated patients with early acute respiratory distress syndrome: a multicenter study. Intensive Care Med 39:1734–1742
7. Slutsky AS, Ranieri VM (2013) Ventilator-induced lung injury. N Engl J Med 369:2126–2136
8. Ijland MM, Heunks LM, van der Hoeven JG (2010) Bench-to-bedside review: hypercapnic acidosis in lung injury – from 'permissive' to 'therapeutic'. Crit Care 14:237
9. Terragni PP, Rosboch G, Tealdi A et al (2007) Tidal hyperinflation during low tidal volume ventilation in acute respiratory distress syndrome. Am J Respir Crit Care Med 175:160–166
10. Hager DN, Krishnan JA, Hayden DL, Brower RG (2005) Tidal volume reduction in patients with acute lung injury when plateau pressures are not high. Am J Respir Crit Care Med 172:1241–1245
11. Brochard L, Roudot-Thoraval F, Roupie E et al (1998) Tidal volume reduction for prevention of ventilator-induced lung injury in acute respiratory distress syndrome. The Multicenter Trail Group on Tidal Volume reduction in ARDS. Am J Respir Crit Care Med 158:1831–1838
12. Pesenti A, Pelizzola A, Mascheroni D et al (1981) Low frequency positive pressure ventilation with extracorporeal CO2 removal (LEPPV-ECCO2R) in acute respiratory failure (ARF): technique. Trans Am Soc Artif Intern Organs 27:263–266

13. Batchinsky AI, Jordan BS, Regn D et al (2011) Respiratory dialysis: reduction in dependence on mechanical ventilation by venovenous extracorporeal CO2 removal. Crit Care Med 39:1382–1387
14. Batchinsky AI, Chung K, Cannon J, Cancio LC (2011) Respiratory dialysis is not extracorporeal membrane oxygenation. The authors answer. Extracorporeal membrane oxygenation and respiratory dialysis: our expending tool box. Crit Care Med 39:2788–2789
15. Terragni PP, Del Sorbo L, Mascia L et al (2009) Tidal volume lower than 6 ml/kg enhances lung protection: role of extracorporeal carbon dioxide removal. Anesthesiology 111:826–835
16. Feihl F, Perret C (1994) Permissive hypercapnia. How permissive should we be? Am J Respir Crit Care Med 150:1722–1737
17. Laffey JG, Kavanagh BP (1999) Carbon dioxide and the critically ill – too little of a good thing? Lancet 354:1283–1286
18. O'Croinin D, Ni Chonghaile M, Higgins B, Laffey JG (2005) Bench-to-bedside review: Permissive hypercapnia. Crit Care 9:51–59
19. Vadasz I, Hubmayr RD, Nin N, Sporn PH, Sznajder JI (2012) Hypercapnia: a nonpermissive environment for the lung. Am J Respir Cell Mol Biol 46:417–421
20. Curley G, Contreras MM, Nichol AD, Higgins BD, Laffey JG (2010) Hypercapnia and acidosis in sepsis: a double-edged sword? Anesthesiology 112:462–472
21. Nichol AD, O'Cronin DF, Howell K et al (2009) Infection-induced lung injury is worsened after renal buffering of hypercapnic acidosis. Crit Care Med 37:2953–2961
22. Briva A, Vadasz I, Lecuona E et al (2007) High CO2 levels impair alveolar epithelial function independently of pH. PLoS One 2:e1238
23. Stengl M, Ledvinova L, Chvojka J et al (2013) Effects of clinically relevant acute hypercapnic and metabolic acidosis on the cardiovascular system: an experimental porcine study. Crit Care 17:R303
24. Morimont P, Lambermont B, Ghuysen A et al (2008) Effective arterial elastance as an index of pulmonary vascular load. Am J Physiol Heart Circ Physiol 294:H2736–H2742
25. Viitanen A, Salmenpera M, Heinonen J (1990) Right ventricular response to hypercarbia after cardiac surgery. Anesthesiology 73:393–400
26. Sagawa KML, Suga H, Sunagawa K (1988) Cardiovascular interaction. In: Sagawa K (ed) Cardiac Contraction and the Pressure–Volume Relationship. Oxford University Press, New York, pp 232–298
27. Morimont P, Lambermont B, Desaive T et al (2013) Right ventriculoarterial coupling in acute respiratory distress syndrome (ARDS) and expected benefits of CO2 removal therapy. J Crit Care 28:e30
28. Weber T, Tschernich H, Sitzwohl C et al (2000) Tromethamine buffer modifies the depressant effect of permissive hypercapnia on myocardial contractility in patients with acute respiratory distress syndrome. Am J Respir Crit Care Med 162:1361–1365
29. Kolobow T, Gattinoni L, Tomlinson T, Pierce JE (1978) An alternative to breathing. J Thorac Cardiovasc Surg 75:261–266
30. Gattinoni L, Agostoni A, Pesenti A et al (1980) Treatment of acute respiratory failure with low-frequency positive-pressure ventilation and extracorporeal removal of CO2. Lancet 2:292–294
31. Terragni P, Maiolo G, Ranieri VM (2012) Role and potentials of low-flow CO(2) removal system in mechanical ventilation. Curr Opin Crit Care 18:93–98
32. Pesenti A, Patroniti N, Fumagalli R (2010) Carbon dioxide dialysis will save the lung. Crit Care Med 38(10 Suppl):S549–S554
33. Peek GJ, Mugford M, Tiruvoipati R et al (2009) Efficacy and economic assessment of conventional ventilatory support versus extracorporeal membrane oxygenation for severe adult respiratory failure (CESAR): a multicentre randomised controlled trial. Lancet 374:1351–1363
34. Del Sorbo L, Ranieri VM (2010) We do not need mechanical ventilation any more. Crit Care Med 38(10 Suppl):S555–S558
35. Barrett KBS, Boitano S, Brooks H (2003) Ganong's Review of Medical Physiology, 23rd edn. Mc Graw Hill, New York, pp 587–607

36. Park M, Costa EL, Maciel AT et al (2013) Determinants of oxygen and carbon dioxide transfer during extracorporeal membrane oxygenation in an experimental model of multiple organ dysfunction syndrome. PLoS One 8:e54954
37. Toomasian JM, Schreiner RJ, Meyer DE (2005) A polymethylpentene fiber gas exchanger for long-term extracorporeal life support. ASAIO J 51:390–397
38. Morimont P, Desaive T, Guiot J et al (2014) Effects of veno-venous CO2 removal therapy on pulmonary circulation in an ARDS model. Intensive Care Medicine Experimental 2(Suppl 1):P45 (abst)
39. Scaravilli V, Kreyer S, Linden K et al (2014) Modular extracorporeal life support: effects of ultrafiltrate recirculation on the performance of an extracorporeal carbon dioxide removal device. ASAIO J 60:335–341
40. Zanella A, Mangili P, Giani M et al (2014) Extracorporeal carbon dioxide removal through ventilation of acidified dialysate: an experimental study. J Heart Lung Transplant 33:536–541
41. Cove ME, MacLaren G, Federspiel WJ, Kellum JA (2012) Bench to bedside review: Extracorporeal carbon dioxide removal, past present and future. Crit Care 16:232
42. Bein T, Weber-Carstens S, Goldmann A et al (2013) Lower tidal volume strategy (approximately 3 ml/kg) combined with extracorporeal CO2 removal versus 'conventional' protective ventilation (6 ml/kg) in severe ARDS: the prospective randomized Xtravent-study. Intensive Care Med 39:847–856
43. Forster C, Schriewer J, John S, Eckardt KU, Willam C (2013) Low-flow CO(2) removal integrated into a renal-replacement circuit can reduce acidosis and decrease vasopressor requirements. Crit Care 17:R154
44. Rousseau AF, Damas P, Renwart L (2014) Use of a pediatric oxygenator integrated in a veno-venous hemofiltration circuit to remove CO: A case report in a severe burn patient with refractory hypercapnia. Burns 40:e47–e50
45. Fitzgerald M, Millar J, Blackwood B et al (2014) Extracorporeal carbon dioxide removal for patients with acute respiratory failure secondary to the acute respiratory distress syndrome: a systematic review. Crit Care 18:222
46. Ranieri VM, Rubenfeld GD, Thompson BT et al (2012) Acute respiratory distress syndrome: the Berlin Definition. JAMA 307:2526–2533
47. Cardenas VJ Jr., Miller L, Lynch JE, Anderson MJ, Zwischenberger JB (2006) Percutaneous venovenous CO2 removal with regional anticoagulation in an ovine model. ASAIO J 52:467–470
48. Larsson M, Rayzman V, Nolte MW et al (2014) A factor XIIa inhibitory antibody provides thromboprotection in extracorporeal circulation without increasing bleeding risk. Sci Transl Med 6:222ra17

Fundamentals and Timing of Tracheostomy: ICU Team and Patient Perspectives

V. Pandian and M. Mirski

Introduction: Historical Background

Tracheostomy is a surgical procedure performed by creating an artificial opening in the anterior aspect of the neck, into the trachea. Tracheostomy is usually performed in patients who require prolonged mechanical ventilation or who have upper airway obstruction caused either by obstructive sleep apnea, bilateral vocal cord paralysis, tumor or glottic stenosis. Often the procedure is also necessary and beneficial in head and neck or maxillofacial trauma with airway compromise, in patients requiring definitive pulmonary toileting, or as an adjunct to head and neck or thoracic surgery where ventilation problems or prolonged intubation is anticipated.

Tracheostomy is not a new medical procedure; it has been reported to have been performed as early as 3600 BC based on Egyptian artifacts [1]. In the 4th century BC, Alexander the Great was given credit for saving a soldier's life by using the tip of his sword to create an opening in the neck. Asclepiades of Persia is reported to have performed the first formal tracheostomy in 100 BC. The term 'tracheostomy' was coined by Lorenz Heister in 1718, and was associated with trepidation during that period, because safe techniques had not yet been established. Hippocrates, in fact, prohibited the performance of tracheostomy for fear of carotid artery laceration and death both from bleeding and infection. There was an increase in awareness of tracheostomy when George Washington died of an upper airway obstruction in 1799 and no one had the courage to perform a tracheostomy. This fear was later overcome when the indications, techniques, and instruments were studied in depth in response to the death of Napoleon Bonaparte's nephew as a result of diphtheria in 1807.

The history of tracheostomy has been divided into five periods [2]: The period of legend (2000 BC–1546 AD); the period of fear (1546–1833); the period of

V. Pandian · M. Mirski ✉
Department of Anesthesiology & Critical Care Medicine, Johns Hopkins Medicine, Baltimore, USA
e-mail: mmirski1@jhmi.edu

J.-L. Vincent (ed.), *Annual Update in Intensive Care and Emergency Medicine 2015*,
DOI 10.1007/978-3-319-13761-2_16

dramatization (1833–1932); period of enthusiasm (1932–1965); and the period of rationalization (1965–present). During the period of fear, only a few brave physicians performed a tracheostomy, usually at the risk of their own reputation. During the period of drama, tracheostomy was performed only in an emergent airway situation. During the period of enthusiasm, it was performed by many; if they thought about a tracheostomy, they did one. In the current period of rationalization, the risks and benefits of a tracheostomy versus continued intubation are more carefully analyzed (we hope!) prior to performing the procedure.

Open Versus Percutaneous Techniques

Chevalier Jackson, father of ear, nose, and throat surgery, standardized the indications, techniques, and the instruments to perform a tracheostomy in the 20th century [3]. Currently, several techniques for performing a tracheostomy exist. The two main categories are the open and the percutaneous techniques.

Open Tracheostomy

The open technique is usually performed in the operating room. However, in some institutions, it may be performed in the intensive care unit (ICU) as well. Primarily, an open technique is reserved for patients who come directly to the operating room for head and neck surgery in whom airway swelling or bleeding is anticipated, or for major thoracic surgery in whom prolonged mechanical ventilation is anticipated. Mechanically ventilated patients in the ICU who require a tracheostomy are occasionally considered for the open technique if they have anatomical variations due to obesity, are at high risk of bleeding, or have high oxygen requirements. With the open technique, the incision is made in the skin, subcutaneous tissue and the trachea itself. Retractors are used to open the surgical incision, the trachea is viewed directly, and a tracheostomy tube is placed. Typically, the open technique is associated with a larger incisional wound than with the percutaneous procedure, and there is believed to be a higher risk of bleeding and infection.

Percutaneous Tracheostomy

While Seldinger introduced the technique of percutaneous guidewire needle placement for various endovascular procedures in 1953, in 1955 Sheldon described using the same technique to perform a tracheostomy [4, 5]. The concept of percutaneous tracheostomy was further formalized by Toye and Weinstein in 1969 [6]. In 1985, Ciaglia et al. described the wire-guided percutaneous technique using multiple dilators [7]. Several variations of percutaneous techniques are currently used:

1. Blue Rhino Technique: This technique uses a single dilator with a bronchoscopic visualization of the airway [8]. A small incision is made on the skin and

the subcutaneous tissue is dilated with a Kelly clamp. A needle is inserted between the second and third tracheal rings. A guidewire is advanced through the needle down towards the carina, and following a quick dilation with the punch dilator, a tapered Blue Rhino tube is used to dilate the stoma to the anticipated measurement of the tracheostomy tube. A tracheostomy tube is then inserted over the guidewire into the trachea.

2. Griggs Technique: In this technique, an incision is made in the neck and an angiocatheter is inserted between the second and third tracheal ring [9]. A guidewire is threaded through the catheter, and a dilator forceps is then used to enlarge the stoma through which the tracheostomy tube is placed.
3. Fantoni's Technique: This is a retrograde percutaneous translaryngeal tracheostomy technique [10]. The safety and feasibility of this technique have been questioned given the complicated nature of the procedure. In this technique, a needle is inserted between the second and tracheal ring and a guidewire is threaded through the needle into the trachea and then directed up toward the head and past the endotracheal tube. A special tracheostomy tube with a tapered end is passed through the mouth into the trachea over the guide wire. The tracheostomy tube is then pulled out gently through the stoma to a certain measurement and then directed down towards the carina.
4. PercTwist Technique: A screw-like device is used to open the trachea and place the tracheostomy tube [11].
5. Dolphin Technique: This technique is very similar to the Blue Rhino technique except that a balloon is used to dilate the stoma instead of a tapered Blue Rhino tube [12].

While the open technique is predominantly used by otolaryngology head and neck and trauma surgeons, the percutaneous technique is often used by non-surgically trained physicians such as intensivists and interventional pulmonologists.

Standardized Approach

Despite the existence of various techniques, the key to successful performance of a tracheostomy and management of patients with a tracheostomy is standardization. It is vital to select one technique and become expert in its use. Similarly, standardization of care with regards to suctioning, stoma care, tube changes, capping and decannulation can also help in decreasing morbidity and mortality.

Suctioning

It is known that suctioning should not be attempted for longer than 10 seconds but there is a lack of data recommending how deep to suction. Practices vary both between and within institutions. Traditionally, it has been taught to advance the suction catheter through the tracheostomy tube into the trachea until resistance is met, then to retract the catheter for a couple of centimeters and then suction. Given the anatomy of the right main bronchus, it is possible that the suction catheter might be advanced past the carina and suctioning limited to the right main stem. Newer teachings are focused on measuring the length of the suction catheters and advancing only 1 cm past the distal tip of the tracheostomy tube. This can be challenging, because not all suction catheters come with pre-labeled measurements. In such situations, the length to be inserted for suctioning can be estimated by using the obturator as a guide. The important take-home message is that we perform tracheal suctioning and not bronchial suctioning to avoid injury to the airway mucosa and prevent airway bleeding. Deep suctioning may be beneficial in non-routine clinical situations where a patient has thick secretions or poor cough reflex. One area of controversy exists concerning the use of saline prior to suctioning. Several studies have shown that saline is detrimental to a patient's respiratory status, whereas others have shown that it decreases the rate of ventilator associated pneumonia (VAP) [13]. Further research is necessary to resolve this controversial topic.

Stoma Care

The stoma should be cleaned at a minimum of every eight hours in the ICU, and as needed to avoid cellulitis and skin breakdown. Clean techniques are sufficient when providing stoma care in home settings; however, in the ICU or when dealing with an immunocompromised patient, it is recommended that sterile techniques be adapted when the stoma is fresh. It is not clear whether placement of a dressing under the tracheostomy tube flange is efficacious. Some institutions prefer non-dressed stoma sites, while in others it may be common practice to place slit gauze dressings to absorb secretions. The basic principles that need to be considered while standardizing such practices is to prevent fray dressings from entering the airway and to use dressings that will absorb secretions away from the stoma.

Tracheostomy Tube Changes

According to the U.S. Federal Drug Administration (FDA) approved manufacturer's guideline, tracheostomy tubes must be changed at least once a month. Unfortunately, some institutions do not change them according to these guidelines for fear of loss of airway, and others change their tracheostomy tubes as frequently as once a week to decrease the risk of infections. The American Academy of Otolaryngology tracheostomy consensus statement recommends first tracheostomy tube change as early as 7 days for open tracheostomies and 14 days for percutaneous tracheostomies [14].

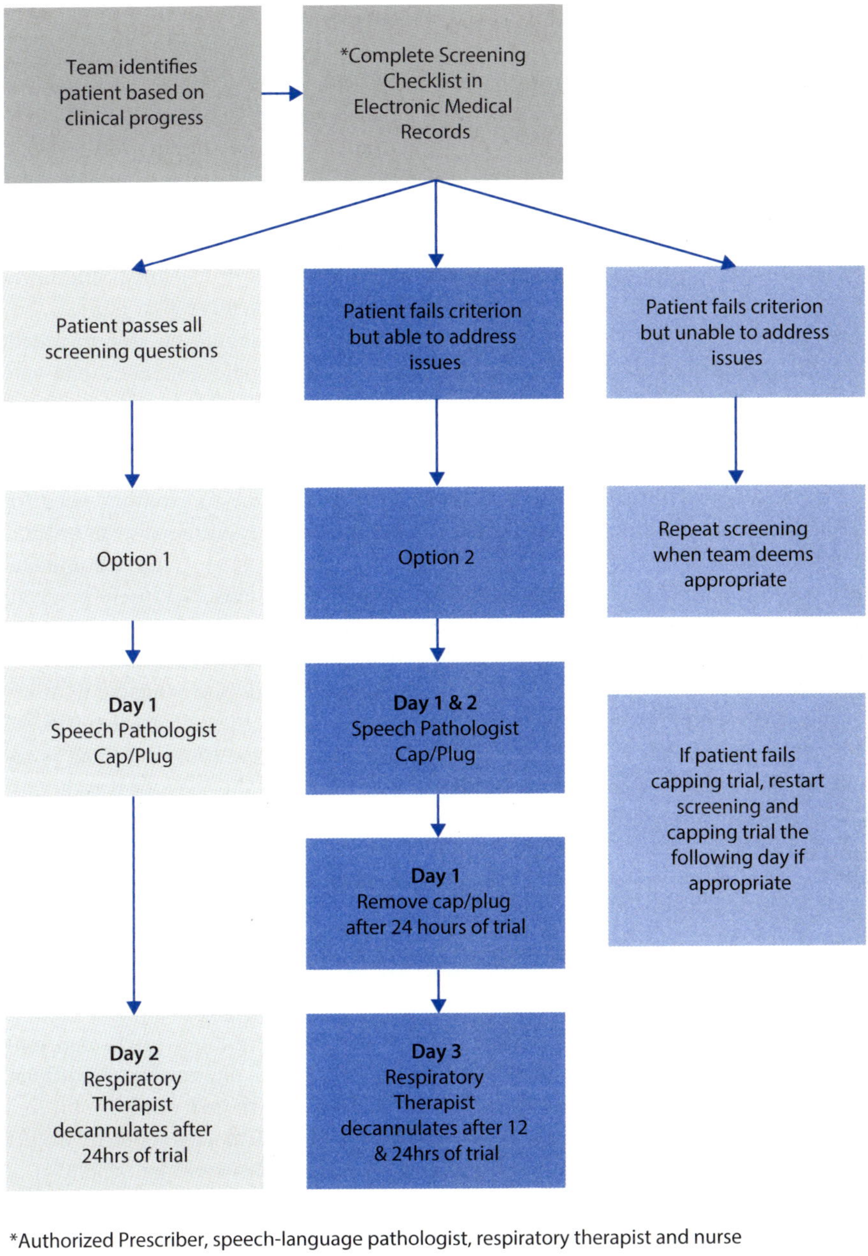

Fig. 1 Flow diagram of capping and decannulation process

Tracheostomy Capping and Decannulation

Once the reasons for a tracheostomy are resolved, a capping trial is performed to ensure the patient can tolerate tracheostomy decannulation. The duration of a capping trial and the type of tracheostomy tube that is used for capping trials varies. The American Academy of Otolaryngology recommended development of a standardized protocol to ensure patient safety during this process. The Johns Hopkins Hospital in the U.S. developed a protocol to guide capping and decannulation of a tracheostomy tube. Pandian et al. also provide criteria to establish eligibility for a capping trial [15]. They recommend using the smallest size cuffless tracheostomy tube for a successful capping trial. Patients should be able to breath comfortably with finger occlusion of the tube for one minute, tolerate a one-way speaking valve while awake, cough up secretions, have stable oxygen saturation, and be alert enough to be able to successfully pass a capping trial. Suctioning requirement should also be less than every four hours. Moreover, there should be no anticipated need for sedation or anesthesia in the near future to avoid the need for an artificial airway after decannulation. Pandian et al. recommend a multidisciplinary approach to capping and decannulation processes [15]. They recommend that speech pathologists, respiratory therapists, and nurses must be closely involved in the screening process to be able to assess the patient from multiple perspectives. A flow diagram of the capping process is shown in Fig. 1.

A patient is considered to have failed a capping trial if he/she is unable to maintain oxygen saturations within ordered parameters, if there is an increase in the oxygen requirement to greater than 40%, and if the tracheostomy cap/plug is removed for any reason, such as suctioning, desaturation, or shortness of breath.

When patients are ready for decannulation, a standardized approach is used. The efficacy of this protocol has been verified in a small pilot study. Larger studies are necessary to establish the feasibility of this protocol.

Multidisciplinary Tracheostomy Service

Multidisciplinary programs have been shown to improve patient safety and outcomes in cases of pain management, palliative care, trauma, and cardiac conditions. Since patients with tracheostomy are usually not located in one ward or unit in a hospital, and they have various needs ranging from pain management to wound care issues, it is believed that a multidisciplinary program would be beneficial to improving outcomes in these patients. Most of the tracheostomy teams or multidisciplinary programs discussed in the literature refer to a team caring for these patients after a tracheostomy tube has been placed. These team approaches have successfully decreased the total tracheostomy time, ICU and hospital lengths of stay, and increased the use of speaking valves.

Mirski and Pandian describe the efficiency of a unique multidisciplinary team approach that is not limited to postoperative care, but includes both pre and intraoperative care of these patients [16, 17]. Educating patients and family members prior to tracheostomy placement can play a significant role in preparing them psychologically for postoperative care expectations and expectations after discharge from the hospital. Mirski and Pandian also describe the importance of a nurse practitioner in the successful functioning of a multidisciplinary program. A nurse practitioner is not only able to provide the postoperative care but is also able to obtain consent for the tracheostomy procedure, and assist during the procedure as well. Being aware of anatomical variations or challenges during tracheostomy tube placement helps anticipate postoperative complications and issues, and manage them prophylactically.

The multidisciplinary team at the Johns Hopkins Hospital is comprised of a clinical coordinator (nurse practitioner), anesthesiologists, credentialed operators (otolaryngology head and neck surgeons, trauma surgeons, and interventional pulmonologists), equipment specialists, nurses, respiratory therapists, and speech-language pathologists. The clinical coordinator schedules the tracheostomy procedure but also follows the patient from the time he/she is identified for a tracheostomy until discharge. If patients are discharged directly to home instead of a rehabilitation or chronic ventilator facility, then they are followed up at the outpatient clinic. Anesthesiologists perform a dual role of providing general anesthesia and performing bronchoscopy during the procedure. As a result of the anesthesiologist's dual role, credentialed operators are able to focus on the procedure without worrying about patient's anesthetic status or the ability to visualize the airway. Equipment specialists take responsibility for setting up the bronchoscope for the tracheostomy procedure and its maintenance after the procedure. Nurses assist in preparing the patient for the procedure, assist with monitoring and supplies during the procedure, and managing patients postoperatively with regards to suctioning and stoma care. Respiratory therapists play a significant role stabilizing the endotracheal tube during the procedure and making changes on the ventilator to accommodate hypoxia and hypoventilation during bronchoscopy. Speech-language pathologists are routinely consulted 48 hours after a tracheostomy, once the stoma has healed to some extent, for speech and swallowing evaluation. In addition to what is described by the Johns Hopkins Hospital in the U.S., the United Kingdom National Tracheostomy Safety Project and the Tracheostomy Review and Management Service in Australia describe the benefits of routine hospital-wide postoperative rounds in managing postoperative issues effectively [18–20].

Outcomes of Patients with Tracheostomy

Patients who undergo a tracheostomy benefit from increased comfort, ability to speak and swallow, and increased mobilization compared to being endotracheally intubated. However, they may also experience poor outcomes depending on the type of postoperative care they receive and the underlying disease process that prompted a tracheostomy.

Hemorrhage

Hemorrhage is one of the most common complications after a tracheostomy. It can occur during the intraoperative, early postoperative, or late postoperative phases. If the bleeding is minimal, the general consensus is to ensure gentle suctioning with a soft rubber catheter instead of tough plastic suction catheters, ensure adequate humidification of the airway, and consider saline prior to suctioning. The use of saline instillation remains controversial, however, and further large scale multi-institutional studies are necessary to understand the effects of saline on respiratory status [13]. If the patient has large amounts of bleeding, it is prudent to save the number of gauzes to quantify the amount of bleeding and control bleeding efficiently. Coagulation status must be checked to ensure that patient coagulation factors are not contributing to bleeding. If the patient is on anticoagulation medications, they should be held temporarily while bleeding is controlled. In addition, if the bleeding source is from the stoma, the stoma should be packed with hemostatic agents. However, in rare situations, patients may develop pulsatile bright red blood emanating from the stoma or through the tracheostomy tube. This is considered a sentinel hemorrhage. In these situations, a computed tomographic angiogram should be done to rule out bleeding from a tracheo-innominate artery fistula if the patient is stable for the diagnostic study [21]. Otherwise, large volume hemorrhage should be treated promptly. The recommendation is to intubate the patient orally or nasally, remove the tracheostomy tube, and apply pressure on the bleeding vessel by placing a finger through the stoma. Often patients with this form of bleeding are taken emergently to the operating room where the bleeding is usually controlled via exploration of the stoma. In rare situations, a sternal incision may be needed to access the bleeding artery for repair.

Infection

Infection is the next most common complication from a tracheostomy. Infection can occur locally and is called stomal cellulitis or can disseminate to the lungs causing pneumonia.

Stomal Cellulitis

Local infection or stomal cellulitis is usually caused by constant leakage of secretions via the stoma from the trachea, and physical irritation of the skin by the tracheostomy tube itself. Stomal cellulitis can be treated locally with good stoma care and frequent change of the tracheostomy tube. If pressure ulcers are anticipated, then applying soft foam dressings to decrease the pressure will be beneficial. Occasionally, local or systemic antibiotics might be necessary to facilitate treatment of the infection.

Ventilator-associated Pneumonia

The rate of VAP ranges between 9 and 27% of all intubated patients [22]. The theoretical premise is that with the placement of a tracheostomy, the risk of VAP decreases as the patient's epiglottis will potentially be able to function after extubation in neurologically intact patients and protect the airway. However, the concept of VAP in patients with a tracheostomy has been actively debated for several years as contradicting findings have been reported. Three studies showed that the rate of VAP was significantly lower in the early tracheostomy group compared to the late tracheostomy group [23–25]. By contrast, five studies showed no difference in the rate of VAP between early vs. late tracheostomy groups [26–30]. Hence, there have been debates on whether performing early tracheostomy provides any added benefit with regards to VAP.

Mortality

While discussing tracheostomy-associated mortality, it is important to recognize that not all deaths of patients with a tracheostomy are caused by the presence of this airway. On post-mortem evaluation, the majority of deaths are related to the underlying disease processes that led to the need for a tracheostomy. Nevertheless, deaths can also be a direct consequence of tracheostomy. Patients may die due to a sentinel bleed from a tracheostomy malposition, loss of airway from accidental decannulation of the tracheostomy tube, or inability to recannulate the stoma. Scales et al. and Combes et al. reported that the rate of mortality was lower in patients who received a tracheostomy compared to patients who did not receive a tracheostomy but remained endotracheally intubated [31, 32]. This is probably because these patients were too sick to even qualify for a tracheostomy. A chart review of 483 patients revealed that patients who received a tracheostomy had a mortality rate of 11% at 2 weeks, 19% at one-month, and 40% at 6 months after tracheostomy [33]. Moreover, in-hospital mortality was found to be 30% in all patients who received a tracheostomy. With regards to early vs. late tracheostomy, several studies have shown that the timing of a tracheostomy is not associated with mortality rate.

Lengths of Stay

Lengths of stay in the ICU and hospital are used as a metric to measure the effectiveness of care provided to patients with a tracheostomy because they directly relate to healthcare costs. Bouderka et al. and Trouillet et al. reported that there were no differences in the ICU length of stay between those who received a tracheostomy and those who remained endotracheally intubated [34, 35]. In contrast, Freeman et al. reported an increase in the ICU and hospital lengths of stay among patients who received a tracheostomy [36]. When comparing patients who received an early vs. late tracheostomy, several studies reported a decrease in ICU and total hospital lengths of stay in patients who received an early tracheostomy. This has been specifically well-documented in patients with a neurological underlying diagnosis in whom a tracheostomy had been placed for airway protection due to loss of oral-pharyngeal-glottic control. A tracheostomy in such patients facilitates discharge from an ICU to the ward, or to a rehabilitation or chronic ventilator facility, thus permitting more rapid transition to a more appropriate care environment.

Ongoing Debate About Timing of Tracheostomy

Discussions about the appropriateness and timing of tracheostomy started with the 'period of rationalization'. Many clinicians tend to wait until all measures have been taken or they have failed to wean a patient from the ventilator. It is often considered as a last resort to help facilitate transfer of the patient out of the hospital. While this might seem prudent, delaying a tracheostomy may place a patient at a risk for VAP, increased discomfort, inability to speak or eat, and decreased mobility. All these issues could slow the ICU progression of clinical care. However, a tracheostomy should not be performed in a person who cannot readily benefit from the advantages that the airway may offer. With the current state of science related to mechanical ventilation and respiratory failure, it is frequently difficult to predict which patient might be a candidate for a tracheostomy. The need for a tracheostomy for airway protection might be quite apparent in patients with neurological pathology having a slow process of recovery. In patients with pneumonia or congestive heart failure, clinicians often rely on medical management, such as antibiotics or diuresis, in the hope of circumventing the need for a tracheostomy. The timing of such a recovery can be challenging, and often the ICU team wrestles with the issue for some time before a decision is made to move forward with a tracheostomy. Investigators in this field rather arbitrarily define early vs. late tracheostomy at 7, 10, or 14 days in light of the fact that the time period during which airway injury secondary to an endotracheal tube may occur is unclear from current pathological studies.

Importance of Patient's Perspective

The fundamental concern in all studies investigating the timing of a tracheostomy is that the metrics have been limited to a few discrete clinical outcomes such as VAP, mortality, and lengths of stay. Few studies have explored the patients' subjective perspectives regarding their experience with a tracheostomy versus endotracheal intubation, and at best are retrospective in nature. Patients are typically interviewed about their experience in the ICU or with a mechanical ventilator after they are discharged from the hospital. Given their critical illness during their ICU period, it is typical that such patients have a very poor recollection of their experience. A recent study by Pandian et al. prospectively surveying awake and interactive, mechanically ventilated ICU patients demonstrated a better quality of life with a tracheostomy compared to being endotracheally intubated [37]. Moreover, patients who received early tracheostomy (within 10 days of being intubated) reported a consequent earlier improvement in their quality of life than those who received one at a later time point or remained endotracheally intubated. This was attributed to improvements in comfort, decreased sedation requirements, greater patient autonomy, and the ability to speak and swallow. The findings from this study are enlightening, as it noted a highly statistically significant difference between early vs. late tracheostomy in the patients' perceived quality of life during this period of ICU care. Such evidence supports the tenet that in addition to the clinical parameters weighing in on the decision to offer a tracheostomy (laryngeal health, pulmonary toilet, neurological status, and lengths of stay), the patient's perspective is equally important to consider.

Conclusion

Tracheostomy is a procedure performed to alleviate airway obstruction or serve as a conduit for chronic mechanical ventilation. There is variation in the techniques used to perform a tracheostomy and how the tracheostomy is cared for. Few evidence-based guidelines are available to direct optimal management of patients with a tracheostomy, and expert opinion often remains the rule of the land. It has been well documented, however, that a tracheostomy does enhance an ICU patient's quality of life while undergoing critical care. The comprehensive goal of ICU airway management is to ensure patient safety and clinical progress while responding to the needs of the patient and family members. Future research is greatly needed in the science of managing a patient with a tracheostomy.

References

1. Durbin CG Jr (2005) Techniques for performing tracheostomy. Respir Care 50:488–496
2. Choby G, Goldenberg D (2011) The history of tracheotomy. Pharos Alpha Omega Alpha Honor Med Soc 74:34–38
3. Jackson C (1909) Tracheostomy. Laryngscope 19:285–290
4. Seldinger DI (1953) Catheter replacement of the needle in percutaneous arteriography. Acta Radiol 39:368–376
5. Sheldon CH, Pudenz RH, Freshwater DB, Crue BL (1957) A new method for tracheotomy. J Neurosurg 12:428–431
6. Toye FJ, Weinstein JD (1969) A percutaneous tracheostomy device. Surgery 65:384–389
7. Ciaglia P, Firsching R, Synieç C (1985) Elective percutaneous dilatational tracheostomy. A new simple bedside procedure; preliminary report. Chest 87:715–719
8. Byhahn C, Lischke V, Halbig S, Scheifler G, Westphal K (2000) Ciaglia blue rhino: a modified technique for percutaneous dilatation tracheostomy. Technique and early clinical results. Anaesthesist 49:202–206
9. Griggs WM, Worthley LI, Gilligan JE, Thomas, Myburg JA (1990) A simple percutaneous tracheostomy technique. Surg Gynecol Obstet 170:543–545
10. Fantoni A, Ripamonti D (1997) A non-derivative, non-surgical tracheostomy: the translaryngeal method. Intensive Care Med 23:386–392
11. Yurtseven N, Aydemir B, Karaca P et al (2007) PercuTwist: a new alternative to Griggs and Ciaglia's techniques. Eur J Anaesthesiol 24:492–497

12. Gromann TW, Birkelbach O, Hetzer R (2009) Ballon dilatational tracheostomy. Technique and first clinical experience with the Ciaglia Blue Dolphin method. Chirurg 80:622–627
13. Caparros AC (2014) Mechanical ventilation and the role of saline instillation in suctioning adult intensive care unit patients: an evidence-based practice review. Dimens Crit Care Nurs 33:246–253
14. Mitchell RB, Hussey HM, Setzen G et al (2013) Clinical consensus statement: tracheostomy care. Otolaryngol Head Neck Surg 248:6–20
15. Pandian V, Miller CR, Schiavi AJ et al (2014) Utilization of a standardized tracheostomy capping and decannulation protocol to improve patient safety. Laryngoscope 124:1794–1800
16. Mirski MA, Pandian V, Bhatti N et al (2012) Safety, efficiency, and cost-effectiveness of a multidisciplinary percutaneous tracheostomy program. Crit Care Med 40:1827–1834
17. Pandian V, Miller CR, Mirski MA et al (2012) Multidisciplinary team approach in the management of tracheostomy patients. Otolaryngol Head Neck Surg 147:684–691
18. Cameron TS, McKinstry A, Burt SK et al (2009) Outcomes of patients with spinal cord injury before and after introduction of an interdisciplinary tracheostomy team. Crit Care Resusc 11:14–19
19. McGrath BA, Bates L, Atkinson D, Moore JA (2012) Multidisciplinary guidelines for the management of tracheostomy and laryngectomy airway emergencies. Anaesthesia 67:1025–1041
20. McGrath BA, Wallace S (2014) The UK National Tracheostomy Safety Project and the role of speech and language therapists. Curr Opin Otolaryngol Head Neck Surg 22:181–187
21. Sung JH, Kim IS, Yang SH, Hong JT, Son BC, Lee SW (2011) Is computerized tomography angiographic surveillance valuable for prevention of tracheoinnominate artery fistula, a life-threatening complication after tracheostomy? J Korean Neurosurg Soc 49:107–111
22. American Thoracic Society (2005) Guidelines for the management of adults with hospital-acquired, ventilator associated, and healthcare-associated pneumonia. Am J Respir Crit Care Med 171:388–416
23. Moller MG, Slaikeu JD, Bonelli P, Davis AT, Hoogeboom JE, Bonnell BW (2005) Early tracheostomy versus late tracheostomy in the surgical intensive care unit. Am J Surg 189:293–296
24. Schauer JM, Engle LL, Maugher DT, Cherry RA (2009) Does acuity matter? – Optimal timing of tracheostomy stratified by injury severity. J Trauma 66:220–225
25. Schneider GT, Christensen N, Doerr TD (2009) Early tracheotomy in elderly patients results in less ventilator-associated pneumonia. Otolaryngol Head Neck Surg 140:250–255
26. Barquist ES, Amortegui J, Hallal A et al (2006) Tracheostomy in ventilator dependent trauma patients: a prospective, randomized intention-to-treat study. J Trauma 60:91–97
27. Kocaeli H, Korfali E, Taskapilioglu O, Ozcan T (2008) Analysis of intracranial pressure changes during early versus late percutaneous tracheostomy in a neuro-intensive care unit. Acta Neurochir (Wien) 150:1263–1267
28. Pinheiro BV, Tostes RO, Brum CI, Carvalho EV, Pinto SP, Oliveira JC (2010) Early versus late tracheostomy in patients with acute severe brain injury. J Bras Pneumol 36:84–91
29. Terragni PP, Antonelli M, Fumagalli R et al (2010) Early vs late tracheotomy for prevention of pneumonia in mechanically ventilated adult ICU patients: a randomized controlled trial. JAMA 303:1483–1489
30. Zagli G, Linden M, Spina R et al (2010) Early tracheostomy in intensive care unit: a retrospective study of 506 cases of video-guided Ciaglia Blue Rhino tracheostomies. J Trauma 68:367–372
31. Scales DC, Thiruchelvam D, Kiss A, Redelmeier DA (2008) The effect of tracheostomy timing during critical illness on long-term survival. Crit Care Med 36:2547–2557
32. Combes A, Luyt CE, Nieszkowska A, Trouillet JL, Gibert C, Chastre J (2007) Is tracheostomy associated with better outcomes for patients requiring long-term mechanical ventilation? Crit Care Med 35:802–807

33. Pandian V, Gilstrap DL, Mirski MA et al (2012) Predictors of short-term mortality in patients undergoing percutaneous dilatational tracheostomy. J Crit Care 27:420–415
34. Bouderka MA, Fakhir B, Bouaggad A, Hmamouchi B, Hamoudi D, Harti A (2004) Early tracheostomy versus prolonged endotracheal intubation in severe head injury. J Trauma 57:251–254
35. Trouillet JL, Luyt CE, Guiguet M et al (2011) Early percutaneous tracheotomy versus prolonged intubation of mechanically ventilated patients after cardiac surgery: a randomized trial. Ann Intern Med 154:373–383
36. Freeman BD, Isabella K, Lin N, Buchman TG (2000) A meta-analysis of prospective trials comparing percutaneous and surgical tracheostomy in critically ill patients. Chest 118:1412–1418
37. Pandian V, Thompson CB, Feller-Kopman DJ, Mirski MA (2015) Development and validation of a quality-of-life questionnaire for mechanically ventilated ICU patients. Crit Care Med 43:142–148

Shared Decision-making to Pursue, Withhold or Withdraw Invasive Mechanical Ventilation in Acute Respiratory Failure

M. E. Wilson, P. R. Bauer, and O. Gajic

Introduction

► **Clinical vignette** A 72-year-old man is admitted to the intensive care unit (ICU) with acute respiratory distress syndrome (ARDS) of unclear etiology. Despite treatment with empiric antibiotics and diuresis, the patient's hypoxia gradually worsened. On hospital admission, he stated that he did not want to be kept permanently alive on machines and because of this he chose a code status of 'do-not-resuscitate and do-not-intubate' (DNR/DNI). For the past 12 hours, he has required non-invasive ventilation (NIV) with a fraction of inspired oxygen (FiO_2) of 100% to maintain an oxygen saturation of 86%. Although his clinical status is not emergently declining, you feel that the patient would benefit from intubation and invasive mechanical ventilation. The patient reconsiders mechanical ventilation and tells you his primary concern is quality of life. He asks you about his chances of going home and getting back to his normal life if he were to be intubated.

Patients with acute respiratory failure, their family members, and clinicians are faced with decisions on whether or not to initiate a trial of life support (invasive mechanical ventilation) and how long to continue that trial. The decisions to initiate or withhold and continue or withdraw mechanical ventilation are preference-sensitive decisions – meaning that the patient's values, preferences, and autonomy may play a role in decision-making [1]. Shared decision-making has been recommended by European and North American critical care societies, as well as a recent international consensus, as a recommended method to approach life support decision-making [2–4]. Shared decision-making is a collaborative process that allows patients and clinicians to evaluate the best scientific evidence available as well as considering the patient's values and preferences in making a healthcare decision together [5].

M. E. Wilson ✉ · P. R. Bauer · O. Gajic
Division of Pulmonary and Critical Care Medicine, Mayo Clinic, Rochester, USA
e-mail: wilson.michael1@mayo.edu

J.-L. Vincent (ed.), *Annual Update in Intensive Care and Emergency Medicine 2015*,
DOI 10.1007/978-3-319-13761-2_17

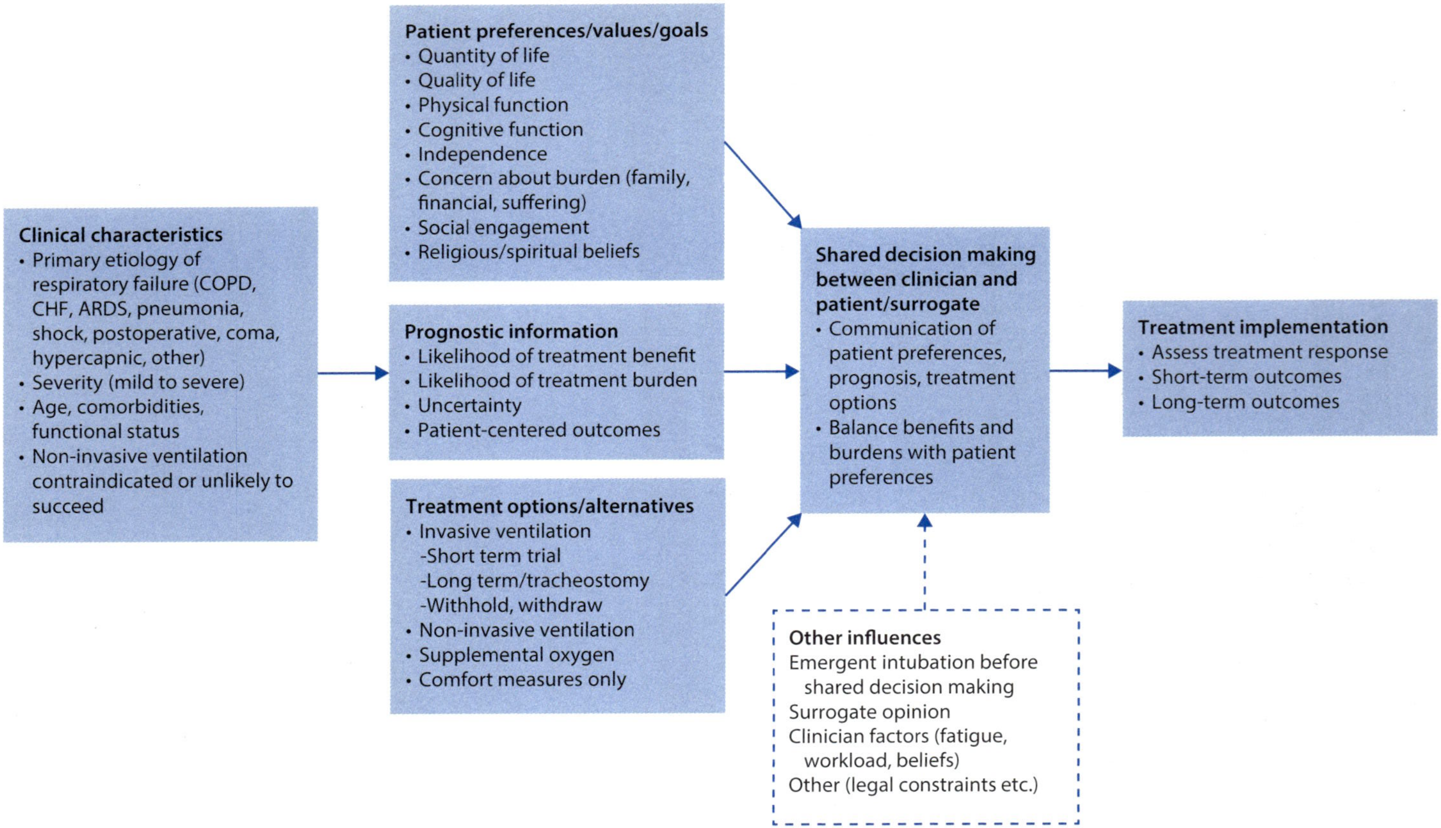

Fig. 1 Conceptual framework for shared decision-making in acute respiratory failure. COPD: chronic obstructive pulmonary disease; CHF: congestive heart failure; ARDS: acute respiratory distress syndrome

One central component of shared decision-making is ensuring that patients understand the available treatment options (and alternatives), the possible benefits and harms of each treatment option and the likelihood of the benefits and harms of each option occurring [6]. When patients have an accurate knowledge of treatment options and prognostic outcomes of those treatment options, patients are more likely to make decisions that are in alignment with their preferences [7, 8]. Thus, obtaining, evaluating, and effectively communicating high quality patient-centered prognostic information to patients, family members, and clinicians is a vital component to optimal shared decision-making. The purpose of this article is to outline the framework for shared decision-making for invasive mechanical ventilation in acute respiratory failure and to highlight the key role of providing patient-centered prognostic information. Figure 1 describes a conceptual framework for this process.

Background

Acute respiratory failure is defined as the potentially life-threatening inability of the respiratory system (lungs, chest wall, respiratory muscles and controllers) to perform ventilation and/or gas exchange (oxygen uptake and/or carbon dioxide elimination) and which develops suddenly (over minutes to hours) [9, 10]. Acute respiratory failure has multiple etiologies and is manifested by hypoxemia and/or hypercapnia in addition to symptoms of respiratory distress such as tachypnea, accessory muscle use, bradypnea and/or respiratory arrest. Acute respiratory failure can also be defined as an acute respiratory condition requiring high-concentration face-mask oxygen or non-invasive or invasive mechanical ventilation [11]. Acute respiratory failure is the most common cause of admission to the ICU [12]. Some patients experience acute-on-chronic respiratory failure in the setting of chronic hypoxemia or hypercapnia due to medical conditions, such as chronic obstructive pulmonary disease (COPD). Possible treatment strategies for acute respiratory failure include a trial of invasive mechanical ventilation, non-invasive ventilation, such as continuous positive airway pressure (CPAP) or bilevel positive airway pressure (BiPAP), supplemental oxygen, high flow oxygen, or comfort measures only. The primary modality for administering supplemental oxygen and treating acute respiratory failure often changes during the course of acute respiratory failure depending on treatment response. Intubation and invasive mechanical ventilation are considered when other therapies, such as high flow oxygen or NIV fail or are contraindicated. Additional treatment strategies, such as antibiotics, steroids, anticoagulation, or diuresis, etc. can be started empirically or based on the underlying etiology.

Decision-making to Pursue Invasive Mechanical Ventilation

The decisions to intubate and pursue invasive mechanical or withhold invasive mechanical and to continue invasive mechanical ventilation or withdraw invasive mechanical ventilation can be made unilaterally by the physician (paternalistic decision-making model), or can be made after considering patient input and values (shared decision-making model). Traditionally, a shared model has been more common in North America, and a paternalistic model has been more common in Europe and throughout the rest of the world [13]. Recent international and European consensus statements strongly recommend a shared decision-making approach, which suggests that attitudes on how to optimally make life-support decisions are evolving towards increased patient involvement [2, 4]. In the past 15 years, several studies have shown that many, but not all, patients, families, and clinicians prefer patient and family involvement in decision-making [14–17]. It is unclear whether a patient and family's desires not to be involved in life-support decision-making is a reflection of true preference or if it is a reflection of societal custom, physician preference, or other underlying concerns, such as inadequate information, mistrust, or dissatisfaction [17].

Shared Decision-making

Shared decision-making is a collaborative process that allows patients, families, and physicians to evaluate the best prognostic evidence and consider the patient's goals, values, and preferences in making a health decision together [5]. The key tenets of shared decision-making for acute respiratory failure are listed in Box 1. Shared decision-making allows a clinician and patient and family to first examine the treatment options and alternatives, the pros and cons of each treatment option and alternatives, and the likelihood of those pros and cons occurring. Clinicians and patients can then discuss the patient's preferences and goals of medical treatment and determine together which treatment options will best achieve the patient's goals. Decision preferences can change overtime and decision-making may involve several conversations. While shared decision-making is a recommended method of discussing preference sensitive decisions, such as life support withdrawal, its widespread implementation is limited [18]. Few decision aids have been developed to help clinicians, patients, and families approach decision-making [19].

Box 1. Shared Decision-making for Invasive Mechanical Ventilation

Prior to the conversation, the clinician:

- Obtains an accurate understanding of the:
  - Medical condition
  - Treatment options and alternatives
  - Highest quality patient-centered prognostic outcomes
  - Treatment burden

During the conversation, the clinician:

- Discusses:
  - The nature of the decision to be made
  - The treatment options
  - The benefits and burdens of each treatment option (prognostic information)
- Elicits:
  - The patient's understanding of information
  - The patient's values, preferences, and goals of medical treatment
  - The patient's preferred role in decision-making
- In consensus with patient:
  - Determines whether treatment can achieve at least one reasonable therapeutic goal
  - Determines whether the patient would want the treatment
  - Determines the treatment decision

After the conversation, the clinician:

- Implements the treatment decision
- Periodically reassesses clinical response, goals, and indications of treatment

When patients and surrogates are involved in the decision-making process for initiating, withholding or withdrawing invasive mechanical ventilation, the following possible treatment preferences include [20]:

- I prefer maximum prolonging treatment without preset limits on advanced life support measures. I prefer a trial of intubation and mechanical ventilation. If a time comes when these treatments do not adequately help my condition or treatment becomes too burdensome, then I prefer comfort measures only.
- I prefer full medical treatment except for intubation and mechanical ventilation (do-not-intubate). If a time comes when these treatments do not adequately help my condition or treatment becomes too burdensome, then I prefer comfort measures only.
- I prefer comfort measures only.
- I am unsure what my preferences are.
- I prefer that somebody else (such as a surrogate or the medical team) make the decision.

Determining Individualized Prognosis

After explaining the possible decision choices, outlining the possible outcomes and the likelihood of those outcomes occurring is a subsequent step in shared decision-making. Information about outcomes of acute respiratory failure is important for patients/families to be able to balance the potential benefits and burdens of treatments. Providing accurate prognostic information has been shown to modify the treatment preferences of hospitalized patients in hypothetical scenarios of acute respiratory failure and other conditions [7, 8]. Information about outcomes of acute respiratory failure is also important for clinicians when making treatment decisions and guiding patients/families through the shared decision-making process.

The qualities of ideal prognostic information are outlined in Box 2, and include providing individualized information regarding patient-centered outcomes communicated in a manner that is understandable and useful. Currently, ideal prognostic information for acute respiratory failure is very limited, as outlined below. The limited prognostic information that is available is difficult for physicians to locate, difficult for physicians to assess in terms of quality and generalizability, and is not found in a format that can easily be shared with patients and families [21]. There is no single source of best available prognostic information for physicians, patients, or surrogates in the ICU. Despite its importance, determining and communicating prognosis is one of the most difficult tasks that critical care physicians face.

Box 2. Ideal Prognostic Information for Decision-making

- Accounts for:
  - Etiology of acute respiratory failure
  - Severity of acute respiratory failure
  - Underlying comorbidities (such as malignancy) or pre-existing poor functional status
  - Likelihood of treatment benefit
  - Likelihood of treatment burden
  - Uncertainty
  - Baseline patient preferences (such as do-not-intubate versus full code)
- Includes patient-centered outcomes (such as quality of life, financial burden in addition to short-term and long-term mortality)
- Applies to the individual patient
- Communicated in a manner that is understandable and useful for patients and families
- Can be reassessed anytime

Three major methods have been used to estimate the prognosis of critically ill patients: Scoring systems, clinician estimation, and outcomes data from clinical trials. Scoring systems (such as the Acute Physiology and Chronic Health Evaluation [APACHE] system, Simplified Acute Physiologic Score [SAPS], Mortality Prediction Model [MPM], and Sequential Organ Failure Assessment score [SOFA]) have been developed to predict hospital mortality. While these scoring systems can reasonably predict mortality in a cohort of ICU patients, their accuracy in prediction of individual risk of mortality has been limited and controversial [22, 23]. Sequential application of scoring systems may improve their utility, although no formal recommendations of how to use scoring systems in routine clinical practice have been developed [24]. In addition to scoring systems, clinician (physician and/or nurse) estimation of ICU outcomes has wide variability and limited accuracy. One recent study showed that physicians are no better than chance at predicting short-term mortality [25, 26].

Randomized controlled trials (RCTs) and cohort studies provide outcome information for patients with acute respiratory failure. For ethical reasons, RCTs cannot assign patients with severe acute respiratory failure to withholding or withdrawing life support. Therefore, RCTs typically exclude patients who are already intubated or need emergent intubation, contributing to limited generalizability. A recent comparative effectiveness review found no short-term mortality benefit to invasive mechanical ventilation compared to NIV, although patients who required emergent intubation were excluded [9]. None of the RCTs assessed patient-centered outcomes, such as health-related quality of life, functional status, or psychological distress. Duration of non-invasive or invasive mechanical ventilation was reported infrequently.

We could find no systematic reviews of cohort studies evaluating the outcomes of patients with acute respiratory failure – either for patients with do-not-intubate preferences or for patients with no life-support treatment limitations (Full Code). Large, multicenter, international, prospective and retrospective cohort studies have described short-term outcomes of patients on invasive mechanical ventilation [27]. Other studies have described mortality for acute respiratory failure in patients with specific comorbidities such as malignancy [28]. In some conditions leading to acute respiratory failure, such as ARDS, many long-term patient-centered outcomes (such as long-term mortality, quality of life, physical impairment, cognitive impairment, psychiatric impairment, subsequent health care utilization, and chronic critical illness) have been described [29, 30]. In patients with acute respiratory failure who do not undergo invasive mechanical ventilation (do-not-resuscitate order), there are limited data on in-hospital mortality and very limited data on patient-centered outcomes, such as quality of life, hospital discharge location, and subsequent health care utilization [31–33]. Nearly all patients who undergo withdrawal of mechanical ventilation die in the hospital, with very limited data on survivors [34]. Major limitations of prognostic information from clinical trial data include the lack of patient-centered outcomes data, including burden of treatment, lack of delineation of the decision-making process and its impact on outcome, variability (location, practice setting) of participating centers, and lack of delineation of the etiology and/or severity of acute respiratory failure.

Patient-centered Outcomes and Burden of Treatment

What prognostic outcomes are important to patients and families when making decisions to pursue, withhold, or withdraw life support? Currently, patient-centered outcomes are not well defined for acute respiratory failure and its treatment options [35–37]. Box 3 lists potentially important patient-centered outcomes, including mortality. Burden of treatment has been shown to impact decision-making in multiple qualitative studies. Many survivors of invasive mechanical ventilation have reported that the pain and discomfort from invasive mechanical ventilation would impact their future decision-making [38]. For many patients, hospital discharge to a skilled nursing facility, not returning to the same occupation, or living with prolonged mechanical ventilation are serious considerations when making decisions about intubation and invasive mechanical ventilation [8, 39]. Many survivors of critical illness say that they would not have pursued the decision to proceed with invasive mechanical ventilation and chronic critical illness had they known the significant financial burden and negative emotional impact their illness would have on their family members. Up to 30% of patients who are treated with NIV discontinue the treatment because of intolerance or other discomfort [9]. In acute respiratory failure, few studies have attempted to systematically quantify and prioritize important patient-centered outcomes or burden of treatment.

Box 3. Patient-centered Outcomes Potentially Important in Acute Respiratory Failure

In-hospital outcomes

- Mortality (hospital, ICU)
- Length of ICU/hospital stay
- Duration of invasive mechanical ventilation, duration of non-invasive ventilation, re-intubation rate, rate of non-invasive ventilation discontinuation due to intolerance
- Symptom control (such as pain, agitation, sedation, dyspnea, confusion, delirium, hunger, thirst, nausea), and associated medication use
- Psychological distress
- Complications (such as deep vein thrombosis, ventilator-associated pneumonia, debility)
- Procedures (such as tracheostomy, chest tube placement, nasogastric tube insertion, cardiopulmonary resuscitation)
- Satisfaction with medical care (support, decision-making, communication with medical team)
- Quality of life during hospitalization (patient inability to communicate, use of restraints, time spent in bed due to debility)
- Quality of death
- Financial burden (direct and indirect cost for the patient/family)
- Burden of treatment modalities

Post-hospital outcomes (for survivors)

- Mortality (long-term)
- Quality of life (satisfaction with life, return to work)
- Health-related quality of life (impact of health and illness on satisfaction with life)
- Functional status (ability to perform the tasks of daily living, exercise capability, ICU acquired weakness)
- Symptom control (such as persistent pain or dyspnea), and associated medication use
- Psychological distress (anxiety, depression, post traumatic distress syndrome)
- Hospital discharge location (home versus skilled nursing facility)
- Subsequent health care utilization and hospitalization
- Cognitive effects
- Quality of death
- Financial burden (direct and indirect cost for the patient/family)
- Home going oxygen, non-invasive ventilation requirements
- Chronic critical illness

Box 3. (Continuation)

Caregiver/family outcomes:

- Quality of life, alteration of lifestyle
- Psychological distress (anxiety, depression, distress, post traumatic distress syndrome)
- Financial burden (direct and indirect cost for the patient/family)

Communicating Prognosis

After the highest quality, patient-specific prognostic information is identified by the clinician, this information must then be communicated to the patient and family in a manner that is understandable and useful. Patients, surrogates, and even physicians find probabilistic information difficult to interpret and explain [40]. It is difficult to translate information from risk prediction models or from clinical trials into individual risk at the bedside. A recent systematic review of methods to communicate risk to patients concluded that although there is no single best method of communicating prognostic information, methods such as visual aids and communication of absolute risk may improve patient comprehension and methods such as number-needed-to-treat may lead to confusion [40]. In addition, despite achieving the goal of providing ideal prognostic information in an ideal format, clinicians will always need to address uncertainty. Even with this uncertainty, patients and their family members desire prognostic information and use this information in decision-making [41].

Patient Preferences, Values and Goals

Once a physician has determined the prognosis and communicated relevant patient-centered prognostic information to the patient and family, an ensuing key step in shared decision-making is assessing the patient's preferences, values, and goals of medical treatment [42]. The purpose of this step is to determine what treatment burdens the patient is willing to endure in an effort to survive and achieve an acceptable quality of life. Seven goals of care of hospitalized patients have been described, ranging from a primary goal to live longer to a primary goal to be comfortable, and include functional ability and cognitive ability (see Box 4) [43]. Patients can have multiple goals at once (for example all patients desire to be comfortable), but it is often helpful to prioritize goals (for example quality of life over quantity of life or vice versa) to guide treatment decisions. Once the goals of medical treatment and patient values for living are assessed, the clinician can integrate this information with prognostic information to help the patient in decision deliberation. Together the clinician and patient can determine if the patient perceives that a treatment (such as invasive mechanical ventilation) is likely to help the patient achieve one or more goals of medical treatment and if the potential benefits of a treatment outweigh the potential burdens.

Box 4. Seven Goals of Treatment of Hospitalized Patients [43]

1. Be cured of disease
2. Live longer
3. Improve or maintain quality of life or function or independence
4. Be comfortable
5. Achieve a particular life goal:
    - Live at home (versus a skilled nursing facility)
    - Strengthen a relationship
    - Special occasion or accomplishment (such as making it to the graduation of a child)
    - Spiritual goal
    - Good death
6. Provide support for family/caregiver
7. Further understand diagnosis or prognosis

Other Decision Determinants

Two major determinants (patient prognosis and patient preferences) should play a role in decision-making for life support [2, 3]. Aside from these factors, other determinants (some of them unwanted) impact decision-making. Culture, geography, religion, laws, and hospital practice setting have been shown to contribute to variability in decisions to withdraw and withhold life-support interventions [4]. There is also significant physician and nurse variability in decision-making, indicating that clinician-level factors play a role. Clinician-level factors, such as fatigue, workload, personal beliefs and biases, personal experiences, specialty training, shift changes, level of experience, and interactions with the patient, such as hearing the patient's wishes firsthand, have all been shown to impact decision-making [34, 44, 45]. In addition, surrogate decision-maker factors, such as disagreement or conflict, trust in the medical system, secondary gain, and experiences also play a role. Finally, sometimes emergent intubation precludes a thoughtful shared decision-making process before treatment implementation occurs. Identifying methods and tools to improve focus on patient prognosis and preferences is one way to overcome unwanted confounding factors.

Conclusion

Shared decision-making is a recommended approach to helping patients, family members, and clinicians make preference sensitive decisions, such as whether or not to pursue invasive mechanical ventilation. When clinicians use a shared decision-making model, they discuss with patients the treatment options as well as the likelihood of the risks and benefits of each option, before assessing patient values and collaboratively making a decision together. Few tools exist to help physicians obtain and communicate high quality patient centered prognostic information about treatment options to patients. Standardized patient-centered outcomes for acute respiratory failure have not been established. A conceptual model of shared decision-making in acute respiratory failure identifies the relationship between key determinants in decision-making (Fig. 1) and identifies key steps in the process (Box 1). In an effort to improve the delivery of high quality patient-centered medical care, novel strategies to improve individual patient risk assessment and implement shared decision-making should be developed.

References

1. Keirns CC, Goold SD (2009) Patient-centered care and preference-sensitive decision making. JAMA 302:1805–1806
2. Carlet J, Thijs LG, Antonelli M et al (2004) Challenges in end-of-life care in the ICU. Statement of the 5th International Consensus Conference in Critical Care: Brussels, Belgium, April 2003. Intensive Care Med 30:770–784
3. Truog RD, Campbell ML, Curtis JR et al (2008) Recommendations for end-of-life care in the intensive care unit: a consensus statement by the American College of Critical Care Medicine. Crit Care Med 36:953–963
4. Sprung CL, Truog RD, Curtis JR et al (2014) Seeking worldwide professional consensus on the principles of end-of-life care for the critically ill: The Welpicus Study. Am J Respir Crit Care Med 190:855–866
5. Informed Medical Decisions Foundation What is Shared Decision Making?. http://www.informedmedicaldecisions.org/what-is-shared-decision-making/. Accessed September 2014
6. Shepherd HL, Barratt A, Trevena LJ et al (2011) Three questions that patients can ask to improve the quality of information physicians give about treatment options: a cross-over trial. Patient Educ Couns 84:379–385
7. Jesus JE, Allen MB, Michael GE et al (2013) Preferences for resuscitation and intubation among patients with do-not-resuscitate/do-not-intubate orders. Mayo Clin Proc 88:658–665
8. Fried TR, Bradley EH, Towle VR, Allore H (2002) Understanding the treatment preferences of seriously ill patients. N Engl J Med 346:1061–1066
9. Williams JW, Cox CE, Hargett CW et al (2012) Noninvasive Positive-Pressure Ventilation (NPPV) for Acute Respiratory Failure. Agency for Healthcare Research and Quality, Rockville, MD
10. British Thoracic Society Standards of Care Committee (2002) Non-invasive ventilation in acute respiratory failure. Thorax 57:192–211
11. Azoulay E, Schlemmer B (2006) Diagnostic strategy in cancer patients with acute respiratory failure. Intensive Care Med 32:808–822
12. Cartin-Ceba R, Kojicic M, Li G et al (2011) Epidemiology of critical care syndromes, organ failures, and life-support interventions in a suburban US community. Chest 140:1447–1455
13. Cook D (2001) Patient autonomy versus parentalism. Crit Care Med 29:N24–N25

14. Heyland DK, Cook DJ, Rocker GM et al (2003) Decision-making in the ICU: perspectives of the substitute decision-maker. Intensive Care Med 29:75–82
15. Johnson SK, Bautista CA, Hong SY, Weissfeld L, White DB (2011) An empirical study of surrogates' preferred level of control over value-laden life support decisions in intensive care units. Am J Respir Crit Care Med 183:915–921
16. Azoulay E, Pochard F, Chevret S et al (2004) Half the family members of intensive care unit patients do not want to share in the decision-making process: a study in 78 French intensive care units. Crit Care Med 32:1832–1838
17. Levy MM (2004) Shared decision-making in the ICU: entering a new era. Crit Care Med 32:1966–1968
18. White DB, Braddock CH, Bereknyei S, Curtis JR (2007) Toward shared decision making at the end of life in intensive care units: opportunities for improvement. Arch Intern Med 167:461–467
19. Cox CE, Lewis CL, Hanson LC et al (2012) Development and pilot testing of a decision aid for surrogates of patients with prolonged mechanical ventilation. Crit Care Med 40:2327–2334
20. Curtis JR, Cook DJ, Sinuff T et al (2007) Noninvasive positive pressure ventilation in critical and palliative care settings: understanding the goals of therapy. Crit Care Med 35:932–939
21. Lamont EB, Christakis NA (2003) Complexities in prognostication in advanced cancer: "to help them live their lives the way they want to". JAMA 290:98–104
22. Rocker G, Cook D, Sjokvist P et al (2004) Clinician predictions of intensive care unit mortality. Crit Care Med 32:1149–1154
23. Kruse JA, Thill-Baharozian MC, Carlson RW (1988) Comparison of clinical assessment with APACHE II for predicting mortality risk in patients admitted to a medical intensive care unit. JAMA 260:1739–1742
24. Ferreira FL, Bota DP, Bross A, Melot C, Vincent JL (2001) Serial evaluation of the SOFA score to predict outcome in critically ill patients. JAMA 286:1754–1758
25. Meadow W, Pohlman A, Frain L et al (2011) Power and limitations of daily prognostications of death in the medical intensive care unit. Crit Care Med 39:474–479
26. Frick S, Uehlinger DE, Zuercher Zenklusen RM (2003) Medical futility: predicting outcome of intensive care unit patients by nurses and doctors – a prospective comparative study. Crit Care Med 31:456–461
27. Esteban A, Anzueto A, Frutos F et al (2002) Characteristics and outcomes in adult patients receiving mechanical ventilation: a 28-day international study. JAMA 287:345–355
28. Azoulay E, Thiery G, Chevret S et al (2004) The prognosis of acute respiratory failure in critically ill cancer patients. Medicine (Baltimore) 83:360–370
29. Herridge MS (2011) Recovery and long-term outcome in acute respiratory distress syndrome. Crit Care Clin 27:685–704
30. Nelson JE, Cox CE, Hope AA, Carson SS (2010) Chronic critical illness. Am J Respir Crit Care Med 182:446–454
31. Azoulay E, Kouatchet A, Jaber S et al (2013) Noninvasive mechanical ventilation in patients having declined tracheal intubation. Intensive Care Med 39:292–301
32. Levy M, Tanios MA, Nelson D et al (2004) Outcomes of patients with do-not-intubate orders treated with noninvasive ventilation. Crit Care Med 32:2002–2007
33. Scarpazza P, Incorvaia C, Amboni P et al (2011) Long-term survival in elderly patients with a do-not-intubate order treated with noninvasive mechanical ventilation. Int J Chron Obstruct Pulmon Dis 6:253–257
34. Cook D, Rocker G, Marshall J et al (2003) Withdrawal of mechanical ventilation in anticipation of death in the intensive care unit. N Engl J Med 349:1123–1132
35. Needham DM (2014) Understanding and improving clinical trial outcome measures in acute respiratory failure. Am J Respir Crit Care Med 189:875–877
36. Curtis JR (1998) The "patient-centered" outcomes of critical care: what are they and how should they be used? New Horiz 6:26–32
37. Peigne V, Chaize M, Falissard B et al (2011) Important questions asked by family members of intensive care unit patients. Crit Care Med 39:1365–1371

38. Mendelsohn AB, Belle SH, Fischhoff B, Wisniewski SR, Degenholtz H, Chelluri L (2002) How patients feel about prolonged mechanical ventilation 1 year later. Crit Care Med 30:1439–1445
39. Rady MY, Johnson DJ (2004) Hospital discharge to care facility: a patient-centered outcome for the evaluation of intensive care for octogenarians. Chest 126:1583–1591
40. Zipkin DA, Umscheid CA, Keating NL et al (2014) Evidence-based risk communication: a systematic review. Ann Intern Med 161:270–280
41. White DB, Engelberg RA, Wenrich MD, Lo B, Curtis JR (2010) The language of prognostication in intensive care units. Med Decis Making 30:76–83
42. Scheunemann LP, Arnold RM, White DB (2012) The facilitated values history: helping surrogates make authentic decisions for incapacitated patients with advanced illness. Am J Respir Crit Care Med 186:480–486
43. Kaldjian LC, Erekson ZD, Haberle TH et al (2009) Code status discussions and goals of care among hospitalised adults. J Med Ethics 35:338–342
44. Cook DJ, Guyatt GH, Jaeschke R et al (1995) Determinants in Canadian health care workers of the decision to withdraw life support from the critically ill. Canadian Critical Care Trials Group. JAMA 273:703–708
45. Wilson ME, Rhudy LM, Ballinger BA, Tescher AN, Pickering BW, Gajic O (2013) Factors that contribute to physician variability in decisions to limit life support in the ICU: a qualitative study. Intensive Care Med 39:1009–1018

Part V
Monitoring

New Fully Non-invasive Hemodynamic Monitoring Technologies: Groovy or Paltry Tools

J. Benes and E. Kasal

Introduction

It is always alluring to dream about the future of medical diagnostics and treatment possibilities to meliorate patient care. Decreasing the distress from invasive procedures, either diagnostic or therapeutic, seems to be one of the possible ways to do so. Decreasing the number of injections, catheters, tubing and large wounds is beginning to be an important part of contemporary medicine. On the other hand, invasive monitoring tools sometimes provide us with very important information hardly obtainable by other means in the critical care environment. Even in this milieu, significant effort has been made to replace highly invasive tools with less-invasive equipment; hemodynamic monitoring being an extraordinary example of this phenomenon.

When in the 1970s the pulmonary artery catheter (PAC) was first used for bedside monitoring of cardiac output, nobody had expected that similar information could be gathered from a finger ring or cuff. The development in technology over recent years has provided clinicians with many different devices based on many different physical principles. However, many uncertainties are still present. The reliability of non-invasively obtained parameters has been questioned by some, but the most important issue is whether we can manage our patients better by using these novel technologies [1]. To answer this question we have to consider two possible fields of new non-invasive hemodynamic monitor use: First, we can use the device to get the same information we already have from invasive monitoring, but without penetrating the skin; and second, because of its non-invasiveness, the device is affordable to use in less severe patients and hence provides us with more information.

J. Benes ✉ · E. Kasal
Department of Anesthesiology and Intensive Care, Charles University Hospital Plzen, Plzen, Czech Republic
e-mail: benesj@fnplzen.cz

J.-L. Vincent (ed.), *Annual Update in Intensive Care and Emergency Medicine 2015*, DOI 10.1007/978-3-319-13761-2_18

Overview of Available Technologies

Ultrasonography and Doppler

Ultrasonography and Doppler-based technologies are long-available monitoring tools for blood flow assessment. Transthoracic and esophageal approaches are widely applied to get the sonographic window and blood vessel alignment. However, only the transthoracic approach can be deemed truly non-invasive. Basic transthoracic echocardiography has become an important part of anesthesiology and critical care education, but due to its intermittent nature is seldom used for minute-to-minute patient management. The Australian USCOM device (USCOM Pty Ltd, Sydney, Australia) simplifies transthoracic echocardiography to one continuous Doppler emitting handheld probe enabling easily performable measurements of blood flow across aortic or pulmonary valves [2]. An important limitation is that no true two-dimensional view of the heart is displayed and that the cross sectional area of the measured heart valves is taken from nomograms. This disadvantage could disappear if a trending assessment were used instead of absolute values of stroke volume, but because of the handheld probe, the position may change slightly over time introducing inter-observation bias and hence also making trending difficult.

Non-invasive Continuous Pressure-based Technologies

Fuelled by the success of less invasive hemodynamic monitoring tools based on pressure wave analysis, several devices were recently marketed enabling totally non-invasive continuous arterial pressure and blood flow assessment. Two of them (ccNexfin/ClearSight, Edwards Lifesciences Inc, Irvine, CA-USA and CNAP; CN-Systems, Graz, Austria) are based on Peňaz's volume clamp/vascular unloading principle. In short, the finger arteries are held under sustained volume (volume clamp) assessed by plethysmography and null transmural pressure (vascular unloading) induced by a fast reacting inflatable cuff over the finger [3]. The pressure inside the cuff is analyzed and using reverse transit function (ccNexfin/ClearSight) or brachial cuff calibration (CNAP) transformed into radial or brachial pressure waveform. The influence of finger soft tissue and changes in vascular tone are eliminated using different algorithms. Validation of these pressure readings has been performed under different conditions by many studies showing promising results, but they are still not interchangeable with invasive standards [4]. Another device (T-Line; Tensys Medical Inc. San Diego, CA, USA) works on the applanation tonometry principle [5]. A transducer incorporated in a wristband is placed over a compressible part of the radial artery. By exerting counter pressure on the vascular wall high enough to induce zero transmural pressure, readings of mean arterial pressure (MAP) and arterial pressure wave are obtained.

The continuous pressure curve obtained by different means is later used for cardiac output assessment either by the device itself (ccNexfin/ClearSight; CNAP; T-Line) or by implementing the monitoring module into another device (LiDCO

Unity, LiDCO, Cambridge, UK). In all these devices, pulse wave analysis is superimposed on the pressure readings enabling stroke volume calculation. Different algorithms are used by these machines, but as with other more invasive pulse wave analysis devices the quality of the primary pressure signal is a pre-requisite for accurate acquisition of hemodynamic variables [3]. In many of these devices, external calibration is possible, but not necessary. However, without correct calibration, the pulse wave analysis results are prone to absolute bias. Nevertheless, the continuous display and blood flow calculation should at least enable monitoring of trends and dynamic variations induced by mechanical ventilation.

Bioimpedance and Bioreactance

Bioimpedance and bioreactance work on the principle of variations in electric conductivity or phase changes induced by the variable amount of fluids (blood) in thorax. Both methods are sensitive to external artefacts, which limits their use in the critical care/operating room environment. Several bioimpedance devices are available from different manufacturers. The bioreactance technology, which is less sensitive to external artefacts, is marketed solely as the NICOM device (Cheetah Medical Inc, Newton, MA, USA) [6]. This device has become more popular recently.

In respiratory monitoring, the multidetector impedance tomography technique (PulmoVista 500, Draeger CO, Lubeck, Germany) is used for bed-side evaluation of lung aeration. From the hemodynamic viewpoint, this might offer a unique opportunity to inspect the heart as well and may lead to interesting joint heart-lung assessment in the future [7].

Pulse Wave Transit Time

The Moen-Kortweg equation-based pulse wave transit time offers a novel and not yet widely clinically inspected hemodynamic monitoring system [8]. A single device (esCCO, Nihon Kohden, Japan) was marketed recently. A usual electrocardiogram (EKG) (R-wave) and pulse oximeter is all that is needed for the pulse wave transit time determination, which makes this technology appealing. However, as with the other non-invasive technologies, the device is based on a mathematical model of circulation with many unmeasured variables (arterial diameter, its wall thickness and elasticity, fluid density etc.), which makes it prone to err. In addition, pulse wave transit time consists of three distinct phases: Pre-ejection period, large conductive vessels and small resistive arteries. Changes in contractility and afterload affect each of these phases in a different way, which may influence both absolute values and trending ability.

Plethysmography

Photoplethysmography is not truly a hemodynamic monitoring technology, but its principle is essentially part of volume clamp and pulse wave transit time methods. In addition, spectrophotometry with use of multiple wavelengths, as for instance in the Massimo Rainbow pulse oximeters (Massimo Corp., Irvine, Ca, USA), enables not only the continuous estimation of oxygen saturation, but also of the hemoglobin concentration itself [9]. In conjunction with non-invasive cardiac output assessment this might in the future allow totally non-invasive continuous monitoring of oxygen delivery. In addition, plethysmography enables assessment of pulse wave amplitude and hence of the change in arteriolar flow throughout the respiratory cycle. The plethysmography variability index (PVI) seems to be a reliable non-invasive substitute of stroke volume variation or other dynamic predictors [10].

What Limits the Use of Non-invasive Technologies

Contemporary non-invasive hemodynamic monitors are based on different physical principles so each of them possesses specific limitations. For example, esophageal Doppler probes are not well tolerated by awake patients; finger cuffs do not work well in patients with peripheral edema; and the applanometric wristband is prone to dislodgement during patient movement. On the other hand, one important limitation is common to all of the devices: These devices are based on mathematical assumptions and models, replacing direct measurement with simplifying calculations. In addition, such models are usually based on many important denominators describing the properties of the vascular tree, body or blood composition. Given their total non-invasiveness, many such denominators are assumed from demographic parameters or other assumptions and embedded models. This makes such calculations demanding in situations when multiple variables change at the same time: For example, during the resuscitative phase of septic shock when fluids, vasopressors and inotropes are all used changing preload, contractility, heart rate, afterload, blood viscosity and water content of the extravascular tissue. For this reason, the performance of non-invasive devices is much better under normal (physiologic) conditions, which are easier to describe by the model and where the denominators are known from population or physiologic studies. The more severe the disease of the patient, the more these influences counteract and may distort the algorithm. In other words, the monitoring accuracy and precision will gradually decrease with increase in patient disease severity (Fig. 1).

Even though not non-invasive in nature, the performance of the Vigileo/FloTrac (Edwards Lifesciences Inc., Irvine, CA, USA) might serve as an excellent example of this problem. Because this system is based on mathematical analysis of the arterial pressure curve without external calibration, all important parameters of arterial compliance and peripheral resistance are calculated from the patient's demographic parameters and statistical analysis of the curve. When these denominators were calculated in a 10-minute long flow window, as was the case for the first genera-

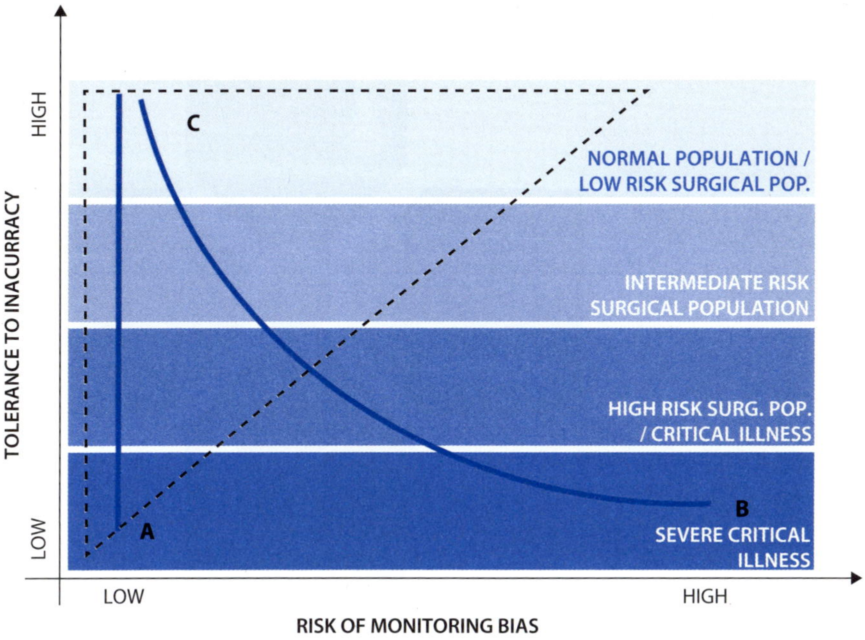

Fig. 1 Illustration of the relationship between risk of and tolerance to false readings. Accurate (and precise) devices (e. g., thermodilution) offer similar performance in all groups of patients (line A). Non-invasive technologies tend to decrease their performance with severity of illness (line B). All monitors could come into consideration for a given case if they fit into the triangle of tolerance (C)

tion software, the performance under steady conditions worked well, but it failed when rapid changes were imposed [11]. When the flow window was shortened to 60 seconds, the performance improved (second generation), but still the model failed to couple with changes in systemic resistance [12]. This means it worked well in normal patients during anesthesia, but not in liver transplant patients or when high doses of pressors were used [13]. After these pathophysiologic features were implemented into the algorithm (so called Dynamic Tone Technology in the third generation software), the device seemed to work well under normo- and hypodynamic conditions (standard or high risk surgery) [14], but still does not reach the reference standard in the most severe patients (septic or cardiogenic shock) [15].

Thanks to the extensive work of Critchley and colleagues [16, 17], we have three statistical instruments in hand to describe a monitor's performance: Accuracy, precision and polar plot methodology – systematic bias, reliability and trending ability. However, these measures are only a statistical base for assessment of the device's performance acceptability. In order to achieve this, we have to also take patient- and situation-dependent factors into consideration (Fig. 1):

1) How probable is the composite risk of a false reading in my patient?
2) How high is the clinical tolerance to such a false reading?

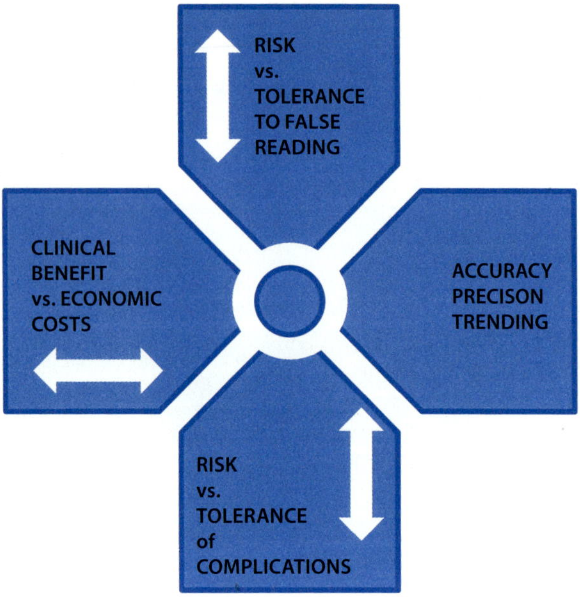

Fig. 2 Factors affecting our monitoring device choice/clinical utility

In addition to these two factors, we have to also consider the risk of monitoring-associated complications and tolerance to them. The risks associated with hemodynamic monitoring using a PAC have been well described in the past [18]; however, less invasive technologies are more common today. The risks of central venous or arterial catheterization are much lower than those associated with a Swan-Ganz catheter. In addition, these monitoring-associated complications are mostly non-severe. In a recent meta-analysis [19], the mean risk of severe catheter-related blood stream infection associated with artery catheterization was $<0.5\%$. Even these complications may be avoided by use of non-invasive monitoring solutions. However, the tolerance to monitoring-associated complications goes in line with disease severity, making some level of complications acceptable for the presumed benefit. For this reason, we can describe four major aspects of a monitor's clinical utility (Fig. 2).

Non-invasive Technologies as Replacement

The first reason to implement new non-invasive technologies is to decrease the monitoring-associated burden by replacing the more invasive alternatives. In order to do so, the performance of the new device in regard of false reading risks/tolerance has to be comparable (optimally non-inferior) to the invasive monitoring tool. For this reason it is important to consider in whom these invasive means are used nowadays. From a practical viewpoint, we can use non-invasive technologies to replace direct arterial pressure and/or advanced hemodynamic monitoring.

Direct arterial pressure monitoring is common during anesthesia in intermediate-to-high-risk surgical cases as well as in the management of most critically ill patients. The most important reason for arterial catheterization is need for accurate and continuous blood pressure monitoring in patients with presumed or existing hemodynamic instability. Once inserted, the catheters offer not only direct arterial pressure wave readings, but the possibility of safe and easily performable blood sampling for biochemical analysis. In most of these cases, rather safe radial artery cannulas are inserted. However, in many situations (mostly in intermediate risk surgery) the need for direct blood monitoring is short-lived and blood samplings are non-frequent. Replacing the invasive catheter by finger cuffs (volume clamp method), wristband (applanation tonometry) or another totally non-invasive interface seems appealing. In order to prove the utility of these non-invasive devices, many studies have been performed in recent years assessing the accuracy and precision of these new methods of blood pressure monitoring (listed in the meta-analysis by Kim and colleagues [4]). In this recently published meta-analysis [4], the mean difference of these non-invasive technologies compared to invasive measurements was 4 ± 9 mmHg for MAP with higher bias for systolic and diastolic pressures. In addition, the performance of some novel non-invasive devices in periods of rapid changes in arterial tone (e. g., anesthesia induction) was unsatisfactory [20]. These two facts delineate the limits of replacing invasive means of blood pressure monitoring. Until these methods are improved significantly, they may replace invasive pressure monitoring in situations where rapid changes of arterial tone are rare and wide limits of agreement (-13 to 21 mmHg) are tolerable.

A similar situation occurs in the case of replacing advanced hemodynamic monitoring by non-invasive tools. In contemporary praxis, hemodynamic monitors are mostly used for management of severely critically ill patients on one hand and for perioperative hemodynamic management on the other. It is important to note that different devices are used in these two populations. Accurate measurements are often necessary in severe patients; in addition, the disease generally affects more aspects of cardiovascular performance decreasing the applicability of mathematical assumptions. From the range of devices, Doppler-based monitoring seems to be the least affected and hence offers tolerable efficiency in this situation [21]. However the utility of non-invasive Doppler in such a scenario has never been tested in large studies.

Minimally invasive devices are generally used for hemodynamic monitoring in less demanding situations, for example, in management of perioperative cases or trauma victims. Uncalibrated pressure wave analysis or esophageal Doppler tools used in protocol fashion were all associated with improved outcome among such patients [22]. The trending ability of the devices and new variables more sensitive to preload, afterload or contractility modulations seem to be more useful than absolute accuracy. New non-invasive monitoring tools might offer similar prospects, but such comparisons have not yet been performed. The limited studies using non-invasive monitoring tools for management of high-risk cases support this notion only in part [23–25].

Non-invasive Technologies as Improvement

The proportion of patients monitored using invasive tools is not negligible, but still patients without continuous or advanced monitoring prevail. However, this does not mean that these patients are without risk of developing hemodynamic instability or complications. In the EuSOS study [26], the mortality of low-risk patients with ASA 1 status (3%) was the same as in the ASA 2 group (3%). Moreover, this rather high mortality in ASA 1 and 2 patients was just a bit lower than in the "intermediate risk" ASA 3 patients (4.7%). The recommendations of the American Society of Anesthesiologists deem 5-minute intervals of intermittent blood pressure readings as the minimum standard for general anesthesia. However, this period may leave periods of hypo- or hypertension undetected. Based on large amounts of retrospective data, even short periods of hypotension (MAP < 55 mmHg) were associated with increased risks of acute myocardial infarction and of acute kidney injury [27]. Two studies were published recently showing that use of continuous non-invasive arterial pressure monitoring offered a safe monitoring alternative by significantly decreasing periods of unknown hypotension [28, 29]. In one study, this effect was translated into the biochemical correlate of better umbilical cord pH values in newborns after Cesarean section delivery managed using continuous non-invasive monitoring [28].

Apart from these hints of positive impact, we have to consider one even more important fact. Non-invasive devices might correct the disproportion in hemodynamic monitoring noted by Jarisch in 1928, that our understanding of the circulation is pressure-oriented given its easy accessibility, as compared to tissues that are, thanks to autoregulation, mostly flow-dependent. However, monitoring the blood flow, even in low-risk patients, would never lead to any benefit if not coupled with correct treatment. Several blood flow-oriented treatments are available: Hemodynamic optimization and goal-directed fluid therapy being the most prominent. Hemodynamic optimization is associated with improvement in high-risk cases, but according to recent data may be redundant in low-risk patients with good exercise tolerance [30]. By contrast, goal-directed fluid management based on functional hemodynamic monitoring or preload responsiveness seems to be better than some other contemporary strategies, at least in intermediate risk patients [23, 24]. Nevertheless, use in general low-risk populations is still debatable and may be affected by a high cost–low benefit ratio.

Conclusion

A wide range of novel non-invasive hemodynamic monitors has been marketed recently. Some of them seem to have promising properties and hence could affect our monitoring and treatment strategies in the near future. In addition, combining some features of several technologies might further improve their performance. However, the efficiency of currently available devices seems to fit more as improvement of care for 'under-monitored' intermediate risk patients or as a substitute for minimally invasive devices in similar populations, than as a replacement for invasive monitoring tools in the critical care setting.

Acknowledgement

The work of JB and EK is supported by the research grant of the Czech Ministry of Education (MSM0021620819) and PRVOUK P36

References

1. Marik PE (2013) Noninvasive cardiac output monitors: a state-of the-art review. J Cardiothorac Vasc Anesth 27:121–134
2. Critchley LAH, Huang L (2014) USCOM-window to the circulation: utility of supra-sternal Doppler in an elderly anaesthetized patient for a robotic cystectomy. J Clin Monit Comput 28:83–93
3. Truijen J, van Lieshout JJ, Wesselink WA, Westerhof BE (2012) Noninvasive continuous hemodynamic monitoring. J Clin Monit Comput 26:267–278
4. Kim SH, Lilot M, Sidhu KS et al (2014) Accuracy and precision of continuous noninvasive arterial pressure monitoring compared with invasive arterial pressure: A systematic review and meta-analysis. Anesthesiology 120:1080–1097
5. Janelle GM, Gravenstein N (2006) An accuracy evaluation of the T-Line Tensymeter (continuous noninvasive blood pressure management device) versus conventional invasive radial artery monitoring in surgical patients. Anesth Analg 102:484–490
6. Keren H, Burkhoff D, Squara P (2007) Evaluation of a noninvasive continuous cardiac output monitoring system based on thoracic bioreactance. Am J Physiol Heart Circ Physiol 293:H583–H589
7. Maisch S, Bohm SH, Solà J et al (2011) Heart-lung interactions measured by electrical impedance tomography. Crit Care Med 39:2173–2176
8. Chen W, Kobayashi T, Ichikawa S, Takeuchi Y, Togawa T (2000) Continuous estimation of systolic blood pressure using the pulse arrival time and intermittent calibration. Med Biol Eng Comput 38:569–574
9. Lamhaut L, Apriotesei R, Combes X, Lejay M, Carli P, Vivien B (2011) Comparison of the accuracy of noninvasive hemoglobin monitoring by spectrophotometry (SpHb) and HemoCue® with automated laboratory hemoglobin measurement. Anesthesiology 115:548–554
10. Sandroni C, Cavallaro F, Marano C, Falcone C, Santis P, Antonelli M (2012) Accuracy of plethysmographic indices as predictors of fluid responsiveness in mechanically ventilated adults: a systematic review and meta-analysis. Intensive Care Med 38:1429–1437
11. Mayer J, Boldt J, Poland R, Peterson A, Manecke GR (2009) Continuous arterial pressure waveform-based cardiac output using the FloTrac/Vigileo: a review and meta-analysis. J Cardiothorac Vasc Anesth 23:401–406
12. Biais M, Nouette-Gaulain K, Cottenceau V et al (2008) Cardiac output measurement in patients undergoing liver transplantation: pulmonary artery catheter versus uncalibrated arterial pressure waveform analysis. Anesth Analg 106:1480–1486
13. Biancofiore G, Critchley LAH, Lee A et al (2009) Evaluation of an uncalibrated arterial pulse contour cardiac output monitoring system in cirrhotic patients undergoing liver surgery. Br J Anaesth 102:47–54
14. Slagt C, Malagon I, Groeneveld ABJ (2014) Systematic review of uncalibrated arterial pressure waveform analysis to determine cardiac output and stroke volume variation. Br J Anaesth 112:626–637

15. De Backer D, Marx G, Tan A et al (2011) Arterial pressure-based cardiac output monitoring: a multicenter validation of the third-generation software in septic patients. Intensive Care Med 37:233–240
16. Critchley LA, Critchley JA (1999) A meta-analysis of studies using bias and precision statistics to compare cardiac output measurement techniques. J Clin Monit Comput 15:85–91
17. Critchley LA, Yang XX, Lee A (2011) Assessment of trending ability of cardiac output monitors by polar plot methodology. J Cardiothorac Vasc Anesth 25:536–546
18. American Society of Anesthesiologists Task Force on Pulmonary Artery Catheterization (2003) Practice guidelines for pulmonary artery catheterization: an updated report by the American Society of Anesthesiologists Task Force on Pulmonary Artery Catheterization. Anesthesiology 99:988–1014
19. Scheer B, Perel A, Pfeiffer UJ (2002) Clinical review: complications and risk factors of peripheral arterial catheters used for haemodynamic monitoring in anaesthesia and intensive care medicine. Crit Care 6:199–204
20. Gayat E, Mongardon N, Tuil O et al (2013) CNAP(®) does not reliably detect minimal or maximal arterial blood pressures during induction of anaesthesia and tracheal intubation. Acta Anaesthesiol Scand 57:468–473
21. Horster S, Stemmler HJ, Strecker N et al (2012) Cardiac output measurements in septic patients: Comparing the accuracy of USCOM to PiCCO. Crit Care Res Pract 2012:270631
22. Hamilton MA, Cecconi M, Rhodes A (2011) A systematic review and meta-analysis on the use of preemptive hemodynamic intervention to improve postoperative outcomes in moderate and high-risk surgical patients. Anesth Analg 112:1392–1402
23. Forget P, Lois F, de Kock M (2010) Goal-directed fluid management based on the pulse oximeter-derived pleth variability index reduces lactate levels and improves fluid management. Anesth Analg 111:910–914
24. Yu Y, Dong J, Xu Z, Shen H, Zheng J (2014) Pleth variability index-directed fluid management in abdominal surgery under combined general and epidural anesthesia. J Clin Monit Comput (in press)
25. Pestaña D, Espinosa E, Eden A et al (2014) Perioperative goal-directed hemodynamic optimization using noninvasive cardiac output monitoring in major abdominal surgery: A prospective, randomized, multicenter, pragmatic trial: POEMAS Study (PeriOperative goal-directed thErapy in Major Abdominal Surgery). Anesth Analg 119:579–587
26. Pearse RM, Moreno RP, Bauer P et al (2012) Mortality after surgery in Europe: a 7 day cohort study. Lancet 380:1059–1065
27. Walsh M, Devereaux PJ, Garg AX et al (2013) Relationship between intraoperative mean arterial pressure and clinical outcomes after noncardiac surgery: toward an empirical definition of hypotension. Anesthesiology 119:507–515
28. Ilies C, Kiskalt H, Siedenhans D et al (2012) Detection of hypotension during Caesarean section with continuous non-invasive arterial pressure device or intermittent oscillometric arterial pressure measurement. Br J Anaesth 109:413–419
29. Benes J, Simanova A, Tovarnicka T et al (2014) Continuous non-invasive monitoring improves blood pressure stability in upright position: randomized controlled trial. J Clin Monit Comput (in press)
30. Challand C, Struthers R, Sneyd JR et al (2012) Randomized controlled trial of intraoperative goal-directed fluid therapy in aerobically fit and unfit patients having major colorectal surgery. Br J Anaesth 108:53–62

Assessing Global Perfusion During Sepsis: SvO_2, Venoarterial PCO_2 Gap or Both?

J.-L. Teboul and X. Monnet

Introduction

Systemic blood flow can be measured easily at the bedside in critically ill patients. However, measuring cardiac output cannot tell much about the adequacy of systemic blood flow for global metabolic conditions. For example, a cardiac output of 5 l/min, which is normal in a healthy human at rest, is abnormally low during exercise or under other conditions of marked increase in oxygen (O_2) demand, such as sepsis. Therefore, the simple measurement of cardiac output cannot provide sufficient information about the need to increase systemic blood flow. The mixed venous blood O_2 saturation (SvO_2) and the difference between mixed venous and arterial blood carbon dioxide (CO_2) pressures (PCO_2 gap) have been proposed to assess the adequacy of cardiac output to metabolic conditions and thus to serve to evaluate the need to increase cardiac output. Since central venous catheters are now more often inserted than pulmonary artery catheters (PACs) in critically ill patients, O_2 saturation measured in a central vein ($ScvO_2$) and the difference between CO_2 pressure in a central vein and arterial CO_2 pressure have been proposed as substitutes for SvO_2 and PCO_2 gap, respectively.

What Does SvO_2 Mean?

Physiological Meaning

The blood flowing through the pulmonary artery comes from the superior and inferior vena cava, and from the coronary sinus. It is thus the mixture of all the venous returns of the body. The amount of O_2 present in the mixed venous blood depends

J.-L. Teboul ✉ · X. Monnet
Service de réanimation médicale, Hôpital de Bicêtre, Hôpitaux Universitaires Paris-Sud, Le Kremlin-Bicêtre, France
e-mail: jean-louis.teboul@bct.aphp.fr

J.-L. Vincent (ed.), *Annual Update in Intensive Care and Emergency Medicine 2015*,
DOI 10.1007/978-3-319-13761-2_19

upon the whole-body O_2 consumption (VO_2) and the amount of O_2 carried from the lungs toward the peripheral tissues by the cardiovascular system (CvO_2). In the vast majority of clinical situations, CvO_2 is linearly correlated with SvO_2, which represents the O_2 saturation (expressed in %) of the hemoglobin contained by the red blood cells of the mixed venous blood. SvO_2 is related to arterial O_2 saturation (SaO_2), VO_2, cardiac output and hemoglobin concentration (Hb) according to the formula derived from the Fick equation applied to O_2:

$$SvO_2 = SaO_2 - [VO_2/(\text{cardiac output} \times \text{Hb} \times 13.4)].$$

The SvO_2 is thus an integrative parameter that reflects the global balance between arterial O_2 delivery (DO_2) and VO_2, because cardiac output, Hb and SaO_2 are the key determinants of DO_2. In healthy subjects at rest with normal SaO_2 and Hb, the value of SvO_2 ranges from 70 to 75%. During exercise, O_2 demand is increased, especially in skeletal muscles. As a consequence, VO_2 will increase because of the increase in cardiac output and of the increase in O_2 extraction of the tissues that occurs especially in the skeletal muscles by redistribution of the intra-organ blood flow. For this reason, SvO_2 values as low as 45% can be observed in healthy subjects during exercise [1]. However, when SvO_2 reaches such a low value, anaerobic metabolism often appears. This point underlines the fact that O_2 extraction has physiological limits. In pathological conditions, SvO_2 is the result of complex interactions between its four major determinants, each of which may be altered by both the disease process and therapeutic agents. Moreover, these determinants are not independent, because compensatory mechanisms occur when one of them is altered. For example, cardiac output should increase in the face of a fall in SaO_2 or in Hb and should decrease after normalization of these latter variables. Thus, it must be kept in mind that SvO_2 changes are rarely linearly correlated to changes in one of its determinants.

The SvO_2 can be measured *in vitro* using a co-oximeter after sampling blood from the distal port of a PAC. Measuring SvO_2 by co-oximetry is time consuming and exposed to errors. It can also lead to complications, such as blood wasting and infections from frequent but necessary manipulations of the PAC. Alternatively, SvO_2 can be measured through fiberoptic PACs by reflectance spectrophotometry, which avoids most of the pitfalls associated with mixed venous blood withdrawal, and allows continuous monitoring of SvO_2. The main inconvenience of this type of catheter is expense when compared to a standard PAC.

Clinical Interpretation of SvO_2

SvO_2 as a Marker of O_2 Extraction

The whole-body O_2 extraction ratio (O_2ER) is defined as the ratio of the whole-body VO_2 to the whole-body DO_2: $O_2ER = VO_2/DO_2$.

As DO_2 equals approximately cardiac output × Hb × 13.4, then $SvO_2 = SaO_2 - (VO_2/DO_2)$. When SaO_2 is close to 1 (100%), SvO_2 can thus be used to estimate O_2ER:

$$SvO_2 = 1 - O_2ER.$$

This can reasonably apply to the majority of critically ill patients that receive mechanical ventilation and in whom arterial oxygenation is controlled by high FiO_2 and/or positive end-expiratory pressure (PEEP). By contrast, in patients with initial severe hypoxemia, changes in SvO_2 are also related to changes in SaO_2 and cannot reflect only changes in O_2ER.

By considering that SvO_2 reflects O_2ER, SvO_2 changes can be interpreted as follows:

- A decrease in SvO_2 means that O_2ER has increased to make the whole-body VO_2 match with the whole-body O_2 demand. This increase in O_2ER can be triggered by either a decrease in DO_2, or an increase in O_2 demand, or both. If, in spite of this normal adaptation, VO_2 does not match O_2 demand, tissue hypoxia and anaerobic metabolism appear [2]. However, no precise value of SvO_2 can be defined as the 'critical' SvO_2 below which tissue hypoxia occurs [2].
- Conversely, an increase in SvO_2 means that O_2ER has decreased as a consequence of either an increase in DO_2 with maintained VO_2 or a decrease in VO_2 with maintained or increased DO_2. This latter situation is typically encountered in hyperdynamic septic shock where the decrease in VO_2 (despite a high whole-body O_2 demand) does not result from a reduced DO_2, but rather from O_2 extraction capacity impairment [3].

These points underline the fact that: 1) SvO_2 cannot be a reliable marker of the adequacy between DO_2 and global O_2 demand in shock states where VO_2 is less than O_2 demand; and 2) interpretation of SvO_2 can be misleading in hyperdynamic states.

Interpretation of SvO_2 in Sepsis

Sepsis results in a complex form of shock. Prior to initial resuscitation, systemic blood flow is often reduced, mostly due to hypovolemia and sometimes to associated myocardial depression [4]. However, in most patients, in whom early correction of volume depletion has resulted in a hyperdynamic circulatory state, oxidative metabolism is still impaired due to inability of tissues to extract sufficient O_2 from the blood [3]. Distributive abnormalities of macrocirculatory and microcirculatory blood flow mainly explain this O_2 extraction impairment [3, 4]. Consequently, the most frequent hemodynamic profile in human septic shock is characterized by high cardiac output and vasodilatation [3, 4], although some clinical studies have reported relatively low values of cardiac output [5–7] either due to insufficient fluid resuscitation and/or to the presence of sepsis-induced myocardial depression.

Since VO_2 is by definition lower than O_2 demand in shock states, SvO_2 cannot serve as a reliable marker of the adequacy between DO_2 and global O_2 demand and thus as a marker of tissue hypoxia. However, knowledge of SvO_2 can be helpful to assess the adequacy of DO_2 relative to global VO_2. Therefore, SvO_2 might take a place in the cardiovascular monitoring of septic shock, by identifying patients in whom DO_2 and mostly cardiac output could be further increased and then by guiding therapy aimed at increasing DO_2 [8]. This point is of particular importance since systematic maximization of cardiac output is no longer recommended in septic shock [9]. A detailed analysis of clinical studies indicated that values of O_2ER ranging from 30% to 35% (or SvO_2 slightly below the range 65–70%) were most often observed in patients who were not optimally resuscitated before entering the study: Some had not yet received any vasoconstrictor to compensate for the non-responsiveness of blood pressure to fluids [10], some had not yet received optimal fluid therapy [11], while others initially had unusually high VO_2 due to increased O_2 demand [12]. Thus, values of SvO_2 below 65–70% in septic patients would mean that initial therapy has not been sufficient and/or that sedation or antipyretic drugs would be used to reduce O_2 demand. Accordingly, targeting a SvO_2 value of at least 65% might be a reasonable goal of treatment in septic shock as recommended by the Surviving Sepsis Campaign [9].

Interpretation of Changes in SvO_2 in Sepsis

In patients with relatively low initial values of SvO_2, following the course of SvO_2 may be helpful to assess the effects on global tissue oxygenation of a therapy given to increase cardiac DO_2. Under conditions of O_2-supply dependence, any increase in cardiac output should be accompanied by an increase in VO_2 so that SvO_2 is expected to increase far less than in the case of O_2-supply independence [8] (Fig. 1). Consequently, unchanged SvO_2 with therapy aimed at increasing DO_2 does not mean that the therapy has failed to reduce O_2 debt. In this case, the therapeutic agent would be maintained and its dose even increased until obtaining a frank increase in SvO_2 that would indicate that the critical level of DO_2 has been passed [8] (Fig. 1). Additionally, SvO_2 monitoring may be helpful to select the appropriate dosage of a therapeutic agent, such as a β1-agonist agent known to exert thermogenic effects resulting in increased O_2 demand and VO_2 [13]. In septic patients without evidence of shock, dobutamine was demonstrated to increase VO_2 at doses higher than 5 µg/kg/min [14]. However, if SvO_2 remains unchanged despite an increase in DO_2 with therapy, differentiating an increase in VO_2 that unmasks an O_2 debt from an increase in VO_2 due to thermogenic effects of the therapy is a difficult challenge, which needs assessment of other metabolic variables such as blood lactate and/or PCO_2 gap.

In patients with SvO_2 higher than 70%, as mentioned above, arguments that suggest that raising DO_2 further would improve tissue oxygenation are lacking. In this regard, Gattinoni et al. [15] reported no reduction in mortality when therapy was targeted at an increase in SvO_2 above 70% in a large population of critically ill patients. Nevertheless, monitoring of SvO_2 may still be useful to detect short-term decreases in SvO_2 that may have prognostic significance by alerting the clinician before patent clinical aggravation occurs [16]. However, to correctly interpret SvO_2 changes in this high range of SvO_2 values, it is necessary to take into consideration the nonlinearity of the relationship between SvO_2 and cardiac output. Indeed,

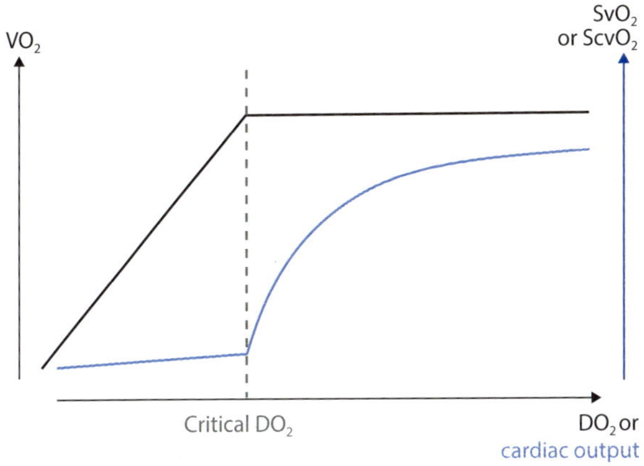

Fig. 1 Relationship between oxygen (O_2) consumption (VO_2), mixed (SvO_2) or central ($ScvO_2$) venous oxygen saturation and oxygen delivery (DO_2). On the left part of the graph, changes in DO_2 are accompanied by significant changes in VO_2 due to DO_2/VO_2 dependence. In case of an increase in cardiac output increasing DO_2, SvO_2 or $ScvO_2$ will remain almost constant until DO_2 reaches a critical value. In the middle part of the graph, changes in DO_2 are not accompanied by changes in VO_2 due to DO_2/VO_2 independence. In case of an increase in cardiac output increasing DO_2, SvO_2 or $ScvO_2$ increases as well. On the right part of the graph, SvO_2 or $ScvO_2$ does not increase in spite of cardiac output increase because the relationship between SvO_2 or $ScvO_2$ and cardiac output is hyperbolic for a constant VO_2

according to the modified Fick equation, for a constant VO_2, SvO_2 is linearly related to cardiac output in the lowest range of cardiac output values, whereas there is a flattening of the SvO_2/cardiac output relationship curve in the highest range of cardiac output values [17] (Fig. 1). It must be kept in mind that the SvO_2/cardiac output relationship also depends on the level of VO_2, so that a family of hyperbolic SvO_2/cardiac output curves can be drawn for various levels of VO_2 (VO_2 isopleths) [17]. As a consequence, interpretation of SvO_2 changes must be particularly cautious under conditions of high systemic blood flow. This point is illustrated by the analysis of data from studies in patients with hyperdynamic sepsis. For example, in the studies by De Backer et al. [14] and Ronco et al. [18], the mean DO_2 in the subgroups of O_2-supply independent patients increased by 36% and 49%, while SvO_2 increased by only 9% (from 70 to 76% and 69 to 75%, respectively) after dobutamine infusion. By comparison, a dobutamine-induced increase in cardiac output of 33% resulted in a 19% increase in SvO_2 in O_2-supply independent patients with low cardiac output and SvO_2 values at baseline [13].

In addition to the nonlinearity of the SvO_2/cardiac output relationship, as mentioned above, SvO_2 can be almost unchanged if the increase in DO_2 is associated with an increase in VO_2 increase in O_2-supply dependent patients [19] (Fig. 1). However, before any definitive interpretation of small changes in SvO_2, one also must take into account the relatively weak precision of reflectance spectrophotometry, because a change in SvO_2 of at least 5% is necessary to affirm that SvO_2 has actually changed [20].

Thus, the following conclusions can be reasonably drawn for clinical practice:

- The fact that monitoring does not detect changes in SvO_2 does not rule out any onset or worsening of global tissue hypoxia. Obviously, this does not support the common idea that SvO_2 monitoring acts as a sensitive warning system in hyperdynamic septic shock. In this regard, benefits may be drawn from the use of PACs allowing for both continuous measurement of cardiac output and SvO_2.
- A decrease in SvO_2 of at least 5% within the 'normal' range (supposed to be between 70% and 75%) should be considered as clinically significant because it indicates a marked fall in DO_2 and/or increase in O_2 demand. This should prompt the checking of Hb, SaO_2, cardiac output, and potential causes of increased O_2 demand, and lead to an appropriate treatment. However, whether application of such rules is superior to simple monitoring of clinical signs and could influence outcomes has never been demonstrated.
- In any shock state (even of septic origin), monitoring of SvO_2 can be helpful since a low value of SvO_2 would incite the clinician to attempt to increase DO_2 in order to improve global tissue oxygenation. On the other hand, a high value of SvO_2 would suggest that attempts to increase DO_2 further have little chance to significantly improve tissue oxygenation and ultimately outcome.
- Finally, it must be underlined that SvO_2 is a flow-weighted average of the venous blood O_2 saturation values from all organs of the body. Organs with high blood flow and low O_2 extraction, such as the kidneys, have a greater influence on SvO_2 than organs with low blood flow and high O_2 extraction, such as the myocardium. In sepsis, the interpretation of SvO_2 is further complicated by the fact that regional and local distribution of blood flow is markedly disturbed.

Physiological and Clinical Meaning of $ScvO_2$

At the beginning of the 21st century, $ScvO_2$ became a popular hemodynamic variable for at least two reasons. First, the use of the PAC, which allows measurements of SvO_2 and PCO_2 gap, was declining [21]. Second, the randomized study by Rivers et al. showed that using a $ScvO_2$ value >70% as an endpoint for the initial resuscitation of patients with severe sepsis or septic shock was associated with an improved outcome [22]. In their study, Rivers et al. used continuous monitoring of $ScvO_2$ with a fiberoptic probe placed in the superior vena cava territory [22]. Following this study, the Surviving Sepsis Campaign recommended targeting an $ScvO_2$ value >70% in the initial phase of resuscitation of severe sepsis and septic shock patients [9]. It is important to underline that this recommendation was made before any validation of $ScvO_2$ as a good substitute for SvO_2 in septic patients. In essence, $ScvO_2$ differs from SvO_2 because the latter results from the mixing of O_2 saturation of all venous territories of the body including the superior vena cava, the inferior vena cava and the coronary sinus. In healthy conditions, $ScvO_2$ is expected to be a little lower than SvO_2. In critically ill patients, $ScvO_2$ was more frequently reported to be higher than SvO_2 [23–28], probably because of a greater rate of O_2 extraction and by the heart or by lower body organs relative to organs draining into the superior vena cava. A positive difference between $ScvO_2$ and SvO_2 was even shown to be associated with a better outcome in critically ill patients [27]. The percentage errors between both parameters have generally been shown to be low [23–26], so that $ScvO_2$ can be considered as an acceptable alternative to SvO_2 [24], although opposite conclusions have also been drawn [23, 25, 26, 28]. More importantly, the simultaneous changes in $ScvO_2$ and in SvO_2 have generally been shown to be well correlated [24, 25], suggesting that monitoring $ScvO_2$ makes sense in critically ill patients.

One indirect confirmation of the relevance of $ScvO_2$ measurements can be drawn from a recent study that replaced SvO_2 by $ScvO_2$ to calculate VO_2 [29]. In this study, including patients with acute circulatory mainly from septic origin, the presence of VO_2/DO_2 dependence during a fluid challenge was associated with hyperlactatemia whereas VO_2/DO_2 independence was associated with normal blood lactate levels [29].

As for SvO_2, $ScvO_2$ can be normal or high in cases of severe sepsis and septic shock because of impairment of O_2 extraction capacities. This is a situation frequently encountered even during the initial phase of resuscitation [30, 31]. As is the case for SvO_2 [32], a high $ScvO_2$ does not exclude an increase in cardiac output after therapy such as fluid challenge [29]. Finally, high $ScvO_2$ and not only low $ScvO_2$ values are associated with a poor outcome in severe sepsis [31].

What Does the PCO_2 Gap Mean?

Physiological Meaning

Under normoxic conditions, CO_2 is normally produced in the cells through the Krebs cycle. CO_2 is thereby a normal terminal product of oxidative metabolism. Under hypoxic conditions, CO_2 can be generated in the cells through buffering of excessively produced protons by local bicarbonates. Protons are generated by two mechanisms: Excessive production of lactic acid owing to an acceleration of anaerobic glycolysis, since pyruvate is no longer cleared by the Krebs cycle; and hydrolysis of ATP and of ADP that occurs in conditions of anaerobiosis.

The Fick equation applied to CO_2 indicates that the CO_2 excretion (equivalent to CO_2 production [VCO_2] in a steady-state) equals the product of cardiac output by the difference between the CO_2 content in the mixed venous blood and in the arterial blood.

The normal relationship between CO_2 content and CO_2 pressure is almost linear over the usual physiological range of CO_2 contents. Thus, by substituting CO_2 pressure for CO_2 content, PCO_2 gap $= k \times VCO_2$/cardiac output, where k is a factor defining the relationship between CO_2 content and CO_2 pressure [33]. Under normal conditions, PCO_2 gap values range between 2 and 6 mmHg [34]. The relationship between cardiac output and CO_2 pressure is explained by the CO_2 stagnation phenomenon that increases venous blood CO_2 pressure relative to arterial blood CO_2 pressure at the peripheral venous level. Thus, a low cardiac output and hence a low efferent venous blood flow should decrease the CO_2 clearance rate and should result in an increased PCO_2 gap for a given VCO_2. Accordingly, in a clinical study performed in normolactatemic patients with low cardiac index at baseline, the increase in cardiac index from 1.6 to 2.2 l/min/m^2 was accompanied by a decrease in PCO_2 gap from 9 to 5 mmHg, while VO_2 (and probably VCO_2) was unchanged [35]

Because of the curvilinear relationship between CO_2 pressure and CO_2 content, k increases with venous hypercapnia [33]. Additionally, metabolic acidosis results in a shift in the CO_2 pressure/CO_2 content relationship so that k increases with metabolic acidosis and tissue hypoxia [33].

Clinical Use of PCO_2 Gap

In case of tissue hypoxia, the determinants of PCO_2 gap can change in opposite directions such that PCO_2 gap can increase, decrease or remain unchanged. On the one hand, the development of local metabolic acidosis shifts the curvilinear relation between CO_2 content and CO_2 pressure so that k increases [33]. This was well illustrated in an experimental study in which tissue hypoxia was induced by cardiac tamponade [36]. The factor k, which can be estimated from independent measurements of PCO_2 gap, cardiac output and VCO_2, increased markedly after induction of tissue hypoxia [36]. On the other hand, VCO_2 decreased along with the decrease in VO_2 [36]. The decrease in VCO_2 during tissue hypoxia strongly suggests that the increased 'anaerobic' production of CO_2 does not compensate for the decreased 'aerobic' CO_2 production. Because VCO_2 must decrease and k must increase during tissue hypoxia, the resultant effect on PCO_2 gap will mainly depend on cardiac output [33]. Clear confirmation of these conceptual aspects was brought by animal studies in which hypoxia (reduced inspired O_2 fraction) and ischemic hypoxia (reduced blood flow) were experimentally created [37, 38]. Therefore, two situations should be distinguished: Tissue hypoxia with reduced blood flow and tissue hypoxia with maintained or high blood flow. In case of tissue hypoxia with reduced systemic blood flow, PCO_2 gap should increase as confirmed by experimental [36] and clinical studies [39, 40]. In case of tissue hypoxia with maintained or high systemic blood flow, PCO_2 gap should be normal or even reduced as confirmed in clinical studies [39–41]. In such conditions, the high venous blood flow can easily remove the low amount of CO_2 produced at the periphery.

The implications for clinical practice can be summarized as follows:

- An increased PCO_2 gap suggests that the cardiac output is not high enough with respect to the global metabolic conditions. Under anaerobic conditions, a high PCO_2 gap could incite the clinician to increase cardiac output with the goal of reducing tissue hypoxia. Under aerobic conditions, this condition can be associated with increased O_2 demand and hence increased VCO_2. In this regard, PCO_2 gap as well as SvO_2 can serve to titrate β1-agonist drugs better than cardiac output because of potential thermogenic effects of these agents [35].

- A normal PCO_2 gap suggests that the cardiac output is high enough to washout the amount of the CO_2 produced from the peripheral tissues. This suggests that increasing cardiac output has little chance of improving global oxygenation even in hypoxic conditions.

Combined Analysis of PCO_2 Gap with Arteriovenous O_2 Content Difference

From the Fick principle, two equations can be written:

$$VCO_2 \times k = \text{cardiac output} \times PCO_2 \text{ gap}$$

$$VO_2 = \text{cardiac output} \times \text{arteriovenous } O_2 \text{ content difference.}$$

During tissue hypoxia, k increases [30] while VCO_2 decreases less than VO_2 [42] because of the generation of anaerobic CO_2. Therefore, the $(VCO_2 \times k)/VO_2$ ratio should increase during tissue hypoxia. Because after eliminating cardiac output present on both the numerator and the denominator, the PCO_2 gap/arteriovenous O_2 content difference ratio equals the $VCO_2 \times k/VO_2$ ratio, the PCO_2 gap/arteriovenous O_2 content difference ratio should increase during hypoxic conditions. This ratio thus could be used to detect global anaerobic metabolism. In a series of critically ill patients (148 measurements), a close correlation was found between blood lactate level and the PCO_2 gap/arteriovenous O_2 content difference ratio, while no correlation was found between blood lactate level and PCO_2 gap alone [43].

Thus, the PCO_2 gap/arteriovenous O_2 content difference ratio could be helpful to detect global anaerobic metabolism whereas PCO_2 gap alone is only an indicator of adequacy of cardiac output.

Is the PCO_2 Gap Determined Using a Central Vein Clinically Relevant?

Since PACs are used less than in the past, the question of substituting the CO_2 pressure measured in the mixed venous blood by the CO_2 pressure measured in a central vein has recently been raised. A good agreement between PCO_2 gap and central PCO_2 gap calculated as the difference between CO_2 pressure in a central vein and arterial CO_2 pressure was reported in clinical studies including critically ill patients [44] and severe sepsis and septic shock patients [45].

Two indirect arguments confirm the clinical relevance of central PCO_2 gap. One argument was made by a study examining the effects of increasing doses of dobutamine in stable septic patients [46] and reporting exactly the same results as those found with PCO_2 gap in a previous study [34]: A decrease in central PCO_2 gap from 0 to 10 μg/kg/min of dobutamine along with an increase in cardiac output and then an unchanged PCO_2 gap for a dose of 15 μg/kg/min in spite of the further increase in cardiac output due to the thermogenic effects of the drug at that dose [46]. Another argument was made by a study including patients with septic shock in whom the central PCO_2 gap/arteriovenous O_2 content difference ratio was shown to predict VO_2 supply dependence after a fluid challenge as accurately as the blood lactate level and far better than $ScvO_2$ [29]. This confirms that the central PCO_2 gap/arteriovenous O_2 content difference ratio, similar to the PCO_2 gap/arteriovenous O_2 content difference ratio [43], can be used as a marker of anaerobic metabolism.

SvO_2 vs. Central PCO_2 Gap

A potential superiority of PCO_2 gap over SvO_2 (and hence of central PCO_2 gap over $ScvO_2$) is that in case of O_2 extraction impairment due to maldistribution of microcirculatory blood flow, PCO_2 gap can keep its property as a marker of the adequacy of cardiac output to the metabolic conditions, whereas SvO_2 inevitably loses it. This could be due to the fact that CO_2 is about 20 times more soluble than O_2 and thus that the likelihood of its diffusion out of ischemic tissues is elevated [47]. Aimed at illustrating this PCO_2 gap property, Vallée et al. included 50 septic shock patients in whom an $ScvO_2$ higher than 70% was achieved [48]. Central PCO_2 gap was abnormally high (>6 mmHg) in half of the population [48]. In that subgroup of patients, blood lactate level tended to be higher and cardiac output to be lower than in patients with a central PCO_2 gap ≤ 6 mmHg. The authors concluded that $ScvO_2$ may not be sufficient to guide therapy and that when the 70% $ScvO_2$ value is reached, the presence of a central PCO_2 gap >6 mmHg might be a useful tool to identify patients who still remain inadequately resuscitated [48]. Another study examined whether patients who normalize both PCO_2 gap and $ScvO_2$ during the first six hours of resuscitation have a greater decrease in blood lactate level than those who only achieve normal $ScvO_2$. The authors found that normalization of both PCO_2 gap and $ScvO_2$ was associated with a greater decrease in blood lactate concentration than normalization of $ScvO_2$ alone [48]. Another study also showed that the combination of $ScvO_2$ and central PCO_2 gap predicted outcome in 172 critically ill patients resuscitated from septic shock better than $ScvO_2$ alone [49]. Patients who met both targets appeared to clear lactate more efficiently [49]. Similar results were reported in another series of septic shock patients [50].

Conclusion

In summary, central PCO_2 gap and $ScvO_2$ (or PCO_2 gap and SvO_2 if a PAC is in place) can complement each other in the management of patients with severe sepsis or septic shock (Fig. 2). Although neither parameter alone can detect global tissue hypoxia, their combination through the calculation of the central PCO_2 gap/arteriovenous O_2 content difference ratio can detect the presence of anaerobic metabolism as does hyperlactatemia. In such a case, a low $ScvO_2$ ($<70\%$) indicates that elevation of DO_2 can be attempted and, if central PCO_2 gap is increased

(> 6 mmHg), that increasing cardiac output should be the reasonable choice for this purpose (Fig. 2). In case of a normal or high $ScvO_2$ ($\geq$ 70%), an increased central PCO_2 gap still indicates that increasing cardiac output can be increased with the aim of reducing O_2 debt (Fig. 2). If $ScvO_2$ is normal or high and central PCO_2 gap is normal in case of global tissue hypoxia, manipulating the macrocirculation will probably fail to reduce O_2 debt (Fig. 2) and this situation, which denotes major microcirculatory and/or O_2 extraction disturbances, is generally associated with a poor outcome.

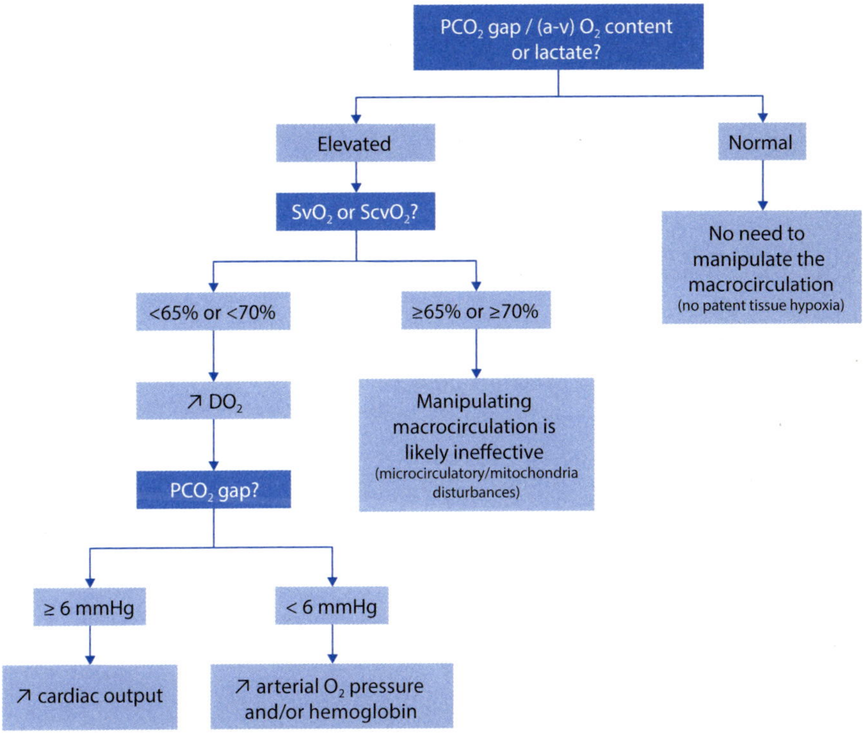

Fig. 2 Therapeutic implications of mixed (SvO_2) and central ($ScvO_2$) venous oxygen saturation, venoarterial carbon dioxide pressure difference (PCO_2 gap) and the ratio between the venoarterial carbon dioxide pressure difference and the arteriovenous difference in oxygen content ([a–v] O_2 content). O_2: oxygen; DO_2: oxygen delivery

References

1. Weber KT, Andrews V, Janicki JS et al (1981) Amrinone and exercice performance in patients with chronic heart failure. Am J Cardiol 48:164–169
2. Kasnitz P, Druger GL, Yorra F, Simmons DH (1976) Mixed venous oxygen tension and hyperlactatemia. JAMA 236:570–574
3. Astiz ME, Rackow EC (1998) Septic shock. Lancet 351:1501–1505
4. Vincent JL, De Backer D (2013) Circulatory shock. N Engl J Med 369:1726–1734
5. Dubin A, Pozo MO, Casabella CA et al (2009) Increasing arterial blood pressure with norepinephrine does not improve microcirculatory blood flow: a prospective study. Crit Care 13:R92
6. Hamzaoui O, Georger JF, Monnet X et al (2010) Early administration of norepinephrine increases cardiac preload and cardiac output in septic patients with life-threatening hypotension. Crit Care 14:R142
7. Monnet X, Jabot J, Maizel J, Richard C, Teboul JL (2011) Norepinephrine increases cardiac preload and reduces preload dependency assessed by passive leg raising in septic shock patients. Crit Care Med 39:689–694
8. Teboul JL, Hamzaoui O, Monnet X (2011) SvO_2 to monitor resuscitation of septic patients: let's just understand the basic physiology. Crit Care 15:1005
9. Dellinger RP, Levy MM, Rhodes A et al (2013) Surviving sepsis campaign: international guidelines for management of severe sepsis and septic shock: 2012. Crit Care Med 41:580–637
10. Yu M, Burchell S, Hasaniya NW, Takanishi DM, Myers SA, Takiguchi SA (1998) Relationship of mortality to increasing oxygen delivery in patients > 50 years of age: A prospective, randomized trial. Crit Care Med 26:1011–1019
11. Friedman G, De Backer D, Shahla M, Vincent JL (1998) Oxygen supply dependency can characterize septic shock. Intensive Care Med 24:118–123
12. Martin C, Viviand X, Vialet ASR, Rougnon T (1999) Effects of norepinephrine plus dobutamine or norepinephrine alone on left ventricular performance of septic shock patients. Crit Care Med 27:1708–1713
13. Teboul JL, Boujdaria R, Graini L, Berton C, Richard C (1993) Cardiac index vs oxygen-derived parameters for rational use of dobutamine in patients with congestive heart failure. Chest 103:81–85
14. De Backer D, Moraine JJ, Berré J, Kahn RJ, Vincent JL (1994) Effects of dobutamine on oxygen consumption in septic patients. Direct versus indirect determinations. Am J Respir Crit Care Med 150:95–100
15. Gattinoni L, Brazzi L, Pelosi P et al (1995) A trial of goal-oriented hemodynamic therapy in critically ill patients. SvO2 Collaborative Group. N Engl J Med 333:1025–1032
16. Krafft P, Steltzer H, Hiesmayr M, Klimscha W, Hammerle AF (1993) Mixed venous oxygen saturation in critically ill septic shock patients. The role of defined events. Chest 103:900–906
17. Jain A, Shroff SG, Janicki JS, Reddy HK, Weber KT (1991) Relation between mixed venous oxygen saturation and cardiac index. Nonlinearity and normalization for oxygen uptake and hemoglobin. Chest 99:1403–1409
18. Ronco JJ, Fenwick JC, Wiggs BR, Phang PT, Russell JA, Tweeddale MG (1993) Oxygen consumption is dependent of increases in oxygen delivery by dobutamine in septic patients who have normal or increased plasma lactate. Am Rev Respir Dis 147:25–31
19. Hayes MA, Timmins AC, Yau EH, Palazzo M, Watson D, Hinds CJ (1997) Oxygen transport patterns in patients with sepsis syndrome or septic shock: Influence of treatment and relationship to outcome. Crit Care Med 25:926–936
20. Scuderi PE, Bowton DL, Meredith JW, Harris LC, Evans JB, Anderson RL (1992) A comparison of three pulmonary artery oximetry catheters in Intensive Care Unit patients. Chest 102:896–905

21. Wiener RS, Welch HG (2007) Trends in the use of the pulmonary artery catheter in the United States, 1993–2004. JAMA 298:423–429
22. Rivers E, Nguyen B, Havstad S et al (2001) Early goal-directed therapy in the treatment of severe sepsis and septic shock. N Engl J Med 345:1368–1377
23. Chawla LS, Zia H, Gutierrez G, Katz NM, Seneff MG, Shah M (2004) Lack of equivalence between central and mixed venous oxygen saturation. Chest 126:1891–1896
24. Reinhart K, Kuhn HJ, Hartog C, Bredle DL (2004) Continuous central venous and pulmonary artery oxygen saturation monitoring in the critically ill. Intensive Care Med 30:1572–1578
25. Dueck MH, Klimek M, Appenrodt S, Weigand C, Boerner U (2005) Trends but not individual values of central venous oxygen saturation agree with mixed venous oxygen saturation during varying hemodynamic conditions. Anesthesiology 103:249–257
26. Varpula M, Karlsson S, Ruokonen E, Pettilä V (2006) Mixed venous oxygen saturation cannot be estimated by central venous oxygen saturation in septic shock. Intensive Care Med 32:1336–1343
27. Gutierrez G, Comignani P, Huespe L et al (2008) Central venous to mixed venous blood oxygen and lactate gradients are associated with outcome in critically ill patients. Intensive Care Med 34:1662–1668
28. van Beest PA, van Ingen J, Boerma EC et al (2010) No agreement of mixed venous and central venous saturation in sepsis, independent of sepsis origin. Crit Care 14:R219
29. Monnet X, Julien F, Ait-Hamou N et al (2013) Lactate and veno-arterial carbon dioxide difference/arterial-venous oxygen difference ratio, but not central venous oxygen saturation, predict increase in oxygen consumption in fluid responders. Crit Care Med 41:1412–1420
30. van Beest PA, Hofstra JJ, Schultz MJ, Boerma EC, Spronk PE, Kuiper MA (2008) The incidence of low venous oxygen saturation on admission to the intensive care unit: a multi-center observational study in The Netherlands. Crit Care 12:R33
31. Pope JV, Jones AE, Gaieski DF, Arnold RC, Trzeciak S, Shapiro NI (2010) Multicenter study of central venous oxygen saturation (ScvO(2)) as a predictor of mortality in patients with sepsis. Ann Emerg Med 55:40–46
32. Velissaris D, Pierrakos C, Scolletta S, De Backer D, Vincent JL (2011) High mixed venous oxygen saturation levels do not exclude fluid responsiveness in critically ill septic patients. Crit Care 15:R177
33. Lamia B, Monnet X, Teboul JL (2006) Meaning of arterio-venous PCO_2 difference in circulatory shock. Minerva Anestesiol 72:597–604
34. Groeneveld AB (1998) Interpreting the venous-arterial PCO_2 difference. Crit Care Med 26:979–980
35. Teboul JL, Mercat A, Lenique F, Berton C, Richard C (1998) Value of the venous-arterial PCO2 gradient to reflect the oxygen supply to demand in humans: effects of dobutamine. Crit Care Med 26:1007–1010
36. Zhang H, Vincent JL (1993) Arteriovenous differences in PCO_2 and pH are good indicators of critical hypoperfusion. Am Rev Respir Dis 148:867–871
37. Vallet B, Teboul JL, Cain S, Curtis S (2000) Venoarterial CO(2) difference during regional ischemic or hypoxic hypoxia. J Appl Physiol 89:1317–1321
38. Nevière R, Chagnon JL, Teboul JL, Vallet B, Wattel F (2002) Small intestine intramucosal PCO(2) and microvascular blood flow during hypoxic and ischemic hypoxia. Crit Care Med 30:379–384
39. Mecher CE, Rackow EC, Astiz ME, Weil MH (1990) Venous hypercarbia associated with severe sepsis and systemic hypoperfusion. Crit Care Med 18:585–589
40. Bakker J, Vincent JL, Gris P, Leon M, Coffernils M, Kahn RJ (1992) Veno-arterial carbon dioxide gradient in human septic shock. Chest 101:509–515
41. Wendon JA, Harrison PM, Keays R, Gimson AE, Alexander G, Williams R (1991) Arterial-venous pH differences and tissue hypoxia in patients with fulminant hepatic failure. Crit Care Med 19:1362–1364

42. Cohen IL, Sheikh FM, Perkins RJ, Feustel PJ, Foster ED (1995) Effect of hemorrhagic shock and reperfusion on the respiratory quotient in swine. Crit Care Med 23:545–552
43. Mekontso-Dessap A, Castelain V, Anguel N et al (2002) Combination of venoarterial PCO_2 difference with arteriovenous O_2 content difference to detect anaerobic metabolism in patients. Intensive Care Med 28:272–277
44. Cuschieri J, Rivers EP, Donnino MW et al (2005) Central venous-arterial carbon dioxide difference as an indicator of cardiac index. Intensive Care Med 31:818–822
45. van Beest PA, Lont MC, Holman ND, Loef B, Kuiper MA, Boerma EC (2013) Central venous-arterial pCO_2 difference as a tool in resuscitation of septic patients. Intensive Care Med 39:1034–1039
46. Mallat J, Benzidi Y, Salleron J et al (2014) Time course of central venous-to-arterial carbon dioxide tension difference in septic shock patients receiving incremental doses of dobutamine. Intensive Care Med 40:404–411
47. Vallet B, Pinsky MR, Cecconi M (2013) Resuscitation of patients with septic shock: please "mind the gap"! Intensive Care Med 39:1653–1655
48. Vallée F, Vallet B, Mathe O et al (2008) Central venous-to-arterial carbon dioxide difference: an additional target for goal-directed therapy in septic shock? Intensive Care Med 34:2218–2225
49. Du W, Liu DW, Wang WT et al (2013) Combining central venous-to-arterial partial pressure of carbon dioxide difference and central venous oxygen saturation to guide resuscitation in septic shock. J Crit Care 28:1110e1–1110e5
50. Mallat J, Pepy F, Lemyze M et al (2014) Central venous-to-arterial carbon dioxide partial pressure difference in early resuscitation from septic shock: a prospective observational study. Eur J Anaesthesiol 31:371–380

An Update on Cerebral Oxygenation Monitoring, an Innovative Application in Cardiac Arrest and Neurological Emergencies

B. Schneider, T. J. Abramo, and G. Albert

Introduction

The aim of this article is to provide an overview on cerebral near infrared spectroscopy (NIRS), now called 'cerebral oximetry'. We will present an overview of recent abstracts and cerebral oximetry studies and discuss its potential impact on critically ill and injured adult and pediatric patients. We will also discuss the capabilities that certain cerebral oximetry machines have of assessing regional blood flow, similar to pulse oximetry's peripheral perfusion index (PPI).

The central nervous system (CNS) is the least monitored end organ in emergency and critical care medicine. CNS monitoring is usually managed by measuring indirect global physiological parameters, such as heart rate, blood pressure and pulse oximetry. While these parameters give a detailed view of peripheral oxygenation, cerebral oxygenation can only be vaguely surmised. In reality, we are able to monitor the cardiovascular and pulmonary systems with some degree of accuracy, but we are not able to determine with certainty the cerebral physiological status of the critically ill and injured adult or child [1, 2]. Although the pathophysiology of brain injury is complex there are two key components:

1. Reduction in oxygen delivery below critical thresholds, and
2. Impaired oxygen utilization leading to cerebral tissue failure [1–4].

Although some cerebral pathophysiological processes are disease specific, the common pathway is cerebral ischemia [2]. This cerebral ischemic event occurs as a result of a mismatch between cerebral regional blood flow and tissue metabolic demand [1–4]. There is a critical time window during which permanent neurologic injury can be minimized or even prevented [1–5]. This opportunity is often missed

B. Schneider · T. J. Abramo ✉
Department of Pediatrics, University of Arkansas School of Medicine, Little Rock, USA
e-mail: TJAbramo@uams.edu

G. Albert
Department of Neurosurgery, University of Arkansas School of Medicine, Little Rock, USA

J.-L. Vincent (ed.), *Annual Update in Intensive Care and Emergency Medicine 2015*,
DOI 10.1007/978-3-319-13761-2_20

because monitoring of cerebral regional tissue hypoxia/ischemia remains misunderstood or ill perceived by the majority of healthcare providers.

Non-invasive CNS monitoring has had its technical difficulties over the last 25 years. In the last 12 years, there has been tremendous success during the critical phase of illness and injury. Most CNS monitors are designed to monitor cerebral hemodynamics or its electrical activity/physiology via invasive methods. None of these monitors give the clinician the true cerebral hemispheric physiology in relationship to its oxygen perfusion, metabolic demands, oxygen extraction, and oxygen debt. Adequacy of tissue oxygenation is a prerequisite of aerobic metabolism and the goal of resuscitative therapy aims to maintain, restore, or optimize tissue oxygenation. There is a challenge in clinically monitoring and assessing tissue oxygenation in the critically ill and injured adult and child. The current global physiological monitoring system does not detect regional ischemia, which is a major contributor to the mortality and morbidity of the critically ill and injured adult and child. Various non-invasive monitoring methods have been investigated to detect this occult regional ischemia in the critically ill and injured patient and to guide therapy to restore this deficiency [1, 4–8].

Cerebral Oximetry Technology

Cerebral oximetry by NIRS is a regional tissue monitoring technique that assesses and trends the regional cerebral tissue oxygen saturation (r_cSO_2). These r_cSO_2 readings provide information regarding the following tissue physiology parameters: Tissue oxygen levels; blood flow; oxygen extraction; and other underlying variables in the brain [1–5]. In comparison, traditional pulse oximetry readings reflect the relative pulsating oxygenated hemoglobin in the arteries while cerebral oximetry reflects the relative regional venous tissue oxygenated hemoglobin. This cerebral oximetry technology has been evaluated and validated in a wide range of adult and pediatric clinical settings, including cardiovascular surgery, neurosurgery and neuro-trauma intensive care units (ICUs). The normal adult and pediatric cerebral r_cSO_2 (%O_2HB) range is 60–70%. Various cerebral oximetry machines have r_cSO_2 ranges from 0–99% or 15–99% [7–9]. In numerous cerebral oximetry studies, the r_cSO_2 values in non-surviving patients were either very low (0 or 15%) or in some instances very high (>95%) [7–9]. Further studies have shown that in reality this 95% reading represented pooled or collected arterial blood in the regional sampling area with no reduction in the oxygen bound to the hemoglobin [7–10]. In certain cerebral oximetry machines in the 'dead cerebral regional tissue' where no metabolism or perfusion is occurring, r_cSO_2 values of 0% were recorded, not representing the true oxygen bounded to hemoglobin. A 15% r_cSO_2 (%O_2Hb) in the INVOS cerebral oximetry system is interpreted as no releasable tissue oxyhemoglobin with either no tissue metabolism or no perfusion [9–11]. This 15% r_cSO_2 represents the region's irreversible or permanent percentage of oxygen bound to hemoglobin. Low or down-trending r_cSO_2 readings indicate hypoxia, and/or decreasing perfusion or increasing oxygen extraction in the cerebral regional tissue sampling area. In pediatric cerebral oximetry studies, it has been validated that r_cSO_2 reading variations correlate with abnormal cerebral physiology in various clinical scenarios in the operating room and in acute care settings [1, 10–12]. Differences between the left or right r_cSO_2 readings or the lower regional r_cSO_2 readings have been show to correlate to radiographically confirmed abnormal cerebral physiology and/or a pathologic lesion (epidural, subdural or intraparenchymal bleed) hematoma in recent adult and pediatric studies [10–12].

The difference between pulse oximetry and cerebral oximetry is that in pulse oximetry the red light transmission is gated by the arterial pulse, while cerebral oximetry is a continuous reading [13]. A cerebral oxygenation signal can be obtained when there is no regional blood flow, as in the non-pulsatile state of cardiac arrest, or even under clinical conditions where there is no cerebral blood flow at all. Pulse oximetry measures oxygen saturation in arterial hemoglobin, whereas cerebral oximetry measures hemoglobin in the regional tissue bed, which includes a mixture of brain tissue, arterial and venous blood. The ratio of arterial:venous blood is 25:75 and primarily measures cerebral venous saturation, reflecting the balance between oxygen supply and demand in the brain. Cerebral oximetry measurements can be affected by changes in blood oxygenation, cerebral blood flow (CBF), hemoglobin concentration and cerebral metabolic rate [1–5, 9–12].

Pulse oximetry can detect relative changes in arterial blood volume by detecting changes in oxygenated hemoglobin passing through the sensors, representing a trend in regional perfusion called the perfusion index. Certain cerebral oximetry machines can, in addition to assessing regional tissue oxygenation saturation by their proprietary internal systems, just like pulse oximetry's PPI system, access the passage of oxygenated hemoglobin through the light source to represent the regional perfusion index. The INVOS NIR cerebral oximetry machine has the similar capability of detecting and trending the regional tissue hemoglobin flow and volume changes expressed as the cerebral blood volume index (CBVI). This CBVI measured by the INVOS 5100 during cardiovascular surgery has been shown to predict blood flow and postoperative ischemia-related cerebral injury. The CBVI is a number displayed from -50 to +50. The -50 value is set by internal calibration by the monitor at startup before patient measurements [12]. This signal strength is proportional to the total percentage of hemoglobin passing through the light path. If there are negative CBVI values, it indicates that very little blood flow is occurring. A positive CBVI value means an increase in regional blood flow has occurred [12]. If the hemoglobin concentration is stable, this signal strength should be proportional to the oxygenated hemoglobin passing through the light path, giving rise to the designated CBVI [12].

Cerebral oximetry with or without CBVI has been evaluated in a wide range of neonatal and pediatric neurological scenarios. In many pediatric cerebral oximetry studies it has been demonstrated that variations in r_cSO_2 readings correlate with abnormal cerebral physiology in various neurological scenarios. Cerebral oximetry and CBVI technology have been used as a non-invasive neurological tool for cerebral pathology and perfusion monitoring in pediatric and adult cardiovascular surgery (for ischemic events and outcomes) [12]. In adult and pediatric neurological emergencies, such as altered mental status, head trauma with epidural or subdural hematomas and more diffuse traumatic brain injuries, cerebral oximetry with CBVI has shown its benefits. In recent adult and pediatric studies, differences between the left or right r_cSO_2 readings and the lower regional r_cSO_2 readings have been demonstrated to correlate to the side of the abnormal cerebral physiology/pathology and radiological pathology [12].

The various cerebral oximetry machines each have their own unique NIRS system. The cerebral oximetry machines use either a narrow or wider regional tissue sampling area. Narrow sampling gives more precise tissue sampling and a greater chance of sampling error by missing broader ischemic areas. This sampling process can give a false negative perspective for regional tissue ischemia. Cerebral oximetry machines with a wider sampling area give a wider regional tissue sampling perspective, which improves the detection of altered regional cerebral physiology compared to the narrow focused cerebral oximetry machine that may completely miss this ischemic cerebral regional physiology.

True cerebral oximetry validation studies in humans are impractical in reality and dangerous to the patient. Cerebral oximetry r_cSO_2 readings have been correlated to jugular venous saturation readings ($SjvO_2$), which have been considered to be the gold standard or the validity test for cerebral oximetry. The inherent sampling error is that the $SjvO_2$ has an undefined portion of a variable cranial venous drainage, which includes the cortical and subcortical tissue, possibly one or both hemispheric venous drainages and with an uncertain extra-cranial component. Thus, correlating a left or right r_cSO_2 reading to the $SjvO_2$ has significant and inherent flaws. A true patient validation of right and left r_cSO_2 is impractical and unethical. To truly find the absolute value of a cerebral r_cSO_2 reading would necessitate placing an oxygen sensing probe into the particular cerebral regional tissue in which the cerebral oximetry sampling area is located and to correlate these two values. Similarly, pulse oximetry can never be truly validated to its reading, but the pulse oximetry reading is extrapolated to the arterial gas finding with the assumption that there is little dis-association of the oxygen from the arterial hemoglobin in the arterial sampling site compared to the pulmonary vascular exchange site [13].

The major focus and use of cerebral oximetry monitoring by healthcare providers and industry has been in the anesthesia, ICU and cardiac ICU realm. Application outside of these arenas has been limited by certain misconceptions by healthcare providers about the technology, interpretation of the readings and trending along with its clinical applications. The difficulty in demonstrating the value of a monitoring device is that the results can prompt a variety of interpretations and clinical responses. If a monitor is used without a concomitant understanding of the interplay of what the monitoring is detecting, then it is likely to be easily misinterpreted. The healthcare provider needs to understand that the readings obtained from the non-invasive monitor are a relative composite value of the regional sampling area as influenced by the regional physiological system and the global physiological effects on the regional sampling area. Healthcare providers tend to focus on absolute values of a new monitoring system versus interpreting all the physiologic parameters producing these values and trends. These non-invasive reading can never be absolute nor absolutely validated because of the sampling area and impractically of obtaining a true sample. Therefore, we extrapolate these non-invasive readings to the patient's regional and global physiological status at the time of the readings in respect to their clinical state. As in pulse oximetry and capnography, the patient's readings are a composite value of the sampling area and can never be a patient's absolute value. This concept must be applied when using cerebral oximetry in any clinical situation.

In numerous clinical cerebral oximetry studies there have been certain misconceptions about cerebral oximetry monitoring systems. Most cerebral oximetry studies have focused on a unilateral regional cerebral oxygenation analysis and have not incorporated the unique physiology of the left and right cerebral hemispheres; therefore, their results have hindered the growth and acceptance of cerebral oximetry for non-invasive neurological monitoring. The primary misconception has been that there is no physiological uniqueness to each cerebral hemisphere and, therefore, each hemisphere does not have its own unique cerebral physiology in response to critical illness. The misconception exists that cerebral oxygenation is uniform in all areas and not specific to each hemisphere. Therefore, in studies utilizing cerebral oximetry, sensors placed in the middle of the forehead were considered the standard for assessing cerebral regional oxygenation. However, we have shown in numerous studies in various disease states that using right and left forehead sensor placement has demonstrated the uniqueness of the left and right frontal cerebral regional physiology. Another misconception is that cerebral lesions in the occipital or parietal area have no effect on the left or right frontal regional tissue physiology. Our cerebral oximetry studies have disproven this cerebral physiology misconception. We have shown that the brain's hemispheric neurovascular and metabolic system is dynamic and does have significant interplay between the two hemispheres and that non-frontal cerebral pathology does affect frontal cerebral physiology. An insult to the occipital area, whether on the ipsilateral or contralateral hemisphere, does have an effect on frontal regional tissue physiology as expressed by the cerebral regional oxygenation values [10–12].

In our cerebral oximetry studies, we have demonstrated that left and right hemispheric cerebral pathology is unique to itself. In hydrocephalus patients with or without increased intracranial pressure (ICP), each patient has unique left and right r_cSO_2 readings. In cerebral oximetry studies, the difference between the right and left r_cSO_2 readings correlated to the ipsilateral cerebral pathology [11]. We have also demonstrated that cerebral pathology causing abnormal cerebral oxygenation can affect the contralateral normal cerebral physiology by lower r_cSO_2 readings [11]. Adult and pediatric oximetry studies in hydrocephalus patients have shown that left and right r_cSO_2 readings are affected by increased ICP [11]. ICP reduction can effectively reverse the regional oxygen debt as expressed by the increase in r_cSO_2 readings [11].

Another facet of NIRS studies has been in the somatic regional tissue sampling in various adult and pediatric clinical scenarios. The overwhelming conclusions of these somatic regional tissue NIRS sampling has been that the greatest consistency is in neonates and patients less than 10 kg. In patients greater than 10 kg there is great variety in the depth of the subcutaneous fat tissue, which greatly hinders accurate somatic regional oxygenation readings. With the varying depth of the subcutaneous fat, the r_cSO_2 readings that are produced are not reflective of true somatic regional tissue oxygenation but more of the perfusion through the fat tissue. There are numerous neonatal cerebral and somatic regional oxygenation monitoring studies demonstrating its significance in various clinical scenarios. Cerebral with somatic regional oximetry has become a standard non-invasive neurological and somatic regional tissue monitoring system in neonatal intensive care, neonatal transport and most recently in neonatal head cooling in patients with hypoxic ischemic encephalopathy.

In summary, in cerebral oximetry monitoring in critically ill and injured adult and pediatric patients, the r_cSO_2 and CBVI readings are composite values of the regional tissue oxygen delivery and demand with varying degrees of influence by global physiological parameters. These r_cSO_2 and CBVI readings must be considered to represent the individual left and right cerebral hemispheric physiologies as well as the cerebral pathologies affecting both the ipsilateral and contralateral hemispheric tissue perfusion, before a neurological clinical decision intervention is utilized [10–12]. The use of single sensor probe analysis in cerebral oximetry has significant air sampling. As such, it does not represent the true uniqueness of left and right cerebral physiology. Using single sensor sampling has significantly delayed the clinical acceptance of cerebral oximetry in critically ill and injured adult and pediatric patients by healthcare providers. The differences between the left and right r_cSO_2 and CBVI readings have shown clinical utility in detecting and locating hemispheric cerebral pathology in adult and pediatric patients [11, 12]. The percentage decrease in r_cSO_2 from a baseline of 15 to 20% seems to be the best threshold indicating occurrence of cerebral ischemia in numerous investigations. For left or right r_cSO_2 values less than 50%, there is a strong association with significant cerebral ischemia, indicating some degree of cerebral pathology [10–12]. Left or right r_cSO_2 readings greater than 85% may represent cerebral pathology as a result of arterial blood pooling or oxygenated stagnant blood, such as in subarachnoid bleeds or epidural hematomas [10–12]. A 0 or 15% r_cSO_2 reading (depending on the cerebral oximetry machine) on either left or right hemispheres reflects no cerebral oxygen perfusion and no cerebral metabolism [10–12].

Through extensive review of cerebral oximetry studies in various clinical situations, our clinical cerebral oximetry pediatric studies and clinical experience with cerebral oximetry in the pediatric emergency department at an academic institution (Arkansas Children's Hospital Pediatric Emergency Department) we have devised a suggested critical thinking analysis of cerebral r_cSO_2 readings, end-tidal CO_2, and other cardiovascular monitoring parameters in pediatric trauma and cardiac arrest (Table 1).

$_cSO_2$ normal values: 60–80%O_2Hb **Adequate regional tissue oxygen present – stable regional oxygen enriched Hb perfusion, oxygen extraction and tissue metabolism**	**r_cSO_2** **Initial Readings and Trends** ***Medical/Trauma Interpretation***	• **15% r_cSO_2 reading represents 25% of oxygen irreversibly bound to Hb (O_2 that is never released from the Hb to the regional tissue)** • **Subdural hematomas produce significant increase in ICP causing significant decrease to regional cerebral perfusion**
MEDICAL/TRAUMA Interpretation **Left and/or right side r_cSO_2 value = 15–20%**	**MEDICAL/TRAUMA Interpretation** **Left and/or right side r_cSO_2 value ≦ 50%**	**MEDICAL/TRAUMA Interpretation** **Left and/or right side r_cSO_2 value ≧ 85%**

• Both sides = 15–20%O_2Hbb
  • Severe ICP, potential for + herniation
Differential diagnoses:
• Bilateral subdural hematomas with or without intraparenchymal bleed
• Unilateral subdural and epidural hematoma causing enough increase in ICP to produce decreased regional tissue perfusion on opposite side producing lower rSO2 value on the opposite side (< 50%)
	• Both sides r_cSO_2 ≦ 50%O_2Hb
	  • Significant increase in ICP causes decreased perfusion, decreased regional tissue perfusion, increased oxygen extraction and increased metabolism
	Differential diagnoses:
	• Bilateral subdural hematomas with or without intraparenchymal bleed
		• Both sides r_cSO_2 ≧ 85% O_2Hb
		  • Stagnant, accumulated/pooled oxygenated blood in the regional cerebral tissue
		  • Little to no O_2 extraction occurring
		Differential diagnoses
		• Bilateral epidural hematomas
		• Subarachnoid bleed

• One side r_cSO_2 = 15–25%O_2Hb
  • Due to significant local increased ICP caused by the hematoma, severe decreases in cerebral tissue perfusion cause increased tissue metabolism and little to no O_2 extraction
  • Severe ICP, potential for + herniation
Differential diagnoses:
• Unilateral subdural hematoma with or without intraparenchymal bleed
	• One side r_cSO_2 ≦ 50%O_2Hb
	  • Due to significant local increased ICP producing decreased regional tissue perfusion, there will be decreased O_2 delivery and increased O_2 extraction and an overall decrease in regional tissue O_2 availability
	Differential diagnoses:
	• Unilateral subdural hematoma with or without intraparenchymal bleed
		• One side r_cSO_2 ≧ 85%O_2Hb
		  • Stagnant, accumulated/pooled oxygenated blood in the regional cerebral tissue
		  • Little to no O_2 extraction occurring
		Differential diagnoses:
		• Unilateral epidural hematoma
		• Unilateral epidural and subdural hematoma
		• Subarachnoid bleed

POSSIBLE THERAPEUTIC INTERVENTIONS
1. Assess for GCS < 13
2. 3% HTS 5 ml/kg peripheral i.v.; may need repeated dose and watch for raises in rSO_2 reading which indicates improved perfusion and O_2Hb delivery
3. If GCS < 10 = possible intubation with ICP precaution:
  a. Lidocaine (1.5 mg/kg)
  b. Etomidate (0.5 mg/kg)
  c. Rocuronium (1 mg/kg)
4. Assess adequacy of MAP and CPP, maintain MAP
5. Maintain patient's head midline and elevate bed to 30° to increase cerebral venous return
6. Decrease overall cerebral metabolism and decreased ICP fluctuations by adequate patient sedation, pain and paralytic and anticonvulsant medications
7. Facilitate faster movement to CT scan of the head, neck and abdomen
	POSSIBLE THERAPEUTIC INTERVENTIONS
	1. Assess for GCS < 13
	2. 3% HTS 5 ml/kg peripheral i.v.
	3. Assess Hb concentration due to bleeding and decreased perfusion
	4. Assess adequacy of MAP and CPP and maintain MAP
	5. If GCS < 10 = possible intubation with ICP precaution:
	  a. Lidocaine (1.5 mg/kg)
	  b. Etomidate (0.5 mg/kg)
	  c. Rocuronium (1 mg/kg)
	6. Maintain patient's head midline and elevate bed to 30° to increase cerebral venous return
	7. Decrease overall cerebral metabolism and decreased ICP fluctuations by adequate patient sedation, pain, and paralytic and anticonvulsant medications
	8. Facilitate faster movement to CT scan of the head, neck and abdomen
		POSSIBLE THERAPEUTIC INTERVENTIONS
		1. Assess for GCS < 13
		2. 3% HTS 5 ml/kg peripheral i.v.
		3. Assess Hb concentration due to bleeding and decreased perfusion
		4. Assess adequacy of MAP and CPP and maintain MAP
		5. If GCS < 10 = possible intubation with ICP precaution:
		  a. Lidocaine (1.5 mg/kg)
		  b. Etomidate (0.5 mg/kg)
		  c. Rocuronium (1 mg/kg)
		6. Maintain patient's head midline and elevate bed to 30° to increase cerebral venous return
		7. Decrease overall cerebral metabolism and decreased ICP fluctuations by adequate patient sedation, pain, and paralytic and anticonvulsant medications
		8. Facilitate faster movement to CT scan of the head, neck and abdomen

Table 1 Critical thinking analysis of regional cerebral tissue oxygen saturation (r_cSO_2) readings, end-tidal CO_2 ($EtCO_2$), and other cardiovascular monitoring parameters in pediatric trauma and cardiac arrest. ICP: intracranial pressure; GCS: Glasgow coma scale; CPP: cerebral perfusion pressure; MAP: mean arterial pressure; CT: computed tomography; Hb: hemoglobin; CPR: cardiopulmonary resuscitation; HTS: hypertonic saline; i.v.: intravenous

$_cSO_2$ normal values: 60–80% O_2Hb **Adequate regional tissue oxygen present – stable regional oxygen enriched Hb perfusion, oxygen extraction and tissue metabolism**	**r_cSO_2** **Initial Readings and Trends** ***Medical/Trauma Interpretation***	• **15% r_cSO_2 reading represents 25% of oxygen irreversibly bound to Hb (O_2 that is never released from the Hb to the regional tissue)** • **Subdural hematomas produce significant increase in ICP causing significant decrease to regional cerebral perfusion**
CPR Interpretation **Left and/or right side r_cSO_2 value = 15–20% O_2Hb** **$EtCO_2$ < 20 mmHg**	**CPR Interpretation** **Left and/or right side r_cSO_2 value = 15–20% O_2Hb** **$EtCO_2$ > 20 mmHg**	**CPR Interpretation** **Left and/or right side r_cSO_2 value ≦ 40% O_2Hb** **$EtCO_2$ > 20 mmHg**
• No metabolism occurring in the cerebral tissue and no blood passing through the pulmonary artery/lungs for CO_2 to be expired. An $EtCO_2$ of < 20 mmHg is the CO_2 in the trachea and large bronchi (physiological dead space) • Low rSO_2 values and $EtCO_2$ values that do not raise above 20 mmHg means no circulation through the brain or systemic perfusion	After 20 minutes of CPR, if $EtCO_2$ is > 20 but r_cSO_2 is 15–20%: • There is no cerebral tissue metabolism, no cerebral tissue perfusion, and no oxygen extraction • There IS blood flow through the pulmonary artery/lungs for CO_2 to be expired • Correlate $EtCO_2$ with chest compressions or with heart rate • These combined readings probably mean there is no cerebral/brain activity but there is systemic perfusion	• There is cerebral tissue metabolism, perfusion and oxygen extraction • There is blood flow through the pulmonary artery/lungs for CO_2 to be expired • These combined readings mean that the brain and systemic perfusion is working
POSSIBLE THERAPEUTIC INTERVENTIONS 1. CPR and airway management, check glucose and K a. If K elevated consider glucose D25 2 ml/kg , HCO_3 2 meq/kg regular insulin 0.1 unit i. v. and possible CaCl 10 mg/kg 2. 3% HTS 5 ml/kg i. v. 3. Intubate and hyperventilate 4. Maintain patient's head midline and elevate bed to 30° to increase cerebral venous return 5. Emergency CT scan 6. Decrease cerebral metabolism 7. Possible need for anticonvulsants, versed, etomidate, or pain medication 8. Consider fluid boluses and epinephrine drip and titrate to improve $EtCO_2$ and r_cSO_2	**POSSIBLE THERAPEUTIC INTERVENTIONS** 1. CPR and airway management, check glucose and K a. If K elevated consider glucose D25 2 ml/kg, HCO_3 2 meq/kg , regular insulin 0.1 unit i. v. and possible CaCl 10 mg/kg 2. 3% HTS 5 ml/kg i. v. 3. Intubate and hyperventilate 4. Maintain patient's head midline and elevate bed to 30° to increase cerebral venous return 5. Emergency CT scan 6. Decrease cerebral metabolism 7. Possible need for anticonvulsants, versed, etomidate, or pain medication 8. Consider fluid boluses and epinephrine drip and titrate to improve $EtCO_2$ and r_cSO_2 9. If $EtCO_2$ and r_cSO_2 improve only with chest compressions, consider emergency ECMO	**POSSIBLE THERAPEUTIC INTERVENTIONS** 1. CPR and airway management, check glucose and K a. If K elevated consider glucose D25 2 ml/kg, HCO_3 2 meq/kg, regular insulin 0.1 unit i. v. and possible CaCl 10 mg/kg 2. 3% HTS 5 ml/kg i. v. 3. Intubate and hyperventilate 4. Maintain patient's head midline and elevate bed to 30° to increase cerebral venous return 5. Emergency CT scan 6. Decrease cerebral metabolism 7. Possible need for anticonvulsants, versed, etomidate, or pain medication 8. Consider fluid boluses and epinephrine drip and titrate to improve $EtCO_2$ and r_cSO_2 9. If $EtCO2_2$ and r_cSO_2 improve only with chest compressions, consider emergency ECMO

Factors DECREASING r_cSO_2 values		**Factors INCREASING r_cSO_2 values**	
Systemic factors: Low MAP/CPP Low cardiac output Systemic hypoxia Hypocapnia – low CO_2	**Intracranial factors:** High ICP/low CPP Seizures	**Systemic factors:** Normal or high MAP/CPP Normal or high cardiac output Hypoxia Normal levels of CO_2	**Intracranial factors:** Metabolic suppression sedatives or hypothermia Normal ICP/CPP Cerebral vasodilation

Table 1 (Continuation)

Cerebral Oximetry and Cardiac Arrest

During cardiac arrest, the brain is hypo-perfused and thus deprived of oxygen. This period of ischemia initiates a cascade of metabolic derangements that ultimately ends in neuronal cell death and irreversible brain damage [14]. The burden of neurologic sequelae in post-cardiac arrest patients looms large even in patients who do achieve return of spontaneous circulation (ROSC) and survive to hospital discharge [15]. The brain is perhaps the most important major end-organ outcome that is not routinely assessed during cardiopulmonary resuscitation (CPR) and little is known of what occurs to cerebrovascular physiology during CPR. Extrapolation of data from animal models suggests significant changes in CBF and metabolic demands in the ensuing 12 hours post-arrest [16]. Cerebral oximetry via NIRS has emerged as a promising and useful adjunct for CPR during cases in which other monitoring modalities (i. e., pulse oximetry, wave form capnography) have little to no information to provide in regards to cerebral physiology [14]. Pulse oximetry, while excellent for providing information concerning oxygenation of peripheral tissues, relies on pulsatile flow, which is conspicuously absent during cardiac arrest and provides no useful information regarding cerebral oxygenation during arrest. Wave capnography is reflective only of the quality of CPR and provides no insight into cerebral physiology during cardiac arrest [17].

Continuous monitoring of cerebral perfusion during cardiac arrest with cerebral oximetry can provide important information about ongoing therapeutic interventions during cardiac arrest in real time. The practicality and utility of non-invasive cerebral oximetry to guide interventions during cardiac arrest is illustrated in a case series published by Abramo et al. [12]. Fourteen patients with malfunctioning ventriculo-peritoneal shunts who suffered cardiac arrest and/or severe bradycardia had ROSC after alleviation of the obstruction by way of shunt tap or shunt externalization by neurosurgery. In each of these cases, r_cSO_2 values were at the lowest level of detection (15%) and rebounded to normal upon alleviation of the increased ICP with improvement in the cardiovascular system [12].

In several studies, researchers have demonstrated that low initial r_cSO_2 correlates with poor outcomes and decreased chances of achieving ROSC [18–20]. Low r_cSO_2 on arrival to the hospital may also predict neurological outcome as demonstrated by Ito et al. [21]· This is not to say that single point measurements should be used to guide resuscitation efforts. Parnia et al. [22] found that while many of their patients had low initial r_cSO_2 values (15–21%) there was a significant difference in r_cSO_2 in the final 5 minutes of resuscitation in patients achieving ROSC. The authors keenly make the point that measurements taken throughout resuscitation may be a better marker to evaluate outcome rather than taking a single measurement as interventions made during continued resuscitation efforts could continue to increase r_cSO_2 and cerebral perfusion. For example, a small case series published by Abramo et al. [23] noted in one case that despite prolonged cardiovascular collapse and pulmonary hemorrhage, which obviated the prognostic value of end-tidal CO_2 measurements, r_cSO_2 values remained constantly in the normal range of 50–70%.

This case series highlights the effectiveness of emergency medical services (EMS) CPR and continuous resuscitative interventions on cardiocerebral resuscitation and the ability of cerebral oximetry to guide resuscitative efforts in cardiac arrest in the case of failure of conventional monitoring methods.

Cerebral oximetry should be continued in the post-arrest period in those patients achieving ROSC. This is a critically important time period during which significant derangement in cerebral metabolism occurs as a result of hypoxic injury to neurons ending ultimately in apoptosis and cerebral edema [14]. Ahn et al. [24] investigated post-arrest r_cSO_2 values and found that median values around 63% in the first 24 hours post-arrest were associated with lower rates of survival, while patients with median values of 70% had improved survival in the post-arrest period. It is important to note that when compared with $SjvO_2$, a widely accepted method of monitoring cerebral oxygenation, similar conclusions were made concerning the level of r_cSO_2 and survival post-arrest [24]. Patients who did not achieve ROSC had low initial r_cSO_2 values and mean r_cSO_2 values remained low throughout the resuscitation period [18–22, 24–26]. It can be concluded that low initial r_cSO_2 values not accompanied by a rapid rise with therapeutic interventions such as CPR portend a poor outcome.

The future of resuscitation lies in grasping the intricacies of cerebral perfusion and ultimately cerebral resuscitation. As such, more attention will be paid to modalities that can achieve this level of insight. Cerebral oximetry via NIRS is a tool that provides valuable insight into cerebral physiology during cardiac arrest and in the inherent differences in cerebral physiology between ROSC and non-ROSC patients. Areas for future study in the field of cerebral oximetry include utilization of r_cSO_2 values for therapeutic intervention during CPR, use of cerebral oximetry as a predictor of neurologic outcomes post-arrest, and use of cerebral oximetry to guide end-point decisions in CPR.

Cerebral Oximetry and Neurologic Emergencies

Cerebral and somatic oximetry has been used for a number of years in critical care medicine to simultaneously monitor cerebral and renal perfusion. The drawback to this strategy is that renal perfusion measures become increasingly less reliable as the size of the patient increases and after the age of 10 become more or less a random number generator. Cerebral oximetry with CBVI, on the other hand, is ideal for cerebral monitoring in patients with neurologic emergencies, because it is continuous, requires few resources after placement of the probes, and is noninvasive. Cerebral oximetry has great potential as a modality for monitoring patients in the emergency room with a variety of neurologic emergencies, including traumatic brain injury (TBI), seizures, increased ICP and stroke. It has even been shown to be useful in patients with malfunctioning ventriculoperitoneal shunts [12]. While these distinct neurologic disease states have differing avenues of preceding pathophysiology, they share at least one common central tenet in that they all feature alterations in unique cerebral physiology (metabolism and blood flow) [11,

27, 28]. It is important to understand that cerebral (metabolism and perfusion) physiology is unique to each cerebral hemisphere and, especially in patients with hydrocephalus, it is uniquely patient and hemisphere specific [11, 27, 28]. For this reason, cerebral oximetry is only useful in these patients if both sides of the cortex are monitored. This observation can aid the clinician in establishing the laterality of an insult and is especially useful in cerebral pathology (epidural, subdural and subarachnoid bleeds), seizure and stroke [11, 27, 28].

It has been known for some time that the rapid increase in neuronal activity that occurs during a seizure causes a significant increase in neuronal metabolism and concomitant alterations in ipsilateral CBF [28]. Through the use of bi-hemispheric NIRS monitoring, relative differences in blood flow can be measured. Suh et al. [29] found that alterations in CBF correlated in a linear fashion with activation of an increasing area of neurons.

'Time is brain' is the popular and oft repeated aphorism in stroke treatment and prevention that summarizes the very realistic concept that cerebral ischemia has irreversible and devastating consequences. Cerebral oximetry with CBVI has the ability to rapidly diagnose alterations in cerebral hemispheric metabolism and perfusion and, therefore, is an excellent modality for diagnosing and treating stroke patients. Cerebral oximetry has been found to be both sensitive and specific for detecting vasospasm and delayed cerebral ischemia in patients with subarachnoid hemorrhage [30]. Abramo et al. [31] found that cerebral oximetry with CBVI was useful for identification of altered cerebral hemispheric physiology and pathology suggestive of cerebral pathology, including subdural and epidural hematomas and especially detecting stroke, in 68 suspected pediatric stroke patients. They also noted that there existed a statistically significant difference between hemorrhagic and ischemic catastrophes in the data provided by cerebral oximetry with CBVI [32]. Cerebral oximetry with CBVI thus has a promising future in cerebrovascular pathology and especially in stroke treatment and possibly prevention.

TBI is a wide reaching diagnosis that causes death and disability across a very wide range of ages. Ischemia in TBI develops as a result of alterations in cerebral perfusion pressure (CPP), which develop at the interplay between hypotension, increasing intracranial pressure and hypoxia. TBI also alters cerebral vascular resistance [4]. Cerebral oximetry can detect these alterations in CPP by measuring changes in the r_cSO_2 and it has been suggested that cerebral oximetry may be a useful adjunct to measuring CPP [4].

Cerebral oximetry, especially with CBVI, is an invaluable tool that can reliably and non-invasively monitor cerebral hemispheric physiology. It has a wide range of applications in a number of different critical care and emergent settings. It is safe, comparatively inexpensive and has been validated across age ranges and disciplines. Cerebral oximetry has a promising future in the world of non-invasive neuro monitoring.

Conclusion

There are several clinical conditions routinely encountered in critical care and emergency medicine that have potential to disrupt the balance between the brain's oxygen supply and demand, exposing the risk of cerebral ischemia and permanent neuronal damage. Standard clinical monitoring tools of O_2 saturation, heart rate, respiratory rate, blood pressure and possibly end-tidal CO_2 do not detect the alteration in the cerebral regional tissue and global cerebral physiology. By the time these alterations are present in the current monitoring systems, significant neurological damage has potentially occurred and not been detected. The effects of these transient alterations in cerebral physiology/metabolism induced by the imbalance between oxygen supply and demand may range from severe neurological complications to acute brain ischemia with serious permanent functional impairment to slight changes in psychosocial profile or cognitive decline after surgery. These alterations in the brain oxygen balance remain totally undiagnosed if we do not specifically monitor them. Monitoring the balance between oxygen supply and demand to the brain tissue using a simple non-invasive device like cerebral oximetry has the potential to optimize our treatment plan to the real needs of the target organ, the neurovascular system. There are increasing numbers of publications supporting the clinical use of cerebral oximetry in the critical care and emergency room. Therefore, future investigative studies of cerebral oximetry must incorporate several components of cerebral oximetry: Comparisons between left and right cerebral hemispheric readings, trends in r_cSO_2 values, variability in r_cSO_2 values, and the response to therapy in relationship to the left and right cerebral/hemispheric pathophysiology.

References

1. Drayna PC, Abramo TJ, Estrada C (2011) Near-infrared spectroscopy in the critical setting. Pediatr Emerg Care 27:432–439
2. Murkin JM, Arango M (2009) Near-infrared spectroscopy as an index of brain and tissue oxygenation. Br J Anaesth 103(Suppl 1):i3–13
3. Scheeren TW, Schober P, Schwarte LA (2012) Monitoring tissue oxygenation by near infrared spectroscopy (NIRS): background and current applications. J Clin Monit Comput 26:279–287
4. Dunham CM, Ransom KJ, Flowers LL, Siegal JD, Kohli CM (2004) Cerebral hypoxia in severely brain-injured patients is associated with admission Glasgow coma scale score, computed tomographic severity, cerebral perfusion pressure, and survival. J Trauma 56:482–491
5. Al-Rawi P, Kirkpatrick P (2006) Tissue oxygen index: thresholds for cerebral ischemia using near-infrared spectroscopy. Stroke 37:2720–2725
6. Lee J, Kibler K, Benni P et al (2009) Cerebrovascular reactivity measured by near infrared spectroscopy. Stroke 40:1820–1826
7. Zweifel C, Castellani G, Czosnyka M et al (2010) Noninvasive monitoring of cerebrovascular reactivity with near infrared spectroscopy in head-injured patients. J Neurotrauma 27:1951–1958
8. Steiner LA, Pfister D, Strebel SP et al (2009) Near-infrared spectroscopy can monitor dynamic cerebral autoregulation in adults. Neurocrit Care 10:122–128

9. Figaji AA, Kent SJ (2010) Brain tissue oxygenation in children diagnosed with brain death. Neurocrit Care 12:56–61
10. Kane I, Abramo T, Meredith M et al (2014) Cerebral oxygen saturation monitoring in pediatric altered mental status patients. Am J Emerg Med 32:356–362
11. Abramo TJ, Zhou C, Estrada C et al (2014) Innovative application of cerebral rSO2 monitoring during shunt tap in pediatric ventricular malfunctioning shunts. Pediatr Emerg Care (in press)
12. Abramo TJ, Meredith M, Jaeger M et al (2014) Cerebral oximetry with blood volume index in asystolic pediatric cerebrospinal fluid malfunctioning shunt patients. Am J Emerg Med 32:1439.e1–7
13. Severinghaus JW (2007) Takuo Aoyagi: discovery of pulse oximetry. Anesth Analg 105(6 Suppl):S1–S4
14. Nolan JP, Neumar RW, Adrie C et al (2008) The post cardiac arrest syndrome: Epidemiology, pathophysiology, treatment, and prognostication. Resuscitation 79:350–379
15. Zheng ZJ, Croft JB, Giles WH, Mensah GA (2001) Sudden cardiac death in the United States, 1989–1998. Circulation 104:2158–2163
16. Lee JK, Brady KM, Mytar JO et al (2011) Cerebral blood flow and cerebrovascular autoregulation in a swine model of pediatric cardiac arrest and hypothermia. Crit Care Med 39:2337–2345
17. Neumar RW, Otto CW, Link MS et al (2010) Part 8: adult advanced cardiovascular life support: 2010 American Heart Association guidelines for cardiopulmonary resuscitation and emergency cardiovascular care. Circulation 122:S729–S767
18. Newman DH, Callaway CW, Greenwald IB, Freed J (2004) Cerebral oximetry in out-of-hospital cardiac arrest: standard CPR rarely provides detectable hemoglobin-oxygen saturation to the frontal cortex. Resuscitation 63:189–194
19. Mullner M, Sterz F, Binder M, Hirschl MM, Janata K, Laggner AN (1995) Near infrared spectroscopy during and after cardiac arrest – preliminary results. Clin Intensive Care 6:107–111
20. McCormick PW, Stewart M, Ray P et al (1991) Measurement of regional cerebrovascular hemoglobin oxygen saturation in cats using optical spectroscopy. Neurol Res 13:65–70
21. Ito N, Nanto S, Nagao K, Hatanaka T, Kai T (2010) Regional cerebral oxygen saturation predicts poor neurologic outcome in patients with out-of-hospital cardiac arrest. Resuscitation 81:1736–1737
22. Parnia S, Nasir A, Shah C, Patel R, Mani A, Richman P (2012) A feasibility study evaluating the role of cerebral oximetry in predicting return of spontaneous circulation in cardiac arrest. Resuscitation 83:982–985
23. Abramo T, Aggarwal N, Kane I, Crossman K, Meredith M (2014) Cerebral oximetry and cerebral blood flow monitoring in 2 pediatric survivors with out-of-hospital cardiac arrest. Am J Emerg Med 32:394.e5–394.e10
24. Ahn A, Yang J, Inigo-Santiago L, Parnia S (2014) A feasibility study of cerebral oximetry monitoring during the post-resuscitation period in comatose patients following cardiac arrest. Resuscitation 85:522–526
25. Takasu A, Yagi K, Ishihrar S et al (1995) Combined continuous monitoring of systemic and cerebral oxygen metabolism after cardiac arrest. Resuscitation 29:189–194
26. Asim K, Gokhan E, Ozlem B et al (2014) Near infrared spectrophotometry (cerebral oximetry) in predicting the return of spontaneous circulation in out-of-hospital cardiac arrest. Am J Emerg Med 32:14–17
27. Kane I, Abramo TJ, Meredith M et al (2014) Cerebral oxygen saturation monitoring in pediatric altered mental status patients. Am J Emerg Med 32:356–62
28. Duncan R (1992) Epilepsy, cerebral blood flow, and cerebral metabolic rate. Cerebrovasc Brain Metab Rev 4:105–121
29. Suh M, Bahar S, Mehta A, Schwarz T (2006) Blood volume and hemoglobin oxygenation response following electrical stimulation of human cortex. Neuroimage 31:66–75

30. Yokose N, Sakatani K, Murata Y et al (2010) Bedside monitoring of cerebral blood oxygenation and hemodynamics after aneurismal subarachnoid hemorrhage by quantitative time-resolved near-infrared spectroscopy. World Neurosurg 73:508–513
31. Abramo T, Jordan L, Harris Z et al (2014) Utility of cerebral oximetry with blood volume index in a pediatric stroke alert system and detecting pediatric strokes. Pediatric Academic Society May 2014, Oral Presentation.
32. Ganne S, Umamaheswara R, Padmaja D (2011) Changing trends in monitoring brain ischemia: from intracranial pressure to cerebral oximetry. Curr Opin Anesthesiol 24:487–494

Part VI
Cardiac Arrest

Out-of-hospital Cardiac Arrest and Survival to Hospital Discharge: A Series of Systemic Reviews and Meta-analyses

M. Vargas, Y. Sutherasan, and P. Pelosi

Introduction

Overall survival rates to hospital discharge after out-of-hospital cardiac arrest (OHCA) range from 8 to 10% [1]. Several factors have been shown to affect hospital outcomes, including cardiopulmonary resuscitation (CPR) of good quality and adequate post-resuscitation care. Standardized algorithms for advanced life support and post-resuscitation care have been implemented in the European guidelines for resuscitation [2]. No updated guidelines have been published since 2010, so we aimed to evaluate the effect of different treatments, as suggested by current guidelines, on survival to hospital discharge after OHCA [2], using a series of new systematic reviews and meta-analyses. The following treatments were analyzed: 1) epinephrine during CPR; 2) vasopressin during CPR; 3) pre-hospital hypothermia after OHCA; 4) in-hospital hypothermia after OHCA; 5) partial pressure of arterial oxygenation (PaO_2) after OHCA; 6) partial pressure of carbon dioxide ($PaCO_2$) after OHCA.

Methodological Issues

We identified all randomized controlled trials (RCTs) assessing survival to hospital discharge. The electronic search strategy applied standard filters for identification of RCTs. The MEDLINE and PUBMED databases were searched (from inception

M. Vargas
Department of Anesthesia and Intensive Care, University of Naples "Federico II", Naples, Italy

Y. Sutherasan
Division of Pulmonary and Critical Care Medicine, Faculty of Medicine, Ramathibodi Hospital, Mahidol University, Bangkok, Thailand

P. Pelosi ✉
IRCCS AOU San Martino-IST, Genoa, Italy
e-mail: ppelosi@hotmail.com

J.-L. Vincent (ed.), *Annual Update in Intensive Care and Emergency Medicine 2015*,
DOI 10.1007/978-3-319-13761-2_21

to April 2014). We applied English language restriction. Our search included the following keywords: cardiac arrest, out of hospital cardiac arrest, circulatory arrest, cardiopulmonary resuscitation, adrenaline, epinephrine, vasopressin, pre-hospital hypothermia, in-hospital hypothermia, induced hypothermia, therapeutic hypothermia, target temperature, oxygenation, hyperoxygenation, hypo-oxygenation, hypercapnia, hypocapnia, normocapnia, mortality at discharge, survival at discharge, humans and randomized clinical trial. We included only published full papers and excluded abstracts. When more than one RCT was not available for each topic, we considered observational clinical studies. Data were independently extracted from each report by two authors (MV and YS) using a data recording form developed for this purpose. After extraction, data were reviewed and compared by a third author (PP). In RCTs, we assessed allocation concealment, baseline similarity of groups and early stopping of treatment. The primary endpoint was survival at hospital discharge after OHCA. The second endpoint was evidence of good neurologic outcome at hospital discharge defined as a cerebral performance category (CPC) of 1 and 2, overall performance category (OPC) of 1 and 2, normal or moderate disability. Studies evaluating in-hospital cardiac arrest were excluded, when possible. Indeed, studies evaluating the role of different levels of PaO_2 and $PaCO_2$ after cardiac arrest reported a mixed cohort of patients with OHCA and in-hospital cardiac arrest. Meta-analysis of risk ratios (RR) was performed with mixed random effect using the DerSimonian and Laird method. Results are graphically represented using Forest plots. The homogeneity assumption was measured by the I^2, which describes the percentage of total variation across studies that is due to heterogeneity rather than chance. A value of 0% indicates no observed heterogeneity, and larger values show increasing heterogeneity. All analyses were conducted with OpenMetaAnalyst (version 6) and SPSS version 20 (IBM SPSS). For all analyses, 2-sided p values less than 0.05 were considered significant. To evaluate potential publication bias, a weighted linear regression was used, with the natural log of the OR as the dependent variable and the inverse of the total sample size as the independent variable. This is a modified Macaskill's test, which gives more balanced type I error rates in the tail probability areas in comparison to other publication bias tests [3].

Effects of Epinephrine on Hospital Survival During CPR

Epinephrine has been reported to increase aortic diastolic pressure, coronary perfusion pressure and coronary blood flow during CPR [4]. However, although epinephrine improved the return to spontaneous circulation (ROSC) rate in OHCA, it did not improve hospital survival [5]. Similar results have been reported when epinephrine was compared with placebo or no drugs during CPR [6, 7]. Furthermore, high-dose epinephrine may be associated with high mortality and poor neurologic outcome [5].

We analyzed 7 RCTs including 4,712 patients with OHCA [6–12]. Table 1 shows the main characteristics of the included studies. From the included studies, standard

Table 1 Study characteristics of included trials for effect of epinephrine on hospital survival during cardiopulmonary resuscitation (CPR) after out-of-hospital cardiac arrest (OHCA)

First Author [ref]	Year	Study design/number of patients	Intervention	Control	Initial rhythm of OHCA
Comparing low- and high-dose epinephrine during CPR					
Brown [8]	1992	RCT/1280	Single dose, LDA: 0.02 mg/kg	Single dose, HDA: 0.2 mg/kg	Asystole/PEA, VF/VT
Callaham [9]	1992	RCT/556	Repeated doses, LDA: 1 mg	Repeated doses, HDA: 5/15 mg	Asystole/PEA, VF/VT
Stiell [12]	1992	RCT/335	Repeated doses, LDA: 1 mg	Repeated doses, HDA: 7 mg	Not reported
Sherman [11]	1997	RCT/140	Repeated doses, LDA: 0.01 mg/kg	Repeated doses, HDA: 0.1 mg/kg	Asystole, VF
Gueugniaud [10]	1998	RCT/3327	Repeated doses, LDA: 1 mg	Repeated doses, HDA: 5 mg	Asystole/PEA, VF
Comparing low dose epinephrine with placebo during CPR					
Jacobs [6]	2011	RCT/534	Repeated doses, 1 mg	Placebo	Asystole/PEA, VF/VT
Comparing low dose epinephrine with no drugs during CPR					
Olasveengen [7]	2009	RCT/851	Repeated dose, 1 mg	No drugs	Asystole/PEA, VF/VT

RCT: randomized clinical trial; LDA: low (standard) dose epinephrine; HDA: high-dose epinephrine; PEA: pulseless electrical activity; VF: ventricular fibrillation; VT: ventricular tachycardia.

or low-dose epinephrine was defined as 1 mg, 0.02 or 0.01 mg/kg and high-dose epinephrine was defined as 0.1 or 0.2 mg/kg, 5 mg, 7 mg, 5–15 mg. Five RCTs compared the effect of low-dose with high-dose epinephrine. One trial compared the effect of low-dose epinephrine with a placebo, and one trial compared the effect of low-dose epinephrine with no drugs administered during CPR. We found no difference in survival to hospital discharge when low-dose epinephrine was compared with high-dose epinephrine (RR 1.037, 95% CI 0.758–1.417, $I^2 = 0\%$, $p = 0.808$), even if epinephrine doses were administered in the pre-hospital setting or emergency room (Fig. 1) (pre-hospital: RR 1.036, 95% CI 0.754–1.423, $I^2 = 0\%$, $p = 0.450$; emergency room: RR 1.071, 95% CI 0.187–6.125, $I^2 = 0\%$, $p = 0.930$). Furthermore, we found no difference in survival to hospital discharge when low-dose epinephrine was compared with placebo or no drugs (Fig. 1, RR 1.280, 95% CI 0.796–2.058, $I^2 = 15\%$, $p = 0.278$). There was no difference in good neurologic outcome when comparing low-dose and high-dose epinephrine (RR 1.203, 95% CI 0.739–1.959, $I^2 = 0\%$, $p = 0.332$) or low-dose epinephrine vs placebo or no drugs (RR 1.243, 95% CI 0.940–1.643, $I^2 = 0\%$, $p = 0.532$).

A. Studies	Estimate (95% CI)		LDA	HDA
Brown 1992 [8]	0.860	(0.517, 1.431)	26/632	31/648
Callaham 1992 [9]	0.636	(0.153, 2.634)	3/270	5/286
Stiehl 1992 [12]	1.030	(0.147, 7.229)	2/165	2/170
Sherman 1997 [11]	1.254	(0.025, 62.317)	0/62	0/78
Gueugniaud 1998 [10]	1.230	(0.805, 1.880)	46/1650	38/1677
Overall (I^2=0%, p=0.808)	**1.037**	**(0.758, 1.417)**	**77/2779**	**76/2859**

$Tau^2 = 0.000$; $Q (df = 4) = 1.607$; $I^2 = 0\%$; $p = 0.821$

B. Studies: Pre-hospital	Estimate (95% CI)		LDA	HDA
Brown 1992 [8]	0.860	(0.517, 1.431)	26/632	31/648
Callaham 1992 [9]	0.636	(0.153, 2.634)	3/270	5/286
Gueugniaud 1998 [10]	1.230	(0.805, 1.880)	46/1650	38/1677
Overall (I^2=0%, p=0.450)	**1.036**	**(0.754, 1.423)**	**75/2552**	**74/2611**

$Tau^2 = 0.000$; $Q (df = 2) = 1.598$; $I^2 = 0\%$; $p = 0.829$

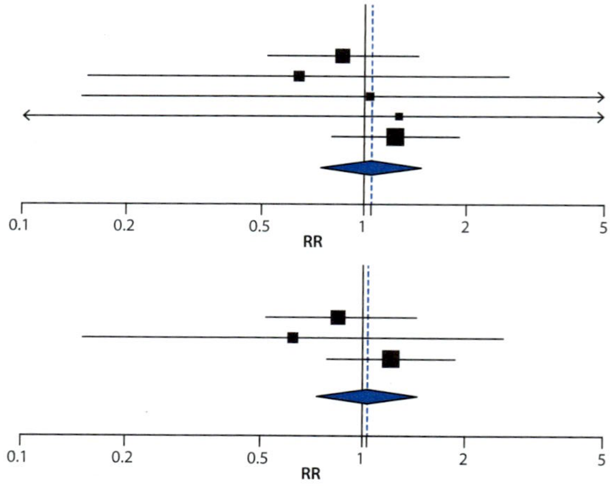

Fig. 1 Epinephrine administration during cardiopulmonary resuscitation (CPR) for out-of-hospital cardiac arrest (OHCA). *A*: Forest plot showing risk ratio (RR) of survival to hospital discharge. Weights: Brown: 37.6%; Callaham: 4.8%; Stiel 5.6%; Sherman: 0.7%; Gueugniaud: 54.3%. *B*: Forest plot showing RR of survival to hospital discharge including studies with pre-hospital administration of epinephrine. Weights: Brown: 38.9%; Callaham: 5%; Gueugniaud: 56.1%. *C*: Forest plot showing RR of survival to hospital discharge including studies with emergency room administration of epinephrine. Weights: %; Stiel 80%; Sherman: 20%. *D*: Forest plot showing RR of survival to hospital discharge including studies comparing low-dose epinephrine (LDA) versus placebo or no drugs. Weights: Olasveengen: 81.2%, Jacobs: 18.8%. HDA: high-dose epinephrine; CI: confidence interval

C. Studies: Emergency room	Estimate (95% CI)		LDA	HDA
Stiehl 1992 [12]	1.030	(0.147, 7.229)	2/165	2/170
Sherman 1997 [11]	1.254	(0.025, 62.317)	0/62	0/78
Overall (I^2=0%, p=0.930)	**1.071**	**(0.187, 6.125)**	**2/227**	**2/248**

$Tau^2 = 0.006$; Q (df = 1) = 0.008; $I^2 = 0\%$; p = 0.938

D. Studies	Estimate (95% CI)		LDA	No drugs
Olasveengen 2009 [7]	1.139	(0.759, 1.711)	44/418	40/433
Jacobs 2001 [6]	2.119	(0.746, 6.016)	11/272	5/262
Overall (I^2=0%, p=0.278)	**1.280**	**(0.796, 2.058)**	**55/690**	**45/695**

$Tau^2 = 0.029$; Q (df = 1) = 1.179; $I^2 = 15\%$; p = 0.308

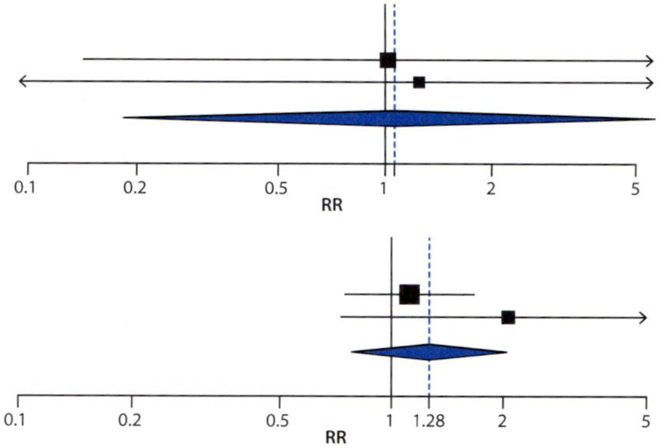

Fig. 1 (Continuation)

Hence, we found that, after OHCA:

1) the use of low-dose or high-dose epinephrine during CPR did not improve survival at hospital discharge or incidence of good neurologic outcome, even if administered in the pre-hospital setting or emergency room;
2) the use of low-dose epinephrine during CPR compared with placebo or no drugs did not improve survival at hospital discharge.

To our knowledge, this is the first meta-analysis reporting these results in studies divided into pre-hospital setting or emergency room administration of epinephrine, and comparing epinephrine with placebo and no drugs. Lin et al. performed a subgroup analysis of RR dividing the included studies into low-dose epinephrine vs. placebo, low-dose vs. high-dose epinephrine, vasopressin vs. epinephrine and vasopressin vs. placebo [13]. However, they did not include in the analysis the study by Olasveengen et al. [7] and did not divide the studies according to the intervention location [13]. Furthermore, the authors did not find any difference in survival to hospital discharge or neurological outcome comparing low-dose to high-dose epinephrine [13]. Patanwala et al. conducted a meta-analysis including two RCTs and eight observational studies comparing the effects of epinephrine vs no epinephrine or placebo [14]. In this study, epinephrine was not associated with improved survival at hospital discharge and it may have worsened long-term outcomes [14]. Atiksawedparit et al. performed a meta-analysis, including one RCT and 14 observational trials, to compare the effect on short- and long-term outcomes of epinephrine vs. no epinephrine or placebo [15]. Also in this study, epinephrine was not effective at increasing survival at hospital discharge [15].

Current guidelines on cardiac arrest state that it is reasonable to consider administering a 1 mg dose of epinephrine every 3 to 5 minutes during adult cardiac arrest (Class IIb, Level of Evidence A) mainly due to the increase in incidence of ROSC [2]. Our meta-analysis confirmed the failure of low- or high-dose epinephrine administered in a pre-hospital setting or emergency room to improve survival at hospital discharge. Interestingly, even when considering RCTs with low-dose epinephrine compared with no epinephrine or placebo, there was no improvement in survival at hospital discharge. Epinephrine as a short-acting cardiovascular stimulant may be useful to induce ROSC but seems to have no effect on survival to hospital discharge.

Effects of Vasopressin on Hospital Survival During CPR

Vasopressin is a potent vasoconstrictor, promoting the contraction of vascular smooth muscle and increasing smooth muscle response to catecholamines [16]. Use of vasopressin (40 international units [IU]) as replacement for the first or second dose of epinephrine during CPR was suggested by the most recent advanced cardiovascular life support guidelines (level of evidence A) [17]. Vasopressin may be administered in a single dose of 40 IU or up 2 doses of 40 IU, according to the literature.

Table 2 Study characteristics of included trials for vasopressin effect on hospital survival during cardiopulmonary resuscitation (CPR) after out-of-hospital cardiac arrest (OHCA)

First Author [ref]	Year	Study design/Number of patients	Intervention	Control	Initial rhythm of OHCA
Lindner [21]	1997	RCT/40	Vasopressin 40 IU (single dose) + Epinephrine 1 mg	Epinephrine 1 mg + Placebo	VF
Wenzel [24]	2004	RCT/1166	Vasopressin 40 IU (2 doses) + Epinephrine 1 mg	Epinephrine 1 mg + Placebo	Asystole/PEA, VF
Callaway [18]	2006	RCT/325	Vasopressin 40 IU (2 doses) + Epinephrine 1 mg	Epinephrine 1 mg + Placebo	Asystole/PEA, VF
Gueugniaud [20]	2008	RCT/2887	Vasopressin 40 IU (2 doses) + Epinephrine 1 mg	Epinephrine 1 mg + Placebo	Asystole/PEA, VF
Mukoyama [22]	2009	RCT/336	Vasopressin 40 IU (4 doses)	Epinephrine 1 mg	Asystole/PEA, VF
Ducros [19]	2010	RCT/44	Vasopressin 40 IU (3 doses) + Epinephrine 1 mg +/− nitroglycerin 300 μg	Epinephrine 1 mg + Placebos	Asystole/PEA, VF
Ong [23]	2012	RCT/727	Vasopressin 40 IU (single dose)	Epinephrine 1 mg	Asystole/PEA, VF/VT

RCT: randomized clinical trial; PEA: pulseless electrical activity; VF: ventricular fibrillation; VT: ventricular tachycardia.

We analyzed 7 RCTs including 5,525 patients with OHCA [18–24]. Table 2 shows the characteristics of the included studies. We found no difference in survival to hospital discharge comparing vasopressin plus epinephrine vs epinephrine alone (RR 1.032, 85% CI 0.785–1.404, $I^2 = 15\%$, $p = 0.317$), even when vasopressin was administered in pre-hospital settings or in the emergency room (pre-hospital: RR 1.009, 95% CI 0.443–2.298, $I^2 = 49\%$, $p = 0.118$; emergency room: RR 1.071, 95% CI 0.787–1.456, $I^2 = 49\%$, $p = 0.692$) (Fig. 2). There was no difference in rate of good neurologic outcome when comparing vasopressin plus epinephrine vs epinephrine alone (RR 0.815, 95% CI 0.566–1.175, $I^2 = 0\%$, $p = 0.624$). Vasopressin had no beneficial effect on survival to hospital discharge (RR 1.042, 95% CI 0.726–1.496, $I^2 = 28\%$, $p = 0.222$) (Fig. 3) or rate of good neurologic outcome (RR 0.811, 95% CI 0.559–1.176, $I^2 = \%$, $p = 0.482$) when it was administered more than 10 minutes after OHCA.

A. Studies	Estimate (95% CI)		Vasopressin	Control
Lindner 1997 [21]	2.667	(0.825, 8.620)	8/20	3/20
Wenzel 2004 [24]	1.000	(0.707, 1.415)	57/578	58/588
Callaway 2006 [18]	1.183	(0.323, 4.325)	5/167	4/158
Gueugniaud 2008 [20]	0.732	(0.435, 1.232)	24/1439	33/1448
Mukoyama 2009 [22]	1.479	(0.550, 3.978)	10/178	6/158
Ducros 2010 [19]	0.117	(0.006, 2.301)	0/28	2/16
Ong 2012 [23]	1.298	(0.528, 2.189)	11/374	8/353
Overall ($I^2 = 15\%$, $p = 0.317$)	**1.032**	**(0.758, 1.404)**	**115/2784**	**114/2741**

$Tau^2 = 0.027$; $Q\ (df = 6) = 7.042$; $I^2 = 15\%$; $p = 0.842$

B. Studies: Pre-hospital	Estimate (95% CI)		Vasopressin	Control
Lindner 1997 [21]	2.667	(0.825, 8.620)	8/20	3/20
Callaway 2006 [18]	1.183	(0.323, 4.325)	5/167	4/158
Gueugniaud 2008 [20]	0.732	(0.435, 1.232)	24/1439	33/1448
Ducros 2010 [19]	0.117	(0.006, 2.301)	0/28	2/16
Overall ($I^2 = 49\%$, $p = 0.118$)	**1.009**	**(0.443, 2.298)**	**37/1654**	**42/1642**

$Tau^2 = 0.326$; $Q\ (df = 3) = 5.869$; $I^2 = 49\%$; $p = 0.938$

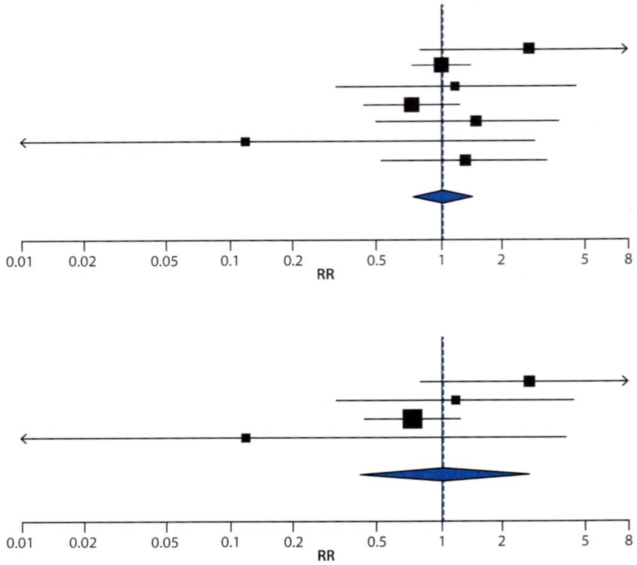

Fig. 2 Vasopressin administration during cardiopulmonary resuscitation (CPR) for out-of-hospital cardiac arrest (OHCA). *A*: Forest plot showing risk ratio (*RR*) of survival to hospital discharge. Weights: Lindner: 6.4%; Wenzel: 42.6%; Callaway: 5.3%; Gueugniaud: 25.4%; Mukoyama: 8.8%; Ducros: 1%; Ong: 10.4%. *B*: Forest plot showing RR of survival to hospital discharge including studies with pre-hospital administration of vasopressin. Weights: Lindner: 25.7; Callaway: 23%; Gueugniaud: 44.5%; Ducros: 7%. *C*: Forest plot showing RR of survival to hospital discharge including studies with emergency room administration of vasopressin. Weights: Wenzel: 78.6%; Mukoyama: 9.7%; Ong: 11.7%

C. Studies:

Emergency room	Estimate (95% CI)		Vasopressin	Control
Wenzel 2004 [24]	1.000	(0.707, 1.415)	57/578	58/588
Mukoyama 2009 [22]	1.479	(0.550, 3.978)	10/178	6/158
Ong 2012 [23]	1.298	(0.528, 2.189)	11/374	8/353
Overall ($I^2 = 0\%$, $p = 0.692$)	**1.071**	**(0.787, 1.456)**	**78/1130**	**72/1099**

$Tau^2 = 0.000$; $Q\ (df = 2) = 7.763$; $I^2 = 0\%$; $p = 0.664$

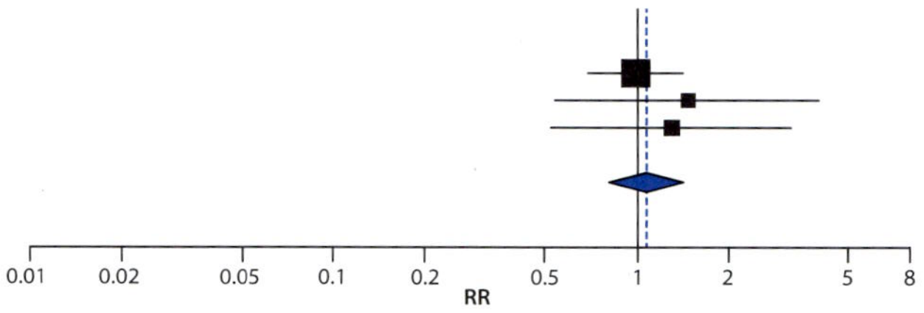

Fig. 2 (Continuation)

Studies:
Vasopressin administration
> 10 minute

	Estimate (95% CI)		Vasopressin	Control
Lindner 1997 [21]	2.667	(0.825, 8.620)	8/20	3/20
Wenzel 2004 [24]	1.000	(0.707, 1.415)	57/578	58/588
Gueugniaud 2008 [20]	0.732	(0.435, 1.232)	24/1439	33/1448
Mukoyama 2009 [22]	1.479	(0.550, 3.978)	10/178	6/158
Ducros 2010 [19]	0.117	(0.006, 2.301)	0/28	2/16
Ong 2012 [23]	1.298	(0.528, 2.189)	11/374	8/353
Overall (I^2 = 28%, p = 0.222)	**1.042**	**(0.756, 1.496)**	**110/2617**	**110/2583**

Tau² = 0.055; Q (df = 5) = 6.982; I^2 = 28%; p = 0.822

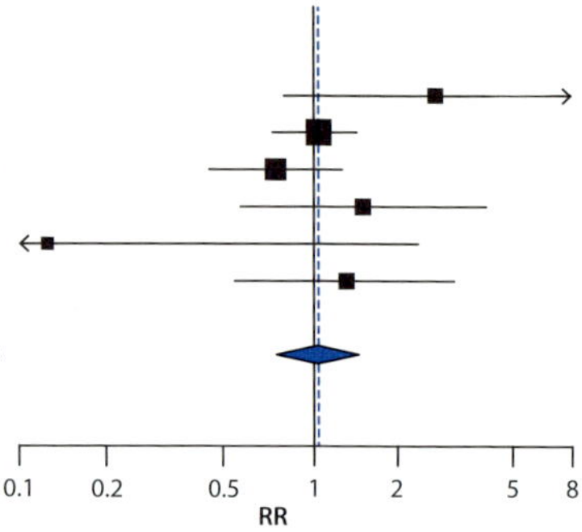

Fig. 3 Vasopressin administration during 10 minutes for out-of-hospital cardiac arrest (OHCA). Forest plot showing risk ratio (*RR*) of survival to hospital discharge including studies with vasopressin administered more than 10 minutes after OHCA. Weights: Lindner: 8.2%, Wenzel 39.4%, Gueugniaud 27.1%, Mukoyama 11%, Ducros 1.5%, Ong 12.8%

Hence, we found that after OHCA:

1) single or repeated doses of vasopressin plus epinephrine vs. epinephrine alone did not improve survival to hospital discharge, even if they were administered in the pre-hospital setting or emergency room;
2) when single or repeated doses of vasopressin plus epinephrine were administered more than 10 minutes after OHCA they did not improve survival to hospital discharge.

This is the first meta-analysis reporting the results in studies divided according to pre-hospital setting or emergency room administration of vasopressin and of studies administering vasopressin more than 10 minutes after OHCA. Wyer et al. summarized the results of a meta-analysis and 3 RCTs on vasopressin vs. epinephrine, and found no reduction in mortality at hospital discharge or improvement in neurologic outcome [25]. A recent meta-analysis also did not find any beneficial effect in terms of short- and long-terms outcome of vasopressin compared with epinephrine [26]. Indeed none of the included RCTs reported a statistical significance in survival to hospital discharge in the vasopressin group over epinephrine [18–24]. Timing of drug administration may have a significant effect on the impact of vasopressin and epinephrine use. Layek et al., choosing 10 min as a cut-off point of delay in vasopressin administration, showed a better survival to hospital discharge when vasopressin was administered in less than 10 minutes. However, the authors combined RCTs with in-hospital and out-of-hospital cardiac arrest. Furthermore, they did not find any beneficial effects on hospital discharge or good neurologic outcome when vasopressin was administered after more than 10 minutes [26]. We found only one RCT [18] using vasopressin within 10 minutes of OHCA with a RR 1.183 (95% CI 0.323–4.323), but no increase in survival at hospital discharge when vasopressin was used after 10 minutes. We believe that, as supported by the majority of RCTs [19–24], the administration of vasopressin more than 10 minutes after OHCA may be reasonable in the pre-hospital setting of cardiac arrest. By contrast, OHCA patients may be difficult to reach within 10 minutes. Current guidelines on cardiac arrest state that the effects of vasopressin do not differ from those of epinephrine in cardiac arrest, but one dose of vasopressin 40 IU may replace either the first or second dose of epinephrine in the treatment of cardiac arrest (Class IIb, level of evidence A) [2]. We believe that further studies are needed to evaluate the right dose and timing of vasopressin for OHCA.

Effects of Pre-hospital Hypothermia on Hospital Survival After OHCA

The impact of the timing of induced hypothermia after cardiac arrest is not yet understood [2]. Animal studies showed beneficial effects when hypothermia was induced in less than 10 or 20 minutes, but this effect disappeared when hypothermia was delayed [2]. Therefore, the induction of hypothermia in pre-hospital settings for OHCA may be useful to improve short- and long-term outcomes.

We analyzed 6 RCTs including 2,118 patients with OHCA [27–32] (Table 3). At hospital admission, the group treated with pre-hospital hypothermia had a temperature $<35\,°C$, ranging from 34.1 to 34.7 °C, whereas the control group had a temperature $>35\,°C$, ranging from 35.1 to 35.7 °C [27–32]. Pre-hospital hypothermia was obtained with infusion of cold solution in 5 studies and with transnasal evaporative cooling in 1 study [27–32]. We found no difference in survival to hospital discharge when pre-hospital hypothermia was compared with the control (RR 1.002, 95% CI 0.894–1.124, $I^2=0\%$, $p=0.810$) (Fig. 4). We found no improvement in survival to hospital discharge even if pre-hospital hypothermia followed by no in-hospital cooling (P+/I-) was compared with no pre-hospital or in-hospital hypothermia (P-/I-) (RR 1.077, 95% CI 0.703–1.650, $I^2=0\%$, $p=0.677$), and if pre-hospital hypothermia and in-hospital cooling (P+/I+) was compared with no pre-hospital hypothermia and in-hospital cooling (P-/I+) (RR 0.997, 95% CI 0.886–1.122, $I^2=0\%$, $p=0.575$). There was also no improvement in the rate of good neurologic outcome when comparing pre-hospital hypothermia with control (RR 0.959, 95% CI 0.830–1.108, $I^2=0\%$, $p=0.745$).

Hence, we found that after OHCA:

1) pre-hospital hypothermia did not improve survival or incidence of good neurologic outcome at hospital discharge;
2) pre-hospital hypothermia without in-hospital cooling did not increase hospital survival compared with no pre-hospital hypothermia and no in-hospital cooling; and
3) pre-hospital hypothermia and in-hospital cooling did not improve survival at hospital discharge compared with no pre-hospital hypothermia and in-hospital cooling.

This is the first meta-analysis reporting the results from RCTs about pre-hospital hypothermia alone and with in-hospital cooling compared with a control group without pre-hospital hypothermia associated or not with in-hospital cooling. Current guidelines on cardiac arrest recommended the use of hypothermia between 32–

Table 3 Study characteristics of included trials for effect of pre-hospital hypothermia on hospital survival after out-of-hospital cardiac arrest (OHCA)

First Author	Year	Study design/ Number of patients	Intervention	Control	Initial rhythm of OHCA
Kim [32]	2007	RCT/125	Pre-hospital infusion of 4 °C normal saline, in-hospital standard care and no cooling	Pre-hospital no cooling and in-hospital standard care	Asystole/PEA, VF/VT
Kamarainen [30]	2009	RCT/37	Pre-hospital infusion of 4 °C Ringer's acetate, in-hospital standard care and no cooling	Pre-hospital no cooling and in-hospital standard care	Asystole/PEA, VF/VT
Bernard [27]	2010	RCT/234	Pre-hospital infusion of ice cold Ringer's solution and in-hospital surface cooling	Pre-hospital no cooling and in-hospital surface cooling	VF
Castren [29]	2010	RCT/200	Pre-hospital and in-hospital transnasal evaporative cooling	Pre-hospital no cooling and in-hospital transnasal evaporative cooling	Asystole/PEA, VF/VT
Bernard [28]	2012	RCT/163	Pre-hospital infusion of ice cold Ringer's solution and in-hospital surface cooling	Pre-hospital no cooling and in-hospital surface cooling	Asystole/PEA
Kim [31]	2014	RCT/1359	Pre-hospital infusion 4 °C normal saline and in-hospital cooling	Pre-hospital no cooling and in-hospital cooling	Asystole/PEA, VF/VT

RCT: randomized clinical trial; PEA: pulseless electrical activity; VF: ventricular fibrillation; VT: ventricular tachycardia.

34 °C after ventricular fibrillation (VF) OHCA (Class I, level of evidence B) [2]. Furthermore, hypothermia may also be considered for OHCA with initial asystole or pulseless electric activity (PEA) (Class IIb, level of evidence A) [2].

Diao et al. reported no benefit of pre-hospital hypothermia even in a subgroup of patients with VF [33]. Interestingly, none of the included studies reported a clear improvement in short- or long-term outcomes using pre-hospital cooling [27–32]. It is likely that we did not find any beneficial effects of pre-hospital hypothermia because the temperature of the interventional and control groups at hospital arrival or in the emergency room was not sufficiently different. Indeed, the temperature difference was only about 1 °C in each study [27–32]. However, the quality of the RCTs was generally good with a low risk of bias, even if only Kim et al. included a

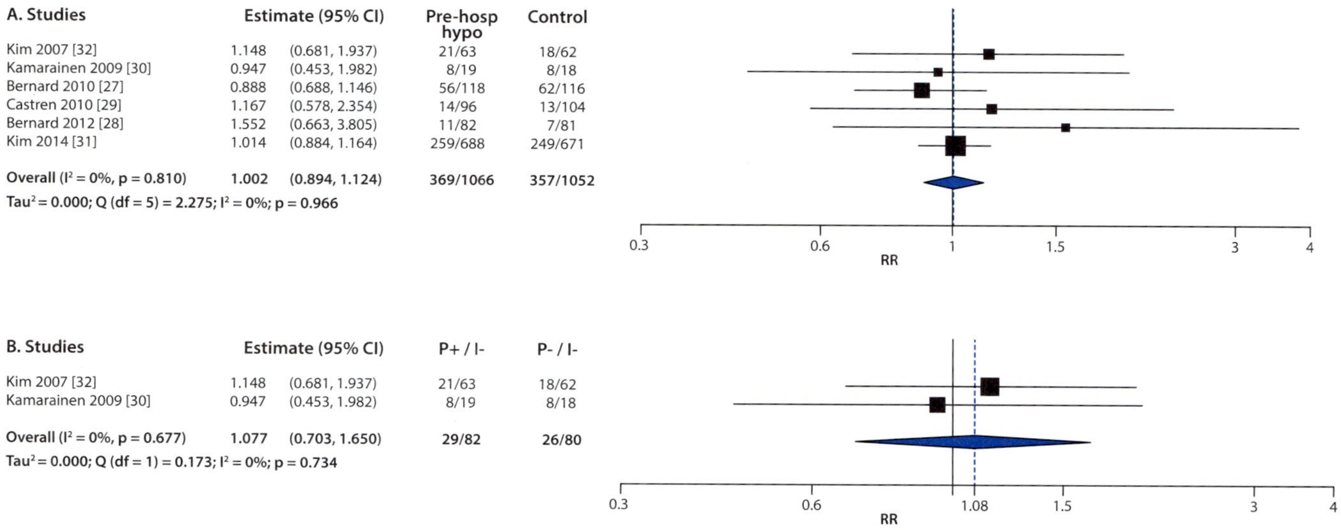

Fig. 4 Pre-hospital hypothermia for out-of-hospital cardiac arrest (OHCA). *A*: Forest plot showing risk ratio (RR) of survival to hospital discharge. Weights: Kim: 4.7%; Kamarainen: 2.4%; Bernard: 20%; Castren: 2.6%; Bernard: 1.6%; Kim: 68.5%. *B*: Forest plot showing RR of survival to hospital discharge including studies evaluating pre-hospital hypothermia (P+) and in-hospital no cooling (I-) versus no pre-hospital hypothermia (P-) and in-hospital no cooling (I-). Weights: Kim: 66.6%; Kamarainen: 33.4%. *C*: Forest plot showing RR of survival to hospital discharge including studies evaluating pre-hospital hypothermia (P+) and in-hospital cooling (I+) versus no pre-hospital hypothermia (P-) and in-hospital cooling (I+). Weights: Bernard: 21.5%; Castren: 2.8%; Bernard: 1.7%; Kim: 73.8%

C. Studies	Estimate (95% CI)		P+ / I+	P- / I+
Bernard 2010 [27]	0.888	(0.688, 1.146)	56/118	62/116
Castren 2010 [29]	1.167	(0.578, 2.354)	14/96	13/104
Bernard 2012 [28]	1.552	(0.663, 3.805)	11/82	7/81
Kim 2014 [31]	1.014	(0.884, 1.164)	259/688	249/671
Overall ($I^2 = 0\%$, $p = 0.575$)	**0.997**	**(0.886, 1.122)**	**340/984**	**331/972**

$Tau^2 = 0.000$; Q (df = 3) = 1.985; $I^2 = 0\%$; $p = 0.960$

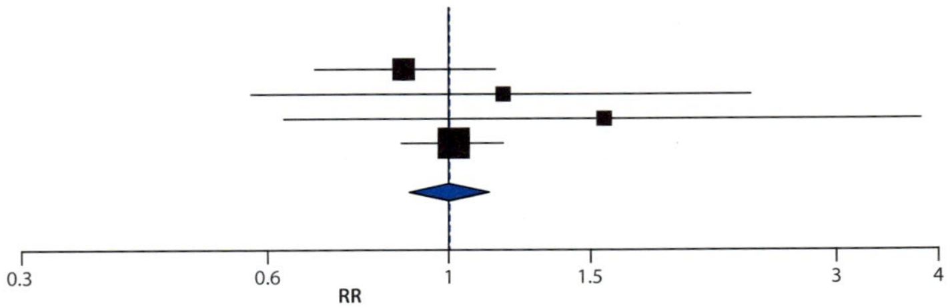

Fig. 4 (Continuation)

large number of patients (1,359 patients) [31]. The timing of cooling was different between the RCTs. In the study by Castren et al. [29], pre-hospital hypothermia was started within 20 minutes from OHCA while in the other RCTs it was started as soon as possible following ROSC [27, 28, 30–32]. However, Castren et al. did not find significant improvements in survival and neurological outcome despite starting cooling earlier than in the other studies [29]. RCTs and meta-analyses do not support routine use of pre-hospital hypothermia to improve clinical outcome. Furthermore, rapid infusion of cold fluid may increase clinical instability and make management more difficult during transport of OHCA patients [31]. We believe that future studies on this topic should at least have a more efficient cooling protocol with increased difference in temperature between interventional and control groups and standardized timing of cooling.

Effects of In-hospital Hypothermia on Hospital Survival After OHCA

Two pivotal trials published in 2002 reported a favorable neurologic outcome and reduced mortality in patients treated with mild hypothermia [34, 35]. In these studies, mild therapeutic hypothermia was set at about 33 °C with the control at above 36 °C [34, 35]. The latest guidelines on resuscitation after cardiac arrest recommend cooling to between 32 to 34 °C for adult patients with ROSC after OHCA of any rhythm [2]. Recently, the target temperature management (TTM) trial showed that hypothermia at a targeted temperature of 33 °C was not associated with a beneficial effect on survival and neurologic outcomes compared with a targeted temperature of 36 °C [36].

We analyzed 5 RCTs including 1,363 patients with OHCA [34–38] (Table 4). In the in-hospital hypothermia group, the target temperature was set at <34 °C while in the control group it was >36 °C [34–38]. The duration of cooling ranged from 8 to 28 hours [34–38]. There was no beneficial effect on survival to hospital discharge when comparing in-hospital hypothermia with a control group (RR 1.024, 95% CI 0.832–1.261, $I^2=47\%$, $p=0.111$) (Fig. 5). Furthermore, when comparing studies in which the hypothermia was set at 33 °C and the control at ≥ 36 °C we were not able to find any improvement in considered outcomes (RR 0.972, 95% CI 0.712–1.327, $I^2=81\%$, $p=0.005$). There was no significant improvement in rate of good neurologic outcome when comparing in-hospital hypothermia vs control (RR 0.788, 95% CI 0.556–1.116, $I^2=70\%$, $p=0.018$) and T. 33 °C vs $T \geq 36$ °C (RR 1.249, 95% CI 0.877–1.780, $I^2=78\%$, $p=0.010$).

Hence, we found that after OHCA:

1) in-hospital therapeutic hypothermia did not improve survival at hospital discharge; and
2) even comparing a targeted temperature of 33 °C with a temperature ≥ 36 °C, we did not find any beneficial effect on survival. Similar results were found for rates of good neurologic outcome.

This is the first meta-analysis to include the TTM trial and to compare data from a targeted group at 33 °C vs. a targeted group ≥ 36 °C. The possible beneficial effects

Table 4 Study characteristics of included trials for effect of in-hospital hypothermia on hospital survival after out-of-hospital cardiac arrest (OHCA)

First Author	Year	Study design/Number of patients	Intervention	Control	Initial rhythm of OHCA
Hachimi-Idrissi [37]	2001	RCT/32	In-hospital cooling with helmet device, T 34 °C	No cooling	Asystole/PEA
Bernard [34]	2002	RCT/77	In-hospital cooling with ice pack, T 33 °C	No cooling, controlled T 36 °C	VF
Holzer [35]	2002	RCT/275	In-hospital external cooling device, T 33 °C	No cooling, controlled T 36 °C	VF/VT
Laurent [38]	2005	RCT/42	In-hospital cooling with hemofiltration, T 32 °C	No cooling, controlled T 37 °C	Asystole, VF/VT
Nielsen [36]	2013	RCT/937	In-hospital surface and intravascular cooling, T 33 °C	No cooling, controlled T 36 °C	Asystole/PEA, VF/VT

RCT: randomized clinical trial; T: temperature; PEA: pulseless electrical activity; VF: ventricular fibrillation; VT: ventricular tachycardia.

of in-hospital therapeutic hypothermia on survival were investigated in two previous meta-analyses by the Cochrane library [39, 40]. Surprisingly these meta-analyses, using a fixed effect model, concluded that mild therapeutic in-hospital hypothermia seemed to improve survival and neurologic outcome after OHCA, supporting the best medical practice of the International Resuscitation Guidelines. Accordingly, current guidelines also suggest the use of hypothermia after OHCA (Class I, level of evidence B, Class IIb level of evidence B) [2]. Our meta-analysis, using a random effect model, was not able to confirm the data reported by the Cochrane group [39] concerning survival to hospital discharge. Furthermore, our meta-analysis, including the TTM trial with a large sample size and 90% power to detect possible beneficial effects of outcome, had a lower risk of bias compared with previously published Cochrane meta-analyses that also included abstracts in the analysis. Our results, showing no beneficial effect of in-hospital therapeutic hypothermia on hospital survival, were in line with those reported by the TTM trial. In the TTM trial, the temperature in the two groups was targeted at different levels (33 °C vs 36 °C), so there was also a close control of fever [36]. In the study by Bernard et al. [34] the temperature of the control group was targeted at 37 °C, whereas in the other studies it was not controlled [35, 37, 38]. The duration of cooling and the type of cooling were also different between the studies. The duration of cooling varied from 8 to 28 hours and the type of cooling was external, internal or both [27, 34–38]. Accordingly, we found a moderate heterogeneity in our results ($I^2 = 47\%$ and $I^2 = 81\%$, Fig. 5). In-hospital therapeutic hypothermia is still debated and higher quality research investigating the effect of lower and higher controlled temperature is needed to establish best medical practice.

A. Studies	Estimate	(95% CI)	Hypothermia	Control
Hachimi 2001 [37]	1.000	(0.236, 4.231)	3/16	3/16
Bernard 2002 [34]	0.662	(0.373, 1.176)	11/34	21/43
Holzer 2002 [35]	1.289	(1.043, 1.592)	87/137	68/138
Laurent 2005 [38]	0.808	(0.387, 1.685)	8/22	9/20
Nielsen 2013 [36]	0.988	(0.883, 1.106)	265/473	263/464
Overall ($I^2 = 47\%$, $p = 0.111$)	**1.024**	**(0.832, 1.261)**	**374/682**	**364/681**

$Tau^2 = 0.021$; $Q (df = 4) = 7.512$; $I^2 = 47\%$; $p = 0.823$

B. Studies	Estimate	(95% CI)	T. 33°C	T. 36°C
Bernard 2002 [34]	0.524	(0.301, 0.911)	11/34	21/34
Holzer 2002 [35]	1.289	(1.043, 1.592)	87/137	68/138
Nielsen 2013 [36]	0.993	(0.887, 1.111)	265/473	263/466
Overall ($I^2 = 81\%$, $p = 0.005$)	**0.972**	**(0.712, 1.327)**	**363/644**	**352/638**

$Tau^2 = 0.055$; $Q (df = 2) = 10.456$; $I^2 = 81\%$; $p = 0.859$

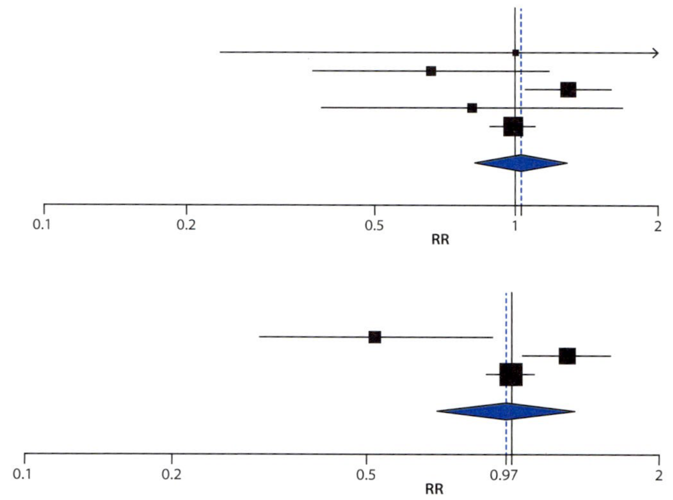

Fig. 5 In-hospital hypothermia for out-of-hospital cardiac arrest (OHCA). *A*: Forest plot showing risk ratio (RR) of survival to hospital discharge. Weights: Hachimi: 2%; Bernard: 10.5%; Holzer: 34.4%; Laurent: 7%; Nielsen: 46.1%. *B*: Forest plot showing risk ratio of survival to hospital discharge for studies evaluating temperature of 33 °C (T. 33 °C) versus temperature of 36 °C (T. 36 °C) after the cooling period. Weights: Bernard: 18.7%; Holzer: 37.9%; Nielsen: 43.3%

Effects of PaO_2 on Survival to Hospital Discharge

In post-cardiac arrest after ROSC, controlling PaO_2 and $PaCO_2$ levels has significant effects on cerebrovascular regulation. Hypoxia leads to anoxic brain injury. On the other hand, regarding systemic ischemic-reperfusion syndrome, hyperoxia may have detrimental effects on the brain and other vital organs via several mechanisms: 1) increase in reactive oxygen species, which associates with ischemic-reperfusion injury; 2) increase in lipid peroxidation of neuronal cells causing mitochondrial injury; 3) increase in cellular injury and apoptosis; and 4) promotion of cerebral vasoconstriction [41]. In experimental models, 100% oxygen administration was associated with worse neurological outcome [42] compared with lower oxygen concentrations. From recent observational studies, even though hypoxia was definitely associated with in-hospital mortality, there were conflicting results about the possible association of hyperoxia and mortality [43, 44].

We identified 8 observational studies in adults investigating the effect of PaO_2 level on survival at hospital discharge [43–50]. We categorized oxygenation as follows: PaO_2 of ≥ 300 mmHg as hyperoxia, $PaO_2 < 60$ mmHg as hypoxia and PaO_2 60–300 mmHg as normoxia. Four studies were excluded because there was no outcome of interest evaluated. Overall, we analyzed 4 studies including 23,482 patients [43–46]. The characteristics of the studies included in our meta-analysis are shown

Table 5 Study characteristics of included studies for effect of oxygen tension after out-of-hospital cardiac arrest (OHCA)

First Author	Year	Study design/number of patients	Timing of PaO_2 measurement	Cut off value of PaO_2 Hyperoxia/Hypoxia/ Normoxia	Initial rhythm of OHCA
Kilgannon [44]	2010	Cohort/6326	First ABG	≥ 300 mmHg/< 60 mmHg or PaO_2/FiO_2ratio < 300/PaO_2 60–300 mmHg	Non-traumatic cardiac arrest
Kilgannon [43]	2011	Cohort/4464	Highest PaO_2 over the 1st 24 hours in the ICU	≥ 300 mmHg	Non-traumatic cardiac arrest
Bellomo [45]	2011	Cohort/12108	Lowest PaO_2 with highest A-a gradient over the 1st 24 hours	≥ 300 mmHg/< 60 mmHg, or PaO_2/FiO_2ratio < 300/≥ 60 to 300 mmHg	Non-traumatic cardiac arrest
Ihle [46]	2013	Retrospective analysis of prospective cohort/581	The worst PaO_2 level in the first 24 hours of ICU stay	≥ 300 mmHg/< 60 mmHg/ 60–299 mmHg	VF

ABG: arterial blood gas; VF: ventricular fibrillation.

A. Studies	Estimate (95% CI)		Hypoxia	Normoxia
Kilgannon 2010 [44]	0.780	(0.732, 0.831)	1702/3999	639/1171
Bellomo 2011 [45]	0.770	(0.733, 0.809)	3601/8904	1008/1919
Ihle 2013 [46]	0.808	(0.612, 1.068)	27/55	300/494
Overall ($I^2 = 0\%$, $p = 0.908$)	**0.774**	**(0.745, 0.805)**	**5330/12958**	**1947/3584**

$Tau^2 = 0.000$; Q (df = 2) = 0.193; $I^2 = 0\%$; $p < 0.001$

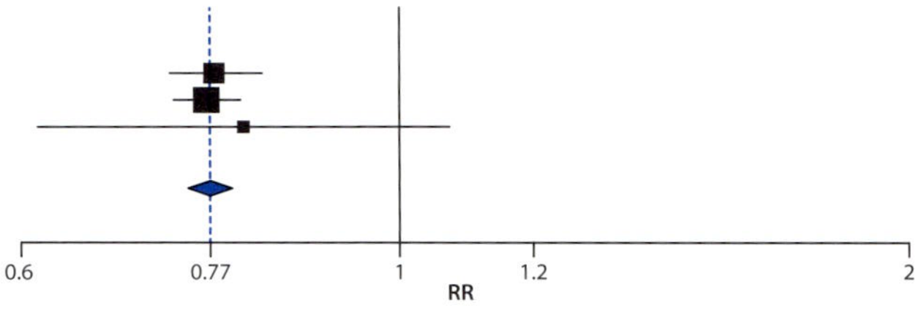

B. Studies	Estimate (95% CI)		Hyperoxia	Normoxia
Kilgannon 2010 [44]	0.672	(0.613, 0.737)	424/1156	639/1171
Bellomo 2011 [45]	0.787	(0.728, 0.850)	531/1285	1008/1919
Kilgannon 2011 [43]	0.687	(0.635, 0.745)	510/1525	1430/2939
Ihle 2013 [46]	0.894	(0.654, 1.221)	19/35	300/494
Overall ($I^2 = 71\%$, $p = 0.017$)	**0.727**	**(0.660, 0.802)**	**1484/4001**	**3377/6523**

$Tau^2 = 0.006$; Q (df = 3) = 10.248; $I^2 = 71\%$; $p < 0.001$

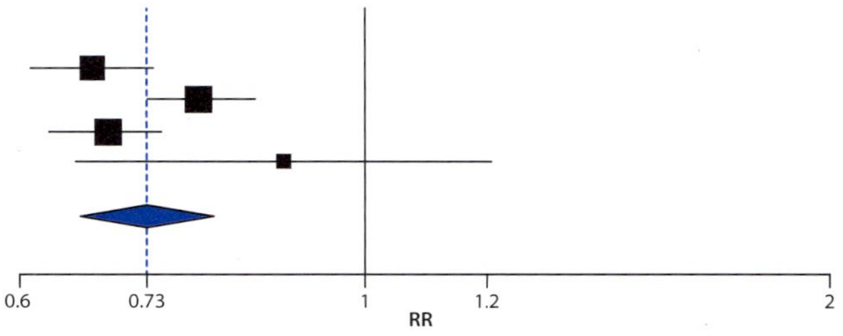

Fig. 6 Different levels of oxygenation for cardiac arrest. *A*: Forest plot showing risk ratio (RR) of survival to hospital discharge comparing hypoxia vs normoxia. Weights: Kilgannon: 37%; Bellomo: 61%; Ihle: 2%. *B*: Forest plot showing RR of survival to hospital discharge comparing hyperoxia vs normoxia. Weights: Kilgannon: 29.3%; Bellomo: 31.6%; Kilgannon: 31.3%; Ihle: 7.8%

in Table 5. Normoxia was associated with a decrease in survival to hospital discharge compared with hyperoxia and hypoxia (RR 0.727, 95% CI 0.660–0.802, $I^2 = 71\%$, $p = 0.017$; RR 0.774, 95% CI 0.745–0.805, $I^2 = 0\%$, $p = 0.908$, respectively) (Fig. 6).

The main aims of post-resuscitation care are to avoid post-anoxic brain injury and post-cardiac arrest syndrome in order to decrease mortality. In an observational study by Kilgannon et al. at least 1/5 of post-cardiac arrest patients were exposed to hyperoxia [44]. In our meta-analysis, we found that normoxia was associated with a decrease in survival to hospital discharge compared with hypoxia and hyperoxia. The results of our meta-analysis are in line with the recent meta-analysis reported by Wang et al. who found that hyperoxia was associated with an increase in in-hospital mortality (OR, 1.40; 95% CI, 1.02–1.93; $I^2 = 69.27\%$) [51]. Therapeutic hypothermia may mitigate hyperoxia-induced injury by providing some protective effects to the brain from reactive oxygen species. Therapeutic hypothermia is not applied as standard therapy in some countries. Only two studies by Janz et al. and Lee et al. [47, 48], not included in this meta-analysis, demonstrated the impact of therapeutic hypothermia on the influence of oxygen exposure. Janz et al. found that in patients treated with therapeutic hypothermia, survivors had a significantly lower maximum PaO_2 (198 mmHg) in the first 24 hours than non-survivors (254 mmHg; $p = 0.022$) [47]. On the other hand, a recent retrospective single-center study measuring the mean PaO_2 in patients treated with mild therapeutic hypothermia demonstrated that mean PaO_2 during therapeutic hypothermia was not associated with in-hospital mortality [48]. Nevertheless, in this study, 97% of PaO_2 values were within the 60–300 mmHg range according to the protocol, which tried to achieve the PaO_2 of 100 mmHg. Due to the limited number of studies, we were not able to create subgroups according to the site of cardiac arrest (out-of-hospital or in-hospital cardiac arrest) or to the initial cardiac rhythm prior to cardiac arrest (VF, PEA or asystole).

In summary, since recent evidence suggests that not only hypoxia but also hyperoxia are associated with mortality and worse neurological performance, physicians should focus their attention on how to monitor oxygenation to keep the PaO_2 at appropriate levels. From recent data, current guidelines recommend achieving an oxygen saturation (SaO_2) 94–96% or 98% (Class I, level of evidence C) [2]. However, pulse oximetry is less sensitive than arterial blood gas analysis due to poor peripheral perfusion during the resuscitation period. Rapidly obtaining an arterial blood gas would help the clinician titrate oxygen supply to safe levels. Because the effects of hyperoxia on mortality are dose-dependent, prospective studies are warranted to determine the appropriate level of optimal PaO_2 [43].

Effects of $PaCO_2$ on Survival to Hospital Discharge

$PaCO_2$ plays an important role in regulating cerebral blood flow. Hypocarbia causes cerebral vasoconstriction, decreased cerebral blood flow with decreased cerebral perfusion and oxygenation, and potentiates anoxic brain injury. On the other hand, hypercapnia may decrease cerebrovascular resistance, and may provide benefit in patients with ischemic brain injury. Mild hypercapnia may improve cerebral perfusion, has an anticonvulsive effect and decreases inflammation as well as oxidative stress. However, severe hypercapnia may worsen neurological performance and affect outcomes because of too much cerebral vasodilatation, increased intracranial blood volume and pressure. The incidence of hypo/hypercarbia is not uncommon and has been observed as unexpectedly high (45%) in OHCA patients treated with mild therapeutic hypothermia regardless of the method of arterial blood gas analysis [52]. Since there is only one observational study that has reported the association between $PaCO_2$ level and survival to hospital discharge [50], we were not able to perform a meta-analysis. In a multicenter cohort study from the ANZICS-APD database in non-traumatic cardiac arrest patients, normocapnia was associated with a decrease in survival to hospital discharge compared with hypocapnia ($PaCO_2 < 35$ mmHg) and hypercapnia ($PaCO_2 > 45$ mmHg) (RR 0.840. 95% CI 0.800–0.880; RR 0.870, 95% CI 0.840–0.910, respectively). Surprisingly, among survivors, the hypercapnia group had a higher rate of discharge home [50]. In line with a recent study by Lee et al. in therapeutic hypothermia patients, hypocarbia was associated with an increase in in-hospital mortality (odds ratio 2.52 95% CI 1.18–5.37) [48]. The mean $PaCO_2$ in survivors was higher than in non-survivors (39 mmHg vs. 37.6 mmHg) [48]. Roberts et al. reported that hypocapnia and hypercapnia exposure during the first 24 hours after ROSC were independent predictors of poor neurological outcome (CPC score ≥ 3) [53]. Hypocapnia ($PaO_2 < 30$ mmHg) and hypercapnia ($PaO_2 > 50$ mmHg were independently associated with worse neurological outcome [41, 53]. Karnatovskaia et al. demonstrated that therapeutic hypothermia compared with standard treatment without therapeutic hypothermia may decrease mechanical ventilator duration and CPC score on discharge with no significant effects on respiratory mechanics [54].

Different methods of $PaCO_2$ measurement were used in the RCTs supporting the evidence that mild therapeutic hypothermia may improve survival and neurological improvement [34, 35]. There are two methods that have been proposed to measure the gas-exchange associated with temperature namely α-stat (non-corrected to body temperature) and pH-stat (corrected to body temperature). In the α-stat method, clinicians set mechanical ventilation to achieve the targeted $PaCO_2$ according to $PaCO_2$ measured at 37 °C not the patient's actual temperature. On the other hand, with the pH-stat method, mechanical ventilation is titrated to achieve the $PaCO_2$ measured at the patient's actual temperature. Despite reduced metabolism during therapeutic hypothermia and increased CO_2 solubility, the $PaCO_2$ level is decreased during therapeutic hypothermia. The pH-stat method reported relatively greater hypoventilation than the α-stat method. In a prospective observational crossover study in OHCA patients with therapeutic hypothermia, Voicu et al. adjusted the $PaCO_2$ using an α-stat strategy vs a pH-stat strategy. The α-stat strategy group showed an increase in internal jugular vein oxygen desaturation and cerebral oxygen extraction compared with the pH-stat strategy group [55]. Among survivors, patients with $PaCO_2$ adjusted by the α-stat strategy method had decreased cerebral blood flow velocities compared to those with the $PaCO_2$ adjusted by the pH-stat strategy [55]. Recent studies have shown that normocapnia has greater beneficial effects than hypocapnia in terms of mortality and both hypocapnia and hypercapnia were associated with worse neurological outcome. Current practice guidelines suggest maintaining normocapnia in the post-resuscitation period with $PaCO_2$ between 40 and 45 mmHg (Class IIb, level of evidence C) [2].

Limitations

This series of systematic reviews and meta-analyses has limitations that need to be addressed. First, we considered only survival to hospital discharge. Second, we evaluated treatments that guidelines for cardiac arrest report are still under debate [56]. Third, we found a heterogeneity > 25% in 5 out of 15 comparisons on survival to hospital discharge. Fourth, the studies on oxygenation and cardiac arrest included both OHCA and in-hospital cardiac arrest patients, so we were not able to consider only OHCA patients for this comparison.

Current Recommendations and Results of Our Series of Systematic Reviews and Meta-Analyses

Guidelines for cardiac arrest published in 2010 suggested a series of treatments to establish ROSC and improve survival and neurologic outcome after cardiac arrest [56]. In the present series of systematic reviews and meta-analyses, we evaluated the effectiveness of six treatments, defined by current guidelines as still debated or promising, to improve survival to hospital discharge. In Fig. 7, we summarize our results regarding the grade and level of evidence for each considered treatment as reported by current guidelines [56].

First, according to current guidelines on adult cardiac arrest [56], it is reasonable to consider administering a 1 mg dose of epinephrine every 3 to 5 minutes (Class IIb, level of evidence A) mainly to increase the incidence of ROSC. In our meta-analysis, we found that low- or high-dose epinephrine during CPR did not improve survival at hospital discharge, even if administered in the pre-hospital setting or emergency room. The use of low-dose epinephrine during CPR did not improve survival at hospital discharge compared with placebo or no drugs. Second, the effects of vasopressin did not differ from those of epinephrine in cardiac arrest, although it is recommended that one dose of vasopressin 40 IU may replace either the first or second dose of epinephrine (Class IIb, level of evidence A) [56]. In our meta-analysis, single or repeated doses of vasopressin 40 IU plus epinephrine vs. epinephrine alone did not improve survival to hospital discharge, even when they were administered in the pre-hospital setting or emergency room. In addition, when single or repeated doses of vasopressin plus epinephrine were administered after 10 minutes of OHCA, they did not improve survival to hospital discharge. Third, current guidelines suggest the use of hypothermia for OHCA in patients with VF (Class I, level of evidence B) and asystole/PEA (Class IIb, level of evidence B). In our meta-analysis, pre-hospital hypothermia did not improve survival at hospital

Level A	• Data from multiple RCTs and meta-analysis including multiple or large population
Level B	• Data from single RCT or non-randomized studies including limited population
Level C	• Consensus opinion, case studies or case series including very limited population
Class I	• Benefit >>> Risk • Should be performed
Class IIa	• Benefit >> Risk • Reasonable to perform
Class IIb	• Benefit ≥ Risk • To consider
Class III	• Risk ≥ benefit • Not helpful or harmful

Level of evidence of treatment suggested by CPR guideline to improve outcomes	Results of this meta-analyses considering treatments suggested by guidelines on survival to hospital discharge
Epinephrine during CPR Class IIb, LOE A	No significant increase of the outcome (7 RCTs, 4712 patients)
Vasopressin during CPR Class IIb LOE A	No significant increase of the outcome (7 RCTs, 5525 patients)
Hypothermia for OHCA and VF patients Class I LOE B	No significant increase of the outcome (6 RCTs, 2118 patients)
Hypothermia after OHCA and asystole or PEA Class IIb LOE B	No significant increase of the outcome (6 RCTs, 1363 patients)
$SaO_2 = 100\%$ correspond to $PaO_2 = 80–500$ mmHg, provide $SaO_2 \geq 94'\%$ Class I LOE C	Normoxia between 60–30 0 mmHg increase the outcome (3 cohort and 1 retrospective studies, 23 482 patients)
- Hyperventilation with hypocapnia Class II LOE C - PaO_2 35–40mmHg or P_{ETCO_2} 35–40mmHG Class IIb LOE C	Normocapnia increase the outcome (RR, 1 cohort study, 9715 patients)

Fig. 7 Summary of the results of this series of systematic reviews and meta-analyses compared to the grade and level of evidence (LOE) from current guidelines on cardiac arrest. On the *left*, we report the grades and the levels of evidence used in the last guidelines on cardiac arrest [56]. On the *right*, we report the grades and the levels of evidence (first column) for each treatment we investigated and the main results (second column) of our meta-analyses. RCT: randomized controlled trial; CPR: cardiorespiratory resuscitation; OHCA: out of hospital cardiac arrest; PEA: pulseless electrical activity; VF: ventricular fibrillation; SaO_2: oxygen saturation; PaO_2: arterial pressure of oxygenation; $PaCO_2$: arterial pressure of carbon dioxide

discharge, even when we analyzed subgroups of patients with or without in-hospital cooling. Furthermore, in-hospital hypothermia had no beneficial effects on survival to hospital discharge even considering a subgroup of studies comparing a targeted temperature of 33 °C with a temperature ≥ 36 °C. Fourth, current guidelines recommend achieving an SaO_2 of 94–96% or 98% (Class I, level of evidence C) [56], because an SaO_2 of 100% corresponds to a PaO_2 between 80–500 mmHg. In our studies, we found that normoxia, defined as PaO_2 between 60–300 mmHg, was associated with an increase in survival to hospital discharge compared with hypoxia and hyperoxia. Fifth, current practice guidelines suggest maintaining normocapnia in the post-resuscitation period with $PaCO_2$ between 40 and 45 mmHg (Class IIb, level of evidence C) [56]. Analyzing the RR from the data of a cohort study, we found that normocapnia decreased survival to hospital discharge compared with hypocapnia ($PaCO_2 < 35$ mmHg) and hypercapnia ($PaCO_2 > 45$ mmHg).

In conclusion, many of the treatments analyzed in this series of systematic reviews and meta-analyses including 45,552 patients showed no beneficial effect on long-term outcome after OHCA; we, therefore, believe that an urgent revision of current guidelines on cardiac arrest care, to include the recent developments in the literature, is needed.

References

1. Schober A, Holzer M, Hochrieser H, Posch M, Schmutz R, Metnitz P (2014) Effect of intensive care after cardiac arrest on patient outcome: a database analysis. Crit Care 18:R84
2. Peberdy MA, Callaway CW, Neumar RW et al (2010) Part 9: post-cardiac arrest care: 2010 American Heart Association Guidelines for Cardiopulmonary Resuscitation and Emergency Cardiovascular Care. Circulation 122:S768–S786
3. Peters JL, Sutton AJ, Jones DR, Abrams KR, Rushton L (2006) Comparison of two methods to detect publication bias in meta-analysis. JAMA 295:676–680
4. Ornato JP (2008) Optimal vasopressor drug therapy during resuscitation. Crit Care 12:123
5. Hagihara A, Hasegawa M, Abe T, Nagata T, Wakata Y, Miyazaki S (2012) Prehospital epinephrine use and survival among patients with out-of-hospital cardiac arrest. JAMA 307:1161–1168
6. Jacobs IG, Finn JC, Jelinek GA, Oxer HF, Thompson PL (2011) Effect of adrenaline on survival in out-of-hospital cardiac arrest: A randomised double-blind placebo-controlled trial. Resuscitation 82:1138–1143
7. Olasveengen TM, Sunde K, Brunborg C, Thowsen J, Steen PA, Wik L (2009) Intravenous drug administration during out-of-hospital cardiac arrest: a randomized trial. JAMA 302:2222–2229
8. Brown CG, Martin DR, Pepe PE et al (1992) A comparison of standard-dose and high-dose epinephrine in cardiac arrest outside the hospital. The Multicenter High-Dose Epinephrine Study Group. N Engl J Med 327:1051–1055
9. Callaham M, Madsen CD, Barton CW, Saunders CE, Pointer J (1992) A randomized clinical trial of high-dose epinephrine and norepinephrine vs standard-dose epinephrine in prehospital cardiac arrest. JAMA 268:2667–2672
10. Gueugniaud PY, Mols P, Goldstein P et al (1998) A comparison of repeated high doses and repeated standard doses of epinephrine for cardiac arrest outside the hospital. European Epinephrine Study Group. N Engl J Med 339:1595–1601
11. Sherman BW, Munger MA, Foulke GE, Rutherford WF, Panacek EA (1997) High-dose versus standard-dose epinephrine treatment of cardiac arrest after failure of standard therapy. Pharmacotherapy 17:242–247
12. Stiell IG, Hebert PC, Weitzman BN et al (1992) High-dose epinephrine in adult cardiac arrest. N Engl J Med 327:1045–1050
13. Lin S, Callaway CW, Shah PS et al (2014) Adrenaline for out-of-hospital cardiac arrest resuscitation: a systematic review and meta-analysis of randomized controlled trials. Resuscitation 85:732–740
14. Patanwala AE, Slack MK, Martin JR, Basken RL, Nolan PE (2014) Effect of epinephrine on survival after cardiac arrest: a systematic review and meta-analysis. Minerva Anestesiol 80:831–843
15. Atiksawedparit P, Rattanasiri S, McEvoy M, Graham CA, Sittichanbuncha Y, Thakkinstian A (2014) Effects of prehospital adrenaline administration on out-of-hospital cardiac arrest outcomes: a systematic review and meta-analysis. Crit Care 18:463
16. Yang G, Xu J, Li T, Ming J, Chen W, Liu L (2010) Role of V1a receptor in AVP-induced restoration of vascular hyporeactivity and its relationship to MLCP-MLC20 phosphorylation pathway. J Surg Res 161:312–320
17. Neumar RW, Otto CW, Link MS et al (2010) Part 8: adult advanced cardiovascular life support: 2010 American Heart Association Guidelines for Cardiopulmonary Resuscitation and Emergency Cardiovascular Care. Circulation 122:S729–S767
18. Callaway CW, Hostler D, Doshi AA et al (2006) Usefulness of vasopressin administered with epinephrine during out-of-hospital cardiac arrest. Am J Cardiol 98:1316–1321
19. Ducros L, Vicaut E, Soleil C et al (2011) Effect of the addition of vasopressin or vasopressin plus nitroglycerin to epinephrine on arterial blood pressure during cardiopulmonary resuscitation in humans. J Emerg Med 41:453–459

20. Gueugniaud PY, David JS, Chanzy E et al (2008) Vasopressin and epinephrine vs. epinephrine alone in cardiopulmonary resuscitation. N Engl J Med 359:21–30
21. Lindner KH, Dirks B, Strohmenger HU, Prengel AW, Lindner IM, Lurie KG (1997) Randomised comparison of epinephrine and vasopressin in patients with out-of-hospital ventricular fibrillation. Lancet 349:535–537
22. Mukoyama T, Kinoshita K, Nagao K, Tanjoh K (2009) Reduced effectiveness of vasopressin in repeated doses for patients undergoing prolonged cardiopulmonary resuscitation. Resuscitation 80:755–761
23. Ong ME, Tiah L, Leong BS et al (2012) A randomised, double-blind, multi-centre trial comparing vasopressin and adrenaline in patients with cardiac arrest presenting to or in the Emergency Department. Resuscitation 83:953–960
24. Wenzel V, Krismer AC, Arntz HR et al (2004) A comparison of vasopressin and epinephrine for out-of-hospital cardiopulmonary resuscitation. N Engl J Med 350:105–113
25. Wyer PC, Perera P, Jin Z et al (2006) Vasopressin or epinephrine for out-of-hospital cardiac arrest. Ann Emerg Med 48:86–97
26. Layek A, Maitra S, Pal S, Bhattacharjee S, Baidya DK (2014) Efficacy of vasopressin during cardio-pulmonary resuscitation in adult patients: a meta-analysis. Resuscitation 85:855–863
27. Bernard SA, Smith K, Cameron P et al (2010) Induction of therapeutic hypothermia by paramedics after resuscitation from out-of-hospital ventricular fibrillation cardiac arrest: a randomized controlled trial. Circulation 122:737–742
28. Bernard SA, Smith K, Cameron P et al (2012) Induction of prehospital therapeutic hypothermia after resuscitation from nonventricular fibrillation cardiac arrest. Crit Care Med 40:747–753
29. Castren M, Nordberg P, Svensson L et al (2010) Intra-arrest transnasal evaporative cooling: a randomized, prehospital, multicenter study (PRINCE: Pre-ROSC IntraNasal Cooling Effectiveness). Circulation 122:729–736
30. Kamarainen A, Virkkunen I, Tenhunen J, Yli-Hankala A, Silfvast T (2009) Prehospital therapeutic hypothermia for comatose survivors of cardiac arrest: a randomized controlled trial. Acta Anaesthesiol Scand 53:900–907
31. Kim F, Nichol G, Maynard C et al (2014) Effect of prehospital induction of mild hypothermia on survival and neurological status among adults with cardiac arrest: a randomized clinical trial. JAMA 311:45–52
32. Kim F, Olsufka M, Longstreth WT Jr et al (2007) Pilot randomized clinical trial of prehospital induction of mild hypothermia in out-of-hospital cardiac arrest patients with a rapid infusion of 4 degrees C normal saline. Circulation 115:3064–3070
33. Diao M, Huang F, Guan J et al (2013) Prehospital therapeutic hypothermia after cardiac arrest: a systematic review and meta-analysis of randomized controlled trials. Resuscitation 84:1021–1028
34. Bernard SA, Gray TW, Buist MD et al (2002) Treatment of comatose survivors of out-of-hospital cardiac arrest with induced hypothermia. N Engl J Med 346:557–563
35. Hypothermia after Cardiac Arrest Study G (2002) Mild therapeutic hypothermia to improve the neurologic outcome after cardiac arrest. N Engl J Med 346:549–556
36. Nielsen N, Wetterslev J, Cronberg T et al (2013) Targeted temperature management at 33 degrees C versus 36 degrees C after cardiac arrest. N Engl J Med 369:2197–2206
37. Hachimi-Idrissi S, Corne L, Ebinger G, Michotte Y, Huyghens L (2001) Mild hypothermia induced by a helmet device: a clinical feasibility study. Resuscitation 51:275–281
38. Laurent I, Adrie C, Vinsonneau C et al (2005) High-volume hemofiltration after out-of-hospital cardiac arrest: a randomized study. J Am Coll Cardiol 46:432–437
39. Arrich J, Holzer M, Havel C, Mullner M, Herkner H (2012) Hypothermia for neuroprotection in adults after cardiopulmonary resuscitation. Cochrane Database Syst Rev 9:CD004128
40. Arrich J, Holzer M, Herkner H, Mullner M (2009) Hypothermia for neuroprotection in adults after cardiopulmonary resuscitation. Cochrane Database Syst Rev CD004128
41. Sutherasan Y, Vargas M, Brunetti I, Pelosi P (2014) Ventilatory targets after cardiac arrest. Minerva Anestesiol (in press)

42. Pilcher J, Weatherall M, Shirtcliffe P, Bellomo R, Young P, Beasley R (2012) The effect of hyperoxia following cardiac arrest – A systematic review and meta-analysis of animal trials. Resuscitation 83:417–422
43. Kilgannon JH, Jones AE, Parrillo JE et al (2011) Relationship between supranormal oxygen tension and outcome after resuscitation from cardiac arrest. Circulation 123:2717–2722
44. Kilgannon JH, Jones AE, Shapiro NI et al (2010) Association between arterial hyperoxia following resuscitation from cardiac arrest and in-hospital mortality. JAMA 303:2165–2171
45. Bellomo R, Bailey M, Eastwood GM et al (2011) Arterial hyperoxia and in-hospital mortality after resuscitation from cardiac arrest. Crit Care 15:R90
46. Ihle JF, Bernard S, Bailey MJ, Pilcher DV, Smith K, Scheinkestel CD (2013) Hyperoxia in the intensive care unit and outcome after out-of-hospital ventricular fibrillation cardiac arrest. Crit Care Resusc 15:186–190
47. Janz DR, Hollenbeck RD, Pollock JS, McPherson JA, Rice TW (2012) Hyperoxia is associated with increased mortality in patients treated with mild therapeutic hypothermia after sudden cardiac arrest. Crit Care Med 40:3135–3139
48. Lee BK, Jeung KW, Lee HY et al (2014) Association between mean arterial blood gas tension and outcome in cardiac arrest patients treated with therapeutic hypothermia. Am J Emerg Med 32:55–60
49. Nelskyla A, Parr MJ, Skrifvars MB (2013) Prevalence and factors correlating with hyperoxia exposure following cardiac arrest – an observational single centre study. Scand J Trauma Resusc Emerg Med 21:35
50. Schneider AG, Eastwood GM, Bellomo R et al (2013) Arterial carbon dioxide tension and outcome in patients admitted to the intensive care unit after cardiac arrest. Resuscitation 84:927–934
51. Wang CH, Chang WT, Huang CH et al (2014) The effect of hyperoxia on survival following adult cardiac arrest: A systematic review and meta-analysis of observational studies. Resuscitation 85:1142–1148
52. Falkenbach P, Kamarainen A, Makela A et al (2009) Incidence of iatrogenic dyscarbia during mild therapeutic hypothermia after successful resuscitation from out-of-hospital cardiac arrest. Resuscitation 80:990–993
53. Roberts BW, Kilgannon JH, Chansky ME, Trzeciak S (2014) Association between initial prescribed minute ventilation and post-resuscitation partial pressure of arterial carbon dioxide in patients with post-cardiac arrest syndrome. Ann Intensive Care 4:9
54. Karnatovskaia LV, Festic E, Freeman WD, Lee AS (2014) Effect of therapeutic hypothermia on gas exchange and respiratory mechanics: a retrospective cohort study. Ther Hypothermia Temp Manag 4:88–95
55. Voicu S, Deye N, Malissin I et al (2014) Influence of alpha-stat and pH-stat blood gas management strategies on cerebral blood flow and oxygenation in patients treated with therapeutic hypothermia after out-of-hospital cardiac arrest: a crossover study. Crit Care Med 42:1849–1861
56. Field JM, Hazinski MF, Sayre MR et al (2010) Part 1: executive summary: 2010 American Heart Association Guidelines for Cardiopulmonary Resuscitation and Emergency Cardiovascular Care. Circulation 122:S640–S656

Cooling Techniques for Targeted Temperature Management Post-cardiac Arrest

C. Vaity, N. Al-Subaie, and M. Cecconi

Introduction

The use of hypothermia for clinical purposes dates back to antiquity. For example, Hippocrates advocated packing wounded patients in snow and ice to reduce hemorrhage [1]. The concept that hypothermia can provide neuroprotection also has roots in the past where it was observed that infants abandoned and exposed to cold often remained viable for prolonged periods. In modern medicine, clinical interest in hypothermia developed in the 1930s and 1940s with case reports of successful resuscitation of drowning victims despite prolonged asphyxia. The first scientific paper on the clinical application of hypothermia in severe head injury patients, was published in 1943 [2]. Clinical trials on hypothermia were first started in the 1960s [3, 4] but they were soon discontinued because of adverse effects and unclear benefits. Very deep hypothermia (30 °C or lower) was used in most of these studies. Renewed interest in hypothermia developed in the 1980s when animal studies demonstrated that there was some benefit when mild hypothermia (32–35 °C) was used.

Severe neurological injury is now a recognized consequence of cardiac arrest following successful resuscitation. In post-cardiac arrest patients who survive to admission to the intensive care unit (ICU) but subsequently die, irreversible brain injury is the most common cause of death [5]. Cerebral damage occurs not only during cardiac arrest but also during the phase of reperfusion due to generation of free radicals and other mediators [6]. Randomized controlled trials (RCTs) using pharmacological interventions, such as thiopental [7], corticosteroids [8], lidoflazine [9] and nimodipine [10], found no benefit in improvement of neurological outcome. Targeted temperature management has been demonstrated in major studies to be a potent neuroprotective measure in post-resuscitation care following cardiac arrest

C. Vaity · N. Al-Subaie · M. Cecconi ✉
Intensive Care Unit, St George's Hospital, London, UK
e-mail: m.cecconi@nhs.net

J.-L. Vincent (ed.), *Annual Update in Intensive Care and Emergency Medicine 2015*,
DOI 10.1007/978-3-319-13761-2_22

[11, 12]. The mechanism by which targeted temperature management works is complex and still not fully understood.

Hyperthermia following cardiac arrest has been shown to be associated with unfavorable neurological outcome. For each degree rise in temperature above 37 °C there was an increased association with severe disability, coma or persistent vegetative state [13]. The mechanism of hyperthermia remains to be defined but several have been proposed, including increased heat production due to increased production of endogenous catecholamines, decreased heat loss or altered distribution of body heat due to vasoconstriction [14]. Loss of thermoregulatory mechanisms is seen in patients with stroke due to lesions in the anterior region of the hypothalamus [15]. One other cause of hyperthermia after cardiopulmonary resuscitation (CPR) can be infection. Infection can be secondary to pulmonary aspiration or gut translocation of bacteria and toxins following global ischemia during and after CPR [16, 17].

The mechanism by which hyperthermia affects the ischemic brain is known from various animal studies. The release of neurotransmitters is increased by hyperthermia and decreased by hypothermia [18]. An additional mechanism is production of oxygen radicals during the reperfusion period. There is a 4- to 5-fold increase in oxygen radicals during the hyperthermic phase [19, 20]. Hyperthermia also influences brain metabolism by adenosine triphosphate (ATP) depletion and by adenylate energy changes in cortical and subcortical regions. These changes in ATP metabolism in combination with metabolic insults are highly correlated with the release of endogenous glutamate and aspartate [21]. Hyperthermia also markedly enhances calpain activation, which is a calcium-sensitive cysteine protease, and spectrin (microtubule-associated protein-2) proteolysis in cortical pyramidal neurons soon after the onset of reperfusion, an effect that becomes marked by 4 and 24 hours, in association with morphological evidence of irreversible neuronal injury [22].

There are several mechanisms by which targeted temperature management may improve neurological outcome when used after reperfusion. Hypothermia reduces the cerebral metabolic rate for oxygen ($CMRO_2$) by 6% for every 1 °C reduction in brain temperature >28 °C. This effect is partly due to reduced normal electrical activity [23]. Targeted temperature management is thought to suppress many of the chemical reactions associated with reperfusion injury. These reactions, as mentioned previously, are associated with hyperthermia and include free radical production, excitatory amino acid release, and calcium shifts, which can in turn lead to mitochondrial damage and apoptosis. Hypothermia attenuates pro-apoptotic signals, such as cytochrome c release, *Fas* and *Bax* up-regulation, and caspase activation and activates anti-apoptotic mechanisms, such as the Erk1/2 pathway and the *Akt* pathway [24]. The expression of p53 is enhanced by hypothermia, promoting repair after focal ischemia [25]. The levels of neuron-specific enolase, a marker of neuron death, are also reduced in patients treated with hypothermia following CPR [26].

Rapid rewarming exaggerates neural injury partly by modulating cellular and molecular mechanisms, as discussed above. In experimental models of traumatic brain injury (TBI) and stroke, rapid rewarming led to loss of cerebral autoregulation. Controlled rewarming, as in targeted temperature management, protects vascular reactivity and also reduces the oxygen radical-mediated endothelial and smooth muscle cell injury in brain vessels [27, 28].

Targeted temperature management aims to attenuate this secondary cascade of events and to prevent or minimize the impact of this secondary injury mechanism [29–31]. Targeted temperature management has become standard therapy following cardiac arrest. It is recommended by major organizations providing resuscitation guidelines, including the European Resuscitation Council, International Liaison Committee on Resuscitation (ILCOR) and American Heart Association [32, 33].

The term 'targeted temperature management' has replaced 'therapeutic hypothermia' or 'mild hypothermia' to emphasize the importance of defining a complete temperature profile. Manipulating the body temperature, intentionally, has become one of the treatment strategies with an impact on outcome post-cardiac arrest. Targeted temperature management can be divided into three phases:

1) intentional change from current temperature to lower temperature – 'induction';
2) maintenance of that temperature for a time – 'maintenance'; and
3) change to a new temperature value by increase in temperature at a specific rate to a normothermic target – 'rewarming'.

In earlier studies, there was emphasis on rapid introduction of cooling [34], but a recent RCT did not demonstrate any benefit in terms of speed to achieve therapeutic hypothermia in comparison to targeted temperature management [11]. Induction of hypothermia is not easy and can be associated with complications, including decreased cardiac output, arrhythmias, bleeding diathesis, electrolyte disturbances, and insulin resistance. Therefore, cooling should be achieved in an easy, controllable manner. The emphasis of targeted temperature management is tight maintenance of temperature.

Cooling Techniques

Currently available cooling techniques can be divided into three main categories:

1) Conventional cooling techniques
2) Surface cooling systems
3) Intravascular cooling systems.

Conventional Cooling Systems

Cold saline, crushed ice or ice bags have been used as the easiest way to induce hypothermia. Cold saline infusion has been shown to be effective in inducing hypothermia but not so effective in maintaining target temperature [35]. The main advantages of cold intravenous fluid are its easy availability and low cost. Volumes of up to two liters of intravenous fluids can be safely administered post-cardiac arrest [36]. Some studies have shown that saline or Ringer's lactate in combination with ice bags can achieve acceptable reductions in temperature [37].

Conventional cooling methods, in addition to being useful and cost-effective for the induction of hypothermia, can be used as adjuncts to other more advanced cooling devices [38]. The disadvantages of using conventional cooling techniques are that they are labor intensive; moreover, unintentional cooling below target temperature is common and can have deleterious effects [39]. Conventional cooling systems are also less effective at maintaining temperature when compared to surface or intravascular cooling systems [40].

Surface Cooling Systems

Surface cooling systems work by circulating cold fluid or cold air through blankets or pads that are wrapped around the patient. There is a range of products currently available, including cooling blankets (Curewrap™ with CritiCool by MTRE, Yavne, Israel; Kool-Kit® with Blanketrol III, by Cincinnati Sub-Zero, Cincinnati, OH) and surface pads (InnerCool STX by Philips, Best, Netherlands; Artic Sun® by Medivance, Louisville, CO) (Table 1). A study comparing the Cincinnati Sub-Zero system, a water-circulating cooling blanket, to the Medivance Artic Sun® hydrogel-coated water-circulating energy transfer pads, showed that the pads were superior in controlling fever in critically ill neurologic patients [41]. A study comparing the Arctic Sun surface system with the invasive intravascular Coolgard (Zoll, Chelmsford, MA) system in post-cardiac arrest patients showed similar survival to hospital discharge and comparable neurologic function at follow-up. Interpretation of device efficacy (cooling/rate), though, was limited by concurrent use of cold saline and ice bags [42]. The EMCOOLS cooling system (Vienna, Austria) uses adhesive non-invasive HypoCarbon® pads with a carbon-based cooling gel and provides cooling rates of 3.5 °C/h. There is no feedback system or computer control. The technology uses the thermal conductivity properties of the carbon-based gel to provide a highly effective cooling rate. Because if its ease of application and high cooling rate it can be used in the pre-hospital setting [43].

Table 1 Surface cooling devices

Company	Device	Type of cooling	Salient feature	Auto-feedback
MTRE	CritiCool	Surface blanket	Water-filled body shaped wrap covers the skin	Yes
Philips	InnerCool STX	Surface pads	Non-adhesive surface pads	Yes
EMCOOLS	Flexipads	Surface pads	Hypocarbon-based pads	No
C.R. Bard	ArticSun	Surface pads	Adhesive pads	Yes

This table shows commonly available devices and is by no means complete.

The advantages with using surface systems are ease of application and rapid initiation of treatment. Most of the devices have computerized auto-feedback mechanisms allowing the user to set target temperature and the system modifies the water temperature using the feedback from patient's skin and core temperature sensors.

The disadvantages of these systems are rare risk of skin burns and skin irritation [44]. The initiation of hypothermia varies between different devices and can range from 2–8 hours. Maintenance of temperature may also be difficult. Shivering is more commonly seen with surface systems than with other systems [41], which may necessitate the use of muscle relaxants.

Intravascular Cooling Systems

There are two devices currently available on the market: Thermoguard XP temperature management system (Zoll) and InnerCool RTx with Accutrol catheter (Philips).

The Thermoguard XP system uses percutaneously placed central venous catheters, which can be placed in subclavian, internal jugular or femoral veins. Temperature control is achieved by circulating cool or warm saline in a closed loop through the catheter's balloon [45]. Zoll offers different types of catheters, which can be used to adapt to different clinical needs (Table 2).

The InnerCool RTx endovascular cooling system uses a specific catheter, Accutrol, which has an integrated temperature sensor for precise control of temperature in all three phases of temperature management, without the possibility of lag in core temperature measurement that may be inherent with rectal or bladder temperature probes. There is no additional central venous access provided with the catheter [46].

Both these systems have computerized temperature control with an auto-feedback mechanism. The intravascular cooling systems provide precise temperature control during maintenance and rewarming phases of temperature management. There are fewer incidences of failure to reach target temperature and less overcooling than with other systems. There is also less shivering compared to surface devices [47]. Despite these advantages, however, there was no difference in out-

Table 2 Catheter specifications for the Thermoguard XP system (Zoll)

Catheter Name	Cool Line®	Solex®	ICY®	Quattro®
Number of heat exchange balloons	2	Serpentine balloon	3	4
Number of infusion lumens	3	3	3	3
Insertion site	Subclavian Internal jugular Femoral	Internal jugular	Femoral	Femoral
Length	22 cm	25 cm	38 cm	45 cm

Adapted from Zoll Catheter Specification Sheet [45].

come when compared to surface cooling systems [48]. There is an added risk of catheter-related bloodstream infection, venous thrombosis and complications related to insertion of intravascular lines.

Other Cooling Methods

An extracorporeal cooling method using KTEK-3 (Kawasumi, Tokyo, Japan) has been used in post-cardiac arrest patients in Japan [49]. This technique can only be employed in places where an extracorporeal device is available and needs trained personnel to deliver care. RhinoChill® is a novel intranasal cooling system, designed to provide early and rapid initiation of patient cooling [50]. It was shown to effectively reduce temperature in pre-hospital intra-arrest patients [51]. There is no temperature feedback mechanism and the main application of this device is in the pre-hospital setting for induction of hypothermia.

There have been case reports on the use of continuous renal replacement therapy (CRRT) for induction and maintenance of hypothermia [52, 53]. Selective brain cooling by hypothermic retrograde jugular vein flush and intranasally has been investigated in animal models and this may be relevant in conditions where whole body hypothermia may be detrimental, such as cardiac arrest associated with polytrauma [54, 55]. Further investigations are being conducted into use of intra-pulmonary perflurochemical fluids for induction and maintenance of hypothermia and also to support gas exchange and pulmonary structure [56]. The esophageal route is also being investigated, because of the close proximity of the esophagus to blood flow from the heart and great vessels. Initial animal and mathematical studies have shown that the esophageal route is safe and effective for inducing, maintaining and reversing hypothermia [57, 58].

Conclusion

Various cooling methods and techniques are currently available to achieve targeted temperature management. There are three phases of targeted temperature management: Induction, maintenance and rewarming. Different cooling methods vary in their effectiveness for each phase of cooling. The most beneficial time to commence hypothermia is debatable. The current recommendation by ILCOR is to start hypothermia as soon as possible and to aim for a temperature between 32–34 °C. However, a recently concluded RCT showed no evidence to support inducing hypothermia, but an emphasis on maintenance of temperature and avoiding pyrexia; there was also no association of time to target temperature and neurological outcome [11].

A study comparing different cooling methods in ICU patients concluded that water circulating blankets, gel-pads and intravascular devices are almost equivalent for inducing hypothermia but intravascular devices are superior in maintaining target temperature [40]. The performances of the different devices may change as technology evolves; however, each method has its own limitations and the combination of conventional methods and automatic computer-processed feedback devices seems a safe option.

Temperature management is no longer just a question of whether a patient is cool, but has evolved into a complex treatment management procedure. It is, therefore, paramount to ensure precise control of temperature during all three phases of temperature management, especially during the phase of rewarming during which a passive, uncontrolled rise in temperature can be deleterious to the patient. The development of different devices aimed at greater precision in monitoring and managing temperature in cardiac arrest patients will help to make treatment safe and easy.

This review on the different cooling methods is written at a time where news on targeted temperature management breaks daily and, therefore, cannot claim to be complete but rather a snap shot in a rapidly developing field. With so many different devices available and the likelihood of new devices emerging, the device used should be selected according to its ability to effectively maintain temperature within the therapeutic range with the fewest possible adverse effects while being as minimally invasive as possible.

References

1. Hippocrates (460–375 BC) De Vetere Medicina.
2. Fay T (1943) Observations on generalized refrigeration in cases of severe cerebral trauma. Assoc Res Nerv Ment Dis Proc 24:611–619
3. Rosomoff HL, Safar P (1965) Management of the comatose patient. Clin Anes 1:244–258
4. Lazorthes G, Campan L (1964) Moderate hypothermia in the treatment of head injuries. Clin Neurosurg 12:293–299
5. Laver S, Farrow C, Turner D, Nolan J (2004) Mode of death after admission to an intensive care unit following cardiac arrest. Intensive Care Med 30:2126–2128
6. Negovsky VA (1988) Postresuscitation disease. Crit Care Med 16:942–946
7. Brain Resuscitation Clinical Trial I Study Group (1986) Randomized clinical study of thiopental loading in comatose survivors of cardiac arrest. N Engl J Med 314:397–403
8. Jastremski M, Sutton-Tyrrell K, Vaagenes P (1989) Glucocorticoid treatment does not improve neurological recovery following cardiac arrest. JAMA 262:3427–3430
9. Abramson N (1991) A randomized clinical-study of a calcium-entry blocker (lidoflazine) in the treatment of comatose survivors of cardiac-arrest. N Engl J Med 324:1225–1231
10. Roine R, Kaste M, Kinnunen A et al (1990) Nimodipine after resuscitation from out-of-hospital ventricular-fibrillation – a placebo-controlled, double-blind randomized trial. JAMA 264:3171–3177
11. Nielsen N, Wetterslev J, Cronberg T (2013) Targeted temperature management at 33 C versus 36 C after cardiac arrest. N Engl J Med 369:2197–2206
12. The Hypothermia after Cardiac Arrest Study Group (2002) Mild therapeutic hypothermia to improve the neurologic outcome after cardiac arrest. N Engl J Med 346:549–556
13. Zeiner A, Holzer M, Sterz F (2001) Hyperthermia after cardiac arrest is associated with an unfavorable neurologic outcome. Arch Intern Med 161:2007–2012
14. Safar P (1988) Resuscitation from clinical death: pathophysiologic limits and therapeutic potentials. Crit Care Med 16:923–941
15. Powers JH, Scheld WM (1996) Fever in neurologic diseases. Infect Dis Clin North Am 10:45–66

16. Sterz F, Safar P, Diven W et al (1993) Detoxification with hemabsorption after cardiac arrest does not improve neurologic recovery. Review and outcome study in dogs. Resuscitation 25:137–160
17. Stone BJ, Chantler PJ, Baskett PJF (1998) The incidence of regurgitation during cardiopulmonary resuscitation: a comparison between the bag valve mask and laryngeal mask airway. Resuscitation 38:3–6
18. Sternau L, Globus MYT, Dietrich WD, Martinez E, Busto R, Ginsberg MD (1992) Ischemia-induced neurotransmitter release: effects of mild intraischemic hyperthermia. In: Globus M, Dietrich WD (eds) The Role of Neurotransmitters in Brain Injury. Plenum Press, New York, pp 33–38
19. Globus MY, Busto R, Lin B et al (1995) Detection of free radical activity during transient global ischemia and recirculation: Effects of intraischemic brain temperature modulation. J Neurochem 65:1250–1256
20. Kil HY, Zhang J, Piantadosi CA (1996) Brain temperature alters hydroxyl radical production during cerebral ischemia/reperfusion in rats. J Cereb Blood Flow Metab 16:100–106
21. Madl JE, Allen DL (1995) Hyperthermia depletes adenosine triphosphate and decreases glutamate uptake in rat hippocampal slices. Neuroscience 69:395–405
22. Morimoto T, Ginsberg MD, Dietrich WD, Zhao W (1997) Hyperthermia enhances spectrin breakdown in transient focal cerebral ischemia. Brain Res 746:43–51
23. Steen PA, Newberg L, Milde JH, Michenfelder JD (1983) Hypothermia and barbiturates: individual and combined effects on canine cerebral oxygen consumption. Anesthesiology 58:527–532
24. Han HS, Park J, Kim J, Suk K (2012) Molecular and cellular pathways as a target of therapeutic hypothermia: pharmacological aspect. Curr Neuropharmacol 10:80–87
25. Tomasevic G, Kamme F, Stubberöd P et al (1999) The tumor suppressor p53 and its response gene p21WAF1/Cip1 are not markers of neuronal death following transient global cerebral ischemia. Neuroscience 90:781–792
26. Rundgren M, Karlsson T, Nielsen N et al (2009) Neuron specific enolase and S-100B as predictors of outcome after cardiac arrest and induced hypothermia. Resuscitation 80:784–789
27. Povlishock JT, Wei EP (2009) Posthypothermic rewarming considerations following traumatic brain injury. J. Neurotrauma 26:333–340
28. Linares G, Mayer SA (2009) Hypothermia for the treatment of ischemic and hemorrhagic stroke. Crit Care Med 37:S243–S249
29. Andrews PJD, Sinclair HL, Battison CG et al (2011) European society of intensive care medicine study of therapeutic hypothermia (32–35 °C) for intracranial pressure reduction after traumatic brain injury (the Eurotherm3235Trial). Trials 12:8
30. Benz-Woerner J, Delodder F, Benz R, Cueni-Villoz N (2012) Body temperature regulation and outcome after cardiac arrest and therapeutic hypothermia. Resuscitation 83:338–342
31. Polderman KH, Herold I (2009) Therapeutic hypothermia and controlled normothermia in the intensive care unit: Practical considerations, side effects, and cooling methods. Crit Care Med 37:1101–1120
32. Peberdy MA, Callaway CW, Neumar RW et al (2010) Part 9: post-cardiac arrest care: 2010 American Heart Association Guidelines for Cardiopulmonary Resuscitation and Emergency Cardiovascular Care. Circulation 122:S768–S786
33. Nolan JP, Neumar RW, Adrie C et al (2008) Post-cardiac arrest syndrome: Epidemiology, pathophysiology, treatment, and prognostication. Resuscitation 79:350–379
34. Bernard SA, Mac Jones BC, Horne MK (1997) Clinical trial of induced hypothermia in comatose survivors of out-of-hospital cardiac arrest. Ann Emerg Med 30:146–153
35. Kliegel A, Janata A, Wandaller C et al (2007) Cold infusions alone are effective for induction of therapeutic hypothermia but do not keep patients cool after cardiac arrest. Resuscitation 73:46–53
36. Kim F, Olsufka M, Carlbom D et al (2005) Pilot study of rapid infusion of 2 L of 4 C normal saline for induction of mild hypothermia in hospitalized, comatose survivors of out-of-hospital cardiac arrest. Circulation 112:715–719

37. Larsson I, Wallin E, Rubertsson S (2010) Cold saline infusion and ice packs alone are effective in inducing and maintaining therapeutic hypothermia after cardiac arrest. Resuscitation 81:15–19
38. Kliegel A, Losert H, Sterz F et al (2005) Cold simple intravenous infusions preceding special endovascular cooling for faster induction of mild hypothermia after cardiac arrest – a feasibility study. Resuscitation 64:347–351
39. Merchant RM, Abella BS, Peberdy MA et al (2006) Therapeutic hypothermia after cardiac arrest: Unintentional overcooling is common using ice packs and conventional cooling blankets. Critical Care Medicine 34:S490–S494
40. Hoedemaekers C, Ezzahti M, Gerritsen A (2007) Comparison of cooling methods to induce and maintain normo-and hypothermia in intensive care unit patients: a prospective intervention study. Crit Care 11:R91
41. Mayer SA, Kowalski RG, Presciutti M et al (2004) Clinical trial of a novel surface cooling system for fever control in neurocritical care patients. Crit Care Med 32:2508–2515
42. Tømte Ø, Drægni T, Mangschau A et al (2011) A comparison of intravascular and surface cooling techniques in comatose cardiac arrest survivors. Crit Care Med 39:443–449
43. EMCOOL. Available at: http://www.emcools.com/en/home.aspx
44. Varon J, Acosta P, Wintz R, Mendoza N (2008) Unusual side effect from hydrogel pads during therapeutic hypothermia. Resuscitation 78:248–249
45. IVTM Intravascular Temperature Management Catheter Specifications. http://www.zoll.com/uploadedFiles/Public_Site/Products/Catheters/Catheters_spec_sheet.pdf. Accessed Nov 2014
46. High performance temperature management RTx Endovascular and STx Surface Cooling Systems. http://incenter.medical.philips.com/doclib/enc/6293662/Philips_InnerCool_Advanced_Temperature_Modulation_Therapy_-_Enhancing_patient_care.pdf%3ffunc%3ddoc.Fetch%26nodeid%3d6293662%26vernum%3d4. Accessed Nov 2014
47. Lyden, Allgren RL, Ng K et al (2005) Intravascular cooling in the treatment of stroke (ICTuS): Early clinical experience. J Stroke Cerebrovasc Dis 14:107–114
48. Gillies M, Pratt R, Whiteley C et al (2010) Therapeutic hypothermia after cardiac arrest: a retrospective comparison of surface and endovascular cooling techniques. Resuscitation 81:1117–1122
49. Soga T, Nagao K, Kikushima K et al (2006) Mild therapeutic hypothermia using extracorporeal cooling method in comatose survivors after out-of-hospital cardiac arrest. Circulation 114:II_1190
50. Rhinochill Advantage. Available at: http://www.benechill.com/wp/rhinochill-trade/ems-use/. Accessed Nov 2014.
51. Castrén M, Nordberg P, Svensson L et al (2010) Intra-arrest transnasal evaporative cooling: a randomized, prehospital, multicenter study (PRINCE: Pre-ROSC IntraNasal Cooling Effectiveness. Circulation 122:729–736
52. Ma Y, Ning B, Cao W et al (2013) Good neurologic recovery after cardiac arrest using hypothermia through continuous renal replacement therapy. Am J Emerg Med 31:1720.e1–1720.e3
53. Karacan H, Valentin A, Carl P (2009) Mild therapeutic hypothermia after cardiac arrest through continuous dialysis. Ugeskr Laeger 171:1396–1400
54. Wen Y, Huang M, Lin M (2005) Rapid brain cooling by hypothermic retrograde jugular vein flush. J Trauma 58:577–581
55. Covaciu L, Allers M, Enblad P, Lunderquist A (2008) Intranasal selective brain cooling in pigs. Resuscitation 76:83–88
56. Yang S, Jeng M, McShane R et al (2005) Cold perfluorochemical-induced hypothermia protects lung integrity in normal rabbits. Biol Neonate 87:60–65
57. Kulstad E, Metzger A, Courtney D, Rees J (2013) Induction, maintenance, and reversal of therapeutic hypothermia with an esophageal heat transfer device. Resuscitation 84:1619–1624
58. Vaicys V, Eason A, Schieber J, Kulstad E (2012) Therapeutic hypothermia induction via an esophageal route – a computer simulation. Am J Emerg Med 30:932–935

Part VII
Fluids

How Does Volume Make the Blood Go Around?

S. Magder

Introduction

The initial response to the question, "How does volume make the blood go around?", is usually something like: Volume stretches the left ventricular wall and the greater the stretch the greater the stroke output from the left heart because of an increase in preload as first described by Otto Frank and Ernest Starling. While this is true, it is just part of the role that volume plays in the generation of flow around the circulation. At the beginning of the last century, Ernst Starling appreciated the fundamental point that the heart only can pump out what it receives and factors that affect the return of blood to the heart play a key role in what comes back to the heart [1]. The basic principle in this chapter is that the elastic properties of vascular structures are key determinants of the distribution and movement of the blood volume around the circulation. The discussion will revolve around how the distribution of compliances in the circulation, the concepts of stressed and unstressed volume [2, 3], and Sagawa's concept of time varying elastance of the ventricles [4] explain how much blood flows around the circulation for a given amount of blood volume. Many of the concepts in this paper are derived from a computerized computational model that we have applied to the circulation [5, 6] as well as measurements in animal studies [7–9]. Although a computational analysis does not indicate exactly what goes on in a living organism, its advantage is that one variable can be changed at a time, which allows an analysis of changes in the mechanical properties of the vasculature in steady states. The real-life situation is a composite of these isolated mechanical changes.

S. Magder ✉
Department of Critical Care, McGill University Health Center, Montreal, Canada
e-mail: sheldon.magder@muhc.mcgill.ca

J.-L. Vincent (ed.), *Annual Update in Intensive Care and Emergency Medicine 2015*,
DOI 10.1007/978-3-319-13761-2_23

Compliance and Vascular Volume

Vascular compliance is defined as the change in volume for a change in pressure [10]. Its inverse is elastance, which is defined as the tendency of a substance to return to its original (or relaxed) position after an applied force. In the vasculature, elastance of vessels is given by the change in pressure for a change in volume. This indicates the tension created in the elastic walls of vessels, including the heart, due to the distention of the chamber walls by the contained volume. This tension creates an elastic recoil pressure that sets the pressure of the volume in the region. The term compliance makes it seem that the pressure determines the volume. However, the total volume in the vasculature is relatively fixed and the volume determines the pressure in the different parts of the vasculature. On the other hand, the pressure difference between one elastic region and the next determines the movement of volume through the system. In the steady state, equilibrium is reached when the volumes distribute based on the compliances of the regions and the resistances between them.

The circulation is a system with multiple compliant regions in series (Fig. 1). These different vascular compartments can be lumped into six major regions: Four that have a static fixed compliance, which includes the pulmonary arterial and venous vessels and the systemic arterial and venous vessels, and two that have dynamic time varying elastances, which are the right and left hearts. In a system with compliances in series, total compliance is simply the sum of all the compliances of all the parts (Fig. 1).

A fundamental point is that, although volume constantly moves in and out of the circulation due to filtration into the interstitial space, renal tubules and gastrointestinal tract, vascular volume remains relatively constant under steady state conditions. When there is no flow around the circuit, the pressure is the same everywhere in the vasculature. Since total vascular volume is a fixed value (at least over the short-term), and compliance of vascular structures is a property of the walls that does not change significantly, the pressure at zero flow is simply determined by the total volume and the total compliance of all parts of the circulation. This pressure is called the mean circulatory filling pressure (MCFP) and normally is most likely in the range of 8 to 9 mmHg. I say 'likely' because this cannot readily be measured in an intact normal person. Arthur Guyton obtained this value in dogs by first putting the animals into ventricular fibrillation and then rapidly pumping arterial blood into the venous compartment until the pressures were equal in arteries and veins. This had to be done rapidly to avoid reflex adjustments and a loss of volume from vascular leak [11]. This clearly is not feasible in humans but based on some measurements in humans the value is likely similar [2].

When there is no blood flow, volume distributes in the circulation based solely on regional compliances. The compliance of systemic veins and venules is much larger than that of any other region and accounts for 70% of the total vascular compliance (Fig. 1). Accordingly, 70% of blood volume resides in the veins and venules in the no-flow state. This region is critical for the determination of cardiac output because

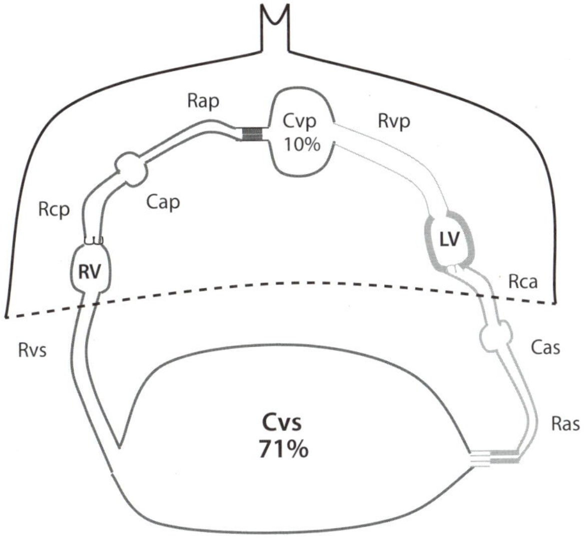

Fig. 1 General schema of the circulation with 6 lumped compliant regions in series and resistances between them. The regions are roughly drawn in proportion to their relative sizes. Regions above the *dotted line* are in the thorax. C refers to compliance and R to resistance, RV = right ventricle and LV = left ventricle, vs = systemic venous compartment, ap = pulmonary arterial compartment, vp = pulmonary venous compartment, as = systemic arterial compartment. When there is no flow, 71% of stressed volume is in the systemic venous compartment (for a total stressed volume of 1,400 ml this is 1,022 ml), and 10% in the pulmonary venous compartment (137 ml). The total compliance (Ctotal) is the sum of the compliances of the 6 regions and this value is dominated by Cvs

it is upstream from the right heart and determines the gradient for right heart filling. Even more so, the pressure gradient from this region to the right heart is only in the range of 3 to 5 mmHg so that small changes in the gradient for venous return can have important effects. The pressure of the volume that is specifically in systemic veins is called the mean systemic filling pressure (MSFP in contrast to MCFP). The total compliance of the pulmonary arteries and veins is around one eighth that of the total vascular compliance and normally accounts for about 12–14% of total blood volume. Systemic arterial compliance is less than 3% of the total vascular compliance but because of the high pressure in this region during flow conditions it can accumulate volume out of proportion to its fraction of total compliance.

When there is blood flow in the circulation, pressure gradients develop between the different compliant regions and vascular volume redistributes among the different compliant regions. The pressure gradients occur because the dynamic right and left heart regions have transient increases in the elastance of their walls, which increases the pressure of the volume they contain (diastolic volume). This creates a pressure gradient to the next downstream region and allows the volume to flow out of the ventricle and into the next compliant region (the systemic arterial compartment), which is what we recognize as stroke volume. On the right side of the heart, the flow out of the heart also allows roughly the same volume to flow in from the systemic venous compartment. This equal volume-in versus volume-out means that the heart cannot add or take up much volume from the systemic circulation except by altering the distribution of blood volume between the systemic and pulmonary vascular compartments. Under flow conditions, volume still distributes based on the compliance of each region but distribution is also affected by the inflow and outflow resistance of each region. The redistribution of volume during flow conditions reduces the systemic venous volume to about 60% of blood volume as compared to 70% during the no-flow state. However, the MSFP is still only about 1 mmHg less than MCFP with normal cardiac function. This is because the systemic venous system is so compliant that the loss of volume produces only a small pressure change.

MSFP can be more easily assessed than MCFP by processes that transiently stop the heart, such as transient arrest of the heart when testing an artificial pacemaker to look for an escape rhythm or when testing the function of an implantable defibrillator during its insertion [12, 13]. MSFP can also be mathematically estimated from the right atrial pressure, blood pressure, and estimates of venous resistance [14, 15] or through respiratory maneuvers [16]. MCFP describes the overall capacity for flow in the system whereas MSFP gives an indication of the upstream pressure driving volume back to the heart. However, the relationship between MSFP and MCFP changes when there are changes in the relative functions of the right and left hearts, changes in distribution of cardiac output and changes in arterial and venous resistances. Thus, the significance of MSFP becomes more limited as a clinical tool, but it is still a useful general descriptive parameter of the circulation for understanding broad physiological changes.

The presence of separate right and left ventricles allows the same flow to occur through the pulmonary circuit as the flow in the systemic circuit but at a much lower pressure. This protects delicate alveoli. Because pressures in the pulmonary compartment are much lower than systemic pressures and the pulmonary compliance is much higher than that of the systemic compartment, less volume accumulates in the pulmonary compartment than in the systemic circulation under flow conditions. The advantage of this is a lower risk of pulmonary edema. However, the distribution changes dramatically when there is left ventricular dysfunction and elevated left ventricular diastolic pressure. Much more volume accumulates in the pulmonary circuit, increasing the risk of pulmonary edema with infusion of volume (Fig. 2).

The principle that volume has a fixed value during steady state conditions raises an important difference between electrical models and hydrodynamic models of the circulation. In an electrical model, the voltage, which is the equivalent of a pressure drop, is kept constant and the 'volume' of electrons is determined by the voltage and the current or flow of electrons. The input 'volume' of electrons is essentially infinite. The 'pressure' determines the total 'volume' of electrons. In a hydrodynamic system with a closed loop, as is the case with the circulation, the volume is

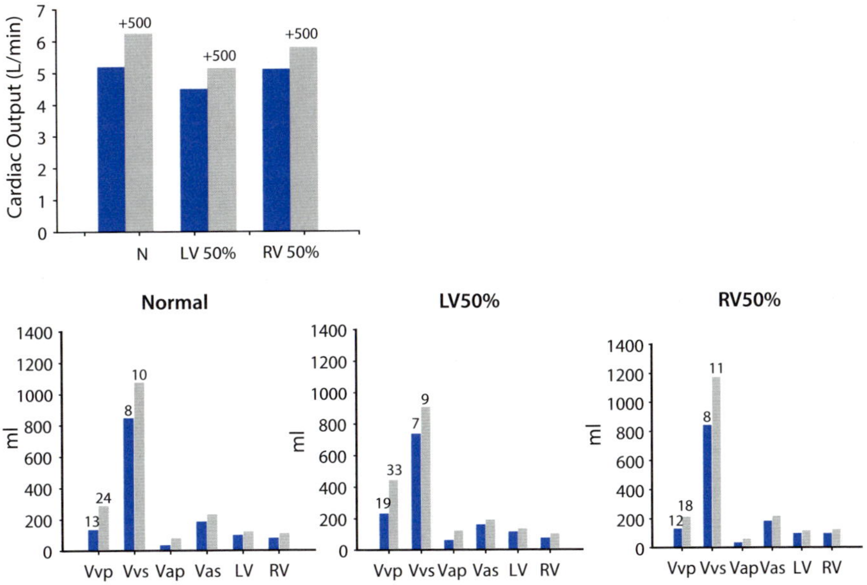

Fig. 2 Changes in cardiac output and distributions of volume with addition of 500 ml stressed volume. The *top graph* shows cardiac output (l/min) before (*dark blue bars*) and after (*light blue bars*) addition of volume with normal (N) cardiac function, a 50% decrease in left ventricular function (LV50%) (decreased end-systolic elastance), and decreased RV function (RV50%). The *bottom three graphs* show the volumes (V) in the pulmonary venous compartment (vp), systemic venous compartment (vs), pulmonary arterial compartment (ap), systemic arterial compartment (as) and the right and left ventricles with a normal heart, LV50%, RV50% before and after (*light blue bars*) addition of 500 ml stressed volume. The numbers above the bars indicate the pressures in the regions. Note the much larger increase in pressure in Vvp and smaller increase in Vvs with volume infusion in LV50% than in the normal or RV50% conditions. The values were calculated using the computational model in [5]

constant and the pressure varies based on the elasticity of the walls of the system and the distribution of the volume. The input force is a cyclic change in elasticity in two regions but the overall volume remains constant. Importantly, the regulation of arterial pressure comes from control of cardiac output and systemic vascular resistance and the arterial pressure does not determine the cardiac output. Thus, hydrodynamic models are preferred over electrical models. However, if one is examining flow in a regional vasculature or flow across a heart valve, electrical models are useful, because the blood pressure is a regulated variable in the circulation and regional flows vary depending upon the downstream resistance as in an electrical circuit.

Stressed and Unstressed Volume

The blood volume of a 70 kg man is in the range of 5.5 l but not all the volume distends the vascular walls and produces the recoil pressure that drives fluid from one compliant region to the next. A large proportion of the volume just fills out the interiors of the cylindrical vascular structures and, accordingly, is called *unstressed* volume because it does not stretch the vessel wall. The volume that actually stretches the walls is called *stressed* volume and is in the range of 25 to 30% of total blood volume under resting conditions, or about 1.4 l [2]. The significance of this is that a much smaller amount of volume than often appreciated is responsible for making the blood go around. This volume is a mixture of red cells and plasma as indicated by the hematocrit so that the actual non-red cell component of stressed volume is less than 1 l. In hydrodynamics, the total volume for static pressure is called capacitance. (Note that in electrical circuits, capacitance is used to describe the relationship of change in total amount of charge, an equivalent of volume, to voltage, an equivalent of pressure, and thus capacitance in electrical models is the equivalent of compliance in hydrodynamics). A strong sympathetic discharge can recruit up to ~ 18 ml/kg of unstressed volume into stressed volume [3 8, 17] although a more common upper limit is likely around 10 ml/kg. If the initial stressed volume is 1.4 l, this would produce a 50% increase in stress volume in just seconds because it is a reflex response. At least 2 l of a saline solution would be needed to have the same effect. Importantly, not all this recruited volume will remain in the systemic veins but will be redistributed throughout the vasculature as described below for the infusion of 500 ml of normal saline. This assumes that all the volume remains in the vasculature but the consequent increase in capillary pressure will also increase microcirculatory filtration and some volume will be lost.

Heart Rate and Time Constants of Drainage

The product of a resistance draining a region and the compliance of the region gives what is called a time constant. This is the time it takes to reach 63% of the new steady state value after a step change in the flow going into a region or a step change in the inflow pressure [8]. The time constant is important because flow into and out of the heart is pulsatile and thus the entry and exit times for filling and emptying the two sides of the heart are fixed by the rhythmicity of the pulsations. When the cycle length, the inverse of heart rate, becomes shorter than the time needed to reach complete emptying or filling of a region during the cycle, cardiac cycle length limits the flow into or out of the cardiac regions and thus total flow in the system. This can change the distribution of volume throughout the system depending upon the upstream and downstream time constants. Just to emphasize this again, at least over short periods and in the steady state, total blood volume is constant so that when it accumulates in an upstream region, it must decrease the volume and thus elastic recoil of the downstream region and flow out of that region because the downstream region must loose volume for total volume to be constant.

Cardiac Factors

The cardiac chambers contribute to the distribution of blood volume by the relative functions of the left and right sides of the heart during systole and during diastole as well as by setting the periodicity of the cyclic nature of the cardiac cycle, which impacts on filling and ejection as explained above because of the time constants of the various compartments.

As elegantly described by Sagawa [4], ejection of blood during systole by the heart is based on what they called a time-varying elastance. What this means is that during systole the interaction of actin and myosin makes the heart progressively stiffer (greater elastance). This continues as long as intracellular calcium remains elevated inside the cytoplasm of myocytes and allows the interaction of actin and myosin. Calcium is removed from the cytoplasm at the end of the cardiac cell action potential, which ends the increase in elastance (contraction). During the phase of increased elastance, the pressure of the blood volume in the heart is markedly increased, which creates the pressure gradient between the left heart and aorta or the right heart and the pulmonary artery. This allows blood to flow into the downstream elastic chamber. At the end of the cycle, the elastance decreases meaning that cardiac muscle cells relax and can again hold volume at a lower pressure which ends up being below the MSFP. This allows the cardiac chambers to refill. In the normal resting physiological state, peak elastance of the right heart is about one third that of the left heart. Changes in the contractile function of cardiac chambers are the equivalent of changes in the maximum elastance at the end of systole [4]. Changes in the relative values of the maximal elastance of the right and left sides of the heart, alter the distribution of blood volume between the systemic and pulmonary compartments. A decrease in right-sided function results in a decrease in pulmonary blood volume and an increase in systemic blood volume (Fig. 2). A decrease in left-sided function results in an increase in pulmonary volume relative to systemic volume. In modeling studies in which volume is fixed so that total volume does not change, and there are no reflex adaptations, a marked decrease in left ventricular systolic function leads to a large shift of volume from the systemic compartment to the pulmonary compartment. This results in a decrease in MSFP and actually contributes to the decrease in cardiac output [5]. In this situation, not only does less blood go out because of the weaker ejection force but less also comes back because the upstream systemic venous elastic recoil force is decreased due to the displacement of blood volume to the pulmonary compartment. Ironically, right-sided filling pressure is decreased. This is not usually evident clinically because homeostatic mechanisms retain volume and restore MSFP and if there is not enough time for this to happen, clinicians often restore the systemic volume when they see the low right atrial pressure!

Changes in diastolic function are represented by changes in diastolic compliance. These have the same effects on volume distribution as changes in systolic function but to a much smaller degree likely because the pressure differences during the cycle are so much smaller. Based on our modeling studies, under basal conditions the effect of decreases in diastolic function would be hardly noticeable. However, what does become very important is the volume in the ventricles at which the diastolic passive filling curve becomes steep for this creates a limit to the volume that can fill the ventricle and thus a limit to stroke volume. This is seen as the flat part of the cardiac function curve. This limit can be reached when the heart rate is not sufficient to allow the timely ejection of the returning blood [18]. It also occurs when ejection is insufficient and end-systolic volume increases so that the returning blood can reach the steep part of the diastolic passive filling curve.

Effects of Giving Volume

As is the case with baseline volume distribution, volume added to the vasculature, whether by normal oral intake, reabsorption from the interstitial space or recruitment from unstressed volume, distributes according to the regional compliances and the resistances separating them. If there is no change in regional venous and arterial resistances, the volume redistributes in proportion close to but not the same as in the baseline state. As shown in Fig. 2, model calculations predict that at baseline cardiac output of 5.2 l/min and a stressed volume of 1.4 l, 61% of the volume resides in the systemic veins and 10% in the pulmonary veins. With a 500 ml increase in stressed volume, 45% of the increase would go to systemic veins and 30% would go to pulmonary veins. In life, this redistribution is further distorted because the increased cardiac output initiates baroreceptor reflex adjustments to local resistances to try to maintain arterial pressure constant. There are also myogenic responses that likely vary among the various vascular regions which will result in some further variable changes in local resistances and critical closing pressures [19, 20].

If left ventricular function is decreased by 50% and right ventricular function is unchanged, pulmonary veins would get 42% of the 500 ml increase in stressed volume and the systemic veins would only get 33% of the increase in volume. Accordingly, in the failing heart the increase in cardiac output with volume infusion is much less than the increase in the normal situation because of the smaller increase in MSFP (Fig. 2).

As discussed in the previous section, alterations in the relative functions of the right and left sides of the heart change the distribution of volume between systemic and pulmonary circuits compared to baseline conditions [6]. If the primary problem is decreased left ventricular function, a greater proportion of the added volume will end up in the pulmonary compartment and produce a greater increase in pulmonary hydrostatic pressure than in a normal heart (Fig. 2). If the primary problem is decreased right heart function, a smaller proportion of volume will end up in the pulmonary compartment and it will be relatively protected. More will accumulate in this case in the systemic veins. If there is right heart limitation because the right heart is functioning on the flat part of the cardiac function curve, there may be almost no change in the volume of the pulmonary compartments and thus almost no change in output from the right, and consequently, left heart [21].

Changes in cardiac output also affect the distribution of blood volume, but first one must consider how the cardiac output can increase. Cardiac output can increase due to an increase in cardiac function or an increase in the return function. An increase in cardiac function occurs when there is an increase in heart rate, increase in contractility or decrease in afterload. With all three of these there is no need for a change in stressed volume as long as there is no flow limitation for the venous return due to the development of a vascular waterfall as the great veins enter the thorax [22, 23]. With a rise in cardiac function due an increase in heart rate or contractility, arterial pressure too would increase unless there are reflex adjustments in arterial vascular resistance. The rise in pressure would result in some accumulation of blood volume in the systemic arterial system as well as in the pulmonary circuit, the latter because of the increase in left ventricular afterload. This accumulated volume must come at the expense of the systemic venous compartment, but since the compliance of the systemic venous compartment is about forty times that of the systemic arteries, the loss of volume from this region is small. Furthermore, reflex adjustments in vascular resistance are rapid and modulate the rise in arterial pressure so that there should not be large changes in regional volume distribution. When the increase in cardiac function occurs because of a decrease in left ventricular afterload, i.e., decrease in arterial pressure, the improved ventricular ejection allows more of the pulmonary volume to drain to the left ventricle. The decrease in arterial outflow resistance also leads to decreased arterial volume. Together, these produce a small increase in the volume in the systemic veins. An increase in cardiac output due to changes in circuit factors can come from a primary decrease in the resistance to venous return or to an increase in stressed volume [5]. An increase in stressed volume has the same effect as giving volume, which was discussed above. The volume will redistribute according to baseline conditions with some modification due to baroreceptor-induced changes in systemic resistance in response to the increase in arterial pressure. If cardiac output increases because of a decrease in the resistance to venous return there will be a shift in volume from the systemic compartment to the pulmonary compartment. This means that volume infusions will have a greater than normal effect on the pulmonary venous pressures when venous resistance is low. This likely is the situation in sepsis, because the high cardiac output means that resistance to venous return must be decreased to allow the high flow. Accordingly, a greater proportion of the infused volume will settle in the pulmonary circuit and raise pulmonary hydrostatic pressures in the face of increased capillary leak and, thereby, increase pulmonary edema.

Ventilatory Effects

The distribution of volume is also affected by ventilation. The fall in pleural pressure with a spontaneous inspiratory effort increases the gradient for venous return and acts the same way as increasing MSFP by giving volume as long as there is no flow limitation in the veins as they enter the thorax [24, 25]. On the left side, the negative pleural pressure increases the afterload on the left ventricle during systole and can further increase the shift of volume to the pulmonary compartments [26]. The net effect will depend upon the initial right atrial pressure, because that determines how much right atrial pressure can fall before in-flow is limited; the frequency and depth of breaths; and, on the left side, the steepness of the end-systolic pressure-volume relationship, because that determines how well the left heart will handle the increase in afterload [26]. Positive pleural pressure decreases the volume in the pulmonary compartments because the small gradient for venous return is decreased. It also helps left ventricular ejection but this effect is small and the benefit on the left side is likely more from preventing the increase in afterload with spontaneous efforts. The situation becomes more complicated when lung inflation creates West Zone II conditions in the pulmonary veins. When that happens, the outflow pressure from pulmonary veins to the left heart becomes alveolar pressure and this pressure increases throughout the breath. This results in increased blood volume in the pulmonary compartment [6]. The net effect from the increase in pleural pressure and the creation of zone II conditions will depend upon the magnitude of the change in pleural pressure relative to atmosphere, the extent of regions with zone II conditions and the magnitude of the transpulmonary gradient.

Use of Monitoring of MCFP and MSFP

MCFP and MSFP have been proposed as potential values to follow the management of hemodynamic instability [14, 15, 27, 28]. The concept of MCFP and MSFP as developed by Arthur Guyton [29, 30] has been extremely useful for understanding the relative roles of factors returning blood to the heart and the factors ejecting the blood. They indicate why the static mechanical property, compliance, and the consequent elastic recoil pressure are such important determinants of cardiac output. They also indicate the importance of changes in stressed volume through changes in capacitance. However, I do not find them to be useful for the management of patients. MCFP is an important determinant of the capacity of the system to generate flow but it is not really possible to precisely measure it in an intact person. Because the gradient for venous return is so small, even small errors in the measurement of MCFP would greatly limit the usefulness of the value. What is usually estimated or measured is MSFP but this differs from MCFP under pathological conditions in ways that are not easy to predict without detailed knowledge of all parts of the circulation, including something not discussed in this paper, which is the distribution between venous regions with larger or smaller compliances [7, 8, 23]. Another limitation is that the pressure difference from MSFP to the right atrium is very small so that when MSFP is being estimated from the right atrium under conditions in which there is still output from the heart, changes in venous resistance, even from diaphragmatic contractions can have significant effects on the measurement [31]. MSFP certainly has little value without a measure of cardiac output. For example, in pure severe left ventricular dysfunction without adding stressed volume to the system, MSFP will decrease and there will appear to be a volume problem [5]. Much more value is obtained by examining the changes in patterns of right atrial pressure and cardiac output for this allows an assessment of how the return function is interacting with the cardiac function and where primary therapeutic interventions can be made [29].

Conclusion

Transient changes in the elastance of the ventricles raises and lowers the pressure of the volume within them and allows the flow of volume into and out of the left and right sides of the heart. Importantly, the force for filling the right and left sides of the heart is there even when there is no flow. Filling can occur because emptying of the ventricles from the transient increase in elastance during systole lowers the pressure in the cardiac chambers and allows them to fill. The volume ejected by the heart in systole is passed through the compliant regions of the circulation. Under steady state flow conditions, the volume redistributes from the baseline distribution of volume in the initial static state to a new steady state based on the distribution of regional compliances and resistances separating them. Although volume is a critical determinant of cardiac output, the changes in vascular volume alter cardiac output over a much smaller range than often appreciated. This is partly because of the limited capacity to increase the end-diastolic volume of the ventricles, but also because the volume is distributed throughout the vasculature and a smaller percent of the total volume given goes to the venous compartment, which is upstream from the right heart. Furthermore, decreases in left ventricular function relative to right ventricular function result in a greater proportion of the volume going to the pulmonary venous compartments and have a greater potential to increase pulmonary edema. Use of fluid to augment cardiac output needs to be considered in the context of left and right ventricular function and reserves in ventricular filling as well as the distribution of resistances and compliances in the vasculature.

References

1. Starling EH (1918) The Linacre Lecture of the Law of the Heart. Longmans, Green & Co, London
2. Magder S, De Varennes B (1998) Clinical death and the measurement of stressed vascular volume. Crit Care Med 26:1061–1064
3. Rothe CF (1983) Reflex control of veins and vascular capacitance. Physiol Rev 63:1281–1295
4. Sagawa K (1978) The ventricular pressure-volume diagram revisited. Circ Res 43:677–687
5. Magder S, Veerassamy S, Bates JH (2009) A further analysis of why pulmonary venous pressure rises after the onset of LV dysfunction. J Appl Physiol 106:81–90
6. Magder S, Guerard B (2012) Heart-lung interactions and pulmonary buffering: Lessons from a computational modeling study. Respir Physiol Neurobiol 182:60–70
7. Deschamps A, Magder S (1994) Effects of heat stress on vascular capacitance. Am J Physiol 266:H2122–H2129
8. Deschamps A, Magder S (1992) Baroreflex control of regional capacitance and blood flow distribution with or without alpha adrenergic blockade. J Appl Physiol 263:H1755–H1763
9. Deschamps A, Fournier A, Magder S (1994) Influence of neuropeptide Y on regional vascular capacitance in dogs. Am J Physiol 266:H165–H170
10. Green JF (1987) Fundamental Cardiovascular and Pulmonary Physiology, 2nd edn. Lea and Febiger, Philadelphia
11. Guyton AC, Polizo D, Armstrong GG (1954) Mean circulatory filling pressure measured immediately after cessation of heart pumping. Am J Physiol 179:261–267
12. Jellinek H, Krenn H, Oczenski W, Veit F, Schwarz S, Fitzgerald RD (2000) Influence of positive airway pressure on the pressure gradient for venous return in humans. J Appl Physiol 88:926–932

13. Schipke JD, Heusch G, Sanii AP, Gams E, Winter J (2003) Static filling pressure in patients during induced ventricular fibrillation. Am J Physiol Heart Circ Physiol 285(6):H2510–H2515
14. Parkin WG, Leaning MS (2008) Therapeutic control of the circulation. J Clin Monit Comput 22:391–400
15. Parkin WG (1999) Volume state control – a new approach. Crit Care Resusc 1:311–21
16. Persichini R, Silva S, Teboul JL et al (2012) Effects of norepinephrine on mean systemic pressure and venous return in human septic shock. Crit Care Med 40:3146–3153
17. Rothe CF, Drees JA (1976) Vascular capacitance and fluid shifts in dogs during prolonged hemorrhagic hypotension. Circ Res 38:347–356
18. Magder SA (2012) The ups and downs of heart rate. Crit Care Med 40(1):239–45
19. Shrier I, Magder S (1993) Response of arterial resistance and critical closing pressure to change in perfusion pressure in canine hindlimb. Am J Physiol 265:H1939–H1945
20. Shrier I, Hussain SNA, Magder SA (1993) Carotid sinus stimulation influences both arterial resistance and critical closing pressure of the isolated hindlimb vascular bed. Am J Physiol 33:H1560–H1566
21. Magder S (2013) Is all on the level? Hemodynamics during supine versus prone ventilation. Am J Respir Crit Care Med 188:1390–1391
22. Permutt S, Riley S (1963) Hemodynamics of collapsible vessels with tone: the vascular waterfall. J Appl Physiol 18:924–932
23. Magder S, Scharf SM (2001) Venous return. In: Scharf SM, Pinsky MR, Magder SA (eds) Respiratory-Circulatory Interactions in Health and Diseas, 2nd edn. Marcel Dekker Inc, New York, pp 93–112
24. Magder S (2011) Hemodynamic monitoring in the mechanically ventilated patient. Curr Opin Crit Care 17:36–42
25. Magder S (2010) Mechanical interactions between the respiratory and circulatory systems. In: Bradley TD, Floras JS (eds) Sleep Apnea: Implications in Ccardiovascular and Cerebrovascular Disease. Informa Health Care USA, Inc, New York, pp 40–60
26. Magder SA, Lichtenstein S, Adelman AG (1983) Effects of negative pleural pressure on left ventricular hemodynamics. Am J Cardiol 52:588–593
27. Jansen JR, Maas JJ, Pinsky MR (2010) Bedside assessment of mean systemic filling pressure. Curr Opin Crit Care 16:231–236
28. Maas JJ, Geerts BF, van den Berg PC, Pinsky MR, Jansen JR (2009) Assessment of venous return curve and mean systemic filling pressure in postoperative cardiac surgery patients. Crit Care Med 37:912–918
29. Magder S (2012) An approach to hemodynamic monitoring: Guyton at the beside. Crit Care 16:236–243
30. Guyton AC (1955) Determination of cardiac output by equating venous return curves with cardiac response curves. Physiol Rev 35:123–129
31. Fessler HE, Brower RG, Wise RA, Permutt S (1992) Effects of positive end-expiratory pressure on the gradient for venous return. Am Rev Respir Dis 146:4–10

Clinical Implications from Dynamic Modeling of Crystalloid Fluids

R. G. Hahn

Introduction

The role of colloid fluid is increasingly being questioned as the cornerstone of volume resuscitation, so many anesthetists and intensive care physicians are turning to crystalloid electrolyte solutions with the hope of improving patient outcomes. Clinicians may, therefore, be surprised to find that virtually no information about the clinical pharmacology of these fluids is to be found in medical textbooks. To allow optimal dosing and timing of crystalloid infusions there is a need for data on their distribution and elimination, as well as about adverse effects and limitations.

The understanding of how these fluids behave in the body is hampered by a conservative attachment to static study methods that disregard the effect of *time* on the assessment. Dynamic study models are much more informative and also provide more assistance with regard to how crystalloid fluid therapy can be optimized.

This review aims to illustrate what can be gained from applying a dynamic study model instead of maintaining a static view on the turnover of crystalloid fluids.

The Static Model

Crystalloid fluid is usually described as being evenly distributed in the extracellular fluid space, which amounts to 15 liters in an adult male weighing 75 kg. Distribution across this space is assumed to occur almost immediately because the capillaries are remarkably permeable to water. As the plasma volume is about 3 liters, the fluid efficiency (plasma volume expansion divided by the infused volume) is said to be 0.2. The conclusion usually made is that five units of crystalloid have to be infused to expand the plasma volume by one unit. The picture sketched above dominates

R. G. Hahn ✉
Research Unit, Södertälje Hospital, Södertälje; and the Department of Anesthesiology, Faculty of Health Sciences, Linköping University, Linköping, Sweden
e-mail: r.hahn@telia.com

J.-L. Vincent (ed.), *Annual Update in Intensive Care and Emergency Medicine 2015*,
DOI 10.1007/978-3-319-13761-2_24

medical textbooks and has also been promoted by a long range of scientists from the 1960 s [1] to the present day [2].

This *static* view of the behavior of crystalloid fluid in the body is based on tracer studies, by which an agent (sometimes radioactive) is injected into the body, its concentration measured repeatedly, and the volume of distribution extrapolated by backward extrapolation to zero time. Tracer methods must be applied during a period of steady state with regard to fluid distribution, which is hardly ever at hand when used by an anesthetist or an intensivist. If there is no steady state, the backward extrapolation will provide an erroneous answer. In short, if plasma volume increases gradually during the measurement period, the indicated plasma volume will be too small. If there is a decrease, which is a more likely scenario, the extrapolation will indicate too large a volume.

Tracers with a rapid elimination are cardiac output-dependent, as the time from injection to the site of elimination (usually the liver) is variable. Correction for this confounder is never performed, despite the fact that fluid infusions change cardiac output. In these cases, extrapolation to time zero provides a too small plasma volume. The average magnitude of this error seems to be 25% [3].

More serious objections to static methods include that they do not acknowledge changes in the relationship between plasma volume expansion and infused volume over time. This can result in suboptimal or frankly erroneous advice about how crystalloid should be used.

For more than 50 years, pharmacologists have understood that a single plasma concentration of a drug given intravenously tells us very little about the appropriate dosing and timing of clinically used medications. Neither would the drug industry or regulatory authorities dream about using anything other than *dynamic* models when analyzing and simulating the physiological behavior of their products.

The Dynamic Model

The dynamic approach is particularly important when studying crystalloid fluids, as they have a marked distribution function as well as a situation-dependent and a quite variable turnover time. This presentation is based mainly on information provided by a dynamic model called volume kinetics. This model is a pharmacokinetic analysis of serial measurements of the hemodilution during and after a fluid infusion, sometimes together with the urinary excretion [4]. About 50 studies using this methodology have been published so far. The vast majority of them deal with how crystalloid fluids behave in healthy volunteers and during anesthesia and surgery.

The key model is shown in Fig. 1. The key assumption of volume kinetics, except for those given by the model, is that the hemoglobin molecules sampled from a vein or artery are evenly distributed in a well-confined body fluid space on average during an experiment, which usually lasts from 150–240 min. The existence of a blood volume *per se* is not a prerequisite for the model.

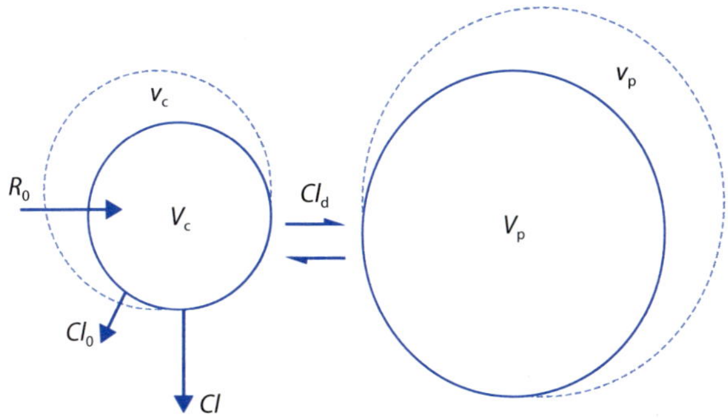

Fig. 1 Kinetic model for analysis of the distribution and elimination of crystalloid infusion fluids. Fluid is infused at a rate R_0 into the plasma volume V_c, which is then expanded to v_c. Fluid is eliminated by a baseline rate Cl_0 and a dilution-dependent clearance mechanism, *Cl*. Fluid is also exchanged with the interstitial fluid space, V_p, at a rate governed by the intercompartmental clearance, Cl_d

The Distribution Function

Volume kinetics shows that distribution of infused crystalloid fluid from the plasma to the interstitial fluid space does not occur immediately if the whole body is considered. The distribution half-life is 8 min, which is quite constant in conscious volunteers and anesthetized patients [5–7]. As a distribution requires four half-lives to be completed, the intensivist can assume that the boosting effect of distribution on the plasma volume has subsided 30 min after an infusion has been turned off.

The impact of distribution on fluid efficiency is profound. As can be seen in Fig. 2, the efficiency is close to 100% when a crystalloid infusion begins, which is no surprise because the fluid is infused intravenously. As the infusion continues, the efficiency decreases, but after 30 min it still amounts to 50%. For an infusion lasting for the average surgical operating time (45 min), the average fluid efficiency is 50–70%, which is three times higher than we have learned from the textbooks. This view was corroborated by a multiple regression model applied every 10 min during 30 operations performed under general anesthesia, which showed that 60% of the infused crystalloid fluid still remained in the bloodstream [8].

This means that a crystalloid fluid is a more efficient plasma volume expander as long as the infusion continues, which is the case during most surgeries and in intensive care. When the infusion is turned off, the plasma volume expansion subsides and about 30 min later it arrives at the figures mentioned in our medical textbooks. There is no evidence that the distribution function illustrated in Fig. 2 is markedly changed because the infusion volume differs (within reasonable limits).

This type of simulation, based on volume kinetic parameters, can also be used to show that a bolus has lower efficiency than a continuous infusion. The same conclusion is valid for all drugs that have an exponential distribution and elimination, which is virtually all of the drugs we know about.

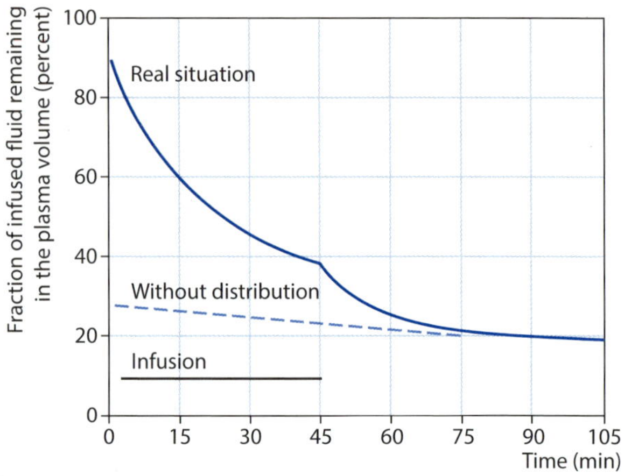

Fig. 2 Fluid efficiency during and after a crystalloid infusion. Note the profound effect of distribution on the plasma volume expansion

Altered Rate of Distribution

Volume kinetics also shows that distribution of crystalloid fluid occurs much more slowly when there has been a sudden reduction in the arterial pressure. A typical situation is induction of anesthesia. Due to blunting of the sympathetic system, the capillary hydrostatic pressure in the Starling equation decreases along with the arterial pressure, which promotes accumulation of infused fluid in the bloodstream.

A decrease in the mean arterial pressure (MAP) by 20% is sufficient to arrest the distribution [4] and further reductions even promote fluid efficiency exceeding 100% [9]. This reduction is calculated from a pre-induction hemodynamic steady state to the new steady state, which is reached approximately 30 min after anesthesia has been induced (Fig. 3). A very important conclusion can be made from such data, namely, that there is no reason to infuse a colloid fluid to compensate for the vasodilatation that occurs during induction of anesthesia. A crystalloid fluid is very effective in this situation.

The fluid efficiency decreases gradually as more fluid is infused until a new Starling equilibrium is reached, which perhaps require 15–30 min if the crystalloid fluid infusion is continued. Measurements performed during ongoing surgery show that the ordinary distribution half-life of approximately 8 min has then been regained [6].

Inflammation increases the capillary permeability and might be a condition associated with more rapid distribution of crystalloid fluid. Pre-eclamptic women had twice as fast a distribution and elimination of Ringer's acetate compared to gestation-age matched pregnant controls [10]. The glycocalyx breakdown associated with inflammation is currently widely promoted as the cause of rapid colloid fluid distribution [11]. Hardly any dynamic data in whole-body humans quantify the effect of inflammation on the distribution and elimination of infusion fluids. On the other hand, data on how much the capillary leakage of colloid macromolecules (such as albumin) increases in sepsis have been available since the 1980 s [12], the rate correlating closely with the reduction in the plasma volume expansion [13].

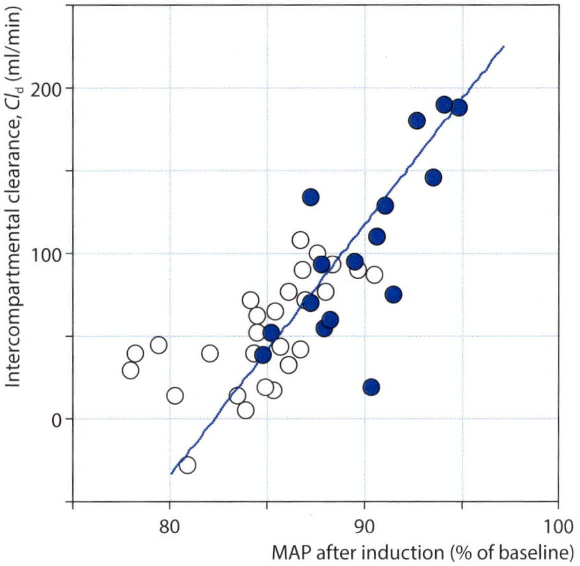

Fig. 3 Distribution of crystalloid fluid occurs more slowly when the arterial pressure has decreased. Zero distribution ($Cl_d = 0$) implies that the fluid efficiency is 100%. Data from [32]. *Open circles*: general anesthesia. *Closed circles*: epidural anesthesia

Volume of Distribution

The volume of the central compartment (V_c) in volume kinetics usually varies between 2.5 and 4 liters (Fig. 1). The smaller volume is found during anesthesia and the higher is in conscious volunteers. V_c is believed to correspond to the plasma volume, possibly with the addition of the highly permeable perivascular spaces in the liver.

The peripheral fluid volume (V_p) is not 12–13 liters, which one may guess after reading tracer studies of the physiological fluid spaces. Measurements with volume kinetics show that V_p is about 6–8 liters. The difference can be explained by the fact that tracers do not expand the fluid spaces into which they are distributed. However, volume kinetics indicates the size of the volumes that actually become expanded by fluid. Some parts of the interstitium, such as the skull, bones, and internal organs with tight capsules, cannot be expanded. This non-expandable part of the interstitial fluid space apparently makes up 1/3 of its total volume.

After distribution, the amount of crystalloid fluid that resides in the plasma is simply $V_c/(V_c + V_p)$, i. e., approximately one third.

Hemorrhage

The recommendation to replace blood loss by five times the hemorrhaged volume with crystalloid fluid also stems from the tracer studies that do not distinguish between expandable and non-expandable body fluid spaces. The clinically adopted 3 : 1 rule is more correct, although there are two reasons to suggest why this rule should be used with caution.

Fig. 4 Plasma volume expansion when Ringer's acetate is used to replace a hemorrhage of 450 ml in the proportion 3 : 1. Titration is needed to avoid hypervolemia. Based on volume kinetic data from [5]

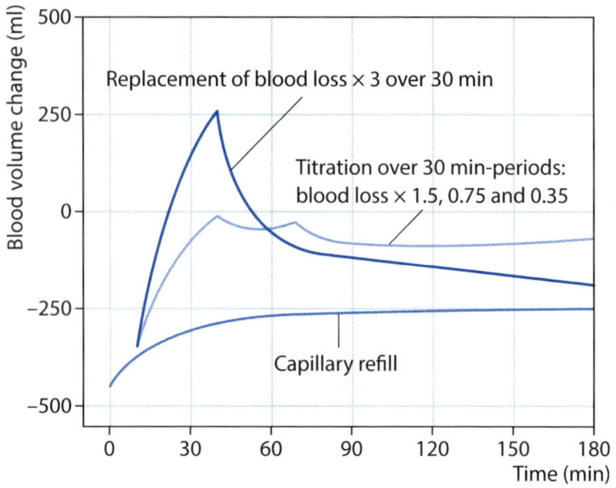

First, the impact of distribution on the plasma volume necessitates a titration procedure if hypervolemia is to be avoided. To maintain normovolemia, simulations show that the bled volume should be replaced by 1.5 times the bled volume over 30 min, reduced by 50% over each of the other two subsequent 30-min periods (Fig. 4). To overlook the effect of distribution is frankly dangerous in situations where the hemorrhage has not yet been arrested surgically, as any increase in blood flow rate might cause rebleeding and, possibly, death [14].

Second, the 3 : 1 rule disregards the effect of capillary refill on the plasma volume. This is a spontaneous process acting to restore the blood volume after hemorrhage. In sheep, 35% of the hemorrhaged volume was corrected within 30 min, regardless of whether the bleeding caused hypotension to develop [15]. The restoration follows an exponential function, and the entire process is not completed until the next day [1]. However, capillary refill might not operate as well during general anesthesia as in conscious patients because of the blunting of the sympathetic nervous system [15].

Capillary refill makes it sufficient to replace blood loss with only twice the bled amount with crystalloid fluid, provided that the patient has a reasonably well preserved sympathetic tone and the volume loading starts with some delay (15–30 min) after the hemorrhage. This can be shown by volume kinetics, and has been corroborated by physiological methods in conscious volunteers [16].

Elimination of Crystalloid Fluid

There is one additional factor affecting crystalloid fluid efficiency in volunteers and during anesthesia and surgery, and that is elimination. This factor reduces the fluid efficiency after distribution is complete to the 15–25% percentage often reported in tracer studies.

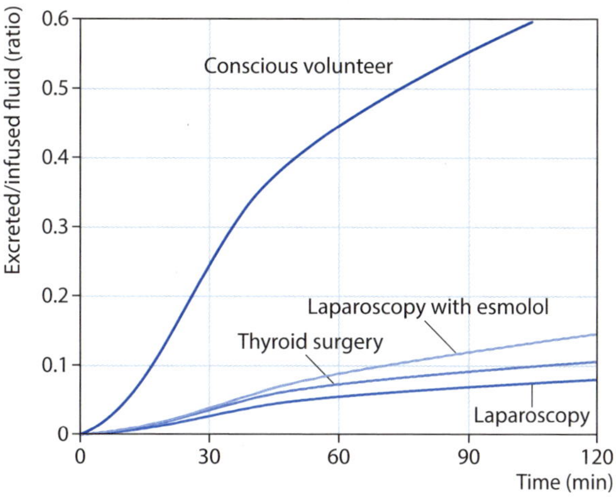

Fig. 5 Elimination of crystalloid fluid is greatly retarded during surgery. Computer simulations of infusions with 25 ml/kg of Ringer's acetate over 30 min based on volume kinetic data from [5, 6, 17, 19, 22]

The rate of crystalloid fluid elimination varies enormously. Half-lives from less than 10 min to approximately 500 min have been reported. Crystalloid fluid is fairly quickly eliminated in conscious volunteers, and the half-life is usually 15–30 min [4, 5]. If two liters are infused rapidly, more than half is then eliminated within one hour. This is very different from the situation during surgery, where the anesthetist is content when recording a urinary excretion of 100 ml per hour, i. e., only 10% as much [6, 17]. Hence, there is a remarkable reduction in the rate of elimination, which is not fully explained to date (Fig. 5). Here we discuss a few more or less well-known mechanisms.

The elimination of crystalloid fluid is increased by alpha-1-adrenergic receptor stimulation and inhibited by beta-1-adrenergic receptor stimulation [18]. Infusion of drugs acting directly or indirectly on these receptors and during surgery results in tripled urinary excretion, but this is still far from being the same as in conscious volunteers [19].

Isoflurane anesthesia without surgery in volunteers reduced the elimination of crystalloid fluid by 50%, probably by virtue of lowered arterial pressure and increased plasma concentrations of renin and aldosterone [20]. Although vasopressin may play a role in fluid retention during surgery, excretion of this hormone is not stimulated by isoflurane anesthesia alone [20].

Animal experiments show that even a short period (5 min) of bleeding-induced hypotension reduces the rate of crystalloid fluid elimination by 50% when assessed over the subsequent 3-hour period [21]. Non-hypotensive hemorrhage of up to 900 ml in volunteers had the same effect [5].

The slow elimination of fluid by urinary excretion makes ambitious administration of crystalloid fluid unnecessary during anesthesia and surgery. How much then should be infused to maintain normovolemia? A simulation based on kinetic data from thyroid surgery under isoflurane anesthesia [6] showed that steady state for the plasma volume was maintained if the infusion rate of Ringers's acetate was 1.85 ml/kg/hour (unpublished calculation). Larger volumes are needed if bleeding is more than minimal.

Adverse Effects

The three principal crystalloid electrolyte solutions on the market are Ringer's lactate, Ringer's acetate, and isotonic saline. In recent years, PlasmaLyte, which is a modification of Ringer's acetate, has also become widely available. There is no evidence that the rate of distribution differs between the crystalloid fluids, but saline has a longer half-life than the two Ringer solutions [22]. The reason appears to be renal vasoconstriction due to the surplus of chloride ions, which also causes mild metabolic acidosis [23]. Saline gives rise to more adverse events when infused in volunteers [24] and during surgery [25], and prolongs the time of acidosis when a crystalloid is used to reverse diabetic ketoacidosis [26]. Although used more widely than the Ringer solutions, the drawbacks of isotonic saline make this classical composition a second-line choice for fluid resuscitation [27]. The only situations where saline holds its place as the first-choice crystalloid is after vomiting and in hyponatremic patients.

There is only one study about interactions between infusion fluids. In volunteers, the elimination of Ringer's acetate was greatly retarded if preceded by hydroxyethyl starch 130/0.4 (Voluven), even when the time lapse between the two infusions was as long as 100 min [28]. Possible explanations include that the saline base of Voluven causes renal vasoconstriction, but a contributing factor could also be the rise in plasma colloid osmotic pressure (+10%) caused by Voluven.

The Ringer solutions contain calcium, which may cause coagulation in the infusion line if given together with citrated erythrocytes. PlasmaLyte avoids this problem by being devoid of calcium. PlasmaLyte also has an osmolality of 295 mosmol/kg while the two Ringer solutions are slightly hypo-osmotic (approximately 270 mosmol/kg), which makes them questionable for use in head trauma patients.

The two buffers in the Ringer solutions, lactate and acetate, are both vasodilators in high concentrations, but differ very little in clinical practice. The main difference is that acetate is a slightly more effective buffer than is lactate.

Overuse of the crystalloid fluids causes adverse effects. More than three liters prolongs the gastrointestinal recovery time [29]. The risk of pulmonary edema, poor wound healing, and infection is increased when six liters have been provided [30]. More than 10 liters on the day of surgery further increases the risk of pulmonary edema, which can be fatal and even occur several days after the surgery [31].

There is no study on the volume kinetic properties of crystalloid fluid in the intensive care setting. This is unfortunate, because crystalloid therapy is very common and the timing and dosing are likely to affect outcome.

Conclusion

Volume kinetics is a dynamic method of studying the turnover of infusion fluids that provides much more information than static methods based on tracer techniques. Dynamic analyses show that distribution of a crystalloid fluid requires 30 min to be completed, which means that the plasma volume is expanded by 60–70% of the infused amount during an ongoing infusion. This differs greatly from the 20% mentioned in medical textbooks. The marked effect of distribution emphasizes that crystalloids need to be titrated to avoid hypervolemia when used to replace blood loss.

Distribution is completely arrested when there is arterial hypotension, which means that all the infused fluid remains in the bloodstream. The elimination half-life of crystalloid fluid is 15–30 min in conscious volunteers but 10 times longer during anesthesia and surgery, which highlights that the body's capacity to excrete a fluid overload is very poor in this setting. A steady state plasma volume during ongoing surgery with minimum evaporation and hemorrhage is maintained by crystalloid fluid infused at a rate of 1.85 ml/kg/hour.

References

1. Moore FD, Dagher FJ, Boyden CM, Lee CJ, Lyons JH (1966) Hemorrhage in normal man: I. Distribution and dispersal of saline infusions following acute blood loss. Ann Surg 163:485–504
2. Jacob M, Chappell D, Hofmann-Kiefer K et al (2012) The intravascular volume effect of Ringer's lactate is below 20%: a prospective study in humans. Crit Care 16:R86
3. Polidori D, Rowley C (2014) Optimal back-extrapolation method for estimating plasma volume in humans using the indocyanine green dilution method. Theor Biol Med Model 11:33
4. Hahn RG (2010) Volume kinetics of infusion fluids. Anesthesiology 113:470–481
5. Drobin D, Hahn RG (1999) Volume kinetics of Ringer's solution in hypovolemic volunteers. Anesthesiology 90:81–91
6. Ewaldsson CA, Hahn RG (2005) Kinetics and extravascular retention of acetated Ringer's solution during isoflurane and propofol anesthesia for thyroid surgery. Anesthesiology 103:460–469
7. Törnudd M, Hahn RG, Zdolsek JH (2014) Fluid distribution kinetics during cardiopulmonary bypass. Clinics 69:535–541
8. Hahn RG (1998) Volume effect of Ringer's solution in the blood during general anaesthesia. Eur J Anaesthesiol 15:427–432
9. Li Y, He R, Ying X, Hahn RG (2014) Dehydration, haemodynamics and fluid volume optimization after induction of general anaesthesia. Clinics (in press)
10. Drobin RG, Hahn RG (2004) Distribution and elimination of crystalloid fluid in pre-eclampsia. Clin Sci 106:307–313
11. Chappell D, Jacob M (2014) Role of the glycocalyx in fluid management: small things matter. Best Pract Res Clin Anaesthesiol 28:227–234
12. Fleck A, Raines G, Hawker F et al (1985) Increased vascular permeability: a major cause of hypoalbuminaemia in disease and injury. Lancet 1:781–784
13. Hedin A, Hahn RG (2005) Volume expansion and plasma protein clearance during intravenous infusion of 5% albumin and autologous plasma. Clin Sci 106:217–224
14. Hahn RG (2013) Fluid therapy in uncontrolled hemorrhage – what experimental models have taught us. Acta Anaesthesiol Scand 57:16–28
15. Hahn RG, Brauer L, Rodhe P, Svensén CH, Prough DS (2006) Isoflurane inhibits compensatory intravascular volume expansion after hemorrhage in sheep. Anesth Analg 103:350–358
16. Riddez L, Hahn RG, Brismar B, Strandberg Å, Svensén C, Hedenstierna G (1997) Central and regional hemodynamics during acute hypovolemia and volume substitution in volunteers. Crit Care Med 25:635–640

17. Olsson J, Svensén CH, Hahn RG (2004) The volume kinetics of acetated Ringer's solution during laparoscopic cholecystectomy. Anesth Analg 99:1854–1860
18. Ewaldsson CA, Vane LA, Kramer GC, Hahn RG (2006) Adrenergic drugs alter both the fluid kinetics and the hemodynamic responses to volume expansion in sheep. J Surg Res 131:7–14
19. Li Y, Zhu HB, Zheng X, Chen HJ, Shao L, Hahn RG (2012) Low doses of esmolol and phenylephrine act as diuretics during intravenous anesthesia. Crit Care 16:R18
20. Norberg Å, Hahn RG, Li H et al (2007) Population volume kinetics predicts retention of 0.9% saline infused in awake and isoflurane-anesthetized volunteers. Anesthesiology 107:24–32
21. Norberg A, Brauer KI, Prough DS et al (2005) Volume turnover kinetics of fluid shifts after hemorrhage, fluid infusion, and the combination of hemorrhage and fluid infusion in sheep. Anesthesiology 102:985–994
22. Drobin D, Hahn RG (2002) Kinetics of isotonic and hypertonic plasma volume expanders. Anesthesiology 96:1371–1380
23. Chowdhury AH, Cox EF, Francis ST, Lobo DN (2012) A randomized, controlled, double-blind crossover study on the effects of 2-L infusions of 0.9% saline and Plasma-Lyte 148 on renal blood flow velocity and renal cortical tissue perfusion in healthy volunteers. Ann Surg 256:18–24
24. Williams EL, Hildebrand KL, McCormick SA, Bedel MJ (1999) The effect of intravenous lactated Ringer's solution versus 0.9% sodium chloride solution on serum osmolality in human volunteers. Anesth Analg 88:999–1003
25. Wilkes NJ, Woolf R, Mutch M et al (2001) The effects of balanced versus saline-based hetastarch and crystalloid solutions on acid-base and electrolyte status and gastric mucosal perfusion in elderly surgical patients. Anesth Analg 93:811–816
26. Chua H-R, Venkatesh B, Stachowski E et al (2012) Plasma-Lyte 148 vs 0.9% saline for fluid resuscitation in diabetic ketoacidosis. J Crit Care 27:138–145
27. Hahn RG (2014) Should anaesthetists stop infusing isotonic saline? Br J Anaesth 112:4–6
28. Hahn RG, Bergek C, Gebäck T, Zdolsek J (2013) Interactions between the volume effects of hydroxyethyl starch 130/0.4 and Ringer's acetate. Crit Care 17:R104
29. Varadhan KK, Lobo DN (2010) Symposium 3: A meta-analysis of randomised controlled trials of intravenous fluid therapy in major elective open abdominal surgery: getting the balance right. Proc Nutr Soc 69:488–498
30. Brandstrup B, Tonnesen H, Beier-Holgersen R et al (2003) Effects of intravenous fluid restriction on postoperative complications: comparison of two perioperative fluid regimens. A randomized assessor-blinded multicenter trial. Ann Surg 238:641–648
31. Arieff AI (1999) Fatal postoperative pulmonary edema. Pathogenesis and literature review. Chest 115:1371–1377
32. Li Y, Zhu S, Hahn RG (2007) The kinetics of Ringer's solution in young and elderly patients during induction of general and epidural anesthesia. Acta Anaesth Scand 51:880–887

Part VIII
Renal Injury

Urinary Electrolyte Monitoring in the Critically Ill: Revisiting Renal Physiology

P. Caironi, T. Langer, and M. Ferrari

Introduction

The kidney, being one of the most fascinating and commonly studied organs within human physiology, has a crucial role in maintaining the homeostasis of our organism from several different perspectives, from clearing of cellular catabolism products, to body fluids and electrolyte content regulation, hemodynamic stability and acid-base equilibrium [1]. Consequently, despite the existence of many strategies to support its function, the renal system is often the focus of our attention during the clinical management of the critically ill, because its function is frequently altered in this category of patients [2].

Looking with more detail at the physiology regulating the renal system, we need to recognize that it has a peculiarity that differentiates it from other organs, i.e., the production of a 'waste matter', urine, which may be collected, analyzed and examined, and that can provide information on what the kidney is doing. Measurements of urinary volumes, electrolyte concentration, pH, osmolality, and, in recent years, biomarkers, have been the key features of the understanding of renal physiology, as well as a crucial aspect in the diagnosis and management of a variety of diseases, both local as well as systemic [3]. Nonetheless, as renal function is far from being entirely unveiled, and normal ranges for urinary parameters are widely variable and fixed with uncertainty, the routine assessment of urinary parameters in clinical practice has not yet obtained proper attention [4]. Such considerations gain more importance when considering critically ill patients, and, in general, patients in 'emergency' conditions. Apart from a few studies investigating urinary electrolyte concentrations in relation to alterations in acid-base equilibrium [5] or the effects of diuretic therapies [6], scarce data are available on the potential role of urinary monitoring for the clinical management of the critically ill [7].

P. Caironi ✉ · T. Langer · M. Ferrari
Dipartimento di Fisiopatologia Medico-Chirurgica e dei Trapianti, Fondazione IRCCS Ca' Granda, Ospedale Maggiore Policlinico, Università degli Studi di Milano, Milan, Italy
e-mail: pietro.caironi@unimi.it

J.-L. Vincent (ed.), *Annual Update in Intensive Care and Emergency Medicine 2015*,
DOI 10.1007/978-3-319-13761-2_25

In the last few years, we have developed a urinary analyzer (Kidney Instant Monitoring – K.IN.G.®, Kardia s.r.l., Milan, Italy), which allows quasi-continuous and non-invasive measurements of urinary pH, and urinary concentration of sodium (Na^+), chloride (Cl^-), potassium (K^+), and ammonium (NH_4^+) [8]. Although still a prototype applied only in experimental settings, this monitoring system has allowed us to zoom in on several aspects of renal function in critically ill patients, unveiling, in our opinion, important features of its physiological and pathophysiological function. In this chapter, we will first summarize and highlight some principles of renal physiology that appear crucial for the understanding of urinary monitoring in the critically ill, with a particular attention to the renal handling of Na^+, Cl^-, and K^+. We will then review the mechanisms regulating the renal production of NH_4^+, and the potential clinical relevance of monitoring urinary anion gap. Finally, we will discuss the physiological role of the renal system in regulating the effective circulating blood volume, and the possible role of urinary monitoring in assessing its adequacy.

Physiological Principles of Urinary Electrolyte Excretion and Monitoring

Considering the physiological principles that regulate renal function, two main premises are necessary. First, among the different objectives that the renal system normally accomplishes, the regulation of acid-base equilibrium is one of the most crucial tasks of the kidney, when dealing with critically ill patients [4]. According to Stewart's approach to acid-base equilibrium, the renal system plays a major role in homeostasis by actively regulating one of three independent determinants: the strong ion difference (SID), defined as the difference between the strong cations (mainly Na^+ and K^+) and the strong anions (mainly Cl^-) [9]. In fact, by actively regulating Na^+, K^+ and Cl^- urinary excretion, it provides the only way of modifying their concentration in the extracellular fluid (and, therefore, in plasma) [10]. This property may potentially have a great impact on the compensatory mechanisms reacting to the increase in hydrogen ion (H^+) concentration during metabolic acidosis [11]. In fact, in the attempt to compensate for such an increase, the system will mainly react to modify the independent determinants of acid-base equilibrium that are adjustable, i.e., carbon dioxide content (through alveolar ventilation) and the SID (through the renal system).

Second, the renal system has the peculiar characteristic of excreting a highly rearranged and 'concentrated' fluid, as compared to plasma. In normal conditions, starting from about 120 ml/min of plasma filtrate, only about 1 ml/min 'remains' as urine at the end of the renal system. This characteristic has two main consequences. On one hand, it underlines the low efficiency, in terms of rapidity, of the renal system to restore alterations occurring at the level of plasma. In fact, given the great size of the extracellular compartment (about 16 l), even small variations in the concentration of a strong ion at the level of plasma will actually correspond to a great modification in its absolute amount. In order to restore plasma SID to a normal level, the renal system should excrete (or reabsorb) the quantity in excess (or deficit) of that strong ion through the urine, which, in contrast to the extracellular compartment, has a very low volume (about 1.5 l). On the other hand, the highly concentrative power of the kidney grants it the peculiar characteristic of working as an 'amplifier' of what is occurring at the level of the plasma. In fact, although the time the renal system needs to determine a change in plasma is long, at the level of urine every small variation in excretion of a strong ion will be reflected by a great variation in its concentration. Thus, when the renal system starts reacting to a process occurring in the plasma, although that reaction will not immediately be 'visible' *per se* at the level of plasma, it will be in the urine.

Renal Sodium and Chloride Handling

Classically, the kidney is considered one of the main organs responsible for the regulation of acid-base equilibrium, mainly through its ability to excrete about 100 mEq of H^+ per day (which is the daily load of H^+ in a healthy human), and to maintain plasma bicarbonate (HCO_3^-) concentration constant [12]. These objectives are achieved on the one hand through the excretion of H^+ either as urinary buffer molecules (so-called titratable acidity) or as transformed in urinary NH_4^+ [13], and on the other through the reabsorption of most of the filtered HCO_3^- [14].

Considering Stewart's theory on acid-base equilibrium [15], the kidney actively acts to regulate pH by its ability to modify plasma SID (or the SID of the extracellular space) through a fine regulation of the excretion of the main electrolytes determining plasma SID, i.e., Na^+, Cl^- and K^+ [10]. At the same time, it is worth noting that electrical neutrality must hold true for every aqueous solution, therefore also for urine. It follows, therefore, that every time a cation is excreted with urine, it should be associated with an anion. Nonetheless, as long as a strong cation (such as Na^+) is excreted in urine associated with a strong anion (such as Cl^-), the ability of the renal system to modify the plasma SID remains limited, although a slight increase in SID theoretically occurs. It follows, therefore, that to increase its efficiency in modifying the SID of the extracellular space, the kidney has only two possibilities: 1) to eliminate (or reabsorb) a strong cation (such as Na^+) associated with a weak anion (such as HCO_3^-); 2) to exchange a strong anion (for instance Cl^-) with a weak anion (such as HCO_3^-). This observation gains even more importance when considering that the renal system usually handles Na^+ and Cl^- excretion/reabsorption for most of the anatomical part of the nephron as associated with each other [16]. Nonetheless, as will see below, the kidney is able, in two particular segments of the nephron, to dissociate Na^+ excretion/reabsorption from that of Cl^-, exactly as we have discussed here, thereby finely regulating the SID of the extracellular space.

Let us therefore focus our attention first on the renal handling of Na^+ and Cl^-. Considering the entire nephron of a normal kidney, there are only two specific loci in which the kidney dissociates the reabsorption of Na^+ from that of Cl^-: 1) the proximal tubule, and 2) the distal collecting tubules, specifically in the B-type in-

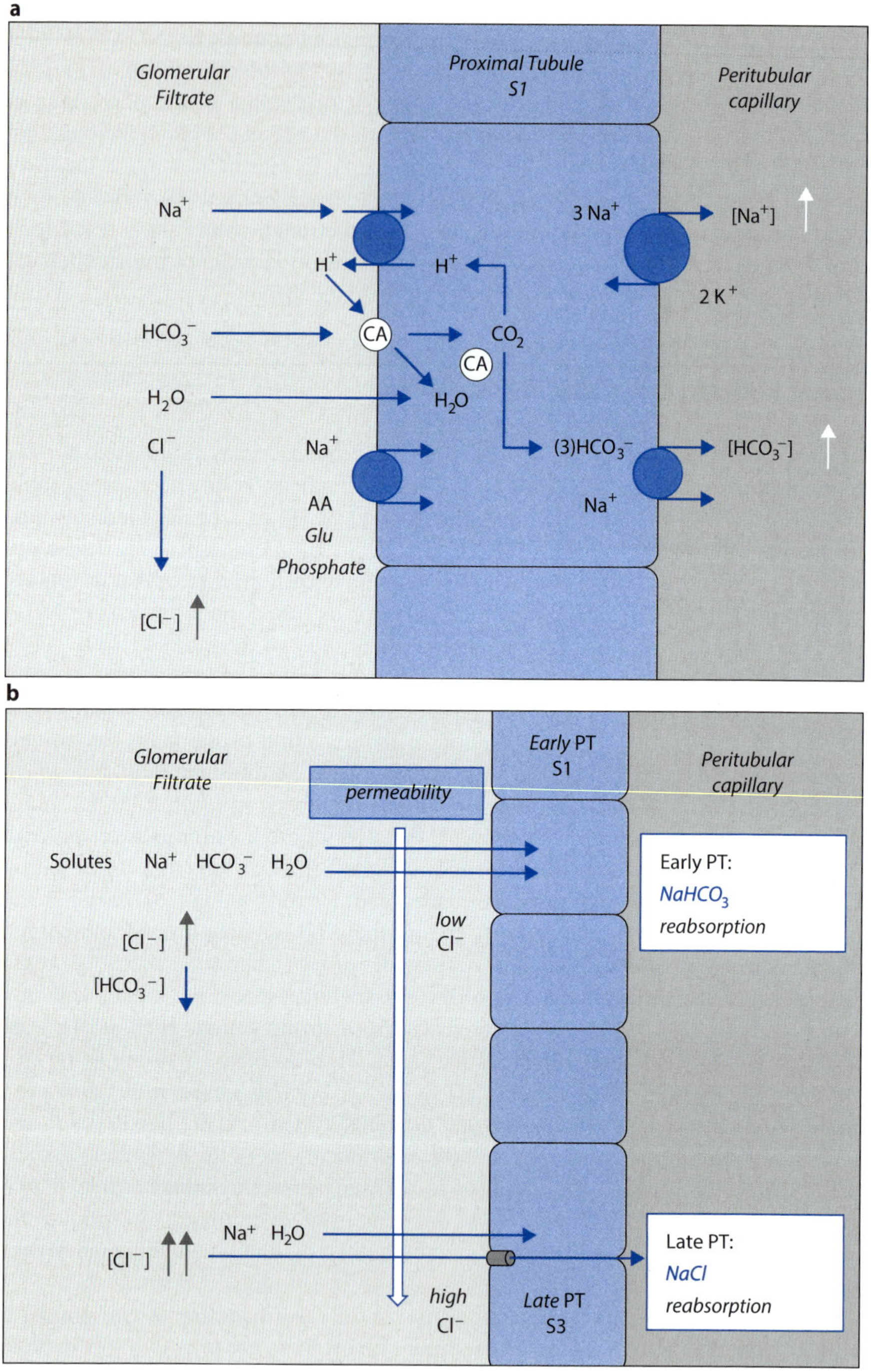
a
Glomerular Filtrate
Proximal Tubule S1
Peritubular capillary
Na+
H+
H+
3 Na+
[Na+]
2 K+
HCO3−
CA
CO2
CA
H2O
H2O
Cl−
Na+
(3)HCO3−
[HCO3−]
AA
Glu
Phosphate
Na+
[Cl−]
b
Glomerular Filtrate
permeability
Early PT S1
Peritubular capillary
Solutes Na+ HCO3− H2O
Early PT: NaHCO3 reabsorption
low Cl−
[Cl−]
[HCO3−]
Na+ H2O
[Cl−]
Late PT: NaCl reabsorption
high Cl−
Late PT S3

Fig. 1 Mechanisms regulating sodium and chloride reabsorption in the proximal tubule. The figures shows the cellular mechanisms regulating Na^+ reabsorption in association with HCO_3^- and solutes in the first part (segment S1) of the proximal tubule (panel **a**), as well as the mechanisms regulating Na^+ reabsorption as associated with Cl^- in the last part (segment S3) of the proximal tubule (panel **b**). Of note, whereas in the first segment Na^+ is actively reabsorbed depending on the activity of the Na^+/K^+-ATPase pump, and Na^+/H^+ exchanger (NHE), in association with HCO_3^-, in the third segment, due to the progressive increase in the permeability of the luminal membrane to Cl^-, Na^+ is passively reabsorbed with Cl^-. See text for further details. PT: proximal tubule

tercalated cells. In healthy conditions, the main function of the proximal tubule is the reabsorption of about 55–60% of the filtrate (glomerular filtration rate [GFR]) [17]. To accomplish this objective, three specific processes mainly take place: First, active transport and reabsorption of Na^+; second, passive reabsorption of water and several solutes; third, active secretion of H^+ [18]. A further crucial aspect of the anatomical structure of the proximal tubule relies on the specific characteristics of its early part (segment S1), the early-convoluted segment, the middle part (segment S2), the late convoluted segment and early pars recta, and the last part (segment S3), the remaining portion of the pars recta. It is sufficient to remember here that these three different portions of the proximal tubule differ, in addition to other specific properties, in their permeability to Cl^- [19]. Consequently, whereas the first S1 segment is mainly characterized by the reabsorption of Na^+, HCO_3^-, and most of the filtered solutes, with the exception of Cl^-, the last S3 segment is characterized by intercellular tight junctions, which are permeable to Cl^-. Thus, while the initial part of the proximal tubule is responsible for the reabsorption of Na^+ associated with HCO_3^-, the last part is responsible for the reabsorption of Na^+ associated with Cl^- (see Fig. 1).

In more detail, the key process for the efficient reabsorption of water and solutes in the early proximal tubule is Na^+ entrance into the cell, which strictly depends on the following processes:

1) the activity of the Na^+/K^+-ATPase pump at the basolateral cell membrane, which actively maintains intracellular concentration of Na^+ equal to 20–30 mEq/l;
2) the action of co-transporters, which passively transport Na^+ associated with glucose, aminoacids and phosphate, into the cell;
3) the action of a Na^+/H^+ exchanger, promoting Na^+ reabsorption and H^+ excretion into the lumen, thereby ultimately leading to HCO_3^- reabsorption (see Fig. 1).

In parallel, the lesser absorption of Cl^- in the early part of the proximal tubule determines a progressive increase in Cl^- concentration within the tubular lumen, which subsequently determines a passive reabsorption of Cl^- associated with Na^+ (and water) in the last part of the proximal tubule through permeable tight junctions (segment S3) [20]. This process provides the rationale for an HCO_3-dependent NaCl reabsorption. As NaCl reabsorption in the last part of the proximal tubule is passive, thus strictly depending on the generation of a Cl-gradient from the tubular lumen to the peritubular capillaries, it follows that the lower the HCO_3^- filtered in the S1–S2 proximal tubule segments, the lower the hyperchloremia developing down to the S3 PT segment and the passive reabsorption of Cl^- will be. This is, actually, what may occur during the development of metabolic acidosis, in which the plasma concentration of HCO_3^- is reduced, and so is the filtered HCO_3^- concentration [21]. From Stewart's perspective, this is a mechanism by which the renal system reacts to the acidosis through the increase in urinary excretion of Cl^- (by reducing its reabsorption), thereby leading to an increase in plasma SID [10].

At the level of the distal collecting tubules, there are two different types of cells, with different properties: The principal cells, mainly responsible for Na^+ reabsorption associated with Cl^-, or exchanged with K^+ (due to aldosterone-sensitive K^+ channels) [22], and the intercalated cells [23]. Intercalated cells are characterized by the presence of two specific structures, which, according to the specific type (either A-type or B-type), have different polarities [24]. In type-A intercalated cells, a H^+-ATPase pump (or H^+/K^+-ATPase exchanger) excretes H^+ into the tubular lumen, whereas a Cl^-/HCO_3^- exchanger (pendrin) is responsible for HCO_3^- reabsorption into the peritubular capillaries, under the stimulation of acidemia and/or aldosterone. Type-B intercalated cells have a reverse polarity, thereby leading to the reabsorption of Cl^- as exchanged with HCO_3^- (Fig. 2). Overall, these types of cell (especially type-B intercalated cells) establish a second structure in which dissociation between Na^+ and Cl^+ reabsorption (or excretion) is possible.

Renal Potassium Handling

Differently to Na^+ and Cl^-, the total body content of K^+ is essentially stored in the intracellular space, amounting, in normal conditions, to about 50–55 mEq/kg body weight. The peculiar compartmentalization of K^+ depends strictly on the activity of Na^+/K^+-ATPase pumps, highly represented throughout the entire organism, which are able to maintain very low K^+ concentrations in the extracellular space by pumping Na^+ out of and K^+ into the cells in a 3 to 2 ratio [25].

The renal system plays a major role in the homeostasis of K^+ content and concentrations, being the most efficient way of excretion (through urine) and, therefore, balancing K^+ dietary intake (about 40–120 mEq/day). This function is mainly performed at the level of the distal collecting tubules, especially in the principle and intercalated cells [26]. In fact, while about 90% of the K^+ filtered is reabsorbed in the proximal tubule (with a passive mechanism) and in the loop of Henle (active process), in the principle and intercalated cells the active reabsorption of Na^+ (under the stimulation of aldosterone) takes place with an exchange with either H^+ or K^+, which are, therefore, excreted into the lumen. Reabsorption of K^+ in the proximal tubule follows the aforementioned passive reabsorption of $NaHCO_3$ and water [27], while the active reabsorption in the medullary portion of the nephron is mediated by the Na^+-K^+-$2Cl^-$ carrier of the luminal membrane in the thick ascending limb of Henle's loop (the site of action of loop diuretics) [28]. Indeed, the synthesis and production of aldosterone and, therefore, its activation of K^+ channels

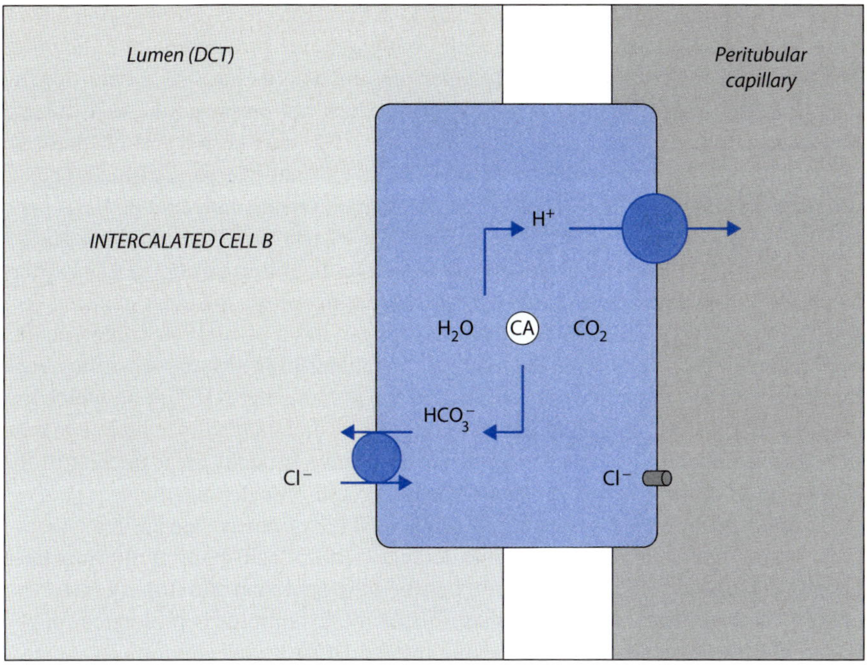

Fig. 2 Mechanisms regulating chloride-bicarbonate exchange in the distal collecting tubule (DCT). The figure shows the cellular mechanisms regulating the Cl^--HCO_3^- exchanger in the B-type intercalated cells of the distal collecting tubule. Of note, the possibility of reabsorbing strong anions, such as Cl^-, in exchange with a weak anion (HCO_3^-) allows dissociation between Na^+ and Cl^- reabsorption/excretion. See text for further details

(and Na^+/K^+ and Na^+/H^+ exchangers) occurs in response to variations in plasma K^+ concentration (which is kept in a tight low range) and of the effective circulating blood volume (as we will see below) [29, 30]. Therefore, in general, the regulation of urinary K^+ excretion has little to do with most of the regulation of acid-base equilibrium. In fact, it is worth noting that the quantitative role of its concentration in the extracellular space in affecting the SID is minimal, as compared to the main effect of Na^+ and Cl^- concentration. Thus, it is conceivable that the monitoring of urinary K^+ concentration does not have any relevant meaning in relation to the variation in acid-base equilibrium, whereas it may have a role in relation to the assessment of the adequacy of hemodynamics.

Renal Ammonium Production and Monitoring

The importance of ammonia (NH_3) in the maintenance of acid-base homeostasis lies in its capacity to bind with H^+ to form NH_4^+. In normal conditions, ammonia is produced in the kidney by a two-step de-amination of glutamine into glutamic acid and α-ketoglutaric acid [31]. The ability of the kidneys to increase ammonia production more than four-fold following an acid load has been clearly demonstrated [32]. Such a response involves an increase in both glutamine production and glutamine uptake by the kidney. Theoretically, once ammonia spills into the tubular lumen, it is 'trapped' in the form of NH_4^+, as NH_4^+ does not permeate the cell luminal membrane. In the luminal electrolyte scenario, NH_4^+ serves as a sort of 'dummy' positive charge allowing both the elimination of Cl^- and the parallel maintenance of electrical neutrality (see below). The elimination of one molecule of NH_4^+ with Cl^- will necessarily lead to the net reabsorption of one positive ion (either Na^+ or K^+) with HCO_3^-. Recently, a novel complex system of transmembrane transporters has been identified as responsible for NH_4^+ handling along different nephron segments (in which NHE3, the PT Na^+/H^+ exchanger, has a pivotal role), allowing the establishment of a cortico-medullary NH_4^+ gradient [33]. Moreover, it has been hypothesized that the kidney is supplied with a pre-existing NH_4^+ pool, which undergoes continuous countercurrent recycling, and which is readily available in case of acid-base alterations [34]. Such discoveries have brought great interest in the investigation of the kinetics of renal response to acid-base derangements.

Routine laboratory assessment of urinary NH_4^+ is costly and difficult to obtain. Studies conducted during chronic derangements of acid-base equilibrium have already established a tight association between the acid load and urinary NH_4^+ excretion. It has been demonstrated that if the acidotic stimulus is prolonged (days), the renal system is capable of preserving plasma HCO_3^- concentration by increasing the excretion of NH_4^+ in urine [32]. Conversely, data regarding the renal response to acute variation of acid-base equilibrium are scarce. This is mainly due to the lack of monitoring devices. It is, in fact, conceivable that the renal activation to modulate urinary NH_4^+ excretion may be rapid enough to be detected in its initial phase. For this purpose, in our center, we have designed a study investigating such a hypothesis. Patients admitted to a postoperative intensive care unit (ICU) after major surgery and still under sedation and paralysis were connected to the urinary analyzer, K.IN.G.®, which allows quasi-continuous measurement of urinary NH_4^+ concentration. During a two-hour study period, patients underwent either an increase or a reduction in minute ventilation, thereby causing either a slight respiratory alkalosis or a slight respiratory acidosis, respectively. The study, still ongoing, is showing interesting preliminary results [35]. Urinary excretion of NH_4^+ following respiratory modifications of acid-base equilibrium appears to be very sensitive to minimal stimuli (within a variation of arterial pH ranging between 7.35 and 7.45), and quite rapid.

Physiological and Clinical Significance of Urinary Anion Gap

In parallel with the definition and the role of plasma SID, or of the SID of the extracellular space, we can also define for urine a difference between measurable strong cations (mainly urinary Na^+ and K^+) and measurable strong anions (mainly Cl^-), i.e., the urinary anion gap. As urine may also be considered as an aqueous solution, the significance of the urinary anion gap does not differ from that of plasma SID, under the perspective of Stewart's approach [9]. Nonetheless, it is worth noting that in urine not all the strong ions are measurable. Therefore, to cope with electrical neutrality, urinary anion gap (defined as the difference between urinary Na^+, K^+ and Cl^-) equals the difference between unmeasured anions (mainly SO_4^{2-}, derived from the metabolism of sulfur amino acids) and unmeasured cations (mainly NH_4^+, as described above) [10]. At the same time, it seems reasonable to focus urinary monitoring on the electrolytes that play a major role in the regulation of plasma acid-base equilibrium, therefore Na^+, K^+ and Cl^-. An example may help to clarify the clinical significance of urinary anion gap. During metabolic acidosis, as we have described above, the renal system may react, in order to correct the acid-base derangement, by increasing urinary excretion of Cl^-, aimed at decreasing plasma SID. At the level of the urine, such an increase in urinary Cl^- excretion will determine a decrease in urinary anion gap, which consequently must be accompanied by a parallel increase in the urinary excretion of unmeasured cations. This is normally accomplished by increasing the excretion rate of NH_4^+, which, therefore, may be considered as a way to excrete Cl^- without Na^+ [36, 37].

From a clinical perspective, and based upon the reasoning described above, urinary anion gap has been proposed in the last few decades as a rough estimate of urinary excretion of NH_4^+, and, therefore, as an estimate of one of the main mechanisms by which the renal system is able to compensate for an increased acid load. In 46 patients with hyperchloremic metabolic acidosis, Batlle and colleagues investigated the value of urinary anion gap to distinguish a subgroup of patients with acidosis associated with diarrhea (and, therefore, with a preserved ability to excrete H^+ as NH_4^+), from those with renal tubular acidosis (characterized by the inability to excrete NH_4^+) [11]. As expected, the former group showed significantly lower values of urinary anion gap (higher urinary Cl^- concentration) associated with higher values of urinary NH_4^+, as compared to patients with renal tubular acidosis. Therefore, the authors concluded that urinary anion gap might be employed as a rough estimate of urinary NH_4^+, and may help as a first assessment of metabolic acidosis.

Despite these data and their scarce clinical application, it is important to highlight that the inclusion of urinary K^+ concentration within the definition of urinary anion gap may be misleading. In fact, as we have discussed above, although urinary K^+ concentration may reach high concentrations, this is not true for the plasma, in which the K^+ concentration affects plasma SID only slightly. Moreover, urinary K^+ excretion is regulated by principles other than the regulation of acid-base equilibrium. Thus, it may be reasonable to consider the difference in Na and Cl^-, without including urinary K^+ concentration, as parameters estimating how the renal system reacts to alterations in plasma acid-base equilibrium, unveiling once again the potential dissociation ongoing in the kidney between Na^+ and Cl^- excretion [35].

Renal Function and the Effective Circulating Blood Volume

Maintenance of tissue perfusion, oxygen delivery and removal of waste products is the key target of the cardiovascular system. For this purpose, three independent variables are responsible for the correct functioning of the circulation: Myocardial contractility, vascular tone, and intravascular volume, i.e., volemia [38]. The resulting cardiac output and arterial blood pressure will determine the amount of oxygen delivery to the tissues necessary to cope with the metabolic requirements of the system. In theory, among the determinants of tissue perfusion, volemia, and in its context, the effective circulating blood volume (ECBV) [1] appears to be the best candidate for easy and continuous monitoring in critically ill patients [39].

In addition to clinical examination, many different invasive and non-invasive techniques have been proposed to assess the hemodynamic/volemic status of critically ill patients. Among them, much attention has been paid to the cardiovascular preload and, in particular, to its assessment through measurements of central venous pressure (CVP) and/or pulmonary artery occlusion pressure (PAOP) [40, 41]. Unfortunately, in addition to a generally recognized low level of accuracy of CVP measurements, preload assessment has been widely reported as not being strictly related to the ability of increasing cardiac output after its augmentation, i.e., the fluid responsiveness [42]. Recently, novel techniques based on the assessment of dynamic variations of arterial pressure (i.e., pulse pressure or systolic pressure variation) have been proposed, but here also several limitations have been recognized [43]. Overall, despite the recognition of the pivotal importance of assessing the ECBV [44], none of the proposed techniques, in fact, performs such an assessment.

When considering the entire overview of the cardiovascular system and its physiology, the kidney appears to have peculiar characteristics, which grant it a main role in regulating the ECBV. First, the kidney is interposed within the 'arterial side' of the systemic circulation, thereby being strictly linked to the ECBV. Moreover, the kidney represents the common pathway of response to alterations of different components of the extracellular space (cardiac pre-load, extra-cellular fluid volume, plasma volume, cardiac output, osmolarity). Involved receptors may either respond to pressure (baroreceptors located at the aortic arch and carotid bodies), to volume or distension/stretch (mechanoreceptors, located in the right atrium), or to osmolarity, osmoreceptors of the hypothalamus. All the mediators with a role in hemodynamic homeostasis act either through an increase in vascular tone (norepinephrine and endothelin), through an increase in Na^+ and water reabsorption (renin-angiotensin-aldosterone-system, RAAS; atrial or brain natriuretic peptide, ANP/BNP), or through a combination of these functions (vasopressin). Overall, all these bio-humoral pathways act to restore the ECBV, and an adequate blood pressure/perfusion. Table 1 summarizes the receptors, mediators and ensuing reactions of the cardiovascular system.

In an attempt to exploit the abovementioned characteristics of the kidney to be a 'monitor' of the adequacy of the ECBV, we have developed the "sodium-bicarbonate test". Indeed, as the kidney mainly regulates the ECBV by handling

Table 1 Effects of physiological bio-humoral systems on regulation of the effective circulating blood volume

Bio-humoral system	Kidney		Cardiovascular system	
	Receptors	Effect	Receptors	Effect
RAAS				
Angiotensin (AT) II	$AT_1 - AT_2$	↑ Na^+ and H_2O reabsorption	AT_1	↑↑ arteriolar tone
Aldosterone	nuclear		–	–
Endothelin	ET-B	↓ Na^+ and H_2O reabsorption	ET-A	↑↑ arteriolar tone
Vasopressin	V_2	↑↑ H_2O reabsorption	V_1	↑ arteriolar tone
Catecholamines				
Norepinephrine	α_1	↑ Na^+ reabsorption	$\alpha_{1,2}$	↑↑ arterial and venous tone
Epinephrine	α_1	↑ Na^+ reabsorption	$\beta_{1,2}$	↑↑ cardiac output and heart rate
Dopamine	D	↓ Na^+ reabsorption	α, β	↑↑ arterial tone and heart rate
ANP/BNP		↓ Na^+ reabsorption	–	–

RAAS: renin-angiotensin-aldosterone-system.

Na^+ balance and, therefore, urinary Na^+ excretion [45], we hypothesized that intravenous administration of a controlled amount of $NaHCO_3$ would unveil the adequacy of ECBV by 'perturbing' the system. In fact, $NaHCO_3$ administration adds an extra amount of Na^+ to the plasma (and the extracellular fluid volume), which acutely reaches the kidney. If the renal system is conditioned by a reduction in ECBV, the extra amount of Na^+ would be entirely reabsorbed, thereby not being excreted through the urine. In contrast, if the system is characterized by a normal or increased ECBV, the added Na^+ would be almost entirely excreted. The extra amount of urinary Na^+ would in turn determine an increase in urinary anion gap, and it would, therefore, lead to a consensual increase in urinary pH. The evaluation of the "sodium-bicarbonate test" is still ongoing, but preliminary results are very promising [46].

Conclusion

Renal physiology has a fundamental role in determining several pathophysiologic processes in critically ill patients, and in funding the rationale for many aspects of their clinical treatment. Consequently, urinary monitoring may provide several pieces of information, potentially of paramount clinical relevance. As far as the assessment of acid-base equilibrium is concerned, the measurement of urinary Na-Cl concentration difference may provide more accurate information compared to the classical assessment of urinary anion gap, because urinary K^+ excretion has minimal relation with plasma acid-base regulation. Moreover, variation in urinary NH_4^+ excretion rate in response to acid-base alterations appears to be more rapid than usually thought and, therefore, its assessment may provide accurate and timely indications of plasma acid-base equilibrium. Finally, the renal system, by handling Na^+ excretion/reabsorption, is crucial for the regulation of the adequacy of the ECBV. Therefore, semi-continuous monitoring of urinary Na^+ excretion may establish a useful minute-by-minute assessment of the adequacy of hemodynamics.

References

1. Schrier RW (1990) Body fluid volume regulation in health and disease: a unifying hypothesis. Ann Intern Med 113:155–159
2. Gomez H, Ince C, De Backer D et al (2014) A unified theory of sepsis-induced acute kidney injury: inflammation, microcirculatory dysfunction, bioenergetics, and the tubular cell adaptation to injury. Shock 41:3–11
3. Kirschbaum B, Sica D, Anderson FP (1999) Urine electrolytes and the urine anion and osmolar gaps. J Lab Clin Med 133:597–604
4. Honore PM, Joannes-Boyau O, Boer W, Rose T (2010) Real-time non-invasive follow-up of acid-base correction by the kidney: a step closer. Minerva Anestesiol 76:307–308
5. Moviat M, Terpstra AM, van der Hoeven JG, Pickkers P (2012) Impaired renal function is associated with greater urinary strong ion differences in critically ill patients with metabolic acidosis. J Crit Care 27:255–260
6. Moviat M, Pickkers P, van der Voort PH, van der Hoeven JG (2006) Acetazolamide-mediated decrease in strong ion difference accounts for the correction of metabolic alkalosis in critically ill patients. Crit Care 10:R14
7. Maciel AT, Park M, Macedo E (2012) Urinary electrolyte monitoring in critically ill patients: a preliminary observational study. Rev Bras Ter Intensiva 24:236–245
8. Caironi P, Langer T, Taccone P et al (2010) Kidney instant monitoring (K.IN.G): a new analyzer to monitor kidney function. Minerva Anestesiol 76:316–324
9. Fencl V, Leith DE (1993) Stewart's quantitative acid-base chemistry: applications in biology and medicine. Respir Physiol 91:1–16
10. Gattinoni L, Carlesso E, Cadringher P, Caironi P (2006) Strong ion difference in urine: new perspectives in acid-base assessment. Crit Care 10:137
11. Batlle DC, Hizon M, Cohen E, Gutterman C, Gupta R (1988) The use of the urinary anion gap in the diagnosis of hyperchloremic metabolic acidosis. N Engl J Med 318:594–599
12. Halperin ML, Jungas RL (1983) Metabolic production and renal disposal of hydrogen ions. Kidney Int 24:709–713
13. Hamm LL, Simon EE (1987) Roles and mechanisms of urinary buffer excretion. Am J Physiol 253:F595–F605
14. Cogan MG, Alpern RJ (1984) Regulation of proximal bicarbonate reabsorption. Am J Physiol 247:F387–F395
15. Stewart PA (1983) Modern quantitative acid-base chemistry. Can J Physiol Pharmacol 61:1444–1461
16. Sherman RA, Eisinger RP (1982) The use (and misuse) of urinary sodium and chloride measurements. JAMA 247:3121–3124
17. Maddox DA, Gennari FJ (1987) The early proximal tubule: a high-capacity delivery-responsive reabsorptive site. Am J Physiol 252:F573–F584
18. Rector FC Jr (1983) Sodium, bicarbonate, and chloride absorption by the proximal tubule. Am J Physiol 244:F461–F471
19. Helbert MJ, Dauwe SE, Van der Biest I, Nouwen EJ, De Broe ME (1997) Immunodissection of the human proximal nephron: flow sorting of S1S2S3, S1S2 and S3 proximal tubular cells. Kidney Int 52:414–428

20. Neumann KH, Rector FC Jr (1976) Mechanism of NaCl and water reabsorption in the proximal convoluted tubule of rat kidney. J Clin Invest 58:1110–1118
21. Cogan MG, Rector FC Jr (1982) Proximal reabsorption during metabolic acidosis in the rat. Am J Physiol 242:F499–F507
22. Sauer M, Flemmer A, Thurau K, Beck FX (1990) Sodium entry routes in principal and intercalated cells of the isolated perfused cortical collecting duct. Pflugers Arch 416:88–93
23. Madsen KM, Tisher CC (1986) Structural-functional relationships along the distal nephron. Am J Physiol 250:F1–F15
24. Kim J, Kim YH, Cha JH, Tisher CC, Madsen KM (1999) Intercalated cell subtypes in connecting tubule and cortical collecting duct of rat and mouse. J Am Soc Nephrol 10:1–12
25. Doucet A (1988) Function and control of Na-K-ATPase in single nephron segments of the mammalian kidney. Kidney Int 34:749–760
26. Giebisch G, Wang W (1996) Potassium transport: from clearance to channels and pumps. Kidney Int 49:1624–1631
27. Kaufman JS, Hamburger RJ (1985) Passive potassium transport in the proximal convoluted tubule. Am J Physiol 248:F228–F232
28. Greger R, Gogelein H (1987) Role of K+ conductive pathways in the nephron. Kidney Int 31:1055–1064
29. Stanton BA (1987) Regulation of Na+ and K+ transport by mineralocorticoids. Semin Nephrol 7:82–90
30. Rabinowitz L (1996) Aldosterone and potassium homeostasis. Kidney Int 49:1738–1742
31. Pitts RF (1972) Symposium on acid-base homeostasis. Control of renal production of ammonia. Kidney Int 1:297–305
32. Welbourne T, Weber M, Bank N (1972) The effect of glutamine administration on urinary ammonium excretion in normal subjects and patients with renal disease. J Clin Invest 51:1852–1860
33. Weiner ID, Verlander JW (2011) Role of NH3 and NH4+ transporters in renal acid-base transport. Am J Physiol Renal Physiol 300:F11–F23
34. DuBose TD Jr., Good DW, Hamm LL, Wall SM (1991) Ammonium transport in the kidney: new physiological concepts and their clinical implications. J Am Soc Nephrol 1:1193–1203
35. Ferrari M, Scotti E, Chiodi M et al (2014) Changes is urinary electrolytes during acute respiratory acid-base modification. Crit Care 18:P430
36. Ring T, Frische S, Nielsen S (2005) Clinical review: Renal tubular acidosis – a physicochemical approach. Crit Care 9:573–580
37. Kellum JA (2000) Determinants of blood pH in health and disease. Crit Care 4:6–14
38. Schrier RW, Niederberger M (1994) Paradoxes of body fluid volume regulation in health and disease. A unifying hypothesis. West J Med 161:393–408
39. Antonelli M, Levy M, Andrews PJ et al (2007) Hemodynamic monitoring in shock and implications for management. International Consensus Conference, Paris, France, 27–28 April 2006. Intensive Care Med 33:575–590
40. Pinsky MR, Teboul JL (2005) Assessment of indices of preload and volume responsiveness. Curr Opin Crit Care 11:235–239
41. Vincent JL, Weil MH (2006) Fluid challenge revisited. Crit Care Med 34:1333–1337
42. Michard F, Teboul JL (2002) Predicting fluid responsiveness in ICU patients: a critical analysis of the evidence. Chest 121:2000–2008
43. Bendjelid K, Romand JA (2003) Fluid responsiveness in mechanically ventilated patients: a review of indices used in intensive care. Intensive Care Med 29:352–360
44. Rivers E, Nguyen B, Havstad S et al (2001) Early goal-directed therapy in the treatment of severe sepsis and septic shock. N Engl J Med 345:1368–1377
45. Schrier RW (1979) Nephrology forum: acute renal failure. Kidney Int 15:205–216
46. Caironi P, Langer T, Bruzzone P, Taccone P, Marenghi C, Gattinoni L (2009) Analysis of urinary pH after sodium-bicarbonate infusion: a novel method for the evaluation of volemia. Intensive Care Med 35:S282

Management of AKI: The Role of Biomarkers

Z. Ricci, G. Villa, and C. Ronco

Introduction: Definition and Diagnosis of AKI

Acute kidney injury (AKI) is a common complication in hospitalized patients, mainly during critical illness. Patients affected by AKI usually require admission to the intensive care unit (ICU) and are typically burdened by longer ICU and in-hospital lengths of stay as well as worse short- and long-term outcomes.

A more accurate understanding of the pathophysiology of AKI is essential to develop new clinical tools for earlier diagnosis, monitoring, treatment and follow up of this syndrome and thus to improve clinical practice and the outcome of AKI patients. The definition, diagnosis and staging of AKI is currently obtained through the application of indices based on the glomerular filtration rate (GFR), such as serum creatinine and/or urinary output. In 2004, the Acute Dialysis Quality Initiative (ADQI) attempted to standardize AKI definition, summarizing different stages of severity and outcome into the RIFLE (an acronym indicating different severity classes: Risk, Injury, Failure, Loss of Function and End Stage kidney Disease) classification. In 2007, the Acute Kidney Injury Network (AKIN) modified this classification, suggesting the use of smaller variation in serum creatinine in order to earlier identify AKI. These classifications were finally summarized in 2012 into the KDIGO (Kidney Disease Improving Global Outcomes) classification. All these clinical classifications are based on alteration of serum creatinine and/or urinary output in order to identify an acute reduction of the GFR [1].

However, although widely available and easily achieved in routine clinical practice, these markers are far from ideal. Hydration status, for example, may affect both urinary output and serum creatinine concentration in critical care patients. In

Z. Ricci ✉
Department of Cardiology and Cardiac Surgery, Pediatric Cardiac Intensive Care Unit, Bambino Gesù Children's Hospital, IRCCS, Rome, Italy
e-mail: zaccaria.ricci@gmail.com

G. Villa · C. Ronco
International Renal Research Institute, San Bortolo Hospital, Vicenza, Italy

J.-L. Vincent (ed.), *Annual Update in Intensive Care and Emergency Medicine 2015*,
DOI 10.1007/978-3-319-13761-2_26

the same manner, drugs (such as diuretics) or the concomitant presence of tubular damage may reduce the sensitivity and specificity of urinary output in detecting AKI, as well as the lack of a urinary catheter, mainly outside the ICU. On the other hand, serum creatinine also depends on non-renal factors, such as age, sex and muscle mass. The metabolism of creatinine varies during AKI as does its clearance during treatment with several drugs (e.g., cimetidine). Moreover, during acute impairment of renal function, the lack of a steady state reduces the clinical correlation of serum creatinine concentration with GFR, which requires more stable conditions to be estimated. Finally, the renal functional reserve allows the serum creatinine concentration to be maintained within the normal range until at least 50% of nephrons have been lost, mainly through recruitment and hyperfiltration of undamaged nephrons.

Biomarkers of AKI have been actively evaluated in order to obtain a novel sensitive and specific parameter, unaffected by other clinical features and possibly able to timely detect this clinical syndrome and/or to establish its prognosis.

A Comprehensive Definition of Acute Kidney Syndrome

In order to understand the clinical implications of the use of biomarkers on AKI management, it is critically important to remark their connection with pathophysiology of AKI. If a 'functional' stressor (e.g., hypovolemia) or a 'metabolic' stressor (such as iodinated contrast media, nephrotoxic drugs, mediators of systemic inflammation during sepsis, etc.) is applied to a healthy kidney, the reduction in GFR (kidney dysfunction) or the organic insult of the kidney (kidney damage) could be detectable through the subsequent alteration in serum creatinine and/or urinary output. A 'clinical AKI' is thus diagnosed and classified according to the RIFLE, AKIN or KDIGO classifications. On the other hand, if a 'renal stressor', in the early phase, is not associated with increased values of serum creatinine and reduction in urinary output below the threshold for AKI diagnosis, this is classified as 'subclinical AKI'. If the stressor insult is maintained during a long period of time and the kidney damage increases with subsequent repercussion on nephron functions, this condition is finally associated with a reduction in GFR and thus becomes clinically manifest [3].

Subclinical AKI should not be overlooked since it has been shown to be associated with several clinical complications and worsened hard outcomes [4, 5]. If not preventable, these should be identified early and treated according to the specific etiology. Because clinical AKI can hardly be identified through clinical tools, such as the KDIGO classification, a possible way of identifying subclinical AKI is to look for specific early markers of kidney damage [5].

In this context, instead of being identified only as earlier tools in predicting future development of GFR reduction, the biomarkers of AKI could enable a comprehensive definition of the so called 'acute kidney syndrome'. Indeed, the entire spectrum of this syndrome encompasses several clinical pictures including both clinical and subclinical kidney damage and/or dysfunction [6].

A more generic term of "kidney attack" has recently been proposed to underlie the possibility that several clinical and subclinical AKI episodes occur in the clinical picture of critically ill patients and that they are certainly related to patient outcome, mainly in terms of nephron loss and reduction in renal functional reserve [7]. This aspect has recently gained interest also as far as long-term outcomes and renal recovery are concerned [5].

Biomarkers

Transcriptomic and proteomic techniques have identified several potential biomarkers of AKI including, but not limited to, neutrophil gelatinase-associated lipocalin (NGAL), cystatin-C (Cys-C), kidney injury molecule-1 (KIM-1), interleukin 18 (IL-18), liver-type fatty acid binding protein (L-FABP) or N-acetyl-β-D-glucosaminidase (NAG) (Table 1). These are molecules or proteins mainly produced during an insult in the renal parenchyma and/or released in the systemic circulation after extra-renal synthesis [8].

The biological roles of these biomarkers range from a functional enzymatic role, to an adaptative (e.g., inflammatory) and structural one. Moreover, these could be low molecular weight molecules, physiologically filtered through the glomerular barrier and catabolized in the healthy tubular epithelium (e.g., Cys-C) [2]. Specific biomarkers are usually increased according to the specific pathophysiology of the occurring insult. Indeed, particularly during abnormalities in cell signaling (due to cytokines, adhesion molecules, etc.) and microvascular dysfunction, biomarkers, such as NGAL, IL-18 or KIM-1, appear to be strongly over-expressed [9]. However, the clinical importance of these biomarkers is mainly due to the biological mechanism that increases their urine or plasma concentrations. In particular, biomarkers of AKI may be classified into those filtered and reabsorbed in the proximal tubule, and those up-regulated and directly released into the tubules by damaged cells. According to this classification, it is possible to speculate on the mainly glomerular and/or tubular nature of damage occurred to the nephrons [10]. This classification could explain the different curve profiles that can be observed for a specific damage over time.

Neutrophil Gelatinase-associated Lipocalin (NGAL)

NGAL is a protein associated with gelatinase from human neutrophils which exists as a 25 kDa monomer, 45 kDa homodimer and conjugated to gelatinase as a 135 kDa heterodimeric form [11]. The monomeric and heterodimeric forms are mainly produced by tubular epithelial cells, whereas the homodimeric form is mainly produced by activated neutrophils [12]. Circulating NGAL is filtered through the glomerular barrier and reabsorbed through megalin-facilitated endocytosis (Table 1). In the steady state, plasma and urine concentrations are about 20 ng/ml.

Table 1 Clinical feature of the most used biomarkers of acute kidney injury (AKI)

Biomarker	Production and renal clearance	Sample sources	Detection time after renal injury
NGAL	Produced by epithelial tissues throughout the body. Excreted through glomerular barrier and completely reabsorbed in healthy tubular cells. It is also produced in distal tubular segments.	Plasma and urine	2–4 hours after renal insult
Cys-C	Produced by all nucleated human cells. Released into plasma at constant rate independent of sex, race, muscle mass and hydration level. Freely filtered through the glomerulus and completely reabsorbed by proximal tubular cells. It is not secreted by tubular cells and is not detectable in the urine of healthy subjects.	Plasma (as marker of GFR) and urine (as biomarker of kidney insult)	12–24 hours post-renal injury
IL-18	Pro-inflammatory cytokine mainly produced by activated neutrophils. Upregulated and released into the tubule by epithelial cells and activated neutrophils.	Plasma and urine	6–24 hours after renal insult
KIM-1	Upregulated and released by proximal tubular cells into the urine.	Urine	12–24 hours after tubular insult
L-FABP	Produced in liver, intestine, pancreas, lung, nervous system, stomach and proximal tubular cells. Completely filtered through glomerular barrier and reabsorbed in healthy proximal tubular cells.	Plasma and urine	1 hour after tubular injury
NAG	Systemically produced as well as in proximal and distal tubular cells. Too large to undergo glomerular filtration; urinary elevations imply released by epithelial tubular cell damage.	Plasma and urine	12 hours after tubular insult
αGST	Cytoplasmatic enzyme produced in proximal tubule. Limited glomerular filtration; increased urinary levels following tubular injury.	Urine	12 hours
IGFBP-7	Upregulated and released during the very early phases of cell injury. Upregulated and released by proximal tubular cells into the urine.	Urine	NA
TIMP-2	Upregulated and released during the very early phases of cell injury. Upregulated and released by proximal tubular cells into the urine.	Urine	NA

NA: not available; NGAL: neutrophil gelatinase-associated lipocalin; Cys-C: cystatin C; IL-18: interleukin-18; KIM-1: kidney injury molecule-1; L-FABP: liver-type fatty acid binding protein; NAG: N-acetyl-β-D-glucosaminidase; GST: glutathione S-transferase; IGFBP: insulin-like growth factor binding-protein; TIMP: tissue inhibitor of metalloproteinase

Kidney protection characteristics have been recognized for NGAL. In particular, the NGAL released by nephron segments may form a complex with iron-binding siderophores, chelate the Fe^{+} released from damaged tubules and prevent the formation of hydroxyl radicals and superoxide. According to several studies, other than ischemic tubular damage, NGAL is upregulated in experimental models of sepsis and systemic inflammation, suggesting that its release into the urinary system is a major response of the kidney to systemic infection as well as local urogenital infection [13]. This has been considered a major limit of NGAL, especially as far as its diagnostic performance is concerned during septic AKI [12].

Cystatin-C

Cys-C is a 13 kDa protein produced by all nucleated cells. Unbound to plasma proteins, it is completely filtered by the glomerular barrier and thus reabsorbed through megalin-facilitated endocytosis and degraded in the renal proximal tubules. Unlike creatinine, it is not secreted into the urine by the tubules [13]. Consequently, higher urinary values during AKI mainly reflect Cys-C glomerular filtration and a reduced reabsorption by damaged proximal tubules [14] (Table 1). Urine Cys-C appears as an earlier and a more sensitive marker of AKI compared to serum Cys-C. However, the blood concentration of Cys-C mainly correlates with GFR, even in a range in which serum creatinine is not able to detect the change in GFR (60–90 ml/min) [15]. Although the superiority of serum Cys-C when compared to serum creatinine has been established, it is unclear whether its improved performance may have clinical relevance with respect to creatinine's diagnostic capacity. Furthermore, diabetes, large doses of corticosteroids, hypertriglyceridemia, hyperbilirubinemia or rheumatoid factor may affect the analysis of Cys-C [13].

Kidney Injury Molecule-1

KIM-1 is a type I cell membrane glycoprotein whose mRNA levels increase more than any other gene after kidney injury. The soluble ectodomain of KIM-1 (about 90 kDa) is shed by a metalloproteinase-dependent process in *in vitro* and *in vivo* studies, becoming detectable in urine samples during AKI [13]. It is also expressed in immune cells, where it is thought to activate Th2 and Th1 differentiation, as well as in antigen presenting cells [16]. During kidney injury, KIM-1 may facilitate remodeling of injured epithelium. In particular, the KIM-1 expressed in the epithelial cells may increase cellular phagocytosis activity by recognizing apoptotic cells, phosphatidylserine and oxidized lipoproteins [13].

Interleukin-18

IL-18 is an 18 kDa molecule produced by mononuclear cells, macrophages and non-immune cells, including proximal tubule cells. It is an important mediator of acute ischemic AKI in which the source of IL-18 is thought to be the proximal tubule [13]. In an obstructive model of AKI, the deleterious effect of IL-18 is due to its activation of epithelial FasL and to an increased expression of caspase-3 and caspase-8 [17].

N-acetyl-β-D-glucosaminidase

NAG is a large size protein (about 140 kDa), which originates from lysosomes of the proximal tubule cells. Its high molecular weight precludes glomerular filtration and, therefore, high urinary levels are unlikely to originate from a non-renal source. NAG correlates with histological evidence of proximal tubule injury as well as renal recovery during effective treatments. Urinary NAG at ICU admission correlates well with outcome in critically ill patients. However, since urinary NAG has been demonstrated to be a sensitive marker of tubular injury, its specificity may be reduced by the low threshold for the release of tubular enzyme in response to any tubular injury and its prognostic value needs to be assessed. False positive values have been reported during diabetes, rheumatoid arthritis and hyperthyroidism [13].

Biomarkers of Cell-Cycle Arrest

Biomarkers of cell-cycle arrest belong to a recently defined category of biomarkers of AKI first observed by Kashani et al. in a multicenter observational study [18]. These authors examined more than 300 molecules in 522 mixed medical-surgical patients with AKI. Urinary insulin-like growth factor binding-protein 7 (IGFBP-7) and urinary tissue inhibitor of metalloproteinase-2 (TIMP-2) were identified as the most specific and sensitive molecules for detecting AKI [18].

Both these molecules are involved with the phenomenon of G1 cell-cycle arrest during the early phases of cell injury. Similar to other cells, renal tubular cells were demonstrated to enter a short period of cell-cycle arrest following injury in experimental models of sepsis [19] or ischemia [20]. In an injured tissue, this process may prevent cells from dividing when the DNA is damaged. These molecules arrest the process of cell division until the damage can be repaired and thus reduce the possibility of a cell's demise and/or senescence. Furthermore, IGFBP-7 and TIMP-2 both appear to be able to spread the 'alarm' of metabolic stress from the site of injury with autocrine and paracrine effects [18]. In other words, with respect to existing biomarkers that identify the damage occurring to nephron cells (in an early phase), markers such as TIMP-2 and IGFBP-7 may indicate that the renal epithelium has been stressed and has reduced function. In these conditions, the cell may still be able to recover without permanent injury if the stressor mechanism is removed. If potentially able to remove the mechanisms of damage (e.g., nephrotoxic drugs or hypotension), clinicians may avoid the nephron substitution with fibrotic tissue, maintaining the entire number of nephron units and thus the entire renal functional reserve of patient. This particular aspect has still not been considered in the current literature [18].

In the discovery phase, receiver operating characteristic (ROC) areas under the curve (AUC) of 0.77 and 0.75 were obtained for IGFBP-7 and TIMP-2, respectively. Furthermore, these biomarkers were shown to have an additive predictive value when used in combination, ([TIMP-2] · [IGFBP-7]) [18]. The same authors validated the combination of these biomarkers in another prospective cohort (728 critically ill patients in the Sapphire study) and compared their predictive characteristics to those observed for other previous biomarkers [18]. An ROC-AUC of 0.80 for development of AKI was found in this validation phase. This value was significantly greater than for any of the previous existing biomarkers ($p<0.002$). Moreover, the performance of ([TIMP-2] · [IGFBP-7]) in detecting AKI was independent of concomitant severe systemic conditions (such as sepsis) or comorbidities (such as chronic kidney disease). Unlike existing biomarkers, ([TIMP-2] · [IGFBP-7]) showed a clear separation between AKI and non-AKI patients even in the presence of these confounding factors. Interestingly, IGFBP-7 was superior to TIMP-2 in predicting AKI in surgical patients, whereas TIMP-2 was best in predicting sepsis-induced AKI. These differences may reflect the different mechanisms of damage among various etiologies of AKI and that the two biomarkers may be involved in different pathways of cell response [18].

In other studies, biomarkers of cell-cycle arrest have been demonstrated as effective and early predictors of clinical AKI. Furthermore, in an observational study in patients undergoing cardiac surgery, Meersch et al. demonstrated a greater correlation with renal recovery (ROC-AUC of 0.79) compared to existing biomarkers of kidney damage [21]. In this study, the renal functional recovery was defined as serum creatinine value at hospital discharge equal to or lower than the preoperative creatinine value [21].

General Considerations

Several factors may reduce the sensitivity and specificity observed for some of these biomarkers used in clinical practice. Chronic kidney disease, for example, may reduce the detecting capability of several biomarkers to identify AKI. In a prospective observational study on 426 adult cardiac surgical patients, McIlroy et al. found that urine NGAL was a better diagnostic predictor for postoperative AKI in patients with a baseline estimated GFR $\geq 60\,\text{ml/min/1.73}\,\text{m}^2$. Moreover, postoperative NGAL best identified AKI in patients with baseline GFR higher than $90\,\text{ml/min/1.73}\,\text{m}^2$ [22]. Albuminuria may further decrease the diagnostic feature of some biomarkers such as NGAL, Cys-C, L-FABP, $\alpha2$- and $\beta2$-microglobulin, all reabsorbed in the tubule through megalin-facilitated endocytosis. Considering that albumin can be reabsorbed via the same way in the proximal tubule, the presence of albuminuria may competitively inhibit biomarker reabsorption, increasing their urinary excretion [23].

Moreover, systemic illness may affect the detecting capability of biomarkers mainly expressed during an inflammatory stimulus, such as IL-18 or NGAL. For example, Doi et al. reported, in a prospective observation single-center study, a higher median NGAL concentration in septic patients without AKI compared to AKI patients without sepsis (137.8 mcg/ml vs 32.8 mcg/ml) [24]. These results should be interpreted considering the limited ability of the NGAL assay to distinguish between the various molecular forms released by different tissues. In particular, activated neutrophils (as during sepsis or extracorporeal circulation in cardiac surgery) are able to release homodimeric NGAL in the systemic circulation [25]. The higher level of plasma NGAL may increase the filtered load and hence urinary levels, irrespective of any potential kidney damage [12]. On the other hand, stressed kidney epithelium, as well as other extra-renal tissues, mainly produce monomeric NGAL. The entire amount of urinary NGAL during AKI could thus be due to different molecular forms with different cellular origins. Monomeric NGAL could be up-regulated in the tubular cells during damage or derive from an impaired absorption of the filtered load produced in extra-renal tissues. Moreover, homodimeric NGAL may derive from neutrophils infiltrated in the damaged kidney as well as a direct glomerular filtration of NGAL produced by extra-renal activated neutrophils and released in the systemic circulation [12].

The biological features of biomarkers of AKI are quintessential in order to avoid the misinterpretation of results and improve clinical practice.

Clinical Applications

Predicting Clinical AKI

Several studies have examined the role of biomarkers of AKI in early detection of clinical AKI. Most of these studies were performed in patients undergoing cardiac surgery, where the timing of the major insult is well determined. One of the most important studies on this topic was the TRIBE (Translational Research Involving Biomarkers and Endpoints) study, performed on more than 1,200 patients mainly undergoing elective on-pump coronary revascularization [21, 22]. Until the first 6 hours after ICU admission, the authors reported higher concentrations of urinary IL-18 and of urinary and plasma NGAL in patients who would have developed clinical AKI in the following hours. Moreover, these biomarkers were able to identify AKI at least 24 hours before its clinical occurrence with a fair to modest performance for urinary IL-18, urinary and plasma NGAL (ROC-AUC of 0.74, 0.67 and 0.7, respectively). However, the same investigators reported that these biomarkers were able to improve the AKI-detecting capability of clinical prediction models [26, 27].

Similar results were obtained by Cruz et al. in a prospective observational study on 300 patients in a mixed ICU. In particular, the authors showed an ROC-AUC of

0.78 for plasma NGAL in detecting AKI, 48 hours before its clinical diagnosis [28]. Although the rise in biomarkers of AKI after iodinated contrast media is less important than that observed during cardiac surgery, several studies have demonstrated an early increase in urinary and plasma concentration of NGAL and L-FABP after contrast exposure. Similar results have also been reported for urinary IL-18 [29, 30].

Several studies have also tried to identify a possible application of these biomarkers of AKI in a more comprehensive setting of critical illness. In these studies, the biomarker concentrations at ICU admission or at emergency department were predictive for AKI development as well as need for renal replacement therapy (RRT). In this context, during the 10th Acute Dialysis Quality Initiative consensus conference it was proposed that patients considered to be at high risk for AKI on ICU admission (according to comorbidities and presence of renal stressor) should be candidates for testing with AKI biomarkers [2].

Differential Diagnosis

Etiology of AKI should be determined as rapidly as possible, regardless of cause, since an early diagnosis is an important determinant of the response to therapy and long-term prognosis in many types of AKI. The combined use of clinical classification and biomarkers of AKI should enable a more accurate and useful differential diagnosis of etiology and mechanisms of AKI [3]. For example, a functional reduction in kidney function without evidence of kidney damage in terms of biomarker increase, may improve clinical categorization of what is currently identified with the non-specific term of 'pre-renal azotemia' (i.e., a volume-responsive and reversible alteration in kidney function) [31]. Isolated kidney dysfunction without evidence of kidney damage is also recognized in the early phase of 'post-renal' obstructive disease: In this case, the reversibility of the underlining condition before the damage occurs may certainly modify the prognosis of this AKI type [3]. In these circumstances, markers of kidney damage and kidney dysfunction could be effectively applied to identify the underlying pathophysiology and sequence of events during AKI, without restricting the differential diagnosis to merely anatomic pre-, intra- and post-renal categories [3].

Finally, the biological characteristics of each biomarker may help to localize the main nephron damage. When the etiology of AKI mainly affects glomerular function, a change in biomarkers of filtration function (e.g., serum Cys-C) should be observed. On the other hand, if the tubular epithelium is damaged, AKI should first be detected by the increase in biomarkers of tubular injury, such as NGAL and KIM-1 [32].

Staging and Monitoring AKI Severity

Following diagnosis of AKI, establishing the stage of severity is essential to facilitate continued monitoring, promote therapeutic actions and assess prognosis [2]. Currently, there are insufficient data on biomarkers of kidney damage to support staging of AKI. The potential inclusion of markers of kidney damage to establish the staging of AKI will theoretically require the possibility of detecting the phase of disease, the amount of affected renal mass and the magnitude and duration of the specific insult [3].

Although the current staging of AKI is based on clinical evaluation of serum creatinine and/or urinary output changes, biomarkers of AKI may help clinicians to better categorize the amount and etiology of damage. However, cut-off values for these biomarkers are still lacking and these combined criteria for AKI staging should be further tested and validated [3]. Based on the current state of knowledge, the staging of AKI by kidney damage biomarkers alone cannot be justified and the recent ADQI Consensus Conference suggestions, as well as KDIGO recommendations, clearly affirm that serum creatinine and urinary output remain the best markers to be used for AKI diagnosis and monitoring at the bedside for routine clinical purposes [2].

Additionally, a substantial gap in knowledge exists in the area determining the optimal times to measure biomarkers for staging AKI and to measure the evolution of severity over time. Although not exactly standardized, the application of a single measurement of biomarkers of damage has usually been performed several hours after a well-known insult (e.g., cardiac surgery or iodinated contrast media) for AKI staging [2].

Renal and Non-renal Outcomes

According to several studies, biomarkers of kidney damage also provide information above and beyond the simple prediction of AKI. Indeed, additional prognostic information has been provided, such as severity and duration of AKI, need for RRT, delayed or non-recovery of kidney function, and mortality. For example, postoperative evaluation of urinary IL-18 and NGAL were associated with longer ICU length of stay in a group of pediatric patient who underwent cardiac surgery [27]. Similar results were also obtained for duration of postoperative mechanical ventilation [27]. Similarly, Bennett et al. reported, in a prospective observational study, that high concentrations of urinary NGAL just 2 hours after surgery may predict the severity and duration of AKI, prolonged ICU length of stay, requirement for renal support and death [33]. Other biomarkers have been shown to be associated with worsening severity of AKI in surgical patients, including plasma Cys-C, urinary π-glutathione-S-transferase and urinary KIM-1 [34].

Although in all these contexts, the timing of the main injury is well-known, when the measurement of the selected biomarker was not necessarily be performed next to the time of injury, but also at predefined time points, as at ICU or ward admission, biomarkers showed some prognostic utility. In particular, in a prospective study on 500 critically ill patients, urinary NGAL, Cyst-C and IL-18 measured at ICU admission predicted the clinical development of AKI, its worsening and RRT requirement [34]. Few studies have assessed the utility of biomarkers for prediction of timing and extent of renal recovery after an episode of AKI [34]. Srisawat et al. examined serial changes in biomarkers of kidney damage in critically ill non-anuric patients [35]. Although these authors observed a high detecting capability in recognizing RRT-requiring AKI patients who recovered renal function through the use of biomarkers alone (ROC-AUC 0.7-0.8), a very high discrimination rate was obtained by integrating this information with clinical parameters, such as the Charlson comorbidity index or APACHE II score (ROC-AUC 0.9). The authors concluded that a panel of urinary biomarkers can improve clinical risk prediction for non-recovery after AKI [35].

Finally, plasma NGAL levels at hospital discharge after acute heart failure have been observed as a strong predictor of 30-day mortality and re-hospitalization [36]. A greater need for surveillance and monitoring following hospital discharge may be suggested according to NGAL concentration at hospital discharge [34].

Biomarkers and Clinical Decisions

Early initiation of renal support in selected patients with established AKI may have the potential to improve outcome [37]. According to data suggesting their role in predicting RRT requirement, biomarkers could potentially be used to inform the decision to initiate renal support therapy [34]. Although the integration of these biomarkers into clinical decision algorithms could improve our current ability to predict the need for RRT, there remain important challenges to creating and testing biomarker-based strategies for RRT initiation [38]. No consensus has yet been obtained for RRT initiation even during clinical AKI. Furthermore, most analyses have been based on a single specimen collection and variable timing of collection of blood and urine samples has been used in different studies (e.g., ICU admission, nephrology consultation, etc.) [38]. Considering that different biomarkers may have varying kinetics following AKI, timing of specimen collection with respect to the main kidney insult may significantly affect their predictive value. Moreover, the number of days between the increase in biomarkers of kidney damage and RRT initiation has not been reported in several studies and, among studies reporting these data, a broad difference has usually been shown [38]. Finally, no cut-off value for each biomarker has been identified that may specifically suggest the need for RRT in different clinical settings. No recommendation or suggestions have yet been made as to whether biomarkers could help clinicians make an early and appropriate decision to initiate RRT [38].

Conclusion

Biomarkers of AKI allow a comprehensive definition of acute kidney syndrome, which includes both clinical and subclinical AKI. Their biologic features may better characterize the specific nephron damage and may inform on the main pathophysiologic mechanisms of damage. Most of them are clinically useful to identify AKI, at least 24 h before its clinical diagnosis, as well as renal recovery. Correlation with non-renal outcomes, such as ICU and hospital length of stay and prolonged mechanical ventilation, has also been observed. Urinary cell-cycle arrest biomarkers are identified as specific and sensitive markers of early kidney damage and may further improve management of AKI in the near future.

References

1. KDIGO workgroup (2012) Kidney Disease: Improving Global Outcomes (KDIGO) Acute Kidney Injury Work Group: KDIGO clinical practice guideline for acute kidney injury. Kidney Int Suppl 2:1–138
2. McCullough P, Shaw A, Haase M et al (2013) Diagnosis of acute kidney injury using functional and injury biomarkers: workgroup statements from the tenth Acute Dialysis Quality Initiative Consensus Conference. Contrib Nephrol 182:13–29
3. Murray P, Mehta R, Shaw A et al (2014) Potential use of biomarkers in acute kidney injury: report and summary of recommendations from the 10th Acute Dialysis Quality Initiative consensus conference. Kidney Int 85:513–521
4. Ronco C, Kellum J, Haase M (2012) Subclinical AKI is still AKI. Crit Care 16:313–316
5. Ronco C (2013) Kidney Attack : Overdiagnosis of acute kidney injury or comprehensive definition of acute kidney syndromes? Blood Purif 36:65–68
6. Ronco C, McCullough P, Chawla L (2013) Kidney attack versus heart attack: evolution of classification and diagnostic criteria. Lancet 382:939–940
7. Kellum JA, Bellomo R, Ronco C (2012) Kidney attack. JAMA 307:2265–2266
8. McIlroy D, Wagener G, Lee H (2010) Biomarkers of acute kidney injury: an evolving domain. Anesthesiology 112:998–1004
9. Ronco C, Kellum J, Bellomo R, Mehta R (2013) Acute Dialysis Quality Initiative (ADQI. Contrib Nephrol 182:1–4
10. Pickering J, Endre Z (2014) Acute kidney injury urinary biomarker time-courses. PLoS One 9:e101288
11. Kjeldsen L, Johnsen A, Sengeløv H, Borregaard N (1993) Isolation and primary structure of NGAL, a novel protein associated with human neutrophil gelatinase. J Biol Chem 268:10425–10432
12. Mårtensson J, Bellomo R (2014) The rise and fall of NGAL in acute kidney injury. Blood Purif 37:304–310
13. Charlton JR, Portilla D, Okusa MD (2014) A basic science view of acute kidney injury biomarkers. Nephrol Dial Transplant 29:1301–1311
14. Vanmassenhove J, Vanholder R, Nagler E, Van Biesen W (2013) Urinary and serum biomarkers for the diagnosis of acute kidney injury: an in-depth review of the literature. Nephrol Dial Transplant 28:254–273
15. Herget-rosenthal S, Bökenkamp A, Hofmann W (2007) How to estimate GFR-serum creatinine, serum cystatin C or equations? Clin Biochem 40:153–161
16. Ichimura T, Brooks C, Bonventre J (2012) Kim-1/Tim-1 and immune cells: shifting sands. Kidney Int 81:809–811
17. Zhang H, Hile KL, Asanuma H et al (2011) IL-18 mediates proapoptotic signaling in renal tubular cells through a Fas ligand-dependent mechanism. Am J Physiol Ren Physiol 310:171–178

18. Kashani K, Al-khafaji A, Ardiles T et al (2013) Discovery and validation of cell cycle arrest biomarkers in human acute kidney injury. Crit Care 17:R25–R36
19. Yang Q, Liu D, Long Y, Liu H, Chai W, Wang X (2009) Acute renal failure during sepsis: Potential role of cell cycle regulation. J Infect 58:459–464
20. Witzgall R, Brown D, Schwarz C, Bonventre JV (1994) Localization of proliferating cell nuclear antigen, vimentin, c-Fos, and clusterin in the postischemic kidney. J Clin Invest 93:2175–2188
21. Meersch M, Schmidt C, Aken H et al (2014) Urinary TIMP-2 and IGFBP7 as early biomarkers of acute kidney injury and renal recovery following cardiac surgery. PLoS One 9:e93460
22. McIlroy DR, Wagener G, Lee HT (2010) Neutrophil gelatinase-associated lipocalin and acute kidney injury after cardiac surgery: the effect of baseline renal function on diagnostic performance. Clin J Am Soc Nephrol 5:211–219
23. Nejat M, Hill JV, Pickering JW, Edelstein CL, Devarajan P, Endre ZH (2012) Albuminuria increases cystatin C excretion: implications for urinary biomarkers. Nephrol Dial Transplant 27:96–103
24. Doi K, Negishi K, Ishizu T et al (2011) Evaluation of new acute kidney injury biomarkers in a mixed intensive care unit. Crit Care Med 39:2464–2469
25. Cai L, Rubin J, Han W, Venge P, Xu S (2010) The origin of multiple molecular forms in urine of HNL/NGAL. Clin J Am Soc Nephrol 5:2229–2235
26. Parikh CR, Coca SG, Thiessen-philbrook H et al (2011) Postoperative biomarkers predict acute kidney injury and poor outcomes after adult cardiac surgery. J Am Soc Nephrol 22:1748–1757
27. Parikh CR, Devarajan P, Zappitelli M et al (2011) Postoperative biomarkers predict acute kidney injury and poor outcomes after pediatric cardiac surgery. J Am Soc Nephrol 22:1737–1747
28. Cruz D, de Cal M, Garzotto F et al (2010) Plasma neutrophil gelatinase-associated lipocalin is an early biomarker for acute kidney injury in an adult ICU population. Intensive Care Med 36:444–451
29. Bachorzewska-Gajewska H, Malyszko J, Sitniewska E, Malyszko J, Dobrzycki S (2006) Neutrophil-gelatinase-associated lipocalin and renal function after percutaneous coronary interventions. Am J Nephrol 26:287–292
30. Ling W, Zhaohui N, Ben H et al (2008) Urinary IL-18 and NGAL as early predictive biomarkers in contrast-induced nephropathy after coronary angiography. Nephron Clin Pr 108:176–181
31. Himmelfarb J, Ikizler T (2007) Acute kidney injury: changing lexicography, definitions, and epidemiology. Kidney Int 71:971–976
32. Endre Z, Kellum J, Di Somma S et al (2013) Differential diagnosis of AKI in clinical practice by functional and damage biomarkers: workgroup statements from the tenth Acute Dialysis Quality Initiative Consensus Conference. Contrib Nephrol 182:30–44
33. Bennett M, Dent CL, Ma Q et al (2008) Urine NGAL predicts severity of acute kidney injury after cardiac surgery: a prospective study. Clin J Am Soc Nephrol 3:665–673
34. Cruz D, Bagshaw S, Maisel A et al (2013) Use of biomarkers to assess prognosis and guide management of patients with acute kidney injury. Contrib Nephrol 182:45–64
35. Srisawat N, Wen X, Lee M et al (2011) Urinary biomarkers and renal recovery in critically ill patients with renal support. Clin. J Am Soc Nephrol 8:1815–1823
36. Maisel AS, Mueller C, Fitzgerald R et al (2011) Prognostic utility of plasma neutrophil gelatinase- associated lipocalin in patients with acute heart failure: The NGAL EvaLuation Along with B-type NaTriuretic Peptide in acutely decompensated heart failure (GALLANT) trial. Eur J Hear Fail 13:846–851
37. Seabra VF, Balk EM, Liangos O, Sosa MA, Cendoroglo M, Jaber B (2008) Timing of renal replacement therapy initiation in acute renal failure: a meta-analysis. Am J Kidney Dis 52:272–284
38. Cruz DN, De Geus HR, Bagshaw SM (2011) Biomarker strategies to predict need for renal replacement therapy in acute kidney injury. Semin Dial 24:124–131

Bone Morphogenetic Protein 7: An Emerging Therapeutic Target for Sepsis-associated Acute Kidney Injury

X. Chen, X. Wen, and J. A. Kellum

Introduction

Acute kidney injury (AKI) is a common organ dysfunction with poor prognosis. A recent study found that hospital mortality for adults with AKI was 23.9%, and 13.8% in children [1]. A prospective study of patients in the intensive care unit (ICU) with severe AKI (most receiving dialysis) reported a 60% hospital mortality rate, and 13.8% of survivors were dialysis-dependent at the time of hospital discharge [2]. Researchers have focused on preventing AKI and promoting its recovery; however, this has been difficult because the pathophysiological mechanisms responsible for AKI are still unclear.

Transforming growth factor-β (TGF-β)1 is believed to be an important molecule in AKI pathogenesis, especially for fibrosis, and its expression is decreased in chronic kidney disease (CKD) and late AKI [3]. It is generally believed that downregulation of TGF-β1 inhibits the process of fibrosis, but may promote inflammation [4]. Although Hiraki et al. reported that TGF-β1 neutralizing antibody improved survival rates of septic mice [5], modulation of the immune response can be difficult in sepsis especially since one cannot easily pinpoint the immune status at the bedside. Therefore, at the present time, the application of immune modulating therapy, including TGF-β1, is limited.

Another member of the TGF-β superfamily is bone morphogenetic protein (BMP)-7. This molecule is an emerging treatment target for AKI. It is a 35-kDa protein that is widely expressed in kidneys, bone, liver, and intestine in the fetus [6]. Although it gradually decreases in other tissues after birth, BMP-7 expression in the kidney is still active [7] in health, but declines under pathological conditions. BMP-7 often acts as a natural antagonist to TGF-β, on the Smad signaling pathway

X. Chen · X. Wen · J. A. Kellum ✉
The Center of Critical Care Nephrology, Department of Critical Care Medicine, University of Pittsburgh School of Medicine, Pittsburgh, USA
e-mail: kellumja@ccm.upmc.edu

J.-L. Vincent (ed.), *Annual Update in Intensive Care and Emergency Medicine 2015*,
DOI 10.1007/978-3-319-13761-2_27

via its unique receptors in the kidney, playing a role not only as an anti-fibrotic, but also on anti-inflammatory processes [8].

Some authors have speculated that BMP-7 may be used for reversing pathological processes in kidney diseases. Indeed, BMP-7 has been found to be beneficial in restoring kidney function, recovery from injury, inhibiting or reversing fibrosis and improving survival in both acute and chronic kidney injury experimental models [6, 9–11]. Surprisingly, although sepsis is the most frequent cause of AKI among the critically ill, there are few studies focusing on the role of BMP-7 in septic AKI. In this review, we systemically evaluate the possible roles that BMP-7 may play in the course of sepsis-associated AKI, based on *in vitro* and *in vivo* experimental data.

BMP-7 Interacts with TGF-β Through Smad Signaling Pathways via Unique Receptors

BMP-7 interacts with TGF-β on different Smad signaling pathways, counter-regulating each other to maintain the balance of their biological activities, and playing important roles in both acute and chronic kidney diseases [12]. These receptors have distinct activities in different cell types upon activation, antagonizing inflammation and apoptosis via up-regulation of serine/threonine kinase activity [13, 14]. TGF-β1 binds with receptors, TGF-β receptor (TGF-βR) I and TGF-βR II, and triggers Smad2/3 activation and subsequent signaling cascades, whereas BMP-7 binds with BMP receptor type I (BMPRI), including Alk2, Alk3, Alk6 and BMPRII receptors, which activate Smad1/5/8 cascades. With stimulation of Smad4, Smad1/5/8 or Smad2/3, phosphorylated complexes shuttle into the nucleus, and bind to DNA sequences or cofactors to regulate gene transcription (see Fig. 1 and Table 1). Smad4/1/5/8 and Smad4/2/3 induce different gene expression and have different roles in fibrosis and inflammation. For the negative regulation of their signal pathways, Smad7 acts as a general antagonist for the entire TGF-β family, while Smad6 has special inhibitory effects on BMP-7 signaling [12]. Smad3/4 also regulates Smad7 to prevent inflammation by inhibition of nuclear factor-kappa

Table 1 Comparison of differences between bone morphogenetic protein (BMP)-7 and transforming growth factor (TGF)-β1

	BMP-7	TGF-β1
Specific receptors in kidney	BMPRI (including Alk2, Alk3, Alk6) BMPRII	TGF-βR I TGF-βR II
Downstream Smad isoform	Smad2/3	Smad1/5/8
Overall roles in inflammation	Anti-inflammation	Anti-inflammation
Overall roles in fibrosis	Anti-fibrosis	Induce fibrosis
Theoretical best timing for administration	Early and late AKI CKD	Late AKI CKD

TGF-βR: TGFβ receptor; Alk: activin-like kinase; AKI: acute kidney injury; CKD: chronic kidney disease.

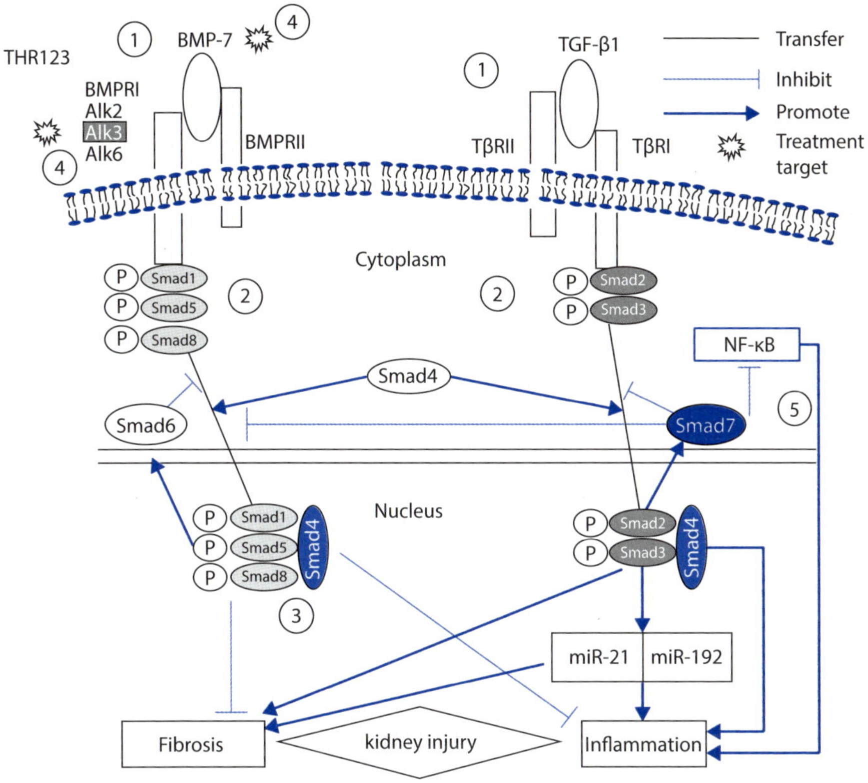

Fig. 1 Bone morphogenetic protein (BMP-7), transforming growth factor (TGF)-β1 signaling pathway and the potential treatment targets in the process of kidney injury. (*1*) TGF-β1 binds with TβR I and TβR II receptors, triggers Smad2/3 activation and subsequent signaling cascades; whereas BMP-7 binds with BMPRI, including Alk2, Alk3, Alk6, and BMPRII receptors, and then activates Smad1/5/8 cascades. (*2*) Activated Smad4, Smad1/5/8 or Smad2/3 form phosphorylated complexes, shuttle into the nucleus, and bind to DNA sequences or cofactors to regulate gene transcription. (*3*) BMP-7 protects kidney from injury by blocking inflammation and fibrosis processes via activated Smad4/1/5/8 complexes. (*4*) Administration of BMP-7 or the agonists of its special receptor in kidneys is the potential treatment target for kidney protection. (*5*) Smad7 inhibits downstream activation of BMP7, TGF-β1, as well as nuclear factor-kappa B (NF-κB) signal. *TβR*: TGFβ receptor; *Alk*: activin-like kinase; *miR*: microribonucleic acid; *P*: phosphorylated

B (NF-κB), thus TGF-β1 has a diverse role in renal fibrosis and inflammation. In addition, manipulating micro-ribonucleic acids (miRs), including upregulating miR-21 and miR-192, or downregulating miR-29 and miR-200, could interfere with the processes of renal fibrosis [15–17] through Smad3/4 complex formation (see Fig. 1). Recently, miR-22 has been identified as a critical miRNA that is positively related to renal fibrosis through the BMP signaling pathway [18]. However, the exact mechanisms for BMP-7 and TGF-β1 in fibrosis and inflammation remain unclear. Overexpression of renal BMP-7 may protect the kidney from TGF-β-

mediated kidney injury by inhibiting TGF-β/Smad3 signaling. On the other hand, renal BMP-7 expression and BMP/Smad signaling can be inhibited by activation of TGF-β/Smad signaling. High-affinity BMPR-II receptors are abundantly expressed in kidney proximal tubular epithelial cells in rats [19].

Protective Roles of BMP-7 in Kidney Injury

By systemically administering exogenous BMP-7 to animal models of kidney injury, investigators found that BMP-7 might be helpful to preserve or regenerate kidney architecture. BMP-7 appears to be an essential morphogenetic protein for renal development, given the fact that BMP-7 knockout mice die of renal failure after birth [20]. Administration of BMP-7 has been shown to alleviate kidney injury [21] in an animal model of bilateral kidney artery occlusion-induced acute kidney failure. Bioavailability studies performed with radioactively-labeled BMP-7 localized the exogenously supplied protein at the kidney; BMP-7 treatment either before or after artery occlusion effectively attenuated the kidney injury. Animals that received BMP-7 demonstrated superior outcomes as measured by improved survival, more favorable blood urea nitrogen and serum creatinine, and less severe changes on histology and immunofluorescence. In other models, such as unilateral ureteral obstruction, diabetic nephropathy, lupus nephritis, Alport's syndrome, and nephrotoxic serum nephritis, administration of BMP-7 has also shown beneficial effects [6, 9–11]. Although in the ICU, patients with sepsis, associated AKI have a remarkably high risk of renal non-recovery and death [22], few studies have focused on applying BMP-7 treatment in this population. To better design future experiments, we will summarize the known roles of BMP-7 in the process of kidney injury and repair in the aspects of inflammation, cellular phenotype trans-differentiation and proliferation, and fibrosis.

Role of BMP-7 in Renal Inflammation

BMP-7 has emerged as a therapeutic target for preventing AKI by regulating inflammation in the kidney. Recent evidence suggested that BMP-7 may play a protective role in AKI by downregulating inflammation. Administration of BMP-7 to experimental animals has been shown to reduce the severity of injury induced by ischemia-reperfusion or obstructive nephropathy, through inhibiting inflammatory cellular infiltration and activation [9, 21]. Specifically it has been found, *in vitro*, that BMP-7 plays a role in blocking macrophage infiltration [23], preventing attachment of monocytes to tubular cells, inhibiting monocyte chemoattractant protein-1 (MCP-1) expression [24], and inhibiting excessive expression of pro-inflammatory factors secreted by proximal tubule epithelial cells in response to stress [25].

Regulation of BMP-7 in Cell Cycle Arrest, Apoptosis, Cellular Phenotype Transition and Proliferation

Renal cell apoptosis, phenotype transdifferentiation and proliferation, and cell cycle arrest are among the several major pathophysiologic changes at the cellular level seen with AKI. BMP-7 plays an opposing role to TGF-β1 in these conditions. BMP-7 may protect tubular epithelial cells from apoptosis [26]. It significantly reduced the proportion of apoptotic tubular epithelial cells through attenuation of caspase-3 activation in animal models of cytotoxicity [27] and unilateral ureteral obstruction [28], and blocked podocyte apoptosis induced by TGF-β1 or high glucose through Smad5 signaling [29].

Renal cell phenotype transdifferentiation, including epithelial-mesenchymal transdifferentiation (EMT) is a pathological cellular response to injury that has been reported in many renal diseases, including diabetic nephropathy, unilateral ureteral obstructive nephropathy, nephrotoxicity, glomerulonephritis and chronic allograft nephropathy [6, 27, 30, 31]. The overall role of BMP-7 in cellular-phenotype transition was controversial, but the majority of studies support the notion that BMP-7 might inhibit cellular transdifferentiation between mature somatic cells [30, 32] in certain pathological circumstances. Specifically, renal tubular epithelial cells may exhibit increased expression of phosphorylated (p)-Smad2/3 during acute or chronic renal allograft rejection but decreased expression of phosphorylated-Smad1/5/8. Indeed, this is the profile associated with EMT; in *in vitro* experiments, in the absence of BMP-7, TGF-β stimulated cells showed a similar pattern of Smad signaling. BMP-7 inhibits TGF-β1-triggered EMT in mouse models of kidney disease demonstrating that BMP-7 could be a key molecule to maintain the phenotype of renal tubular epithelial cells. Importantly, applying BMP-7 to TGF-β-stimulated cells enhanced the expression of pSmad1/5/8 [30]. BMP-7 was also reported to block renal cellular EMT in a cell culture system of cyclosporine-A induced transdifferentiation [31] and in a clinical study of proteinuric nephropathies [33]. Paradoxically, in another study, no effect of BMP-7 was seen on TGF-β1-induced EMT in proximal tubular epithelial cells [34].

BMP-7 also antagonizes TGF-β1 for its effect on cell proliferation, but its exact action varies depending on cell type and on dosage. Yamada et al. reported that BMP-7 induced differentiation and inhibited the proliferation of podocytes through Smad signaling [35]. Conversely, it was reported that reduced induction of BMP-7 may accelerate renal damage after ischemia-reperfusion injury in diabetic kidney; while improved BMP-7 expression by treatment with asialoerythropoietin was accompanied by accelerated tubular proliferation [36]. Interestingly, BMP-7 induced cell proliferation or apoptosis in mouse inner medullary collecting duct cells in a dose-dependent manner: 0.25 nM BMP-7 improved cell proliferation but suppressed cell apoptosis, while 10 nM BMP-7 had the reverse effect via a Smad1-dependent mechanism [37].

Studies on renal cell cycle arrest have emerged in the field of kidney injury including septic AKI in recent years [38]. We recently identified and validated two novel markers for AKI, both inducers of G1 cell cycle arrest, in multicenter human cohort studies [39, 40]. Although no further work has been published on mechanisms at the cellular or subcellular levels regarding sepsis-associated AKI, BMP-7 is reported to induce cell cycle arrest at G1 phase in a variety of cancer studies [41, 42].

Role of BMP-7 in Renal Fibrosis

Fibrosis is a key pathological change in all forms of CKD, including that which may develop from AKI. Renal fibrosis is the final common pathway to terminal renal failure. Experimental data showed that BMP-7 expression in the kidney decreased significantly in fibrous-dominated nephropathies [21, 43]. Administration of recombinant human BMP-7 (rhBMP-7) or overexpressing BMP-7 was beneficial to suppress renal fibrosis in experimental models [6, 9–11, 26]. Blocking endogenous BMP-7 *in vitro* with neutralizing antibodies increased the expression of fibrotic factors, such as fibronectin and collagen III, in cultured renal tubular epithelial cells [43].

Specifically, BMP-7 blocked the activation of both Smad3-dependent and Smad-independent pathways, such as p38, ERK and MAPKs, via the activation of Smad1 and Smad5 in tubular and mesangial cells [43, 44]. Moreover, BMP-7 also prevented Smad3 from binding to the DNA [45], thus reducing TGF-β-triggered fibrotic gene expression. In addition, blockade of macrophages infiltrating the kidney could be another mechanism by which BMP-7 inhibits renal fibrosis [23]. Finally, BMP-7 can antagonize TGF-β1-induced suppression of matrix degradation, such as the production of PAI-1 (plasminogen activator inhibitor-1) [46].

Possible Therapeutic Strategies for BMP-7 in Kidney Diseases

The Advantage of BMP-7 Treatment over TGF-β1 Manipulation

From above, we know that BMP-7 can play a protective role on both renal inflammation and fibrosis. Administration with rhBMP-7 benefits kidney outcomes both in the inflammation stage and in the fibrosis stage in experimental kidney injury models. On the other hand, TGF-β suppresses inflammation in the early stage of AKI, while worsening renal fibrosis in the late stage. Consistently applying TGF-β neutralization antibody reduces the extent of fibrosis in late AKI, but it may be deleterious in the early phase due to severe inflammation [4]. Because of the diverse roles of TGF-β in different stages of AKI, as well as the absence of effective markers for identification of AKI stages, TGF-β targeting treatment is surely a challenge. Specifically, it is difficult to pinpoint the 'sweet spot' between early and late phases of AKI, in order to choose between stimulating or inhibiting TGF-β. By contrast, administration of BMP-7 may be beneficial to kidney outcomes through its anti-inflammatory effects in the early stages of AKI and by its anti-fibrosis effects in later stages of AKI or CKD. Although different effects of BMP-7 may be seen at different doses, there may be no requirement for injury phase identification, and thus easier to adopt compared to TGF-β targeting treatment.

Recombinant BMP-7 Administration

As described above, administration of rhBMP-7 is able to attenuate renal fibrosis and EMT, effectively inhibiting renal inflammation in several animal models of kidney disease. These studies suggest the possibility that BMP-7 exhibits therapeutic efficacy for renal inflammation, fibrosis and apoptosis. Thus it is highly possible that rhBMP-7 may be a therapeutic agent for kidney injury. As mentioned above, rhBMP-7 has been used safely in humans as osteogenic protein-1 (OP-1) paste in the treatment of osteoporosis. However, systemic BMP-7 has not been studied to any significant extent in humans. Importantly, BMP-7 also plays important roles in the physiology and pathophysiology of many other organs, and widely affects disease development in osteoporosis, arthritis, pulmonary hypertension, cerebrovascular disease and cancer. Thus, there is reason to be cautious regarding systemically administered rhBMP-7 because of the possible off-target effects.

BMP-7 Antagonists

Several BMP-7 antagonists have been found to take part in the activity of BMP through binding to their corresponding receptors. BMP-7 interacts with its antagonists to modulate the level of available BMP-7 and its function in kidney pathophysiology. Gremlin, kielin/chordin-like protein (KCP), twisted gastrulation, and uterine sensitization associated gene-1 (USAG-1) are frequently focused on as BMP-7 antagonists in studies of renal disease [47]. For example, USAG-1-knock-out mice are resistant to acute and chronic renal injury due to upregulation of BMP-7 [48]. Inhibiting the antagonists of BMP-7 may represent another therapeutic target in treating renal disease.

miRNAs Related to BMP-7

Accumulating evidence suggests that miRNAs contribute to a myriad of kidney diseases. In a rodent model of kidney fibrosis, miR-22 null mice expressed higher levels of BMP-7 proteins, accompanied by attenuated renal fibrosis compared to wild-type controls [18]. Consistent with these *in vivo* observations, primary renal fibroblasts isolated from miR-22-deficient mice expressed a significantly increased amount of BMP-7 proteins compared to cells obtained from wild-type ones. This phenotype was inhibited when cells were transfected with miR-22 mimics. Interestingly, miR-22 and BMP-7 appear to be in a regulatory feedback circuit, whereby not only miR-22 inhibits BMP-7 but miR-22 itself is induced by BMP-7 [18]. Based on these studies, we suspect that miRNAs are the key mediators of BMP-7 signaling during renal fibrosis or EMT. Targeting miR-22 related to BMP-7 signaling pathways may represent a novel and specific therapy for kidney injury [49].

Treatment with Specific Alk3 Agonist

Considering the widespread expression of BMP receptors in many organs in addition to the kidney, administration of pharmaceutical doses of BMP-7 may cause undesirable off-target effects. Alk3, one of the BMP receptors, is predominantly expressed in kidney epithelial cells. Investigators have found that a specific Alk3 agonist is superior to BMP-7. Sugimoto et al. showed that expression of Alk3 in kidney was increased in both acute and chronic kidney injury animal models [14]. They also found that synthesized THR-123, an Alk3 receptor agonist, could suppress inflammation, apoptosis, and EMT progression, and reverse established fibrosis [14]. Thus, development of a kidney-specific BMP-7 receptor agonist may offer a better therapy for kidney disease.

Future Directions

Until now, the role of endogenous BMP-7 has not been definitively elucidated in mature animals, much less in humans. More research is needed to better understand BMP-7 regulation, the binding proteins that modulate its effects, and the non-renal effects that are unrelated to the treatment goals. Although BMP-7 has been used in various animal disease models, many with positive treatment results, studies in septic AKI are scarce. Sepsis is the most common cause of AKI in critically ill patients, and septic AKI appears to have many different mechanisms compared with ischemic AKI, drug-induced nephropathy and renal dysfunction from other causes.

BMP-7 is emerging as a novel treatment for AKI. Topical application of rhBMP-7 has been approved by the Food and Drug Administration (FDA) as a safe and effective treatment for tibial non-union. To minimize possible off-target effects induced by systemic administration of exogenous BMP-7, it may be useful to examine analogs of BMP-7 that specifically target the kidney. We should also pay attention to the pharmacokinetics of exogenous BMP-7, including its relatively short half-life and dose-dependent actions that may limit its safety or efficacy. Overall, much more work needs to be done in order to properly design and implement BMP-7 treatment in septic AKI.

Conclusion

Clinical studies have established that sepsis-associated AKI is correlated with high morbidity and mortality in critically ill patients. BMP-7 is a key player in the pathogenesis of kidney disease and has emerged as an interesting potential target for treatment. BMP-7 is believed to affect both occurrence and recovery of kidney injury through modulation of inflammation, cellular phenotype transdifferentiation and proliferation, and fibrosis. BMP-7 is a promising novel treatment target for AKI. Further studies are urgently needed to better understand its specific roles in kidney injury in general and in septic AKI in particular.

References

1. Susantitaphong P, Cruz DN, Cerda J et al (2013) World incidence of AKI: A meta-analysis. Clin J Am Soc Nephrol 8:1482–1493
2. Uchino S, Kellum JA, Bellomo R et al (2005) Acute renal failure in critically ill patients: a multinational, multicenter study. JAMA 294:813–818
3. Barrera-Chimal J, Perez-Villalva R, Rodriguez-Romo R et al (2013) Spironolactone prevents chronic kidney disease caused by ischemic acute kidney injury. Kidney Int 83:93–103
4. Meng XM, Huang XR, Xiao J et al (2012) Diverse roles of TGF-beta receptor II in renal fibrosis and inflammation in vivo and in vitro. J Pathol 227:175–188
5. Hiraki S, Ono S, Tsujimoto H et al (2012) Neutralization of interleukin-10 or transforming growth factor-beta decreases the percentages of CD4+ CD25+ Foxp3+ regulatory T cells in septic mice, thereby leading to an improved survival. Surgery 151:313–322
6. Zeisberg M, Hanai J, Sugimoto H et al (2003) BMP-7 counteracts TGF-beta1-induced epithelial-to-mesenchymal transition and reverses chronic renal injury. Nat Med 9:964–968
7. Yanagita M (2007) Balance between bone morphogenetic proteins and their antagonists in kidney injury. Ther Apher Dial 11(Suppl 1):S38–S43
8. Correa-Costa M, Andrade-Oliveira V, Braga TT et al (2014) Activation of platelet-activating factor receptor exacerbates renal inflammation and promotes fibrosis. Lab Invest 94:455–466
9. Hruska KA, Guo G, Wozniak M et al (2000) Osteogenic protein-1 prevents renal fibrogenesis associated with ureteral obstruction. Am J Physiol Renal Physiol 279:F130–F143
10. Zeisberg M, Bottiglio C, Kumar N et al (2003) Bone morphogenic protein-7 inhibits progression of chronic renal fibrosis associated with two genetic mouse models. Am J Physiol Renal Physiol 285:F1060–F1067
11. Ogutmen B, Tuglular S, Cakalagaoglu F, Ozener C, Akoglu E (2006) Transforming growth factor-beta1, vascular endothelial growth factor, and bone morphogenic protein-7 expression in tacrolimus-induced nephrotoxicity in rats. Transplant Proc 38:487–489
12. Meng XM, Chung AC, Lan HY (2013) Role of the TGF-beta/BMP-7/Smad pathways in renal diseases. Clin Sci (Lond) 124:243–254
13. Di GV, Alday A, Chi L, Mishina Y, Rosenblum ND (2011) Alk3 controls nephron number and androgen production via lineage-specific effects in intermediate mesoderm. Development 138:2717–2727
14. Sugimoto H, LeBleu VS, Bosukonda D et al (2012) Activin-like kinase 3 is important for kidney regeneration and reversal of fibrosis. Nat Med 18:396–404
15. Chung AC, Huang XR, Meng X, Lan HY (2010) miR-192 mediates TGF-beta/Smad3-driven renal fibrosis. J Am Soc Nephrol 21:1317–1325
16. Xiao J, Meng XM, Huang XR et al (2012) miR-29 inhibits bleomycin-induced pulmonary fibrosis in mice. Mol Ther 20:1251–1260
17. Zhong X, Chung AC, Chen HY et al (2013) miR-21 is a key therapeutic target for renal injury in a mouse model of type 2 diabetes. Diabetologia 56:663–674
18. Long J, Badal SS, Wang Y, Chang BH, Rodriguez A, Danesh FR (2013) MicroRNA-22 is a master regulator of bone morphogenetic protein-7/6 homeostasis in the kidney. J Biol Chem 288:36202–36214

19. Bosukonda D, Shih MS, Sampath KT, Vukicevic S (2000) Characterization of receptors for osteogenic protein-1/bone morphogenetic protein-7 (OP-1/BMP-7) in rat kidneys. Kidney Int 58:1902–1911
20. Dudley AT, Lyons KM, Robertson EJ (1995) A requirement for bone morphogenetic protein-7 during development of the mammalian kidney and eye. Genes Dev 9:2795–2807
21. Vukicevic S, Basic V, Rogic D et al (1998) Osteogenic protein-1 (bone morphogenetic protein-7) reduces severity of injury after ischemic acute renal failure in rat. J Clin Invest 102:202–214
22. Bellomo R, Kellum JA, Ronco C (2012) Acute kidney injury. Lancet 380:756–766
23. Zhang XL, Selbi W, de la Motte C, Hascall V, Phillips AO (2005) Bone morphogenic protein-7 inhibits monocyte-stimulated TGF-beta1 generation in renal proximal tubular epithelial cells. J Am Soc Nephrol 16:79–89
24. Lee MJ, Yang CW, Jin DC, Chang YS, Bang BK, Kim YS (2003) Bone morphogenetic protein-7 inhibits constitutive and interleukin-1 beta-induced monocyte chemoattractant protein-1 expression in human mesangial cells: role for JNK/AP-1 pathway. J Immunol 170:2557–2563
25. Gould SE, Day M, Jones SS, Dorai H (2002) BMP-7 regulates chemokine, cytokine, and hemodynamic gene expression in proximal tubule cells. Kidney Int 61:51–60
26. Wang S, de Caestecker M, Kopp J, Mitu G, Lapage J, Hirschberg R (2006) Renal bone morphogenetic protein-7 protects against diabetic nephropathy. J Am Soc Nephrol 17:2504–2512
27. Wang Z, Zhao J, Zhang J, Wei J, Zhang J, Huang Y (2010) Protective effect of BMP-7 against aristolochic acid-induced renal tubular epithelial cell injury. Toxicol Lett 198:348–357
28. Kamiura N, Hirahashi J, Matsuzaki Y et al (2013) Basic helix-loop-helix transcriptional factor MyoR regulates BMP-7 in acute kidney injury. Am J Physiol Renal Physiol 304:F1159–F1166
29. De Petris L, Hruska KA, Chiechio S, Liapis H (2007) Bone morphogenetic protein-7 delays podocyte injury due to high glucose. Nephrol Dial Transplant 22:3442–3450
30. Tyler JR, Robertson H, Booth TA, Burt AD, Kirby JA (2006) Chronic allograft nephropathy: intraepithelial signals generated by transforming growth factor-beta and bone morphogenetic protein-7. Am J Transplant 6:1367–1376
31. Xu Y, Wan J, Jiang D, Wu X (2010) BMP-7 blocks the cyclosporine-A-induced epithelial-to-mesenchymal transition in renal tubular epithelial cells. Nephron Exp Nephrol 114:e23–e31
32. Xu Y, Wan J, Jiang D, Wu X (2009) BMP-7 counteracts TGF-beta1-induced epithelial-to-mesenchymal transition in human renal proximal tubular epithelial cells. J Nephrol 22:403–410
33. Rudnicki M, Eder S, Perco P et al (2007) Gene expression profiles of human proximal tubular epithelial cells in proteinuric nephropathies. Kidney Int 71:325–335
34. Dudas PL, Argentieri RL, Farrell FX (2009) BMP-7 fails to attenuate TGF-beta1-induced epithelial-to-mesenchymal transition in human proximal tubule epithelial cells. Nephrol Dial Transplant 24:1406–1416
35. Yamada S, Nakamura J, Asada M et al (2014) Twisted gastrulation, a BMP antagonist, exacerbates podocyte injury. PLoS One 9:e89135
36. Nakazawa J, Isshiki K, Sugimoto T et al (2010) Renoprotective effects of asialoerythropoietin in diabetic mice against ischaemia-reperfusion-induced acute kidney injury. Nephrology (Carlton) 15:93–101
37. Piscione TD, Phan T, Rosenblum ND (2001) BMP7 controls collecting tubule cell proliferation and apoptosis via Smad1-dependent and -independent pathways. Am J Physiol Renal Physiol 280:F19–F33
38. Yang QH, Liu DW, Long Y, Liu HZ, Chai WZ, Wang XT (2009) Acute renal failure during sepsis: potential role of cell cycle regulation. J Infect 58:459–464
39. Kashani K, Al-Khafaji A, Ardiles T et al (2013) Discovery and validation of cell cycle arrest biomarkers in human acute kidney injury. Crit Care 17:R25
40. Bihorac A, Chawla LS, Shaw AD et al (2014) Validation of cell-cycle arrest biomarkers for acute kidney injury using clinical adjudication. Am J Respir Crit Care Med 189:932–939

41. Sakamoto N, Yoshimura M, Kimura T et al (2007) Bone morphogenetic protein-7 and interferon-alpha synergistically suppress hepatitis C virus replicon. Biochem Biophys Res Commun 357:467–473
42. Klose A, Waerzeggers Y, Monfared P et al (2011) Imaging bone morphogenetic protein 7 induced cell cycle arrest in experimental gliomas. Neoplasia 13:276–285
43. Wang SN, Lapage J, Hirschberg R (2001) Loss of tubular bone morphogenetic protein-7 in diabetic nephropathy. J Am Soc Nephrol 12:2392–2399
44. Wang S, Hirschberg R (2004) Bone morphogenetic protein-7 signals opposing transforming growth factor beta in mesangial cells. J Biol Chem 279:23200–23206
45. Luo DD, Phillips A, Fraser D (2010) Bone morphogenetic protein-7 inhibits proximal tubular epithelial cell Smad3 signaling via increased SnoN expression. Am J Pathol 176:1139–1147
46. Wang S, Hirschberg R (2003) BMP7 antagonizes TGF-beta -dependent fibrogenesis in mesangial cells. Am J Physiol Renal Physiol 284:F1006–F1013
47. Yanagita M (2010) Antagonists of bone morphogenetic proteins in kidney disease. Curr Opin Investig Drugs 11:315–322
48. Yanagita M, Okuda T, Endo S et al (2006) Uterine sensitization-associated gene-1 (USAG-1), a novel BMP antagonist expressed in the kidney, accelerates tubular injury. J Clin Invest 116:70–79
49. Chung AC, Yu X, Lan HY (2013) MicroRNA and nephropathy: emerging concepts. Int J Nephrol Renovasc Dis 6:169–179

Long-term Sequelae from Acute Kidney Injury: Potential Mechanisms for the Observed Poor Renal Outcomes

M. Varrier, L. G. Forni, and M. Ostermann

Introduction

Renal disease is a global phenomenon with the incidence of both acute and chronic renal insufficiency continuing to rise [1, 2]. Acute kidney injury (AKI) is a known independent predictor of hospital mortality despite its multifactorial nature. After an episode of AKI, there are four potential outcomes [3]:

i) full recovery of renal function to baseline;
ii) incomplete recovery of renal function resulting in chronic kidney disease (CKD);
iii) exacerbation of pre-existing CKD accelerating progression towards end-stage renal failure (ESRF);
iv) non-recovery of function leading to ESRF.

It was previously assumed that those who recovered kidney function after an episode of AKI were faced with a relatively benign course with favorable outcomes. However, there is now increasing concern that this is not neccesarily the case and these individuals may be at risk of poor long-term outcomes through the development of CKD (including ESRF), further episodes of AKI and an increased risk of premature death. In the following review, we will describe the main pathogenetic links between AKI and CKD and introduce some potential key players.

M. Varrier · M. Ostermann ✉
Department of Critical Care & Nephrology, Guy's & St Thomas' Foundation Hospital, London, UK
King's College London, London, UK
e-mail: Marlies.Ostermann@gstt.nhs.uk

L. G. Forni
Department of Intensive Care Medicine, Surrey Peri-operative Anesthesia Critical Care Collaborative Research group (SPACeR), Royal Surrey County Hospital, Guildford, UK

J.-L. Vincent (ed.), *Annual Update in Intensive Care and Emergency Medicine 2015*,
DOI 10.1007/978-3-319-13761-2_28

Long-term Outcomes After Acute Kidney Injury

The observation that AKI and CKD may be intimately linked has been the subject of several recent studies [4–8]. However, as is often the case, demonstration of a clear association does not necessarily confer causation. Indeed, epidemiological studies often struggle to identify accurate pre-morbid and post-AKI renal function in order to precisely interpret long-term data. For example, in retrospective studies follow-up data may be missing or may have been captured at times of intercurrent illness, hence blunt endpoints, such as dialysis dependence or mortality, are used. In addition, serum creatinine and the derived estimated glomerular filtration rate (eGFR) are the only markers of renal function used in routine clinical practice. Their limitations are well known, and they may not accurately reflect renal function. Critical illness in particular, may be associated with significant decreases in serum creatinine through many potential mechanisms and these changes may persist through to hospital discharge hence confounding assessment of renal function [9]. Moreover, elevated serum creatinine levels at hospital discharge may represent pre-existing CKD rather than non-recovery, depending on the completeness of data availability.

Early studies suggesting a link between AKI and CKD were hindered by sample size as well as selection of population groups but recent studies are based on larger cohorts with longer follow-up data. For example, Lo et al. retrospectively analyzed more than 500,000 patients with a baseline pre-admission eGFR > 45 ml/min^2 who survived a stay in hospital [7]: 343 patients with dialysis-dependent AKI survived their ICU stay and were still dialysis-free at 30 days. Comparison between this cohort and patients without dialysis-require AKI demonstrated an increased risk of CKD stage 4 or 5 of 1.7/100 person-years in the non-AKI group and 47.9/100 person-years in the AKI group (adjusted hazard ratio [HR] 28.1; 95% confidence interval [CI] 21.1–37.6). Of note, 41 patients developed long-term dialysis dependency and all stemmed from the AKI group. Similarily, Wald et al. compared 3,769 adults who received renal support after an episode of AKI to 13,598 matched controls who did not require acute renal replacement therapy (RRT) [10]. After a median follow-up of 3 years, the incidence of chronic dialysis in the AKI cohort was 2.63/100 person-years compared to 0.91/100 person-years among control participants (adjusted HR, 3.23; 95% CI, 2.70–3.86).

Interrogation of large databases continues to support the hypothesis that an AKI event heralds an increased risk of CKD. Using the Medicare database in the US, Ishani et al. identified patients ≥ 67 years old over a 2-year period [11]. More than 200,000 patients who survived to hospital discharge were included with patients categorized as having AKI alone, CKD alone, AKI on background of CKD, or neither. The development of ESRF at 2 years was identified by cross-reference with the US Renal Data System. Predictably, when compared to patients with neither CKD nor AKI, the highest risk of ESRF was for those with acute-on-chronic kidney disease (adjusted HR 41.19; 95% CI 34.58–49.08). Interestingly, patients with AKI alone had a significantly higher risk of developing ESRF than patients with CKD alone (adjusted HR 13.00; 95% CI 10.57–15.99 versus adjusted HR 8.43; 95%

CI 7.39–9.61). However, this study is limited in that it relied on administrative diagnostic coding, which may not have been sufficiently sensitive. For example, the absence of a coded diagnosis for CKD does not reliably indicate normal baseline function.

Existing evidence suggests that the relationship between AKI and risk of CKD depends on the presence and also the severity of AKI. Chawla et al. analyzed the data of 5,351 patients in a Veterans Affairs cohort with normal baseline function admitted with AKI [12]. They developed a number of models to predict the likelihood of developing CKD stage 4 or worse following hospital discharge and showed by multivariate analysis that severity of AKI, whether by RIFLE (Risk – Injury – Failure – Loss – End stage) classification or mean serum creatinine, was a strong predictor of CKD stage 4. Advanced age, low serum albumin and the presence of diabetes were also predictive.

In a meta-analysis of 13 retrospective studies including those cited above, the pooled incidences of CKD and ESRF post-AKI were 25.8/100 person-years and 8.6/100 person-years, respectively [13]. Compared to patients without AKI the adjusted HRs were 8.8 for developing CKD (95% CI 3.1–25.5), 3.1 for ESRF (95% CI 1.9–5.0) and 2.0 for mortality (95% CI 1.3–3.1). Furthermore, 'recovery' of AKI as defined by a recorded eGFR within 90 days post-hospitalization that was at least 90% of the baseline eGFR was still associated with the development of CKD [8]. Cohort patients met strict criteria, including a baseline eGFR >60 ml/min, no history of renal disease (including proteinuria) and an increase of at least 50% in serum creatinine during their index admission. In this single center study, 1,610 patients were matched with 3,652 controls. The risk of *de novo* CKD was nearly doubled (adjusted HR 1.9; 95% CI 1.75–2.09).

To assess these important observations in more detail, there are several ongoing prospective studies focusing on the link between AKI and CKD. The Assessment, Serial Evaluation and Subsequent Sequelae of Acute Kidney Injury (ASSESS-AKI) study is a North American multicenter project including adult and pediatric cohorts [14]. Detailed annual reviews will be conducted for up to 4 years with blood and urinary biomarkers. Similarly, the At Risk in Derby (ARID) study is a UK, single center, case-control study aiming to recruit 1,084 hospitalized patients, again with blood and urine samples collected at designated time points [ISRCTN25405995]. The results of these studies are awaited with interest.

Potential Mechanisms Underlying the Progression of AKI to CKD

In AKI, several processes are initiated in both injured and regenerating tissues, including premature cell-cycle arrest, secretion of bioactive molecules, recruitment of infiltrating inflammatory and stem cells, and activation of myofibroblasts and fibrocytes [4]. Some of these pathways are directly linked to processes that are believed to cause progression of CKD.

Common Risk Factors/Pre-existing Comorbidities

There is intuitively an overlap between risk factors for AKI and progressive CKD. In many patients, the factors that predispose to AKI continue to exist after the episode of AKI has finished. Important risk factors for progressive CKD leading to ESRF include pre-existing CKD and proteinuria. Both signify significant structural and functional changes within glomeruli, tubulo-interstitial compartments and the renal vasculature, which may leave the kidney particularly vulnerable to further injury in the presence of nephrotoxins or intercurrent illness. Importantly, in CKD, the increase in serum creatinine for a given fall in GFR is greater than in patients with normal baseline renal function due to the non-linear relationship between serum creatinine and GFR. As a consequence, the diagnosis of AKI is more likely to be made using conventional consensus criteria.

The importance of proteinuria is apparent in the results described in a prospective cohort of 11,200 participants in the Atherosclerosis Risk in Communities (ARIC) study. The association between baseline urine albumin-to-creatinine ratio and eGFR with hospitalizations or death with AKI was examined [15]. Using a urine albumin-to-creatinine ratio < 10 mg/g as a reference, the relative hazards of AKI after an average of 8-years follow-up, adjusted for age, sex, race, cardiovascular risk factors, and categories of eGFR were 1.9 (95% CI 1.4–2.6), 2.2 (95% CI 1.6–3.0), and 4.8 (95% CI 3.2–7.2) for urine albumin-to-creatinine ratio groups of 11–29 mg/g, 30–299 mg/g, and ≥ 300 mg/g, respectively. There was a similar correlation in risk of AKI with decreasing eGFR groups. The impact of pre-existing CKD and proteinuria was the focus of a Canadian study that retrospectively analyzed outcomes of 920,985 patients who had had their eGFR and urine dipstick recorded between 2002 and 2007 [16]. The authors not only demonstrated that the risk of AKI rose cumulatively with worsening CKD and increased proteinuria but that this risk continued post-AKI with an increased chance of reaching the combined endpoint of ESRF or doubling of the serum creatinine. Harel et al. followed survivors of dialysis-dependent AKI who had recovered renal function [17]. They showed that pre-existing CKD (HR 3.86; 95% CI 2.99–4.98), hypertension (HR 1.82; 95% CI 1.28–2.58) and a higher Charlson comorbidity index score (HR 1.10; 95% CI 1.05–1.15/per unit) were significantly associated with risk of progression to ESRF.

What is clear, is that there is homogeneity among many of the risk factors for both AKI and CKD. For example, the baseline characteristics of patients who develop AKI are often significantly different to those who do not. Hsu et al. compared 1,746 dialysis-requiring AKI patients with 600,820 controls and found that the traditional risk factors for CKD progression (pre-existing CKD, proteinuria, hypertension and diabetes) were all found to be independently associated with risk of severe AKI [18]. Bucaloiu et al. reported that patients with AKI had a significant preponderance of other 'traditional renal risk factors', such as a history of hypertension, coronary artery disease, vascular disease, chronic heart failure, dyslipidemia, chronic lung or liver disease, cancer and hypoalbuminemia [8]. These conditions *per se,* as well as their potential treatments, have the potential to contribute to a decline in kidney function together with, as well as independently of, AKI.

Glomerular Hyperfiltration

In many models of acute renal disease, a loss of nephron mass and resultant hyperfiltration in the remaining glomeruli have been described. Similar to the sequelae following subtotal nephrectomy, it has been postulated that this results in hypertrophy of the residual glomeruli through increased work [4, 6]. As a result, tubular workload and O_2 consumption increase because of the increased flow. This can lead to hypoxic signaling and stimulation of tubulo-interstitial fibrosis, the latter of which is a significant component in the development of CKD [4, 6].

Mitochondrial Dysregulation

Recent findings have revealed striking morphological changes within mitochondria during cell injury. In health, mitochondria constantly undergo fission and fusion [19]. During cell injury, the dynamics are shifted to fission, i.e., the production of short mitochondrial rods or spheres. This type of mitochondrial fragmentation is associated with damage in the outer and inner membranes of the organelles, membrane leakage, decreased function and consequent cell death. Emerging evidence has suggested a pathogenic role of mitochondrial fragmentation in AKI [19, 20]. This may be related to an increase in non-compartmentalized reactive oxygen species (ROS) formation coupled with a loss of competent antioxidant systems. The blockade of mitochondrial fragmentation has a renoprotective effect in both ischemic and cisplatin-induced AKI [20].

While cell death is the predominant effect of mitochondrial dysregulation, mitochondrial fragmentation may have a less dramatic chronic impact under certain circumstances. For example, Funk and Schnellmann demonstrated a persistent disruption of mitochondrial homeostasis after AKI, which in turn may result in suboptimal cellular respiration, reduction in cellular adenosine triphosphate (ATP) and consequent tissue dysfunction, all contributing to the development of chronic damage [21]. It may well be that targeting mitochondrial dynamics for the therapy of AKI and prevention of CKD has a potential role but more preclinical studies are necessary to test this hypothesis.

Endothelial Injury and Reduced Capillary Density

Several different animal models have demonstrated diminished vascular density after an episode of AKI, especially in foci of tubulo-interstitial fibrosis [4, 22–24]. Such vascular rarefaction leads to the activation of hypoxia-inducible pathways and promotion of pro-inflammatory and pro-fibrotic processes [6]. In a vicious circle, capillary rarefaction, hypoxic signaling and tissue hypoxia may mutually reinforce each other leading to further damage and fibrosis.

Tubulo-interstitial Inflammation/Fibrosis

Tubulo-interstitial fibrosis is a predominant feature of CKD following AKI. Tubular hypertrophy and reduced capillary density play an important role in the pathogenesis. In addition, inflammation has been shown to be a key process in both ischemic and septic AKI, characterized by interstitial neutrophil infiltration during the acute phase and monocytic-lymphocytic infiltration in later stages [4, 6]. Monocyte infiltration potentiates injury as well as promoting fibroblast proliferation and consequent fibrosis [6]. Such pro-fibrotic processes are initiated and maintained by ongoing production and secretion of a variety of peptides, including cytokines and growth factors. Although they are necessary for repair and tubule regeneration, these bioactive molecules also have a stimulating effect on perivascular fibroblasts and initiate fibrosis [6].

These cellular and paracrine processes combined with changes in tissue architecture lead to altered anatomical relationships between important structures further promoting fibrosis.

Potential Key Regulators

Transforming Growth Factor β

Transforming growth factor-β (TGF-β) is a key profibrotic cytokine that exerts a broad range of actions in the kidney in both health and disease [25]. AKI is a pro-inflammatory condition involving a complex interaction of cytokines, various renal cell types and infiltrating leukocytes [26, 27]. TGF-β is upregulated in AKI and has a direct, detrimental effect via initiation of renal tubular apoptosis and extracellular matrix deposition [28, 29]. Up-regulation of TGF-β continues into the recovery phase. Animal research using a bilateral ischemia/reperfusion model demonstrated recovery of renal function and normal histology at 4 and 8 weeks post-injury but clear evidence of tubulo-interstitial fibrosis and high levels of TGF-β expression at 40 weeks [30]. Urinary TGF-β levels reflect renal production and are elevated in a wide range of renal disease. Although TGF-β may have a role in AKI, its role in predicting the risk of CKD post-AKI has yet to be defined [31].

Endothelin-1

The kidney is both an important target as well as a source of the potent vasoconstrictor and mitogen, endothelin-1 (ET-1), which is mainly produced by endothelial cells. ET receptors are widely distributed within the human kidney and are present as two sub-types [32]. ET A receptors are localized to vascular smooth muscle notably in the glomeruli, vasa recta and arcuate arteries, and ET B receptors are predominantly localized in the medulla. In AKI, circulating and tissue ET-1 levels rise and ET receptor gene expression increases resulting in both endothelial dysfunction and enhanced vasoconstriction in different vascular beds. Studies which included ET-1 gene deletion, or blockade of the ET receptor, mitigated the *initiation* phase of ischemic, endotoxemic, or rhabdomyolysis-induced AKI [33–35].

However, data are conflicting. At least five studies have shown that ET-1 receptor blockade either conferred no functional protection, or worsened post-ischemic AKI [36–40]. In a more recent ischemia-reperfusion model in mice undergoing unilateral ischemia without contralateral nephrectomy, an increase in intrarenal ET-1 production was observed, along with increased expression of the ET A receptor and evidence of ET-1 gene activation alongside progressive histological changes and a 40% loss of renal mass [41]. Treatment with atrasentan, an ET A receptor antagonist ameliorated microvascular injury and abrogated the loss in renal mass.

The mechanisms underlying the effects of ET-1 and ET receptor blockers remain unclear. ET-1 is known to alter intrarenal vascular tone but may also change systemic hemodynamics and affect oxidative stress and inflammatory processes [32, 42, 43]. Future research may determine the role of ET A and B receptor blockers, either alone or in combination.

Galectin-3

Galectin-3 is a β-galactoside–binding lectin that has emerged as a key regulator of inflammation and fibrosis. It is highly evolutionarily conserved and plays an important role in several diverse biological processes and disease states [44]. Galectin-3 is strongly linked to the development of organ fibrosis in multiple sites [45–49]. The common pathways involve macrophage activation, TGF-β upregulation, fibroblast proliferation and collagen deposition. Galectin-3 knockout mice are resistant to the development of fibrosis, including that in the kidney [45, 47, 50–52].

A retrospective analysis of 2,450 patients who participated in the Framingham Offspring study demonstrated that elevated levels of plasma galectin-3 were associated with increased risks of rapid GFR decline and of incident CKD in the community [53].

There has been intense interest in the setting of chronic heart failure in which galectin-3 has been shown to have an emerging role in the prediction, diagnosis and prognosis of this condition, presumably due to its pathogenic role in cardiac fibrosis [54–62]. Heart failure studies also demonstrated that galectin-3 levels were inversely correlated to GFR [57, 63–65].

The effects of galectin-3 in AKI are far from clear. One group studied two models of AKI in the rat (ischemic and nephrotoxic) and found that galectin-3 was intensely upregulated and prevented chronic tubular injury by limiting apoptosis, enhancing matrix remodeling and attenuating fibrosis [66]. However, another group using an ischemia-reperfusion model in wild-type versus knockout mice demonstrated that in early AKI the knockout mice seemed protected, with lower levels of interleukin-6, fewer ROS, less macrophage infiltration and lower peak concentrations of urea [67]. Using modified citrus pectin to reduce galectin-3 expression in mice, the severity of AKI observed was reduced following nephrotoxic insult [68].

These observations make galectin-3 an attractive candidate molecule to explain the demonstrable link between AKI and CKD. It is upregulated in AKI and serum levels appear to rise with renal impairment. Furthermore, it has pro-fibrotic actions up stream to TGF-β. More research in this area is awaited.

Endothelial Hypoxia-inducible Transcription Factor (HIF)

Chronic renal hypoxia may also play a role in progressive renal disease, in part due to vasoconstriction and reduced capillary density. During periods of renal hypoxia, the kidneys initiate adaptive processes to facilitate endurance and maintain renal oxygenation in order to preserve tubular integrity. Hypoxia also affects the expression of potentially protective genes, which participate in tissue oxygenation, cell metabolism and survival [69]. Proximal tubular cells are highly sensitive to hypoxia because they are principally dependent on oxidative catabolism [69]. In contrast, distal tubular cells are able to use glycolysis and endure severe hypoxic challenges better, provided that transport diminishes [69, 70].

Hypoxia-inducible factors (HIFs) are key regulators of gene expression in response to declining PO_2 [71]. Upon hypoxia, HIF dimers translocate into the nucleus where they activate various genes involved in the relevant adaptive responses. HIF-mediated genes act to ameliorate hypoxia, counteract oxidative stress and improve cell survival. Although HIF protects the kidney against AKI and more than 100 HIF target genes have already been identified, intrinsic HIF activation is submaximal in AKI [72]. There is also some evidence that excessive activation of HIF may be deleterious and induce interstitial fibrosis and cyst formation, suggesting a complex interaction between AKI and CKD via hypoxia and HIF activation [72, 73].

Conclusion

There is a strong intimacy between AKI and CKD. By mutually reinforcing the severity of the other, complex processes lead to the acceleration of disease progression (Fig. 1). Much of the burden of poor outcomes is related to co-morbid disease, which in itself needs correct management. Other important pathogenic mechanisms that pave the road from AKI to CKD include glomerular hyperfiltration and hypertrophy, mitochondrial dysregulation, cellular infiltration and paracrine actions of bioactive molecules, reduced capillary density and promotion of tubulo-interstitial fibrosis. Interestingly, these processes are independent of the original insult or cause of AKI. Endothelin-1, TGF-β, serum galectin-3 and HIF appear to play important roles in these pathways and may be promising target molecules for future intervention studies.

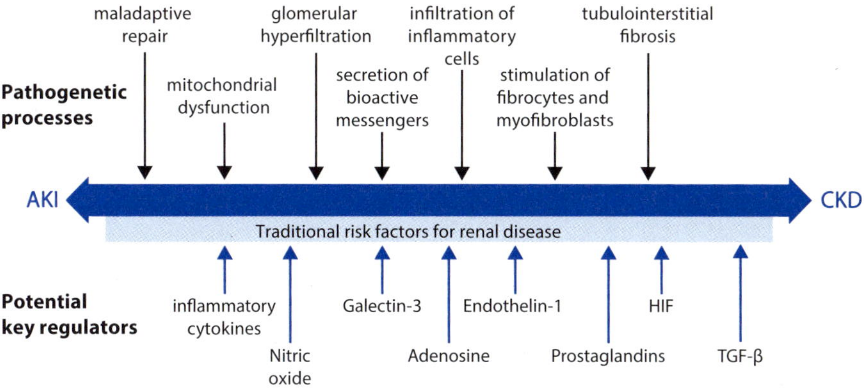

Fig. 1 Pathophysiological processes involved in the acute kidney injury (AKI)-chronic kidney disease (CKD) pathway. HIF: hypoxia-inducible factor; TGF: transforming growth factor

The hope is that future prospective studies will provide further information on the specific risks of CKD after AKI, identify markers of poor outcomes and inform potential preventative strategies. The optimal follow-up and management of patients surviving an episode of AKI have no evidence base to-date. However, measuring a true post-recovery serum creatinine, quantifying degree of proteinuria and identifying any factors that pose a risk of recurrent AKI or progression of CKD seem prudent.

Currently, management is limited to optimization of co-morbid conditions (e.g., diabetes, heart failure, hypertension, fluid balance) and avoidance of nephrotoxic insults. Where impaired eGFR or proteinuria is present, referral to a nephrologist may be appropriate.

References

1. Hsu RK, McCulloch CE, Dudley RA, Lo LJ, Hsu CY (2013) Temporal changes in incidence of dialysis-requiring AKI. J Am Soc Nephrol 24:37–42
2. Hsu CY, Vittinghoff E, Lin F, Shlipak MG (2004) The incidence of end-stage renal disease is increasing faster than the prevalence of chronic renal insufficiency. Ann Intern Med 141:95–101
3. Okusa MD, Chertow GM, Portilla D (2009) The nexus of acute kidney injury, chronic kidney disease, and World Kidney Day 2009. Clin J Am Soc Nephrol 4:520–522
4. Chawla LS, Eggers PW, Star RA, Kimmel PL (2014) Acute kidney injury and chronic kidney disease as interconnected syndromes. N Engl J Med 371:58–66
5. Leung KC, Tonelli M, James MT (2012) Chronic kidney disease following acute kidney injury-risk and outcomes. Nat Rev Nephrol 9:77–85
6. Venkatachalam MA, Griffin KA, Lan R, Geng H, Saikumar P, Bidani AK (2010) Acute kidney injury: a springboard for progression in chronic kidney disease. Am J Physiol Renal Physiol 298:F1078–F1094
7. Lo LJ, Go AS, Chertow GM et al (2009) Dialysis-requiring acute renal failure increases the risk of progressive chronic kidney disease. Kidney Int 76:893–899

8. Bucaloiu ID, Kirchner HL, Norfolk ER, Hartle JE, Perkins RM (2012) Increased risk of death and de novo chronic kidney disease following reversible acute kidney injury. Kidney Int 81:477–485
9. Prowle JR, Kolic I, Purdell-Lewis J, Taylor R, Pearse RM, Kirwan DJ (2014) Serum creatinine changes associated with critical illness and detection of persistent renal dysfunction after AKI. Clin. J Am Soc Nephrol 9:1015–1023
10. Wald R, Quinn RR, Luo J et al (2009) University of Toronto Acute Kidney Injury Research Group: Chronic dialysis and death among survivors of acute kidney injury requiring dialysis. JAMA 302:1179–1185
11. Ishani A, Xue JL, Himmelfarb J et al (2009) Acute kidney injury increases risk of ESRD among elderly. J Am Soc Nephrol 20:223–228
12. Chawla LS, Amdur RL, Amodeo S, Kimmel PL, Palant CE (2011) The severity of acute kidney injury predicts progression to chronic kidney disease. Kidney Int 79:1361–1369
13. Coca SG, Singanamala S, Parikh CR (2012) Chronic kidney disease after acute kidney injury: a systematic review and meta-analysis. Kidney Int 81:442–448
14. Go AS, Parikh CR, Ikizler TA (2010) The assessment, serial evaluation, and subsequent sequelae of acute kidney injury (ASSESS-AKI) study: design and methods. BMC Nephrol 11:22
15. Grams ME, Astor BC, Bash LD, Matsushita K, Wang Y, Coresh (2012) Albuminuria and estimated glomerular filtration rate independently associate with acute kidney injury. J Am Soc Nephrol 21:1757–1764
16. James MT, Hemmelgarn BR, Wiebe N et al (2010) Alberta Kidney Disease Network: Glomerular filtration rate, proteinuria, and the incidence and consequences of acute kidney injury: a cohort study. Lancet 376:2096–2103
17. Harel Z, Bell CM, Dixon SN et al (2014) Predictors of progression to chronic dialysis in survivors of severe acute kidney injury: a competing risk study. BMC Nephrol 15:114
18. Hsu C, Ordonez J, Chertow G, Fan D, McCulloch C, Go A (2008) The risk of acute renal failure in patients with chronic kidney disease. Kidney Int 74:101–107
19. Zhan M, Brooks C, Liu F, Sun L, Dong Z (2013) Mitochondrial dynamics: regulatory mechanisms and emerging role in renal pathophysiology. Kidney Int 83:568–581
20. Brooks C, Wei Q, Cho SG, Dong Z (2009) Regulation of mitochondrial dynamics in acute kidney injury in cell culture and rodent models. J Clin Invest 119:1275–1285
21. Funk JA, Schnellmann RG (2012) Persistent disruption of mitochondrial homeostasis after acute kidney injury. Am J Physiol Renal Physiol 302:F853–F864
22. Horbelt M, Lee SY, Mang HE (2007) Acute and chronic microvascular alterations in a mouse model of ischemic acute kidney injury. Am J Physiol Renal Physiol 293:F688–F695
23. Basile DP, Friedrich JL, Spahic J (2011) Impaired endothelial proliferation and mesenchymal transition contribute to vascular rarefaction following acute kidney injury. Am J Physiol Renal Physiol 300:F721–F733
24. Yuan HT, Li XZ, Pitera JE, Long DA, Woolf AS (2003) Peritubular capillary loss after mouse acute nephrotoxicity correlates with down-regulation of vascular endothelial growth factor-A and hypoxia-inducible factor-1 alpha. Am J Pathol 163:2289–2301
25. Loeffler I, Wolf G (2014) Transforming growth factor-beta and the progression of renal disease. Nephrol Dial Transplant 29(Suppl 1):i37–i45
26. Kinsey GR, Okusa MD (2012) Role of leukocytes in the pathogenesis of acute kidney injury. Crit Care 16:214
27. Kinsey GR, Li L, Okusa MD (2008) Inflammation in acute kidney injury. Nephron Exp Nephrol 109:e102–e107
28. Gentle ME, Shi S, Daehn I (2013) Epithelial cell TGFbeta signaling induces acute tubular injury and interstitial inflammation. J Am Soc Nephrol 24:787–799
29. Gewin L, Vadivelu S, Neelisetty S (2012) Deleting the TGF-beta receptor attenuates acute proximal tubule injury. J Am Soc Nephrol 23:2001–2011
30. Basile DP, Donohoe D, Roethe K, Osborn JL (2001) Renal ischemic injury results in permanent damage to peritubular capillaries and influences long-term function. Am J Physiol Renal Physiol 281:F887–F899

31. Tsakas S, Goumenos DS (2006) Accurate measurement and clinical significance of urinary transforming growth factor-beta1. Am J Nephrol 26:186–193
32. Dhaun N, Webb DJ (2013) The road from AKI to CKD: the role of endothelin. Kidney Int 84:637–638
33. Mino N, Kobayashi M, Nakajima A et al (1992) Protective effect of a selective endothelin receptor antagonist, BQ-123, in ischemic acute renal failure in rats. Eur J Pharmacol 221:77–83
34. Lopez-Farre A, Gomez-Garre D, Bernabeu F, Lopez-Novoa JM (1991) A role for endothelin in the maintenance of post-ischaemic renal failure in the rat. J Physiol 444:513–522
35. Clozel M, Ramuz H, Clozel JP et al (1999) Pharmacology of tezosentan, new endothelin receptor antagonist designed for parenteral use. J Pharmol Exp Ther 290:840–846
36. Abu-Saleh N, Ovcharenko E, Awad H et al (2012) Involvement of the endothelin and nitric oxide systems in the pathogenesis of renal ischemic damage in an experimental diabetic model. Life Sci 91:669–675
37. Forbes JM, Hewitson TD, Becker GJ, Jones CL (2001) Simultaneous blockade of endothelin A and B receptors in ischemic acute renal failure is detrimental to long-term kidney function. Kidney Int 59:1333–1341
38. Forbes JM, Leaker B, Hewitson TD, Becker GJ, Jones CL (1999) Macrophage and myofibroblast involvement in ischemic acute renal failure is attenuated by endothelin receptor antagonists. Kidney Int 55:198–208
39. Fenhammar J, Andersson A, Forestier J et al (2011) Endothelian receptor A antagonism attenuates renal medullary blood flow impairment in endotoxemic pigs. PLoS One 6:e21534
40. Gellai M, Jugus M, Fletcher T, DeWolf R, Nambi P (1994) Reversal of postischemic acute renal failure with a selective endothelin A receptor antagonist in the rat. J Clin Invest 93:900–906
41. Zager RA, Johnson ACM, Andress D, Becker K (2013) Progressive endothelin-1 gene activation initiates chronic/end-stage renal disease following experimental ischemic/reperfusion injury. Kidney Int 84:703–712
42. Arfian N, Emoto N, Vignon-Zellweger N, Nakayama K, Yagi K, Hirata K (2012) ET-1 deletion from endothelial cells protects the kidney during the extension phase of ischemia/reperfusion injury. Biochem Biophys Res Commun 425:443–449
43. Gulmen S, Kiris I, Narin C et al (2009) Tezosentan reduces the renal injury induced by abdominal aortic ischemia-reperfusion in rats. J Surg Res 157:e7–e13
44. Cummings RD, Liu F-T et al (2009) Galectins. In: Varki A, Cummings RD, Esko JD (eds) Essentials of Glycobiology, 2nd edn. Cold Spring Harbor Laboratory Press, New York, pp 475–488
45. Calvier L, Miana M, Reboul P et al (2013) Galectin-3 mediates aldosterone-induced vascular fibrosis. Arterioscler Thromb Vasc Biol 33:67–75
46. Lalancette-Hebert M, Swarup V, Beaulieu JM et al (2012) Galectin-3 is required for resident microglia activation and proliferation in response to ischemic injury. J Neurosci 32:10383–10395
47. Henderson NC, Mackinnon AC, Farnworth SL et al (2006) Galectin-3 regulates myofibroblast activation and hepatic fibrosis. Proc Natl Acad Sci USA 103:5060–5065
48. Nishi Y, Sano H, Kawashima T et al (2007) Role of galectin-3 in human pulmonary fibrosis. Allergol Int 56:57–65
49. Lippert E, Falk W, Bataille F et al (2007) Soluble galectin-3 is a strong, colonic epithelial-cell-derived, lamina propria fibroblast-stimulating factor. Gut 56:43–51
50. Henderson NC, Mackinnon AC, Farnworth SL et al (2008) Galectin-3 expression and secretion links macrophages to the promotion of renal fibrosis. Am J Pathol 172:288–298
51. Mackinnon AC, Gibbons MA, Farnworth SL et al (2012) Regulation of transforming growth factor-beta1-driven lung fibrosis by galectin-3. Am J Respir Crit Care Med 185:537–546
52. Sasaki S, Bao Q, Hughes RC (1999) Galectin-3 modulates rat mesangial cell proliferation and matrix synthesis during experimental glomerulonephritis induced by anti-Thy1.1 antibodies. J Pathol 187:481–489

53. O'Seaghdha CM, Hwang SJ, Ho JE, Vasan RS, Levy D, Fox CS (2013) Elevated galectin-3 precedes the development of CKD. J Am Soc Nephrol 24:1470–1477
54. Chen K, Jiang RJ, Wang CQ et al (2013) Predictive value of plasma galectin-3 in patients with chronic heart failure. Eur Rev Med Pharmacol Sci 17:1005–1011
55. Fermann GJ, Lindsell CJ, Storrow AB et al (2012) Galectin 3 complements BNP in risk stratification in acute heart failure. Biomarkers 17:706–713
56. Gopal DM, Kommineni M, Ayalon N et al (2012) Relationship of plasma galectin-3 to renal function in patients with heart failure: effects of clinical status, pathophysiology of heart failure, and presence or absence of heart failure. J Am Heart Assoc 1:e000760
57. Ho JE, Liu C, Lyass A et al (2012) Galectin-3, a marker of cardiac fibrosis, predicts incident heart failure in the community. J Am Coll Cardiol 60:1249–1256
58. Lok DJ, Klip IT, Lok SI et al (2013) Incremental prognostic power of novel biomarkers (growth-differentiation factor-15, high-sensitivity C-reactive protein, galectin-3, and high-sensitivity troponin-T) in patients with advanced chronic heart failure. Am J Cardiol 112:831–837
59. Tsai TH, Sung PH, Chang LT et al (2012) Value and level of galectin-3 in acute myocardial infarction patients undergoing primary percutaneous coronary intervention. J Atheroscler Thromb 19:1073–1082
60. van der Velde AR, Gullestad L, Ueland T et al (2013) Prognostic value of changes in galectin-3 levels over time in patients with heart failure: data from CORONA and COACH. Circ Heart Fail 6:219–226
61. Weir RA, Petrie CJ, Murphy CA et al (2013) Galectin-3 and cardiac function in survivors of acute myocardial infarction. Circ Heart Fail 6:492–498
62. de Boer RA, Yu L, van Veldhuisen DJ (2010) Galectin-3 in cardiac remodeling and heart failure. Curr Heart Fail Rep 7:1–8
63. Tang WH, Shrestha K, Shao Z et al (2011) Usefulness of plasma galectin-3 levels in systolic heart failure to predict renal insufficiency and survival. Am J Cardiol 108:385–390
64. Lok DJ, Van Der Meer P, de la Porte PW et al (2010) Prognostic value of galectin-3, a novel marker of fibrosis, in patients with chronic heart failure: data from the DEAL-HF study. Clin Res Cardiol 99:323–328
65. Shah RV, Chen-Tournoux AA, Picard MH, Kimmenade RR, Januzzi JL (2010) Galectin-3, cardiac structure and function, and long-term mortality in patients with acutely decompensated heart failure. Eur J Heart Fail 12:311–319
66. Nishiyama J, Kobayashi S, Ishida A et al (2000) Up-regulation of galectin-3 in acute renal failure of the rat. Am J Pathol 157:815–823
67. Fernandes Bertocchi AP, Campanhole G, Wang PH et al (2008) A Role for galectin-3 in renal tissue damage triggered by ischemia and reperfusion injury. Transpl Int 21:999–1007
68. Kolatsi-Joannou M, Price KL, Winyard PJ, Long DA (2011) Modified citrus pectin reduces galectin-3 expression and disease severity in experimental acute kidney injury. PLoS One 6:e18683
69. Heyman SN, Evans RG, Rosen S, Rosenberger C (2012) Cellular adaptive changes in AKI: mitigating renal hypoxic injury. Nephrol Dial Transplant 27:1721–1728
70. Epstein FH (1997) Oxygen and renal metabolism. Kidney Int 51:381–385
71. Gunaratnam L, Bonventre JV (2009) HIF in kidney disease and development. J Am Soc Nephrol 20:1877–1887
72. Nangaku M, Rosenberger C, Heyman SN, Eckardt KU (2013) Regulation of hypoxia-inducible factor in kidney disease. Clin Exp Pharmacol Physiol 40:148–157
73. Schietke RE, Hackenbeck T, Tran M et al (2012) Renal tubular HIF-2α expression requires VHL inactivation and causes fibrosis and cysts. PLoS One 7:e31034

Part IX

Hepatic and Abdominal Issues

Application of the Acute Kidney Injury Network Criteria in Patients with Cirrhosis and Ascites: Benefits and Limitations

P. Angeli, M. Tonon, and S. Piano

Introduction

Acute renal failure is a common complication in patients with cirrhosis, occurring in approximately 20% of hospitalized patients [1]. A prompt diagnosis of acute renal failure is a crucial step in the management of these patients and requires a dynamic evaluation of glomerular filtration rate (GFR). Serum creatinine is the most widely used marker of GFR in the general population. Serum creatinine is a powerful prognostic marker in patients with cirrhosis and it has been included in the model for end-stage liver disease (MELD) score which, since the early 2000s, has replaced the Child–Pugh score in the evaluation of prognosis in these patients [2]. Nevertheless, many limitations affect serum creatinine as a marker of acute renal failure. First, the increase in serum creatinine is delayed compared to renal injury and, therefore, it is a late marker of acute renal failure. Second, serum creatinine is also greatly influenced by numerous non-renal factors, such as body weight, race, age, sex. In particular, many biases and pitfalls affect the interpretation of serum creatinine as well as serum creatinine-based formulas in the setting of liver cirrhosis [3]:

a) the production of creatinine by the liver is reduced in patients with cirrhosis [4];
b) muscle wasting and malnutrition are common in advanced cirrhosis and result in a reduced production of creatinine;
c) patients with cirrhosis have increased tubular secretion of creatinine [5];
d) high values of bilirubin can interfere with laboratory estimation of creatinine [6].

As far as serum creatinine-based formulas are concerned, the Modification of Diet in Renal Disease 6 (MDRD6) equation has greater precision than other equations for assessing GFR in patients with cirrhosis, but its accuracy is less than that reported in other populations, since it overestimates GFR in these patients [3]. Therefore, direct measurement of GFR using exogenous markers remains the reference

P. Angeli ✉ · M. Tonon · S. Piano
Department of Medicine (DIMED), University of Padua, Padua, Italy
e-mail: pangeli@unipd.it

J.-L. Vincent (ed.), *Annual Update in Intensive Care and Emergency Medicine 2015*,
DOI 10.1007/978-3-319-13761-2_29

method to assess GFR in patients with cirrhosis over a period of several hours. This technique is time consuming, costly and potentially invasive if bladder catheterization has to be performed for urine collection. Other techniques used are limited by exposure to radiation and/or costs. In this context, cystatin C (Cys-C) seems to be a promising biomarker of renal function in patients with cirrhosis [7], although it requires further validation. Recently, it has been shown that serum Cys-C could represent an interesting alternative to serum creatinine [8]. In contrast to creatinine, serum Cys-C is independent of sex, age and muscle mass. The dosage is not influenced by serum bilirubin, inflammation or malignancy [7]. A recent meta-analysis has shown that, in non-cirrhotic patients, Cys-C is better correlated with GFR than creatinine [9]. Interestingly, it has been shown that the sensitivity of Cys-C for the diagnosis of impaired renal function, with a cut-off value of 1.25 mg/dl, is similar in cirrhotic patients and in non-cirrhotic patients [10]. Finally, several equations using serum Cys-C have been proposed to estimate GFR [11].

Although serum Cys-C is easy to obtain routinely, it has several limitations. First, the cost of the assay is significantly higher compared to serum creatinine. Second, the assays need further standardization [12]. Third, serum Cys-C is influenced by infection and by some drugs and by the progression of liver fibrosis [13]. Therefore, despite all its limitations, in clinical practice serum creatinine remains the key biomarker in the diagnosis of acute renal failure in patients with cirrhosis [14].

The AKIN Criteria and Their Application in Patients with Cirrhosis

An increase in serum creatinine $\geq$ 50% to a final value $\geq$ 1.5 mg/dl has been the conventional criterion for the diagnosis of acute renal failure in patients with cirrhosis [15–18]. Nevertheless, a rigid cut-off of 1.5 mg/dl could delay the diagnosis and the treatment of acute renal failure in these patients. In recent years, other criteria have been proposed for the diagnosis of acute renal failure. In particular, the Acute Kidney Injury Network (AKIN) recently developed and published a consensus definition of acute kidney injury (AKI), a new term to define acute renal failure. AKI is defined as an abrupt reduction in renal function (within 48 hours) manifest by an absolute increase in serum creatinine of 0.3 mg/dl, a percentage increase in serum creatinine of 50% or more, or a reduction in urine output (documented oliguria of less than 0.5 ml/kg per hour for more than six hours) (Table 1) [19]. As urine collection and output documentation can be inconsistent, in clinical practice the creatinine kinetic becomes the fulcrum of the definition. This is particularly true in patients with cirrhosis and ascites, who can be oliguric as a result of avid renal sodium retention despite a normal GFR [20]. The main innovative aspects introduced by the AKIN criteria with respect to conventional criteria in patients with cirrhosis are the following:

a) an absolute increase in serum creatinine is considered;
b) the threshold of serum creatinine $\geq$ 1.5 mg/dl is no longer taken into account; and

c) a staging system of AKI is based on the entity of the variation in serum creatinine to enable a progression of stage (from an initial AKIN stage to a higher peak AKIN stage) as well as a regression of stage (from an initial AKIN stage to a lower AKIN stage or to recovery of renal function) (Table 1).

The AKIN criteria have been shown to be a good predictor of mortality in large cohorts of hospitalized patients, in particular in intensive care units (ICUs) [21]. Recently, it has been claimed that the use of AKIN criteria could improve the outcome in patients with cirrhosis by facilitating targeted and timely treatment of AKI, but the need to perform clinical studies to validate this possibility was highlighted [22, 23]. To date, the AKIN criteria have been found to be a good predictor of in-hospital mortality in critically ill patients, including critically ill patients with cirrhosis [24, 25]. They were also associated with increased mortality in patients with cirrhosis hospitalized in regular wards, in a stage-dependent fashion [26–28]. Moreover, the progression of AKI to a higher stage was strongly correlated with mortality in these patients [26–28]. Recently, two prospective studies have shown that patients with cirrhosis and AKI may be differentiated into three groups according to AKIN stage and a cut-off serum creatinine of 1.5 mg/dl: Patients with AKI stage 1 and serum creatinine < 1.5 mg/dl who had short term mortality rates comparable to patients without AKI; patients with AKI stage 1 and serum creatinine ≥ 1.5 mg/dl who had a short-term mortality rate higher than patients without AKI; c) patients with AKI stage 2 and stage 3 who had higher mortality rates [26, 27]. However, when AKIN criteria were compared to conventional criteria they did not have greater accuracy as predictors of in-hospital mortality in patients with cirrhosis and ascites [26]. It should be highlighted that this observation does not exclude the possibility that AKIN criteria may improve the prediction of other relevant outcomes, such as mid-term mortality, morbidity and/or re-hospitalization. Indeed, in outpatients with advanced cirrhosis and AKI, a gradual and significant increase in serum creatinine and a gradual reduction in mean arterial pressure (MAP) were observed, associated with a significant reduction in mid-term survival compared with non-AKI patients, despite the resolution of most of the AKI episodes [29].

The main lesson derived from the application of AKIN criteria is that even a small increase in serum creatinine should be managed promptly. Recently, it has been questioned whether a change in the current definition and diagnostic criteria of

Table 1 Acute Kidney Injury Network (AKIN) criteria

Definition of AKI	An abrupt (within 48 hours) increase in serum creatinine ≥ 0.3 mg/dl and/or a percentage increase in serum creatinine of more than or equal to 50%
Staging of AKI*	**Stage 1**: increase in serum creatinine ≥ 0.3 mg/dl or an increase in serum creatinine ≥ 1.5-fold to 2-fold from baseline; **Stage 2**: increase in serum creatinine > 2-fold to 3-fold from baseline; **Stage 3**: increase in serum creatinine > 3-fold from baseline or serum creatinine ≥ 4.0 mg/dl (with an acute increase of at least 0.5 mg/dl)

* Based on the variation in serum creatinine over a slightly longer time frame, arbitrarily set at one week. AKI: acute kidney injury.

renal failure in cirrhosis is needed [30]. Currently, there is no evidence that patients with cirrhosis and AKIN stage 1 and a final value of serum creatinine < 1.5 mg/dl have reduced short-term survival [26, 27]. However, an AKI with these features is associated with an increase in the medium-term mortality in cirrhotic patients [29]. Furthermore we should recognize that for decades hepatologists have been used to treating small increases in serum creatinine with simple measures, such as tapering or withdrawal of diuretics, withdrawal of nephrotoxic drugs and/or non-steroidal anti-inflammatory drugs (NSAIDs), plasma volume expansion in case of dehydration, the treatment of any bacterial infections when diagnosed. On the basis of these observations, it seems there are no reasons to reject some of the most innovative features of AKIN criteria, such as the small increase in serum creatinine and the staging of AKI. Keeping in mind the difference in prognosis of patients with AKI and serum creatinine greater than or equal to 1.5 mg/dl we think that a combination of the conventional criteria and AKIN criteria could be useful in the management of AKI in these patients.

Thus, in order to titrate the management of AKI on the basis of the prognostic meaning derived from its initial AKIN stage, the serum creatinine value at the first fulfillment of AKIN criteria and/or AKIN stage progression, an algorithm has been recently proposed [26]. In the algorithm, the full application of the conventional criterion was implemented with the two most innovative aspects of the AKIN criteria, which are an absolute increase in serum creatinine ≥ 0.3 mg/dl, the AKIN stage classification and the progression of the initial AKIN stage.

Another major contribution of the AKIN criteria in patients with cirrhosis is to have accelerated the revision process of diagnostic criteria for type 1 hepatorenal syndrome (HRS), the phenotype of AKI with the worst prognosis in these patients [31]. It should immediately be clarified that HRS is just one among the different phenotypes of AKI, which include also pre-renal AKI, intrinsic AKI and post-renal AKI, and that, therefore, the terms AKI and HRS should not in any way be confused with each other. According to the proposed algorithm, when acute renal failure is characterized by a negative prognostic profile due to an initial serum creatinine > 1.5 mg/dl, a progression of AKIN stage despite the preliminary therapeutic measures previously mentioned, or an initial AKIN stage > 1, and has satisfied the diagnostic criteria for HRS other than the final value of serum creatinine, it should receive specific treatment, namely terlipressin and albumin. This is justified by the fact that the patient has an abrupt impairment in renal function in progression so, at least from a pathophysiological point of view, the patient has the same flow of type 1 HRS. The further increase in serum creatinine above the current cut-off of 2.5 mg/dl required for the diagnosis of type 1 HRS, in a patient with functional AKI unresponsive to volume expansion, is a function of the duration of vasoconstriction, not of the severity of vasoconstriction. Therefore, we should recognize that the AKIN criteria have contributed towards motivating us to develop more clearly the process for the prompt diagnosis and management of acute renal failure in patients with cirrhosis. In this context, the dynamic definition of acute renal failure has been intensified, which in the past was set aside in favor of a more generic definition of renal failure based on a serum creatinine ≥ 1.5 mg/dl. In addition, it was proposed that the threshold serum creatinine value of 1.5 mg/dl, although not essential for the diagnosis of AKI, increases its negative prognostic value, and should subsequently be used to titrate the treatment. Nevertheless, we should keep an open mind when considering the limitations of the AKIN criteria in patients with cirrhosis by dividing them into methodological and conceptual.

The Methodological Limitations of AKIN Criteria in Patients with Cirrhosis

Let us leave aside, for the moment, the semantic problem related to the choice of the term 'acute kidney injury'. We recognize that it is not really an appropriate term since it evokes an image of damage of renal tissue. However, this is a minor problem, since the important thing is to agree on the meaning of an expression, and this has already been highlighted, because the term AKI does not exclude the possibility of a functional form of acute renal failure such as pre-renal acute renal failure or HRS. The first methodological limit of the AKIN criteria is in its own definition: "an abrupt (within 48 hours) reduction in renal function manifested by an absolute increase in serum creatinine of 0.3 mg/dl, a percentage increase in serum creatinine of 50% or more" and, in particular, to the expression "within 48 hours". If one considers this time interval, the AKIN criteria only serve to diagnose acute renal failure in hospitalized patients using a serum creatinine value on or after admission as baseline. Nonetheless, in previous studies on the application of AKIN criteria in patients with cirrhosis, the interval between serum creatinine measurements used to define AKI ranged from days to months [25–29]. If there is a definition on which these criteria have been validated, the change in the time intervals to evaluate an increase in serum creatinine appears arbitrary and not appropriate for the detection of abrupt changes in renal function. Recently, a panel of experts suggested combining AKIN criteria (increase in serum creatinine of 0.3 mg/dl within 48 hours) with the RIFLE criteria (increase in serum creatinine greater than 50% within 1 week) [32]. However, these criteria still require a serum creatinine value to be evaluated just prior to hospital admission in order to detect community-acquired AKI, which represents almost one third of all cases of AKI [33]. This is a very crucial point, because it introduces the problem of the use of surrogates for baseline serum creatinine with relevant implications for epidemiological studies, clinical trial enrolment, and resource allocation. The use of surrogates for baseline serum creatinine in the diagnosis of community-acquired AKI can introduce methodological pitfalls that limit the interpretation of data [34]. This methodological limit of the AKIN criteria has been refuted in the general population following the argument that the use of any preadmission value for baseline serum creatinine has been shown to result in a lower misclassification of AKI incidence, severity and prognosis compared to using hospital admission and hospital nadir of serum creatinine [34].

Nevertheless, as regards the use of pre-admission values of serum creatinine, this poses a dilemma as to how far back a baseline value can be retrieved and still be expected to be 'valid'. In the general population, it is reasonable to assume that serum creatinine will be stable over several months, so that a serum creatinine obtained 6 months or even 1 year previously would reasonably reflect the patient's baseline [32, 35]. In patients with advanced liver cirrhosis, this time frame seems too long, since these patients represent a particular population. It must first be acknowledged that, in cirrhosis, the initial organ dysfunction occurs in the liver with secondary renal dysfunction. Renal dysfunction involves portal hypertension leading to splanchnic arterial vasodilatation, a reduction in effective circulating volume, the subsequent activation of the renin–angiotensin–aldosterone system (RAAS), the sympathetic nervous system (SNS) and arginine vasopressin (AVP) in order to maintain blood pressure by increasing systemic vascular resistance, along with the secondary increase in cardiac output [36]. While this compensatory neurohumoral activation attenuates hypotension secondary to arterial vasodilatation, renal vasoconstriction with sodium and water retention also occurs. Since the functional renal impairment in cirrhosis progresses gradually from compensated to decompensated with ascites to HRS it is not clear whether a previously obtained serum creatinine would reasonably reflect the patient's baseline. Furthermore, almost all patients with cirrhosis and ascites receive diuretics. Hepatologists are fully aware that fluctuations in serum creatinine in patients with cirrhosis and ascites taking diuretics are quite common. As a consequence, even if one admits the possibility that the increase in serum creatinine may exceed the 48-hour and/or 7-day limit in the application of the AKIN criteria, the question arises as to which outpatient serum creatinine value should be chosen as baseline during the weeks or months before admission: The highest, the lowest or the mean value. Furthermore, we need to ask whether an increase in serum creatinine ≥ 0.3 mg/dl at a distance of two weeks or more without any further progression can still be considered an index of an 'abrupt' impairment in renal function, i.e., an AKI. If the answer is yes, it means that in patients with cirrhosis we should forget what has been said about the contribution of the AKIN criteria in facilitating the revision of the diagnostic criteria and the management of type 1 HRS [37]. In fact, in this clinical scenario, if the patient meets all the other criteria for the diagnosis of HRS, the diagnostic conclusion will be type 2 and not type 1 HRS. Type 2 and type 1 HRS present two quite different clinical complications in patients with cirrhosis in terms of pathophysiology, prognosis and response to treatment [38]. Type 2 HRS is not an acute renal failure, it is related to splanchnic arterial vasodilation and is associated with refractory ascites and poor survival (months) [39]. Type 1 HRS is an acute renal failure that occurs secondarily to a rapid deterioration in circulatory function, often triggered by bacterial infections or other precipitating events, and is associated with extremely poor survival (days or weeks) [38, 40]. Both type 1 and type 2 HRS can be reversed following treatment with vasoconstrictors and albumin. However, the recurrence of renal failure following the discontinuation of treatment is the rule in type 2 HRS and infrequent in type 1 HRS. Another issue that makes it difficult to define a baseline serum creatinine is represented by the variability in the dosage of serum creatinine from laboratory to laboratory or in the same laboratory according, for example, to the fluctuation of serum bilirubin in patients with cirrhosis.

The final consideration concerns those patients who do not have a creatinine value before hospitalization. It would seem logical for these patients to consider the value at admission to hospital or the lowest value during the hospital stay as baseline serum creatinine. Instead, the use of an imputed value of serum creatinine has been suggested, which is calculated by the reverse application of the MDRD formula using a predetermined value of GFR (75 ml/min). However, it is well known that the MDRD formula overestimates the GFR in patients with cirrhosis [3]. As a result, its reverse application can only provide further biases in the diagnosis of AKI in these patients. On the basis of all these considerations, it is difficult to argue in favor of the applicability of an absolute increase in serum creatinine ≥ 0.3 mg/dl to a community-acquired AKI if a baseline serum creatinine acquired in the last week before hospitalization is not available.

The Conceptual Limitation of the AKIN Criteria in Patients with Cirrhosis

There is only one conceptual limitation to the applicability of the AKIN criteria in hospitalized patients with cirrhosis. This is related to the fact that these patients often have dysfunction of organs other than the kidney and, in particular, of the liver (i.e., severe cholestasis or coagulopathy) and of the central nervous system (i.e., portal-systemic encephalopathy) [41]. As recently observed by Arroyo, the recent introduction of the concept of acute-on-chronic liver failure (ACLF) adds a new dimension to the impairment of renal function in these patients [30]. According to the Canonic study, ACLF grade 1 is defined as the presence of renal failure (creatinine ≥ 2 mg/dl) or other single organ failures associated with renal dysfunction (serum creatinine 1.5–1.9 mg/dl) or moderate hepatic encephalopathy (grade 1–2), ACLF-2 by the presence of 2 organ failures, and ACLF-3 by the presence of 3 or more organ failures [41]. The definition of organ failures was based on a sequential organ failure assessment (SOFA) score specifically adapted to cirrhotic patients. The 28-day and 90-day mortality rates were only 1.9% and 9.8%, respectively, in patients without ACLF, and 33% and 51.2% in patients with ACLF (ranging from 23.1% and 40.8% in ACLF-1 to 74% and 78% in ACLF-3), indicating that stratification based on the function of the most important vital organs correlates closely with short- and mid-term mortality [40]. There are three studies assessing AKI and other stratification methods or scores (Child-Pugh, MELD, APACHE II, APACHE III, SOFA) in critically ill cirrhotic patients and they all showed that SOFA was the most accurate method to predict short-term mortality [42–44]. Thus, the prognostic evaluation in patients with cirrhosis who are hospitalized for an acute decompensation requires a more complete clinical evaluation, which also takes into account the failures of organs other than the kidney. More specifically, there are preliminary results showing that the chronic liver failure-SOFA (CLIF-SOFA) score has a better prognostic value than the AKIN criteria in these patients. If these data are confirmed, they will limit the applicability of AKIN criteria in hospitalized patients with cirrhosis to those who present only acute renal failure.

Conclusion

AKI is the most common complication of cirrhosis. The application of AKIN criteria can facilitate early management of AKI in these patients. However, the uncritical application of AKIN criteria may lead to potentially unjustifiable and dangerous therapeutic underpinnings. In this context, a combination of AKIN criteria with conventional criteria may help to titrate the management of AKI in cirrhosis. Several questions remain to be addressed in the near future concerning the selection of baseline serum creatinine for the diagnosis of community-acquired AKI, the prognosis and therapeutic strategy in patients with peak AKIN stage 1 or peak AKIN stage 2 and serum creatinine < 1.5 mg/dl, as well as the impact of the management of AKI according to new algorithms on the outcome of these patients. Nevertheless, the AKIN criteria have renewed the scientific community's interest in the management of AKI in patients with cirrhosis.

References

1. Garcia-Tsao G, Parikh CR, Viola A (2008) Acute kidney injury in cirrhosis. Hepatology 48:2064–2077
2. Kamath PS, Kim WR (2007) Advanced Liver Disease Study Group. The model for end-stage liver disease (MELD). Hepatology 45:797–805
3. Francoz C, Prié D, Abdelrazek W et al (2010) Inaccuracies of creatinine and creatinine-based equations in candidates for liver transplantation with low creatinine: impact on the model for end-stage liver disease score. Liver Transpl 16:1169–1177
4. Sherman DS, Fish DN, Teitelbaum I (2003) Assessing renal function in cirrhotic patients: problems and pitfalls. Am J Kidney Dis 41:269–278
5. Caregaro L, Menon F, Angeli P et al (1994) Limitations of serum creatinine level and creatinine clearance as filtration markers in cirrhosis. Arch Intern Med 154:201–205
6. Spencer K (1986) Analytical reviews in clinical biochemistry: the estimation of creatinine. Ann Clin Biochem 23:1–25
7. Gerbes AL, Gülberg V, Bilzer M, Vogeser M (2002) Evaluation of serum cystatin C concentration as a marker of renal function in patients with cirrhosis of the liver. Gut 50:106–110
8. Stevens LA, Coresh J, Greene T, Levey AS (2006) Assessing kidney function-measured and estimated glomerular filtration rate. N Engl J Med 354:2473–2483
9. Dharnidharka VR, Kwon C, Stevens G (2002) Serum cystatin C is superior to serum creatinine as a marker of kidney function: a meta-analysis. Am J Kidney Dis 40:221–226
10. Orlando R, Mussap M, Plebani M et al (2002) Diagnostic value of plasma cystatin C as a glomerular filtration marker in decompensated liver cirrhosis. Clin Chem 48:850–858
11. Grubb A, Nyman U, Björk J et al (2005) Simple cystatin C-based prediction equations for glomerular filtration rate compared with the modification of diet in renal disease prediction equation for adults and the Schwartz and the Counahan-Barratt prediction equations for children. Clin Chem 51:1420–1431
12. Laterza OF, Price CP, Scott MG (2002) Cystatin C: an improved estimator of glomerular filtration rate? Clin Chem 48:699–707
13. Chu SC, Wang CP, Chang YH et al (2004) Increased cystatin C serum concentrations in patients with hepatic diseases of various severities. Clin Chim Acta 341:133–138
14. Francoz C, Glotz D, Moreau R, Durand F (2010) The evaluation of renal function and disease in patients with cirrhosis. J Hepatol 52:605–613

15. Ginès P, Arroyo V, Vargas V et al (1991) Paracentesis with intravenous infusion of albumin as compared with peritoneovenous shunting in cirrhosis with refractory ascites. N Engl J Med 325:829–835
16. Sort P, Navasa M, Arroyo V et al (1999) Effect of intravenous albumin on renal impairment and mortality in patients with cirrhosis and spontaneous bacterial peritonitis. N Engl J Med 341:403–409
17. Ginès A, Fernández-Esparrach G, Monescillo A et al (1996) Randomized trial comparing albumin, dextran 70, and polygeline in cirrhotic patients with ascites treated by paracentesis. Gastroenterology 111:1002–1010
18. Angeli P, Fasolato S, Mazza E et al (2010) Combined versus sequential diuretic treatment of ascites in non-azotaemic patients with cirrhosis: results of an open randomized clinical trial. Gut 59:98–104
19. Mehta RL, Kellum JA, Shah SV et al (2007) Acute Kidney Injury Network: report of an initiative to improve outcomes in acute kidney injury. Crit Care 11:R31
20. Angeli P, Gatta A, Caregaro L et al (1990) Tubular site of renal sodium retention in ascitic liver cirrhosis evaluated by lithium clearance. Eur J Clin Invest 20:111–117
21. Joannidis M, Metnitz B, Bauer P et al (2009) Acute kidney injury in critically ill patients classified by AKIN versus RIFLE using the SAPS 3 database. Intensive Care Med 35:1692–1702
22. Wong F, Nadim MK, Kellum JA et al (2011) Working Party proposal for a revised classification system of renal dysfunction in patients with cirrhosis. Gut 60:702–709
23. Angeli P, Sanyal A, Moller S et al (2013) Current limits and future challenges in the management of renal dysfunction in patients with cirrhosis: report from the International Club of Ascites. Liver Int 33:16–23
24. Tu KH, Jenq CC, Tsai MH et al (2011) Outcome scoring systems for short-term prognosis in critically ill cirrhotic patients. Shock 36:445–450
25. de Carvalho JR, Villela-Nogueira CA, Luiz RR et al (2012) Acute kidney injury network criteria as a predictor of hospital mortality in cirrhotic patients with ascites. J Clin Gastroenterol 46:e21–e26
26. Piano S, Rosi S, Maresio G et al (2013) Evaluation of the Acute Kidney Injury Network criteria in hospitalized patients with cirrhosis and ascites. J Hepatol 59:482–489
27. Fagundes C, Barreto R, Guevara M et al (2013) A modified acute kidney injury classification for diagnosis and risk stratification of impairment of kidney function in cirrhosis. J Hepatol 59:474–481
28. Belcher JM, Garcia-Tsao G, Sanyal AJ et al (2013) Association of AKI with mortality and complications in hospitalized patients with cirrhosis. Hepatology 57:753–762
29. Tsien CD, Rabie R, Wong F (2013) Acute kidney injury in decompensated cirrhosis. Gut 62:131–137
30. Arroyo V (2013) Acute kidney injury (AKI) in cirrhosis: Should we change current definition and diagnostic criteria of renal failure in cirrhosis? J Hepatol 59:415–417
31. Martín-Llahí M, Guevara M, Torre A et al (2011) Prognostic importance of the cause of renal failure in patients with cirrhosis. Gastroenterology 140:488–496
32. KDIGO (2012) Clinical Practice Guideline for Acute Kidney Injury. Kidney Int Suppl 2:19–36
33. Daher EF, Silva GB Jr, Santos SQ et al (2012) Differences in community, hospital and intensive care unit-acquired acute kidney injury: observational study in a nephrology service of a developing country. Clin Nephrol 78:449–455
34. Siew ED, Matheny ME, Alp Ikizler T et al (2010) Commonly used surrogates for baseline renal function affect the classification and prognosis of acute kidney injury. Kidney Int 77:536–542
35. Bagshaw SM, Uchino S, Cruz D et al (2009) A comparison of observed versus estimated baseline creatinine for determination of RIFLE class in patients with acute kidney injury. Nephrol Dial Transplant 24:2739–2744

36. Schrier RW, Shchekochikhin D, Ginès P (2012) Renal failure in cirrhosis: prerenal azotemia, hepatorenal syndrome and acute tubular necrosis. Nephrol Dial Transplant 27:2625–2628
37. Arroyo V, Gines P, Gerbes AL et al (1996) Definition and diagnostic criteria of refractory ascites and hepatorenal syndrome in cirrhosis. Hepatology 23:164–176
38. Alessandria C, Ozdogan O, Guevara M et al (2005) MELD score and clinical type predict prognosis in hepatorenal syndrome: relevance to liver transplantation. Hepatology 41:1282–1289
39. Ruiz-del-Arbol L, Monescillo A, Arocena C et al (2005) Circulatory function and hepatorenal syndrome in cirrhosis. Hepatology 42:439–447
40. Fasolato S, Angeli P, Dallagnese L et al (2007) Renal failure and bacterial infections in patients with cirrhosis: epidemiology and clinical features. Hepatology 45:223–229
41. Moreau R, Jalan R, Gines P et al (2013) Acute-on-chronic liver failure is a distinct syndrome that develops in patients with acute decompensation of cirrhosis. Gastroenterology 44:1426–1437
42. Cholongitas E, Calvaruso V, Senzolo M et al (2009) RIFLE classification as predictive factor of mortality in patients with cirrhosis admitted to intensive care unit. J Gastroenterol Hepatol 24:1639–1647
43. Pan HC, Jenq CC, Tsai MH et al (2012) Risk models and scoring systems for predicting the prognosis in critically ill cirrhotic patients with acute kidney injury: a prospective validation study. PLoS One 7:e51094
44. Jenq CC, Tsai MH, Tian YC et al (2007) Rifle classification can predict short-term prognosis in critically ill cirrhotic patients. Intensive Care Med 33:1921–1930

Intensive Care Management of Severe Acute Liver Failure

S. Warrillow and R. Bellomo

Introduction

Severe acute liver failure is defined as the development of overt liver failure with encephalopathy over eight weeks or less in previously healthy individuals. In hyperacute liver failure, deterioration occurs in less than 14 days. Whilst it is a relatively uncommon reason for admission to the intensive care unit (ICU), acute liver failure is important because it often occurs in previously well young adults and carries a high mortality. Management of these patients presents considerable challenges within the ICU due to the extreme nature of the associated pathophysiological processes, which affect multiple systems. Integrated management strategies have been poorly studied and treatment is often center-specific [1]. Clinical manifestations include a reduced conscious state, jaundice with abnormal liver function tests (especially elevations in amino acid transferase levels more than 25 times the upper limit of normal) and coagulopathy. Further deterioration can involve marked cerebral edema, hypoglycemia and severe shock with lactic acidosis and multiple organ failure. The use of clinical management guidelines may assist in the treatment of these patients by providing an evidence-based framework for care by staff at the bedside, which ensures that all important priorities are adequately addressed. It is possible that a coordinated combination of specific and general therapies may reduce mortality and the need for liver transplantation. Consideration for transfer to a unit with expertise in liver transplantation may be appropriate in order for this option to be available as a life-saving treatment should supportive care fail to arrest deterioration.

S. Warrillow ✉ · R. Bellomo
Department of Intensive Care, The University of Melbourne, Austin Health, Heidelberg, Australia
e-mail: Stephen.Warrillow@austin.org.au

J.-L. Vincent (ed.), *Annual Update in Intensive Care and Emergency Medicine 2015*,
DOI 10.1007/978-3-319-13761-2_30

Etiology of Severe Acute Liver Failure

Hepatotropic viral infections, drug-induced liver injury, autoimmune processes, metabolic disorders and vascular thrombosis are responsible for most cases of acute liver failure [2] (Table 1). Causes of severe acute liver failure requiring ICU admission vary across regions, with drug-induced liver injury more common in industrialized nations and viral pathogens more common in developing countries. Up to a fifth of cases have no clear cause and may be due to as yet unrecognized viral entities, unusual presentations of autoimmune processes or unrecognized drug complications. Patients in whom critical illness develops rapidly (e.g., hyperacute liver failure from paracetamol [acetaminophen] toxicity) may recover completely without the need for liver transplantation if not overwhelmed by multiple organ failure, severe cerebral edema or complications, such as sepsis. For patients who exhibit a less fulminant course (e.g., as a result of idiosyncratic drug reactions), death is a frequent outcome unless transplantation is undertaken. Severe liver injury can sometimes also occur as a consequence of prolonged shock, where situations of advanced hemodynamic compromise result in ischemic hepatitis and considerable derangement of liver function. In this setting, ICU management is most appropriately directed to addressing the cause of the shocked state and its consequences, with specific liver failure directed therapies rarely required.

Table 1 Etiology of acute liver failure

Major causes of acute liver failure	Examples
Drugs	Dose related: – Paracetamol Idiosyncratic: – Isoniazid – Beta-lactams – NSAIDS – Herbal remedies
Toxins	Amanita mushroom
Viral	HAV, HBV, HEV, HSV, CMV, EBV
Vascular thrombosis	Budd-Chiari syndrome
Inherited metabolic disorders	Wilson's disease
Pregnancy-related	Acute fatty liver of pregnancy
Other	Autoimmune hepatitis Reye Syndrome

NSAID: non-steroidal anti-inflammatory drug; HAV: hepatitis A virus; HBV: hepatitis B virus; HEV: hepatitis E virus; HSV: herpes simplex virus; CMV: cytomegalovirus; EBV: Epstein-Barr virus.

Management Problems

The rapid onset, severity and complexity of organ failure in patients with severe acute liver failure necessitate urgent admission to the ICU in the majority of cases. Patients with acute liver failure exhibiting any combination of encephalopathy, acute renal failure, hypotension, lactic acidemia or hypoglycemia should be admitted to the ICU as fulminant deterioration is likely.

Cerebral Edema and Intracranial Hypertension

Cerebral edema occurs in many patients with high-grade encephalopathy. Brainstem herniation is a common cause of death in acute liver failure and occurs because of severe cerebral swelling causing refractory intracranial hypertension. The pathophysiology of acute liver failure-associated cerebral edema is complex, but the accumulation of metabolic toxins, such as ammonia [3], and the loss of cerebral autoregulation resulting in hyperemia [4] are two key drivers.

Ammonia is a waste product of nitrogen metabolism and undergoes detoxification via the urea cycle. The liver is responsible for most of this detoxification activity and hyperammonemia is a cardinal feature of severe liver failure. Ammonia readily crosses the blood brain barrier and the increasing brain tissue concentrations cause neuroexcitation, astrocyte swelling and disruption of many crucial neuronal processes. A range of crucial astrocyte signaling and intracellular functions are also impacted, causing further central nervous system (CNS) impairment. Ammonia concentrations more than 117 μmol/l are highly associated with the development of severe cerebral edema and intracranial hypertension [5]. Severe acute liver failure also results in the accumulation of false neurotransmitters, CNS depressants, and inflammatory mediators, which may reduce consciousness. Like ammonia, these neurotoxic substances are generally small and water-soluble and may, therefore, be removed by extracorporeal therapy.

Cerebral blood flow is normally tightly regulated across a wide range of systemic arterial pressures. Autoregulation is lost in patients with severe acute liver failure due to abnormal regulation of vasoactive mediators within the CNS. This leads to cerebral hyperemia and vasogenic edema in severely encephalopathic patients.

Features of severe cerebral edema with resultant intracranial hypertension are difficult to detect in critically ill patients with multiple organ failure and regular clinical evaluation is necessary.

Vasodilatory Shock

A vasodilated, hyperdynamic circulation is present in most patients with acute liver failure. Relative or absolute hypovolemia may develop due to poor fluid intake prior to presentation, abnormal external fluid losses, loss of intravascular volume into the interstitium and vasodilatation. Many patients will be shocked and require vasopressor therapy [2]. Occasional patients may exhibit a low cardiac output state, (for example, due to pre-existing cardiac pathology), and require inotropic support. Circulatory failure results in generalized malperfusion ultimately leading to critical dysfunction in multiple organ systems.

Sepsis

Acute liver failure patients with multi-organ dysfunction are at high risk of infective complications [6], especially overwhelming Gram-negative and fungal sepsis. Pathogens may emerge from a patient's own microbiological flora or may be acquired from the hospital environment. Common sites of infection include the lower respiratory tract, the urinary tract and invasive vascular access devices.

Coagulopathy

Coagulopathy is one of the defining features of hepatic decompensation. Hepatic synthesis of clotting factors fails and many patients also develop significant thrombocytopenia. Bleeding may complicate the insertion of invasive devices, or occur spontaneously. While spontaneous intracranial hemorrhage is very rare, the consequences can be devastating. Sometimes, despite severe derangement of measured clotting parameters, a hypercoaguable state develops [7] and may result in thrombotic complications, such as digital ischemia, portal vein thrombosis or lower limb deep venous thrombosis. A patient's clotting profile can be a guide to the severity of their liver failure and normalization of a prolonged prothrombin time or international normalized ratio (INR) in the absence of clotting factor support suggests hepatic regeneration and recovery of synthetic function.

Renal Failure

Whether as a result of the primary pathology that also affects the liver (e.g., paracetamol overdose) or as a consequence of systemic inflammatory response with shock, renal failure is a common problem in patients with acute liver failure. Consequences of renal failure include electrolyte derangement and fluid balance problems, both of which contribute significantly to the complex pathophysiology of acute liver failure. Severe uremia is relatively uncommon due to disruption of the urea cycle.

Fluid and Electrolyte Management

Patients with acute liver failure will tend to accumulate a positive fluid balance and electrolyte abnormalities due to the administration of fluid boluses for circulatory support, clotting factors and various other intravenous therapies, such as antimicrobials. This can have several undesirable consequences including a predisposition to cerebral edema.

Initial Evaluation and Investigations

Critically ill patients with acute liver failure with airway compromise or respiratory failure should be urgently intubated and appropriately ventilated. Shocked patients must be resuscitated with intravenous fluid and vasoactive infusions. Hypoglycemia should be checked for and reversed with prompt parenteral glucose administration. A careful history, clinical examination and series of investigations should follow.

History

It is often necessary to obtain important details from friends and relatives of critically ill patients. Important details include: Previous general health, history of chronic liver disease (to differentiate from decompensated cirrhosis), family history of liver disease, and risk factors for viral hepatitis (illicit drug use, tattoos, sexual history, travel). A comprehensive discussion of drug therapies (prescription and non-prescription pharmaceuticals, herbal remedies, illicit drugs, alcohol use) must occur and a specific history of mushroom ingestion should be sought. Female patients should be asked about the possibility of pregnancy.

Examination

After initial resuscitation, patients must be checked for evidence of chronic liver disease (e.g., wasting, clubbing, leukonychia, gynecomastia, spider nevi, advanced ascites, prominent abdominal wall veins). Encephalopathy can be graded according to the West Haven criteria, but critical care physicians may be more familiar with the Glasgow Coma Scale (GCS) for describing abnormal conscious states. Whichever approach is utilized, a base-line assessment will allow for subsequent repeated appraisal so that deterioration may be detected. The skin should be assessed for herpetic lesions, tattoos and needle tracks. Eye examination should include looking for Kayser-Fleischer rings. Abdominal examination should evaluate liver and spleen size as well as the presence of ascites.

Investigations

All acute liver failure patients should have a full blood examination (including a blood film), electrolyte profile and renal function tests. Blood levels of bilirubin, transaminases, albumin, clotting profile and glucose will help determine the extent of liver injury and function. Arterial blood gas analysis (including lactate) is extremely useful in guiding therapy and assessing the severity of the patient's illness. Serum lipase should be checked to detect associated pancreatitis. Blood ammonia levels may be predictive of encephalopathy and samples should be transported to the pathology laboratory in ice. All of the above investigations should be repeated regularly to guide treatment. Paracetamol levels must be checked in all patients, even in the absence of a documented overdose. Levels of other drugs may also be appropriate depending on circumstances. Viral testing for hepatitis A, B and E as well as Epstein-Barr virus (EBV), herpes simplex virus (HSV) and cytomegalovirus (CMV) should be undertaken. Copper studies, autoimmune testing and an abdominal ultrasound (including Doppler assessment of flow in the hepatic vessels) should be completed early during admission along with pregnancy testing of female patients. In shocked patients on vasoactive infusions, a bed-side hemodynamic assessment using echocardiography may guide the approach to circulatory support. If there is concern about intracranial pathology (e.g., possible head trauma), computed tomography (CT) imaging should be arranged.

Treatments for Specific Causes of Acute Liver Failure

Specific therapies directed towards the cause of acute liver failure have limited utility except in a few instances. N-acetylcysteine (NAC) should be started in all patients with known or suspected paracetamol-induced acute liver failure. Continuation of NAC by infusion is recommended until the resolution of critical illness. Nucleoside analogs are indicated for acute hepatitis B infection and acyclovir for HSV. A trial of corticosteroids may be appropriate for autoimmune hepatitis, although resolution of acute liver failure is rare in this situation. Emergency cesarean section delivery is indicated for critically ill women with acute fatty liver of pregnancy. High doses of intravenous penicillin or silibinin may be useful in amanita mushroom poisoning, although the latter may be difficult to source.

Prevention and Management of Neurological Complications in Acute Liver Failure

The risk of death from cerebral edema and associated refractory intracranial hypertension from acute liver failure is considerable. A number of treatments have been trialed and it may be that the utilization of combination therapy offers the most effective approach. The combination of mild hyperventilation, high dose hemodiafiltration, hypernatremia and mild hypothermia has been termed quadruple-H therapy [8] (Table 2) and may be readily delivered in most ICUs.

Table 2 Summary of quadruple-H interventions and therapeutic targets for acute liver failure patients with severe encephalopathy. From [8] (with permission)

Neuroprotective Intervention	Therapeutic Target	Method of Therapy	Mechanism
Hyperventilation	$PaCO_2 = 35$ mmHg or that achieved by the patient prior to intubation (whichever is lower)	Set mechanical ventilation to achieve sufficient minute ventilation	Attenuates cerebral hyperemia Lowers ICP
Hemodiafiltration	Blood ammonia < 60 μmol/l and even daily fluid balance	High volume CRRT utilizing dialysis and filtration	Reduces blood ammonia concentration Allows precise metabolic, electrolyte and fluid management Cooling effect
Hypernatremia	Serum sodium 145–155 mmol/l	Continuous infusion of concentrated saline via central venous catheter	Increased serum tonicity and reduces cerebral edema
Hypothermia	Core temperature 33–35 °C	CRRT circuit and external cooling blanket	Reduces ammonia production and CNS uptake Attenuates cerebral hyperemia and reduces cerebral metabolic rate Reduces neuro-excitation Anti-inflammatory effects

CRRT: continuous renal replacement therapy; ICP: intracranial pressure; CNS: central nervous system.

Hyperventilation

Even when in an advanced state of coma, patients with acute liver failure tend to hyperventilate [9]. It is important when undertaking intubation and initiating mechanical ventilation that sufficient support is provided in order to target a $PaCO_2$ equivalent to the lower of that achieved by the patient prior to intubation, or at least a value at the low end of the normal range [1]. Hypercarbia must be assiduously avoided. Mild hyperventilation helps attenuate cerebral vasodilatation and associated hyperemia and can be safely guided by regular arterial blood gas analysis and end-tidal exhaled CO_2 ($EtCO_2$) monitoring. Hyperventilation to $PaCO_2$ values significantly lower than the normal range offer little additional benefit and tend to become ineffective over a short time with risk of rebound intracranial hypertension [10]. Aggressive hyperventilation should be reserved for use only as a rescue therapy in cases where severe intracranial hypertension is evident and rapid transplantation is planned.

Hemodiafiltration

All intubated patients with acute liver failure should have urgent placement of a dual lumen vascular access catheter for initiation of continuous renal replacement therapy (CRRT). Clotting factor support may be required to facilitate insertion of large venous catheters. Modalities incorporating both diffusive and convective clearance (e.g., hemodiafiltration) may be more effective than filtration alone. Lactate-free replacement fluid (i.e., bicarbonate buffered) must be used for hemofiltration to avoid contributing to elevations in blood lactate concentrations. Modern integrated CRRT machines used in the ICU have integrated heating mechanisms, which may be turned off or run at the lowest permitted temperatures as a way of lowering the patient's core temperature. Anticoagulation is rarely required, especially if good circuit blood flows can be achieved. The use of an extracorporeal blood purification therapy, such as CRRT, can rapidly lower blood ammonia concentrations and is a key neuroprotective strategy [8]. Ammonia undergoes similar clearance to urea when CRRT is applied and treatment should be given at sufficient intensity to lower levels to near the normal range. Treatment should not be delayed until overt renal failure or uremia is evident. Additional benefits of CRRT include achievement of an even fluid balance, correction of electrolyte disturbances, improvement of acid-base abnormalities and prevention of fever. High dose CRRT may result in hypophosphatemia and measurements should be undertaken at least daily with low serum levels being treated as required. Intermittent dialysis is less preferred in acute liver failure [11] because of the undesirable impact on already compromised hemodynamics and problems associated with discontinuous therapies, such as rebound hyperammonemia.

Hypernatremia

Osmotherapies have a long established role in the management of cerebral edema. The continuous administration of hypertonic saline (e.g., 20% sodium chloride at 5–10 ml/hour) via a central line is an effective and straightforward approach to increasing serum tonicity and inducing dehydration of brain parenchyma [8]. Serum sodium concentrations of 145–155 mmol/l should be targeted and can be readily checked using point-of-care blood gas analysis within the ICU. Additional potential benefits include anti-inflammatory effects, reduced cerebral hyperemia [12] and maintenance of the systemic circulatory volume [13]. Hypertonic saline may be preferred to other osmotherapies, such as mannitol. Mannitol has also been used in acute liver failure-associated intracranial hypertension, but repeat dosing might result in delayed worsening of cerebral edema as it enters into brain tissue through a damaged blood-brain-barrier, inducing a 'reverse' osmotic gradient.

Hypothermia

The therapeutic lowering of core body temperature reduces both ammonia production and its entry into the CNS [14]. CNS inflammation and toxic injury to astrocytes are also attenuated at sub-normal body temperatures. Therapeutic hypothermia is safe to apply in the ICU and most studies have aimed for a core temperature range of 32 to 33 °C, but higher targets of up to 35 °C are also effective [15] and may be safer. Lower temperatures may provide further cerebral protection, but with an increased theoretical risk of complications, such as bleeding, immunosuppression and sepsis. More extreme hypothermia should be relegated to use as a rescue therapy when severe cerebral edema is present and urgent liver transplantation is available. External cooling is usually effective, and servo-controlled cooling blankets using continuous core temperature monitoring are recommended in order to achieve effective temperature regulation.

Other Therapies for Severe Cerebral Edema in Acute Liver Failure

A range of treatments have been proposed for refractory cerebral edema and may be trialed as rescue therapies. In addition to more aggressive application of the quadruple-H measures outlined above, deep sedation (e.g., with propofol) and muscle relaxants may acutely lower intracranial pressure (ICP) [16]. Other options include the administration of indomethacin, which has been shown to transiently reduce cerebral hyperemia and lower ICP [17]. Unless life-saving liver transplantation can be urgently arranged, however, these strategies are unlikely to impact on outcomes.

Quadruple-H neuroprotective therapy should continue for the period of most severe encephalopathy, which generally lasts 4 to 7 days for paracetamol related-acute liver failure, but may persist for significantly longer when the hepatic injury results from other causes. The role of invasive ICP monitoring has been increasingly questioned given a lack of evidence for benefit [18, 19]. The routine application of neuroprotective measures for acute liver failure patients in ICU may render the insertion of ICP monitors unnecessary.

Other Neurological Care

A range of additional ammonia lowering therapies may be considered, but limited evidence of benefit and lack of availability may deter their use. Enteral administration of lactulose can be tried, but may produce significant abdominal distension without substantial benefit in acute liver failure. L-ornithine-L-aspartate [20] and L-ornithine-phenylacetate [21] accelerate ammonia metabolism and have shown promise in limited animal and clinical studies. Complex blood purification technologies such as Coupled Plasma Filtration Adsorption (CPFA) [22], Molecular Adsorbent Recirculation System (MARS) [23], the bio-artificial Extracorporeal Liver

Assist Device (ELAD) and Normothermic Extracorporeal Liver Perfusion (NELP) [24] may have a place, but have yet to be demonstrably beneficial as routine care in the setting of acute liver failure and their use should be confined to clinical trials.

Seizures may occur in the setting of severe acute liver failure-associated cerebral edema and may be difficult to detect clinically [25]. Electroencephalography (EEG) assessment is necessary to establish the diagnosis definitively and guide treatment with anticonvulsants, such as propofol, benzodiazepines or levetiracetam.

Supporting the Circulation in Acute Liver Failure

Patients with severe acute liver failure usually have a vasodilated, hypotensive and hyperdynamic circulation with preservation of cardiac output. Loss of vascular tone results in failure to maintain adequate end-organ perfusion pressure in a manner very similar to advanced states of septic shock. In addition to vasodilatory shock, microvascular dysfunction causes the loss of fluid into the interstitium, intravascular thrombosis and abnormalities of blood flow within capillary beds. While the exact mechanisms underlying the loss of normal hemodynamic homeostasis are incompletely understood, severe inflammation, abnormal neurohormonal control and endothelial injury are all likely to contribute to the evolution of severe shock. Coupled with mitochondrial dysfunction and generalized inflammation, lactic acid levels rise as production increases and clearance (mainly hepatic) decreases [26].

Intra-arterial catheters are required for adequate monitoring in critically ill acute liver failure patients. Central venous access allows assessment of the central venous pressure (CVP) in response to fluid challenges and the safe administration of vasoactive infusions. Given the number of infusions required by critically ill acute liver failure patients, several multi-lumen central venous catheters may be necessary. Continuous or intermittent measurement of cardiac output (e.g., intra-arterial pulse contour measuring technologies) may be useful to guide treatment of severely shocked acute liver failure patients. The insertion of vascular catheters may necessitate the administration of clotting factors to prevent major bleeding related to the procedure. If such administration is provided, the additional volume should be removed by CRRT in order to avoid fluid overload and more cerebral edema and/or acute respiratory distress syndrome (ARDS). Focused bedside hemodynamic assessment using echocardiography is an increasingly available technology, but requires skill and experience to perform reliably.

After adequate fluid resuscitation has been administered, the majority of patients will remain hypotensive and shocked such that vasopressor therapy is indicated. Norepinephrine by continuous infusion through a central venous catheter and titrated to effect is a common approach to supporting the systemic arterial pressure. In situations where large doses of intravenous catecholamine infusions are required (e.g., norepinephrine > 0.5 μg/kg/min), it may be reasonable to commence vasopressin by infusion as a means of improving vascular tone. Concerns that similar drugs can worsen cerebral edema [27] need to be considered against the need to respond to a severely compromised circulation. Moreover, many of these patients are young and a mean arterial pressure (MAP) of 60 mmHg may be acceptable. Of interest, although never formally studied, the hyperemic cerebral edema of acute liver failure may be increased when higher MAP values are targeted.

The administration of large volumes of fluid to critically ill patients is routine during the resuscitation phase of ICU management. Ongoing accumulation of fluid after this period is also common, especially in the setting of multiple drug infusions, clotting factor support and artificial nutrition. Coupled with reduced plasma protein levels, this may lead to severe generalized interstitial fluid overload resulting in a propensity for edema in vulnerable organs such as the lungs and brain. Efforts to carefully manage fluid therapy in order to avoid an escalating positive fluid balance might be beneficial, as may be the utilization of concentrated albumin (e.g., 20% human albumin solution) to maintain intravascular volume without associated fluid overload. Hypotonic solutions (e.g., 5% dextrose) must be carefully avoided in acute liver failure patients in order to minimize the risk of exacerbating cerebral edema.

The exact role of corticosteroid therapy for circulatory support in critical illness currently remains somewhat unresolved. While the use of low dose corticosteroids in septic shock may not impact on patient-centered outcomes, such as mortality, few adverse events have been associated with the administration of relatively low doses in this context. It may be that absolute or relative adrenal insufficiency with potential end-organ cortisol resistance does occur in severe acute liver failure [28], such that corticosteroid administration does have a specific role in this context.

Prolonged infusion of NAC is absolutely indicated in patients with paracetamol-induced acute liver failure, and there could be a role in patients with severe acute liver failure from other causes also. Continuous infusion of NAC may improve hemodynamic parameters and provide other benefits in shocked acute liver failure patients [29] and has few associated risks with extended use.

General Supportive Care in Acute Liver Failure

Critically ill patients with multiple organ failure require carefully coordinated care by all members of the ICU multidisciplinary team. In addition to acute liver failure-specific neurological care and circulatory support, other aspects of management may be influenced by the presence of hepatic dysfunction.

Sepsis

Serious infection is a major cause of death in patients admitted to the ICU with acute liver failure. Nosocomial pneumonia, catheter-related blood stream infections, intra-abdominal sepsis and urinary tract infection commonly develop in the context of acute liver failure-associated multiple organ failure with shock. Gram-negative and fungal pathogens are major culprit organisms and may be acquired from the hospital environment or arise from the patient's own flora. The role of early empiric antimicrobial therapy is not fully established; however, given the high risks of overwhelming sepsis contributing to cerebral edema and circulatory failure, the routine use of early broad spectrum antibiotics and antifungal therapies has been suggested [2]. Stringent surveillance for possible infection should always be undertaken, including chest X-rays and regular cultures of blood, urine and sputum.

Respiratory Support

Patients with advanced encephalopathy (e.g., West Haven grade III or IV or a GCS of < 8) should be intubated to minimize the risk of airway obstruction or aspiration. The need for sufficient minute ventilation required to optimize $PaCO_2$ is an important component of neuroprotective care and hypoventilation must be carefully avoided. Periods of risk include during intubation, the initiation of mechanical ventilation and patient transport (e.g., between hospitals or to the radiology department). Regular arterial blood gas testing and measurement of exhaled $EtCO_2$ is mandatory to guide ventilatory support.

Renal Support

The early initiation of CRRT may more correctly be considered as part of a CNS protective strategy and control of ammonia levels, rather than renal replacement therapy and as such, treatment should not be delayed until problems associated with overt renal dysfunction are evident. The maintenance of high blood flow (e.g., > 250 ml/min), the use of pre-dilution hemofiltration replacement fluid and optimal vascular access are important factors in ensuring adequate circuit life. Anticoagulation treatment may not significantly improve filter life [30] and is best avoided in patients with severe coagulopathy. Hemofiltration fluid exchange rates of 40 to 50 ml/kg/hour may be necessary to achieve adequate ammonia clearance. With high intensity CRRT, close monitoring and replacement of electrolytes (e.g., potassium, phosphate, magnesium) and supplementation of water-soluble vitamins is advisable. Frequent interruptions to CRRT are undesirable and should prompt a careful evaluation for preventable causes. Phosphate supplementation in particular should be started early (within 24 hours of initiation of CRRT) because high volume therapy will remove approximately 1 mmol/l and liver regeneration will also consume significant amounts of phosphate.

Hematological Support

Marked abnormalities in laboratory-based measurements of clotting are a hallmark of severe acute liver failure. Despite sometimes gross prolongation of the prothrombin time, significant hypofibrinogenemia and severe thrombocytopenia, spontaneous major hemorrhage is uncommon. Parenteral vitamin K should be administered to all patients with acute liver failure-associated coagulopathy. Many patients may actually manifest a strong tendency to pro-thrombotic complications and caution is, therefore, warranted regarding the administration of clotting factors except where invasive procedures are necessary or actual bleeding occurs. In the absence of major bleeding events, reasonable targets include an INR of <6, platelet count of $>20/\text{mm}^3$, and a fibrinogen concentration of more than 1.0 g/l. Clotting factor support may include fresh-frozen plasma (FFP), prothrombin concentrate, pooled platelets and cryoprecipitate.

Metabolic, Gastrointestinal Care and Nutritional Support

Hypoglycemia is common in severe acute liver failure and should be immediately corrected as part of initial management. Patients with persisting low blood glucose levels will require the continuous infusion of concentrated glucose (e.g., 25% dextrose solution) via a central venous catheter, aiming for a blood glucose concentration of between 6 and 10 mmol/l. Once hepatic recovery is established, many patients will exhibit a tendency to hyperglycemia and require continuous infusion of short acting insulin to avoid excessive elevations in blood glucose concentrations.

Patients with acute liver failure are at high risk of gastrointestinal hemorrhage. The routine use of H_2-blockers (e.g., ranitidine) or proton-pump-inhibitors (e.g., pantoprazole) is appropriate.

Enteral tube feeding is recommended for patients with acute liver failure and is achievable in most situations. Evidence supporting specific recommendations for the content of enteral feeds in acute liver failure patients is poor. Branch-chain amino acid-enriched formulations are significantly more expensive and may confer little benefit beyond standard formulations used within the ICU.

The Role of Liver Transplantation in Acute Liver Failure

Orthotopic liver transplantation has been shown to be life-saving in some circumstances [31]. For patients with severe acute liver failure from Wilson's disease, autoimmune hepatitis or idiosyncratic drug reactions, survival in the absence of transplantation is rare. Optimal treatment may, however, offer an extension on the period of time available to source a suitable organ for transplantation and maintain patients in a state suitable to undergo the rigors of major surgery. The decision to transplant a patient with acute liver failure is extremely challenging and must involve extensive evaluation by experienced hepatologists, transplant surgeons and intensivists. The development of better prognostic scoring systems is needed [2]. For other causes of severe acute liver failure, such as paracetamol toxicity or viral hepatitis, effective supportive care will ideally result in a live patient discharged from hospital with their own liver fully recovered.

Table 3 General management of patients with severe acute liver failure in the ICU

Intervention	Goals/Approach	Method/Examples
Treatment for specific causes of acute liver failure	Reversal of/prevention of further hepatic injury	NAC infusion for paracetamol overdose Nucleoside analogues for acute HBV Penicillin or silibinin for amanita mushroom poisoning Emergent delivery for AFLP
Circulatory support	Hemodynamic parameters according to patient's clinical progress: CVP 6–10 mmHg MAP 65–70 mmHg Even daily fluid balance	Fluid administration Vasoactive infusions e.g. norepinephrine Low dose corticosteroid administration
Sepsis care	Empiric broad spectrum antibiotics and antifungal therapy Regular culture of blood, urine and sputum Daily CXR	Extended spectrum beta-lactams Liposomal amphotericin
Ventilatory support	See hyperventilation section of Table 2	Intubate patients with advanced encephalopathy Provide adequate ventilation to achieve neuroprotective $PaCO_2$
Renal support	See hemodiafiltration section of Table 2	Run blood flow > 200 ml/min Use pre-dilution to minimize filter clotting Use high exchange rates of lactate free replacement fluid (40–50 ml/kg/h) Turn off heater Monitor electrolytes (especially phosphate, potassium, magnesium)
Hematological support	Hb > 7.0 g/dl INR < 6 Platelet count > $20/mm^3$ Fibrinogen > 1.0 g/l	Do not attempt to normalize abnormal clotting values unless extreme derangement, active bleeding or need for invasive procedures Administer Vitamin K 10 mg i.v. daily Use FFP, platelets and cryoprecipitate if factor support is required
Metabolic/ gastrointestinal/ nutritional support	Blood glucose 6–10 mmol/l Stress ulcer prophylaxis Enteral feeding	Concentrated dextrose infusion via central line H_2-blocker or PPI therapy Enteral feeding via nasogastric tube

CVP: central venous pressure; MAP: mean arterial pressure; CXR: chest X-ray; Hb: hemoglobin; NAC: N-acetylcysteine; HBV: hepatitis B virus; AFLP: acute fatty liver of pregnancy; FFP: fresh frozen plasma; PPI: proton pump inhibitor.

Conclusion

Despite the severe and complex nature of critical illness resulting from acute liver failure, good patient outcomes may be achieved through the use of an integrated management plan (Table 3) that targets specific pathophysiological processes. The combination of quadruple-H therapy and comprehensive general intensive care support can be provided in most critical care settings and may reduce mortality and the need for liver transplantation. In extremely unwell patients, transfer to a major transplant center may be appropriate in order to optimize care, even if need for transplantation is not considered a likely ultimate outcome.

References

1. Stravitz RT, Kramer AH, Davern T et al (2007) Intensive care of patients with acute liver failure: recommendations of the U.S. Acute Liver Failure Study Group. Crit Care Med 35:2498–2508
2. Polson J, Lee WM (2005) AASLD position paper: the management of acute liver failure. Hepatology 41:1179–1197
3. Wendon J, Lee W (2008) Encephalopathy and cerebral edema in the setting of acute liver failure: pathogenesis and management. Neurocrit Care 9:97–102
4. Raghavan M, Marik PE (2006) Therapy of intracranial hypertension in patients with fulminant hepatic failure. Neurocrit Care 4:179–189
5. Clemmesen JO, Larsen FS, Kondrup J, Hansen BA, Ott P (1999) Cerebral herniation in patients with acute liver failure is correlated with arterial ammonia concentration. Hepatology 29:648–653
6. Wasmuth HE, Kunz D, Yagmur E et al (2005) Patients with acute on chronic liver failure display "sepsis-like" immune paralysis. J Hepatol 42:195–201
7. Agarwal B, Wright G, Gatt A et al (2012) Evaluation of coagulation abnormalities in acute liver failure. Journal of hepatology 57:780–786
8. Warrillow SJ, Bellomo R (2014) Preventing cerebral oedema in acute liver failure: the case for quadruple-H therapy. Anaesth Intensive Care 42:78–88
9. Lee WM, Stravitz RT, Larson AM (2012) Introduction to the revised American Association for the Study of Liver Diseases Position Paper on acute liver failure 2011. Hepatology 55:965–967
10. Robertson C (2004) Every breath you take: hyperventilation and intracranial pressure. Cleve Clin J Med 71(Suppl 1):S14–S15
11. Davenport A (2008) Practical guidance for dialyzing a hemodialysis patient following acute brain injury. Hemodial Int 12:307–312
12. Castillo LB, Bugedo GA, Paranhos JL (2009) Mannitol or hypertonic saline for intracranial hypertension? A point of view. Crit Care Resusc 11:151–154
13. Drobin D, Hahn RG (2002) Kinetics of isotonic and hypertonic plasma volume expanders. Anesthesiology 96:1371–1380
14. Stravitz RT, Larsen FS (2009) Therapeutic hypothermia for acute liver failure. Critical care medicine 37:S258–S264
15. Jalan R, Olde Damink SW, Deutz NE et al (2003) Moderate hypothermia prevents cerebral hyperemia and increase in intracranial pressure in patients undergoing liver transplantation for acute liver failure. Transplantation 75:2034–2039
16. Rangel-Castilla L, Gopinath S, Robertson CS (2008) Management of intracranial hypertension. Neurol Clin 26:521–541

17. Tofteng F, Larsen FS (2004) The effect of indomethacin on intracranial pressure, cerebral perfusion and extracellular lactate and glutamate concentrations in patients with fulminant hepatic failure. J Cereb Blood Flow Metab 24:798–804
18. Vaquero J, Fontana RJ, Larson AM et al (2005) Complications and use of intracranial pressure monitoring in patients with acute liver failure and severe encephalopathy. Liver Transpl 11:1581–1589
19. Keays RT, Alexander GJ, Williams R (1993) The safety and value of extradural intracranial pressure monitors in fulminant hepatic failure. J Hepatol 18:205–209
20. Bai M, Yang Z, Qi X, Fan D, Han G (2013) l-ornithine-l-aspartate for hepatic encephalopathy in patients with cirrhosis: a meta-analysis of randomized controlled trials. J Gastroenterol Hepatol 28:783–792
21. Jalan R, Wright G, Davies NA, Hodges SJ (2007) L-Ornithine phenylacetate (OP): a novel treatment for hyperammonemia and hepatic encephalopathy. Med Hypotheses 69:1064–1069
22. Ronco C, Brendolan A, d'Intini V, Ricci Z, Wratten ML, Bellomo R (2003) Coupled plasma filtration adsorption: rationale, technical development and early clinical experience. Blood Purif 21:409–416
23. Tan HK (2004) Molecular adsorbent recirculating system (MARS). Ann Acad Med Singapore 33:329–335
24. Bellomo R, Marino B, Starkey G et al (2013) Normothermic extracorporeal human liver perfusion following donation after cardiac death. Crit Care Resusc 15:78–82
25. Beaumont A, Vespa P (2010) Seizures in fulminant hepatic failure, multiorgan failure, and endocrine crisis. In: Varelas P (ed) Seizures in Critical Care. Humana Press, Clifton, pp 179–201
26. Bernal W, Donaldson N, Wyncoll D, Wendon J (2002) Blood lactate as an early predictor of outcome in paracetamol-induced acute liver failure: a cohort study. Lancet 359:558–563
27. Shawcross DL, Davies NA, Mookerjee RP et al (2004) Worsening of cerebral hyperemia by the administration of terlipressin in acute liver failure with severe encephalopathy. Hepatology 39:471–475
28. Harry R, Auzinger G, Wendon J (2002) The clinical importance of adrenal insufficiency in acute hepatic dysfunction. Hepatology 36:395–402
29. Harrison PM, Wendon JA, Gimson AE, Alexander GJ, Williams R (1991) Improvement by acetylcysteine of hemodynamics and oxygen transport in fulminant hepatic failure. N Engl J Med 324:1852–1857
30. Chua HR, Baldwin I, Bailey M, Subramaniam A, Bellomo R (2012) Circuit lifespan during continuous renal replacement therapy for combined liver and kidney failure. J Crit Care 27:744.e7–744.e15
31. Farmer DG, Anselmo DM, Ghobrial RM et al (2003) Liver transplantation for fulminant hepatic failure: experience with more than 200 patients over a 17-year period. Ann Surg 237:666–675

Human Albumin: An Important Bullet Against Bacterial Infection in Patients with Liver Cirrhosis?

M. Bernardi, M. Domenicali, and P. Caraceni

Introduction

Sepsis represents a common and ominous complication in patients with advanced cirrhosis. In fact, in addition to being exposed to a higher risk of bacterial infections due to invasive procedures and repeated hospitalizations, patients with cirrhosis actually exhibit an increased susceptibility. Several factors contribute to this abnormality, including pathological bacterial translocation from the gut secondary to intestinal bacterial overgrowth and/or dysbiosis and enhanced intestinal permeability, and impaired innate and acquired immunity [1]. Moreover, once infections have been contracted, abnormalities in the systemic inflammatory response along with the peculiar cardiovascular background of cirrhosis make their consequences far more severe than in the general population [2]. Indeed, sepsis in cirrhosis often leads to liver and non-liver related complications, multiorgan failure, and increased mortality. Septic cirrhotic patients need to be hospitalized in regular wards or intensive care units (ICUs), which imposes a heavy burden to healthcare costs. Thus, improvements in the efficacy of treatment of bacterial infections in cirrhosis would be of paramount importance and deserves extensive research activity.

Bacterial Infections in Cirrhosis

Even though some specific conditions are associated with a very high incidence (about 50%) of bacterial infection, such as gastrointestinal bleeding or severe cirrhosis with low (< 1.5 g/dl) ascitic protein level [3, 4], a high prevalence of infections in hospitalized patients is reported irrespective of the direct cause of hospitalization. Indeed, about one third of patients admitted to hospital have a bacterial

M. Bernardi ✉ · M. Domenicali · P. Caraceni
Department of Medical and Surgical Sciences, Alma Mater Studiorum University of Bologna, Bologna, Italy
e-mail: mauro.bernardi@unibo.it

J.-L. Vincent (ed.), *Annual Update in Intensive Care and Emergency Medicine 2015*,
DOI 10.1007/978-3-319-13761-2_31

infection or develop it during hospitalization. The prevalence of nosocomial infections in patients with cirrhosis ranges from 24 to 35%, being relatively stable over the last 15 years and far greater than in the population of non-cirrhotic patients [5, 6].

The outcome of sepsis is greatly influenced by the presence of cirrhosis, as the occurrence of bacterial infections increases patient mortality by 4-fold, with 30% of patients dying within 1 month after the infectious episode and another 30% dying by 1 year [7]. Bacterial infections represent the most common precipitating factor in patients presenting acute-on-chronic liver failure (ACLF) at admission to hospital, being associated with this condition in about one-third of cases, with a prevalence that increases in parallel with the severity of ACLF, reaching about 45% in grade 3 ACLF, which is characterized by a 28-day mortality of 77% [8].

The most common bacterial infection that develops in patients with advanced cirrhosis and ascites is spontaneous bacterial peritonitis (SBP) with a prevalence ranging from 24 to 31% [5], followed by urinary tract infections, pneumonia, bacteremias and soft tissue infections.

Factors Predicting the Outcome of Bacterial Infections in Cirrhosis

The identification of factors associated with the outcome of bacterial infections in patients with cirrhosis is of considerable importance, because it would allow the development of treatment strategies aimed at preventing the progression to severe sepsis and septic shock and the complications that are ultimately responsible for infection-associated mortality.

Among these outcome predictors, acute kidney injury (AKI) holds particular importance, as it occurs in 8% of patients with compensated cirrhosis to one third of patients with cirrhosis and ascites [9–13], and represents a strong independent risk factor for death, with a 40–50% mortality rate. Conversely, among the causes of AKI in cirrhosis, which are also independent outcome predictors, bacterial infections are among those associated with the highest 3-month mortality (69%) [13]. It has to be stressed that infection-induced renal impairment does not always revert with plasma volume expansion and/or the resolution of the infection itself, but can progress, presenting the phenotype of hepatorenal syndrome (HRS) type 1 or acute tubular necrosis [9–13].

The incidence and phenotype of AKI in septic patients with cirrhosis are influenced by the different sites of infection. About one third of patients affected by SBP develop renal impairment, which is progressive, irrespective of the resolution of infection, in most cases (42%), steady in one third of cases and transient in 25% [9]. The independent predictors of SBP-induced AKI at the time of diagnosis of SBP are increased blood urea nitrogen (BUN) or serum creatinine, hyponatremia, increased serum bilirubin, and neutrophilic leukocytosis. Among these variables, BUN and serum sodium concentration independently predicted the development of non-transient AKI [9]. The development of AKI is an independent predictor of in-hospital mortality of SBP, as 42% of patients developing this complication will die, while the mortality of those who do not develop renal impairment is only 7%. Moreover, the AKI phenotype is also a major determinant of in-hospital mortality, ranging from 5% in patients with the transient form, to 31% and 100% in those with steady and progressive renal impairment, respectively [9].

AKI also frequently occurs in patients with bacterial infections other than SBP. In one study that enrolled 106 consecutive patients with cirrhosis and sepsis unrelated to SBP [10], renal impairment developed in 27% of cases compared with only 8% in those without sepsis. The infections that most often led to AKI were culture-negative sepsis (66%) and spontaneous bacteremia (45%), followed by cellulitis, pneumonia and urinary tract infections. Contrary to SBP, however, reversible renal impairment prevailed (76%), a percentage that was not substantially different from that found in patients without sepsis (62%). Interestingly, according to the results of one study, non-reversible renal impairment would only be precipitated by infections located in the sub-diaphragmatic area, such as SBP, biliary or gastrointestinal tract infections and urinary tract infections [11].

As in SBP, AKI strongly influences the outcome of patients with non-SBP bacterial infections, as 43% die during the hospital stay [11] and 66% within 3 months [10], percentages far higher than those seen in patients who did not develop renal impairment (7% and 13%, respectively). The AKI phenotype also influences patient mortality: The non-reversible type invariably led to death within 3 months compared with 55% 3-month mortality in patients with reversible renal impairment [10].

There are several other predictors of mortality in septic patients with cirrhosis in addition to the occurrence of renal failure. A systematic review [7] reported that the independent prognostic indicators of mortality were Child–Pugh and MELD scores, age, BUN/creatinine level, hepatic encephalopathy, gastrointestinal bleeding, shock, serum bilirubin concentration and hepatocellular carcinoma. Another important risk factor for the development of severe sepsis and mortality is represented by nosocomial and healthcare-related infections, which are often due to antibiotic-resistant microorganisms and, therefore, can fail to achieve a prompt resolution [6, 14]. Indeed, a study including 669 infections from two series of patients (2005–2007 and 2010–2011) demonstrated that infections caused by multi-drug resistant bacteria were more common among nosocomial infections and had a poorer prognosis than those caused by susceptible bacteria, with higher rates of treatment failure and septic shock (26% vs. 10% respectively), and higher in-hospital mortality (25% vs. 12% respectively) [6].

Pathophysiology of Sepsis in Cirrhosis (Fig. 1)

The defense mechanisms against bacteria, involving both innate and acquired immunity, are impaired in patients with cirrhosis and lead to an increased susceptibility to infections. Impairment of macrophage Fcγ-receptor-mediated clearance of antibody coated bacteria, deficiencies in the complement system, downregulation of

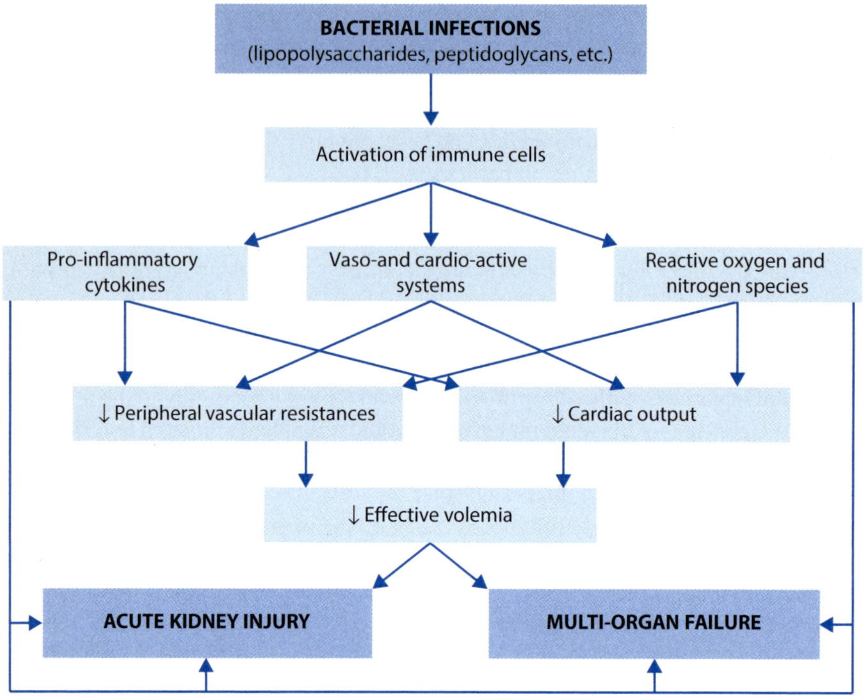

Fig. 1 Effect of bacterial infections in cirrhosis

monocyte HLA-DR expression, depressed neutrophil phagocytic and intracellular killing contribute to these abnormalities [3]. The mechanisms leading to immune suppression in cirrhosis are complex and far from being clarified. Very recent data suggest that increased synthesis of the immunosuppressive prostaglandin, PGE_2, by circulating monocytes and resident macrophages plays a crucial role [15].

Genetic defects likely contribute to the abnormalities in defense mechanisms in cirrhosis [3]: Patients carrying nucleotide-binding oligomerization domain containing 2 (NOD2) variants, which are associated with impairment of recognition of bacterial products, mannose-binding lectin deficiency, inducing a defect in opsonophagocytosis of bacteria, and Toll-like receptor 2 (TLR-2) polymorphisms have a higher risk of bacterial infections, particularly SBP, and reduced survival.

Thus, cirrhosis-associated immune dysfunction involves a state of immunodeficiency, which is coupled, however, with a state of persistent activation of the immune system cells with production of pro-inflammatory cytokines. In fact, the pro-inflammatory host response to bacterial infections is enhanced in patients with cirrhosis, who can exhibit increased circulating pro-inflammatory cytokines even in the absence of infection. Indeed, patients without infection exhibit increased tumor necrosis factor (TNF)-α, interferon (IFN)γ and interleukin (IL)-12 concentrations in blood and ascitic fluid, as well as increased circulating nitric oxide (NO) metabolites, similar to those seen in patients with SBP [16]. These abnormalities are related to a sustained stimulation of the immune system cells by microbial- and damage-associated molecular patterns (MAMPs, DAMPs) [3].

An exaggerated production of pro-inflammatory cytokines, such as TNF-α and IL-6, has long been recognized from the early phase of bacterial infections in cirrhosis, due to an excessive mononuclear cell response to lipopolysaccharide (LPS) and other bacterial products [17]. Such a cytokine cascade leads to the activation of several vasoactive systems, including NO, carbon monoxide, prostaglandins and endocannabinoids, which are likely involved in the development of complications induced by bacterial infections. Cytokines also promote the generation of reactive oxygen species (ROS) by the activated phagocytes, which contribute to tissue damage in severe sepsis. This pro-inflammatory phase can be followed by a prolonged 'immunoparalysis', called compensatory anti-inflammatory response syndrome (CARS) [3, 18], responsible for repeated secondary nosocomial infections, which, in turn, represent a major cause of mortality [19].

The development of AKI in patients affected by SBP is associated with plasma and ascitic fluid pro-inflammatory cytokine levels at diagnosis of infection far higher than in patients without renal impairment. Consistently, IL-6 levels independently predict the occurrence of renal impairment, in addition to increased BUN, serum creatinine and reduced arterial pressure [20].

The cardiovascular complications potentially induced by SBP and, presumably, other bacterial infections in cirrhosis are complex and involve both vascular tone and cardiac function. However, while peripheral vascular resistance (PVR) remains substantially unchanged, possibly as a result of a striking compensatory activation of vasoconstrictor systems, cardiac output significantly declines [21]. The latter can be related not only to chronotropic incompetence – an electrophysiological abnormality of cirrhotic cardiomyopathy [22] – but also to reduced myocardial contractility. Interestingly, in experimental cirrhosis with ascites, reduced cardiac contractility is associated with an increased myocardial expression of TNF-α and inducible NO synthase (iNOS), along with a nuclear translocation of nuclear factor-kappa B (NF-κB) [23]. It can be predicted that these abnormalities are enhanced by bacterial infections.

The cardiovascular abnormalities described above ultimately lead to a striking reduction in effective arterial blood volume, which reduces renal and, more in general, organ perfusion, generating ischemic organ damage. In addition, end-organ damage can also be induced by ROS generation unbalanced by antioxidant systems [24].

In the light of these pathophysiological mechanisms, an ideal treatment strategy aimed at preventing sepsis-induced complications and death in patients with cirrhosis, beside the resolution of infection by antibiotics, should aim at defending effective blood volume and protecting target organs. This could be achieved by increasing plasma volume, PVR, and cardiac output, and/or inhibiting pro-inflammatory cytokine production, and/or blunting cytokine effects by counteracting vasodilators, such as NO, and ROS. Relief of immune suppression by reducing circulating free PGE_2 could also represent a potential perspective.

The Albumin Molecule

Albumin Structure

Human albumin is the main circulating protein in healthy individuals (3.5–5 g/dl), representing about 50% of the total protein content in the plasma. It is a small globular protein, consisting of a single chain of 585 amino acids, with a molecular weight of 66.5 kDa. In the human body, human albumin assumes the tertiary structure of an ellipsoid, formed by 67% of α-helices and organized in three repeated homologous domains (sites I, II, and III), each of which is comprised of two separate sub-domains (A and B). Of the 35 cysteine residues of the molecule, 34 are involved in internal disulfide bonds that stabilize the spatial conformation of the molecule, while the cysteine at position 34 (Cys-34) remains free. The different domains are capable of folding into hydrophobic pockets, which can open and close, and accommodate large insoluble anions, such as fatty acids [25].

Albumin Metabolism

Human albumin is synthesized by hepatocytes and released into the circulation (about 10–15 grams every day) with no or very little intrahepatic storage. Its synthesis is stimulated by hormonal factors, such as insulin, cortisol and growth hormone, while pro-inflammatory mediators exert an inhibitory effect. Once produced, approximately 30–40% is maintained in the blood stream, while the remainder is distributed in the interstitium, where its concentration is low (1.4 g/dl), leaving the vascular compartment at a rate of 5% per hour (transcapillary escape rate) and returning to it via the lymphatic system in an amount comparable to the output. The circulatory half-life of human albumin is approximately 16–18 hours, while its total half-life varies from about 12 to 19 days in healthy young adults. Human albumin is mainly degraded by the muscles, liver and kidneys, although many other tissues can participate in its catabolism [25].

Albumin Properties

Human albumin is the main modulator of fluid distribution in the various compartments of the body, accounting for about 70–80% of the plasma oncotic pressure. Two-thirds of the oncotic capacity is derived from the direct osmotic effect related to its molecular mass and high plasma concentration and one-third from the Gibbs-Donnan effect, due to the negative net charge of the molecule that is consequently able to attract positively charged molecules (i.e., sodium and, therefore, water) into the bloodstream. Thus, most of the clinical use of human albumin is based on the capacity to act as a plasma-expander [26, 27].

Human albumin also has many other biological properties that are unrelated to the regulation of fluid compartmentalization (Fig. 2). Among these non-oncotic

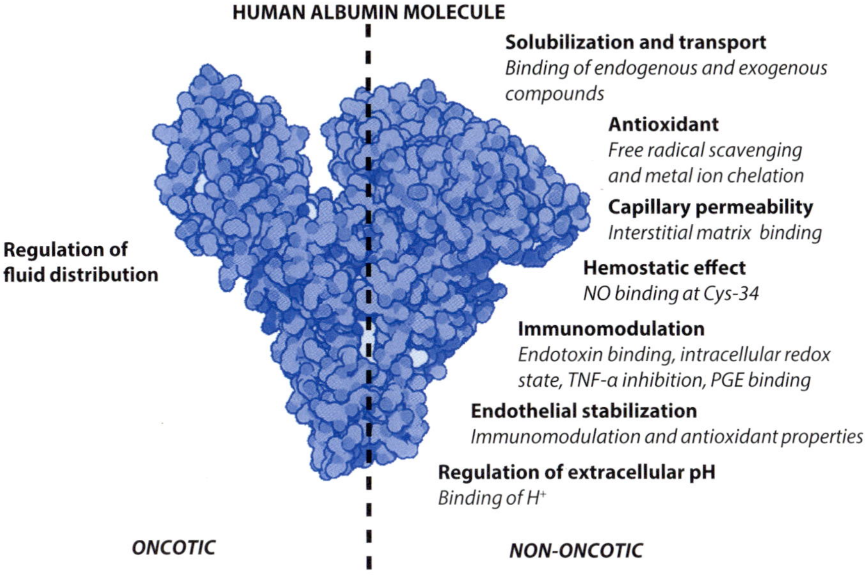

Fig. 2 Oncotic and non-oncotic properties of human albumin. NO: nitric oxide; TNF: tumor necrosis factor; Cys-34: cysteine-34

properties, some assume particular importance in relation to bacterial infections, such as antioxidant and scavenging activities, binding and transport of many endogenous and exogenous substances, and regulation of endothelial function and inflammatory response [26, 27].

Human albumin is the major source of extracellular reduced sulfhydryl groups, mainly located at the cysteine (Cys)-34 free residue, which is mostly in the reduced state, thus acting as a potent ROS-scavenger. As a result, human albumin is the main circulating antioxidant system in the body [28]. Human albumin is also capable of binding, at the N-terminal portion of the molecule, several metal ions, which are therefore inhibited from catalyzing many chemical reactions generating free radicals [29].

A large number of binding sites with different affinities for plasma compounds have been identified in the albumin molecule due to its peculiar and dynamic structure. Human albumin is able to bind and carry a great variety of hydrophobic molecules, including endogenous (i.e., cholesterol, fatty acids, bilirubin, thyroxine) or exogenous (i.e., drugs including many antibiotics) substances, LPS, transition metal ions, and gases (NO), with consequent implications for their solubilization, transport, and metabolism [26, 27].

Human albumin also contributes to the integrity of the microcirculation, by binding the interstitial matrix and interacting with the sub-endothelial space, thus participating in the maintenance of normal capillary permeability. Human albumin may impact positively on endothelial function also by reducing oxidative damage and modulating the signaling systems between neutrophils and endothelial cells. Finally, human albumin carries an anti-thrombotic effect by binding NO at the Cys-34 site, preventing its rapid inactivation and thus prolonging its anti-aggregant effect on platelets [26, 27].

Albumin Alterations in Cirrhosis

Hypoalbuminemia is a long recognized feature of cirrhosis, mainly resulting from decreased hepatocyte synthesis, dilution secondary to total plasma volume expansion, and increased transvascular escape rate. In addition to quantitative changes, human albumin in cirrhosis presents structural and functional changes that affect its non-oncotic properties. It has been demonstrated that extensive post-transcriptional changes in human albumin occur in patients with cirrhosis, involving several sites of the molecule (Fig. 3) and increasing in parallel with disease severity, so that, beside the native, unchanged molecule, the proportion of circulating abnormal isoforms is greatly increased with respect to healthy individuals [30]. Among these alterations, oxidation and truncation of the Cys-34 residue is independently associated with specific clinical complications of the disease, such as ascites, renal failure and bacterial infection [30], and predicts patient survival alone [31] or in combination with concomitant changes at the N-terminal site of the molecule [30].

In addition to structural changes, physiological functions of human albumin also appear to be impaired by cirrhosis. The term ischemia-modified albumin (IMA) is used to define a specific functional alteration represented by the reduced ability of human albumin to chelate cobalt, mostly at the N-terminal region [32]. IMA elevation was described initially during myocardial infarction and then during other ischemic and non-ischemic conditions, such as stroke, mesenteric ischemia, ketoacidosis, or end-stage kidney disease [33]. In a small series of patients with acute decompensation or ACLF, the ratio of IMA to plasma serum albumin (IMAr) was increased above normal levels and, in patients with ACLF, discriminated survivors from non-survivors with good accuracy [29]. Furthermore, preliminary observations indicate that, in patients hospitalized for an acute complication of the disease, the circulating IMA level is specifically associated with the presence of bacterial infection, showing a discriminating performance similar to that of C-reactive protein (CRP) [34]. Furthermore, human albumin from patients with advanced cirrhosis presents an impaired affinity for the fatty acid binding sites, and this abnormality again parallels the severity of the disease [29]. Finally, a reduced binding capacity likely favors the increased circulating concentrations of PGE_2 found in patients with acute decompensation and implicated in cirrhosis-associated immunosuppression [15].

In conclusion, it can be assumed that the pro-inflammatory and pro-oxidant state that characterizes the vascular microenvironment in advanced cirrhosis, represents a predisposing factor for the development of structural alterations of the human albumin molecule. This likely has important relevant functional consequences, which have been only partially investigated so far and whose clinical significance is still debated. It is, thus, time to adopt the concept of 'effective albumin concentration', which implies that the global functions of albumin, resulting from both oncotic and non-oncotic properties, are not only related to its absolute circulating concentration, but also to the preservation of its structural and functional integrity [26, 30].

Albumin Administration in Cirrhotic Patients with Bacterial Infection

Pathophysiology

Due to its oncotic and non-oncotic properties, human albumin would appear to be an ideal tool to counteract the deleterious effects of bacterial infections in patients with cirrhosis. Its colloid-osmotic power makes human albumin a strong plasma volume expander. As reduced effective volemia plays a central pathophysiological role in the development of infection-induced complications, this feature is highly relevant. Several clinical studies have shown that human albumin is superior to synthetic colloids and crystalloids for expanding blood volume in patients with cirrhosis [35, 36].

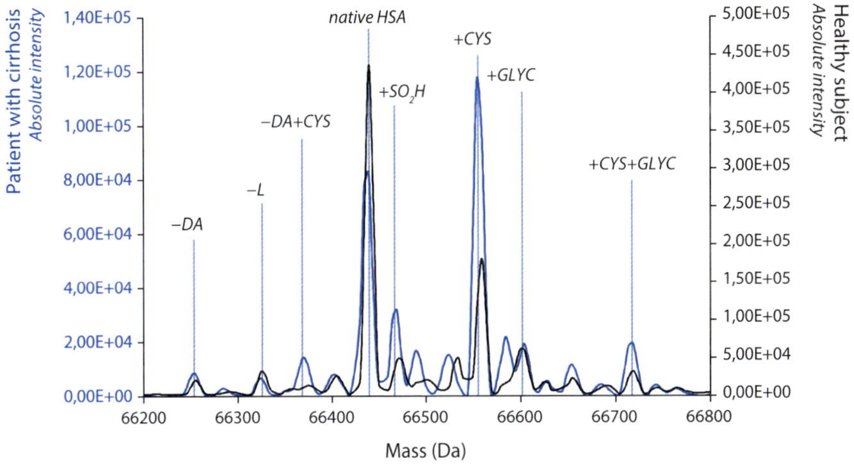

Fig. 3 Representative spectra of serum albumin (HSA) from a cirrhotic patient (*blue*) and a control subject (*black*) obtained with high performance liquid chromatography coupled to electrospray ionization mass spectrometry [30]. In addition to native HSA, which is reduced, an increase in seven HSA isoforms carrying the following structural alterations were detected in cirrhosis: Truncation of the last two aminoacid residues at the N-terminal portion (−DA); truncation of the last aminoacid residue at the C-terminal portion (−L); cysteinylation of the Cys-34 residue (+CYS); sulfinylation of the Cys-34 residue ($+SO_2H$); glycosylation (+GLYC); combination of the cysteinylated with the N-terminal truncated form (−DA+CYS) or the glycosylated form (+CYS+GLYC)

There is mounting evidence that the beneficial effects of human albumin administration are also related to its non-oncotic properties. Indeed, the antioxidant and scavenger activities, along with its capacity to modulate the immune system, stabilize the endothelium, and regulate capillary permeability, could well antagonize the cascade of events promoted by bacterial infection (Fig. 1). Experimental and clinical observations support this assumption. In rats with cirrhosis and ascites, plasma volume expansion with human albumin, but not with hydroxyethyl starch, improved left ventricular function *ex vivo*, counteracting the negative effects of oxidative stress- and TNF-α-induced activation of NF-κB, iNOS pathway and oxidative stress-induced alteration of β-receptor signaling [23]. In patients with cirrhosis and SBP, human albumin, but not hydroxyethyl starch, ameliorated systemic hemodynamics, as witnessed by the significant changes in plasma renin activity and arterial pressure [37]. Along with parameters suggesting total blood volume expansion, such as increases in cardiopulmonary pressures, atrial natriuretic factor and stroke volume, the concomitant striking increase in peripheral vascular resistances can only be related to the non-oncotic properties of albumin. In fact, a significant decrease in the plasma levels of factor VIII and von Willebrand-related antigen was found, suggesting that human albumin was able to attenuate endothelial activation. Furthermore, the significant increase in NO metabolites seen with hydroxyethyl starch was prevented by human albumin administration [37].

As a whole, it appears that human albumin, in addition to direct plasma expansion, can improve effective blood volume by acting on cardiac function and peripheral vascular resistances through its non-oncotic properties.

Clinical Studies: Spontaneous Bacterial Peritonitis

The first controlled clinical trial assessing the effect of human albumin administration in patients with cirrhosis and bacterial infection showed that such a treatment, associated with antibiotic therapy, reduced the incidence of renal failure and in-hospital and 3-month mortality in patients affected by SBP [38]. Namely, 126 patients were randomized to receive human albumin either 1.5 g/kg/bw at diagnosis and 1 g/kg bw on day 3 in addition to cefotaxime or cefotaxime alone. Although resolution of infection was similar in the two groups, the incidence of renal impairment decreased from the expected 33% in patients receiving only cefotaxime to 10% in those treated with cefotaxime plus human albumin. Baseline independent predictors of the development of renal impairment included serum bilirubin and creatinine, and treatment with cefotaxime alone. Confirming that the occurrence of renal failure in the setting of SBP carries a highly adverse prognostic meaning, 29% of patients in the cefotaxime group died in the hospital and 41% within 3 months. These figures were strikingly reduced by albumin administration, as in-hospital and 3-month mortalities were 10% and 22%, respectively. An increase in plasma renin activity occurred over 9 days from diagnosis in the cefotaxime group, especially in those patients who developed renal impairment, which was prevented by human albumin administration. Post-hoc analysis of these data showed that the incidence of renal impairment occurred more often in those with a baseline serum bilirubin ≥ 4 mg/dl (48% in cefotaxime group and 12% in cefotaxime-plus-albumin group) or serum creatinine ≥ 1 mg/dl (32% and 14%, respectively) than in patients with serum bilirubin < 4 mg/dl and serum creatinine < 1 mg/dl (7% and 0%, respectively). This observation raises the question of whether all patients with SBP would need albumin administration. In a preliminary small study, patients with SBP at low risk of developing renal impairment, that is patients with serum bilirubin < 4 mg/dl and serum creatinine < 1 mg/dl, only received antibiotic treatment and none developed renal impairment or died [39].

In a more recent retrospective study [40], episodes of 'low-risk' SBP not treated with human albumin, had a far lower incidence of renal failure before SBP resolution (4.7%) and lower in-hospital (3.1%) and 3-month (7%) mortality with respect to 'high-risk' episodes (25.6%, 38.2% and 47%, respectively). Among the latter, those receiving human albumin had lower in-hospital mortality than those receiving only antibiotics (28.8% vs 46.8%) and a greater 3-month probability of survival (62% vs 45%). The conclusion was that human albumin therapy increases survival of patients who have high-risk episodes of SBP, although it does not seem to be necessary for patients with low risk of death. However, this assumption still waits confirmation in a randomized prospective study.

Similarly, confirmation is needed for the results of a pilot study that assessed whether a lower dose of human albumin could be used [41]. Namely, a reduced dose regimen (1.0 g/kg bw at diagnosis and 0.5 g/kg at day 3) appeared to be as effective as the standard regimen in preventing renal failure in a group of cirrhotic patients with SBP including 77% of 'high-risk' patients. In-hospital (27% vs 21%) and 3-month mortality (36% vs 37%) also did not differ in patients given the reduced or standard albumin dose, respectively.

Finally, a recent meta-analysis of randomized trials substantially confirmed these points: Human albumin infusion prevents renal impairment and reduces mortality among patients with SBP [42]. However, available evidence is still limited on the outcomes of low-risk SBP patients not receiving human albumin as well as on the responsiveness of low-risk patients to human albumin infusion.

Clinical Studies: Non-SBP Bacterial Infections

Whether human albumin administration can also be beneficial in non-SBP bacterial infections is still under investigation. The only published randomized trial [43] enrolled 110 patients affected by pneumonia, urinary tract and skin infections, culture-positive bacteremia; however, in 20% of patients, infection was only suspected. The patients were randomized to receive appropriate antibiotic treatment alone or antibiotic treatment plus human albumin at the 'standard' dose regimen used for SBP. Renal function, as evaluated by serum creatinine and estimated glomerular filtration rate, and circulatory function, as assessed by plasma renin activity, plasma aldosterone, norepinephrine, and atrial natriuretic factor (ANF) levels and mean arterial pressure, only improved in patients receiving human albumin. Although these results indicate that human albumin exerts beneficial effects on effective blood volume also in non-SBP bacterial infections, the occurrence of HRS type 1 and the 3-month mortality (19.6% in the control arm; 17.4% in the albumin arm) did not differ between the two groups. However, multivariate analysis showed that treatment with human albumin was an independent predictive factor for survival when adjusted according to factors with a predictive value of survival, with a 3.4 relative risk of death for patients receiving only antibiotics.

As for SBP, it appears that human albumin administration may also have a beneficial role in other bacterial infections in high-risk patients. Ongoing large, multicenter randomized trials assessing the effect of human albumin administration will hopefully soon provide the information to cover this lack of knowledge.

Conclusion and Perspectives

Bacterial infections are a frequent and potentially fatal complication in advanced cirrhosis. Sepsis-related morbidity and mortality, which assume particular importance in patients listed for liver transplantation, are mainly related to complex immune dysfunction characterized by an immune deficit that predisposes patients to bacterial infection, and to an exaggerated systemic inflammatory response, which primarily affects cardiovascular and, ultimately, end-organ function [3]. Among the latter, AKI, which often presents the phenotype of HRS type 1, is a main determinant of mortality, along with the severity of the underlying liver disease [12].

The oncotic and non-oncotic properties of human albumin potentially make this molecule an ideal tool to defend effective blood volume and neutralize, at least in part, the effects of the sepsis-induced cascade of pro-inflammatory cytokines, ROS generation, and enhanced synthesis of NO and other vasodilating and cardiodepressing substances [26, 27]. Moreover, human albumin infusion may attenuate immune suppression of patients with cirrhosis by increasing the binding sites for PGE_2, an attractive and promising approach [15, 44]. Indeed, several studies have convincingly shown that human albumin administration to patients with cirrhosis and bacterial infections yields favorable effects, even though not all the results are clear-cut and not all the issues related to albumin treatment of septic patients with cirrhosis have been clarified as yet.

The strongest evidence has been obtained in patients with SBP and severe cirrhosis (serum bilirubin ≥ 4 mg/dl) and/or impaired renal function at diagnosis, where few, if any, doubts exist about the beneficial effect of albumin infusion [38]. The suggestion that a reduced dose regimen [41], which would lower costs, could be equally effective with respect to currently employed doses still needs to be substantiated by further studies. Conversely, SBP-induced AKI can still occur despite human albumin administration in 'high risk' patients. In this context, the association with vasoconstrictors or different ways of administering albumin, warrant investigation. Even though data suggesting that human albumin infusion could be avoided in 'low-risk' patients with SBP seem more convincing [40], it should not be disregarded that prospective controlled studies with adequate sample sizes are still lacking.

Data on the effects of human albumin infusion in patients with non-SBP bacterial infections are still inconclusive. The single controlled clinical trial published so far showed that albumin administration was followed by an improvement in effective volemia and renal function, but failed to clearly demonstrate a significant reduction in the incidence of progressive AKI and mortality, the latter only being achieved after adjusting for potentially confounding variables [43]. This disappointing result, however, may be linked to a not entirely appropriate patient selection. Indeed, many patients were affected by pneumonia and skin infections, which more often induce transient rather than steady or progressive AKI [10, 11], and a minority had nosocomial and health-care associated infections, which are most often associated with the development of severe sepsis and mortality [6, 14].

Thus, future studies should address several issues, such as the identification of those patients who are at a higher risk of developing sepsis-induced complications and death, through the assessment of available or specifically tailored prognostic score systems and the identification of early biomarkers predicting the evolution and outcome of bacterial infections. Another most interesting and promising field of research should be devoted to improve our knowledge on the non-oncotic effects following albumin administration to septic patients with cirrhosis, which presumably play an even more important role than volume expansion achieved through the improvement in colloid osmotic pressure, an effect that undoubtedly albumin attains in these patients.

References

1. Tandon P, Garcia-Tsao G (2008) Bacterial infections, sepsis, and multiorgan failure in cirrhosis. Semin Liver Dis 28:26–42
2. Gustot T, Durand F, Lebrec D, Vincent JL, Moreau R (2009) Severe sepsis in cirrhosis. Hepatology 50:2022–2033
3. Jalan R, Fernandez J, Wiest R et al (2014) Bacterial infections in cirrhosis: a position statement based on the EASL Special Conference 2013. J Hepatol 60:1310–1324
4. Fagiuoli S, Colli A, Bruno R et al (2014) Management of infections in cirrhotic patients: report of a Consensus Conference. Dig Liver Dis 46:204–212
5. Fernández J, Navasa M, Gómez J et al (2002) Bacterial infections in cirrhosis: epidemiological changes with invasive procedures and norfloxacin prophylaxis. Hepatology 35:140–148
6. Fernández J, Acevedo J, Castro M et al (2012) Prevalence and risk factors of infections by multiresistant bacteria in cirrhosis: a prospective study. Hepatology 55:1551–1561
7. Arvaniti V, D'Amico G, Fede G et al (2010) Infections in patients with cirrhosis increase mortality four-fold and should be used in determining prognosis. Gastroenterology 139:1246–1256
8. Moreau R, Jalan R, Gines P et al (2013) Acute-on-chronic liver failure is a distinct syndrome that develops in patients with acute decompensation of cirrhosis. Gastroenterology 144:1426–1437
9. Follo A, Llovet JM, Navasa M et al (1994) Renal impairment after spontaneous bacterial peritonitis in cirrhosis: incidence, clinical course, predictive factors and prognosis. Hepatology 20:1495–1501

10. Terra C, Guevara M, Torre A et al (2005) Renal failure in patients with cirrhosis and sepsis unrelated to spontaneous bacterial peritonitis: value of MELD score. Gastroenterology 129:1944–1953
11. Fasolato S, Angeli P, Dallagnese L et al (2007) Renal failure and bacterial infections in patients with cirrhosis: epidemiology and clinical features. Hepatology 45:223–229
12. Tandon P, Garcia-Tsao G (2011) Renal dysfunction is the most important independent predictor of mortality in cirrhotic patients with spontaneous bacterial peritonitis. Clin Gastroenterol Hepatol 9:260–265
13. Martín-Llahí M, Guevara M, Torre A et al (2011) Prognostic importance of the cause of renal failure in patients with cirrhosis. Gastroenterology 140:488–496
14. Merli M, Lucidi C, Giannelli V et al (2010) Cirrhotic patients are at risk for health care-associated bacterial infections. Clin Gastroenterol Hepatol 8:979–985
15. O'Brien AJ, Fullerton JN, Massey KA et al (2014) Immunosuppression in acutely decompensated cirrhosis is mediated by prostaglandin E2. Nat Med 20:518–523
16. Francés R, Zapater P, González-Navajas JM et al (2008) DNA in patients with cirrhosis and non infected ascites mimics the soluble immune response established in patients with spontaneous bacterial peritonitis. Hepatology 7:978–995
17. Byl B, Roucloux I, Crusiaux A, Dupont E, Devière J (1993) Tumor necrosis factor alpha and interleukin-6 plasma levels in infected cirrhotic patients. Gastroenterology 104:1492–1497
18. Wasmuth HE, Kunz D, Yagmur E et al (2005) Patients with acute on chronic liver failure display "sepsis-like" immune paralysis. J Hepatol 42:195–201
19. Bajaj JS, O'Leary JG, Reddy KR et al (2012) Second infections independently increase mortality in hospitalized patients with cirrhosis: the North American consortium for the study of end-stage liver disease (NACSELD) experience. Hepatology 56:2328–2335
20. Navasa M, Follo A, Filella X et al (1998) Tumor necrosis factor and interleukin-6 in spontaneous bacterial peritonitis in cirrhosis: relationship with the development of renal impairment and mortality. Hepatology 27:1227–1232
21. Ruiz-del-Arbol L, Urman J, Fernández J et al (2003) Systemic, renal, and hepatic hemodynamic derangement in cirrhotic patients with spontaneous bacterial peritonitis. Hepatology 38:1210–1218
22. Zambruni A, Trevisani F, Caraceni P, Bernardi M (2006) Cardiac electrophysiological abnormalities in patients with cirrhosis. J Hepatol 44:994–1002
23. Bortoluzzi A, Ceolotto G, Gola E et al (2013) Positive cardiac inotropic effect of albumin infusion in rodents with cirrhosis and ascites: molecular mechanisms. Hepatology 57:266–276
24. Goode HF, Cowley HC, Walker BE, Howdle PD, Webster NR (1995) Decreased antioxidant status and increased lipid peroxidation in patients with septic shock and secondary organ dysfunction. Crit Care Med 23:646–651
25. Fanali G, di Masi A, Trezza V, Marino M, Fasano M, Ascenzi P (2012) Human serum albumin: from bench to bedside. Mol Aspects Med 33:209–290
26. Garcia-Martinez R, Caraceni P, Bernardi M, Gines P, Arroyo V, Jalan R (2013) Albumin: Pathophysiologic basis of its role in the treatment of cirrhosis and its complications. Hepatology 58:1836–1846
27. Arroyo V, García-Martinez R, Salvatella X (2014) Human serum albumin, systemic inflammation, and cirrhosis. J Hepatol 61:396–407
28. Anraku M, Chuang VTG, Maruyama T, Otagiri M (2013) Redox properties of serum albumin. Biochim Biophys Acta 1830:5465–5472
29. Jalan R, Schnurr K, Mookerjee RP et al (2009) Alterations in the functional capacity of albumin in patients with decompensated cirrhosis is associated with increased mortality. Hepatology 50:555–564
30. Domenicali M, Baldassarre M, Giannone FA et al (2014) Post-transcriptional changes of serum albumin: Clinical and prognostic significance in hospitalized patients with cirrhosis. Hepatology 60:1851–1860

31. Oettl K, Birner-Gruenberger R, Spindelboeck W et al (2013) Oxidative albumin damage in chronic liver failure: relation to albumin binding capacity, liver dysfunction and survival. J Hepatol 59:978–983
32. Bar-Or D, Curtis G, Rao N, Bampos N, Lau E (2001) Characterization of the Co(2+) and Ni(2+) binding amino-acid residues of the N-terminus of human albumin. An insight into the mechanism of a new assay for myocardial ischemia. Eur J Biochem 268:42–47
33. Sbarouni E, Georgiadou P, Voudris V (2011) Ischemia modified albumin changes – review and clinical implications. Clin Chem Lab Med 49:177–184
34. Giannone FA, Domenicali M, Baldassarre M et al (2013) Ischemia modified albumin (IMA) as a novel diagnostic marker of bacterial infection in hospitalized patients with cirrhosis. Hepatology 58:860A
35. European Association for the Study of the Liver (2010) EASL clinical practice guidelines on the management of ascites, spontaneous bacterial peritonitis, and hepatorenal syndrome in cirrhosis. J Hepatol 53:397–417
36. Bernardi M, Caraceni P, Navickis RJ, Wilkes MM (2012) Albumin infusion in patients undergoing large-volume paracentesis: a meta-analysis of randomized trials. Hepatology 55:1172–1181
37. Fernández J, Monteagudo J, Bargallo X et al (2005) A randomized unblinded pilot study comparing albumin vs. hydroxyethyl starch in spontaneous bacterial peritonitis. Hepatology 42:627–634
38. Sort P, Navasa M, Arroyo V et al (1999) Effect of intravenous albumin on renal impairment and mortality in patients with cirrhosis and spontaneous bacterial peritonitis. N Engl J Med 341:403–409
39. Sigal SH, Stanca CM, Fernandez J, Arroyo V, Navasa M (2007) Restricted use of albumin for spontaneous bacterial peritonitis. Gut 56:597–599
40. Poca M, Concepción M, Casas M et al (2012) Role of albumin treatment in patients with spontaneous bacterial peritonitis. Clin Gastroenterol Hepatol 10:309–315
41. De Araujo A, De Barros Lopes A, Rossi G et al (2012) Low-dose albumin in the treatment of spontaneous bacterial peritonitis: should we change the standard treatment? Gut 61:1371–1372
42. Salerno F, Navickis RJ, Wilkes MM (2013) Albumin infusion improves outcomes of patients with spontaneous bacterial peritonitis: a meta-analysis of randomized trials. Clin Gastroenterol Hepatol 11:123–130
43. Guevara M, Terra C, Nazar A et al (2012) Albumin for bacterial infections other than spontaneous bacterial peritonitis in cirrhosis. A randomized, controlled study. J Hepatol 57:759–765
44. Arroyo V, Moreau R (2014) Tying up PGE2 with albumin to relieve immunosuppression in cirrhosis. Nat Med 20:467–469

Open Abdomen Management: Challenges and Solutions for the ICU Team

J. J. De Waele and M. L. N. G. Malbrain

Introduction

Open abdomen management – indications, temporary abdominal closure (TAC) techniques as well as critical care management – has changed considerably in the last decade. As a result of better insight into intra-abdominal hypertension (IAH) and abdominal compartment syndrome (ACS), greater experience and improvements in TAC techniques, outcomes of patients requiring open abdomen management have improved, despite increased severity of illness and more severe underlying abdominal conditions.

The open abdomen has always been an intensivist's (and patient's) worst nightmare, mostly because the conditions requiring open abdomen management were difficult to handle from a surgical perspective, often with a protracted stay in the intensive care unit (ICU), uncontrolled septic sources and persistent multiple organ dysfunction syndrome (MODS). It is now clear that opening a patient's abdomen and leaving it open no longer means the beginning of a lengthy disease leaving the patient with a giant hernia and fistulas requiring a long stay in the ICU and multiple surgical procedures. In this chapter, we will highlight the recent advances in this field and discuss remaining challenges in critically ill patients requiring an open abdomen.

J. J. De Waele ✉
Dept. of Critical Care Medicine, Ghent University Hospital, Ghent, Belgium
e-mail: Jan.DeWaele@UGent.be

M. L. N. G. Malbrain
ICU and High Care Burn Unit, Ziekenhuis Netwerk Antwerpen, ZNA Stuivenberg, Antwerp, Belgium

J.-L. Vincent (ed.), *Annual Update in Intensive Care and Emergency Medicine 2015*,
DOI 10.1007/978-3-319-13761-2_32

Contemporary Indications for Open Abdomen Management

All current indications for open abdomen treatment fall into the same main category: The patient's abdomen is left open because of ACS, which was either present before the intervention (in which case the patient underwent a decompressive laparotomy) or that was highly likely to occur postoperatively, because of the presence of risk factors such as emergency surgery, hypotension, coagulopathy and massive transfusion. Whereas the abdomen used to be left open in severely ill patients with abdominal sepsis to allow re-exploration and planned re-laparotomy, recent studies do not show any evidence for this approach and it should, therefore, be discouraged.

Typically, patients will have been treated or operated on for abdominal catastrophes, such as severe peritonitis, ruptured aortic aneurysms, severe acute pancreatitis, intestinal ischemia. However, ACS may also develop in patients with medical conditions [1, 2]. When medical therapy of IAH does not improve the patient's condition, decompressive laparotomy and open abdomen management may also be considered in this patient category. A rare indication may be the patient with necrotizing infection of the abdominal wall that requires extensive resection and leaves a significant defect in the abdominal wall musculature. Primary fascial closure is of course not an option, and more advanced reconstructive techniques should be applied.

Open Abdomen Classification

The recent consensus definitions from the World Society of the Abdominal Compartment Syndrome (WSACS, www.wsacs.org) has defined the open abdomen as one that requires a TAC due to the skin and fascia not being closed after laparotomy [3]. A classification of the open abdomen has been recently developed based on the level of adherence between bowel loops, and the presence of contamination [3, 4]; higher levels represent more challenging cases. Lateralization of the abdominal wall is defined as a phenomenon where the musculature and fascia of the abdominal wall, most exemplified by the rectus abdominis muscles and their enveloping fascia, move laterally away from the midline with time. The consensus statement regarding grading of the open abdomen is shown in Box 1. The grade will not directly affect critical care interventions; open abdomen grades 3 and 4 are, however, different, because they are very difficult to close primarily, and a protracted clinical course can be expected.

Box 1. Classification of the open abdomen (based on [4])

Grade	Description
1A	Clean open abdomen without adherence between bowel and abdominal wall or fixity (lateralization of the abdominal wall)
1B	Contaminated open abdomen without adherence/fixity
2A	Clean open abdomen developing adherence/fixity
2B	Contaminated open abdomen developing adherence/fixity
3	Open abdomen complicated by fistula formation
4	Frozen open abdomen with adherent/fixed bowel, unable to close surgically, with or without fistula

Temporary Abdominal Closure Techniques

The ideal TAC probably does not exist but some important features are listed hereafter: Control of abdominal organs, quantification of peritoneal fluid, prevention of visceral adherence, prevention of fascial retraction, active removal of cytokines, control and prevention of enteric fistulae, prevention of organ dysfunction or failure, and facilitation of functional abdominal closure.

The goal of the initial techniques for TAC was primarily to cover and contain the abdominal contents. These first generation abdominal closure techniques that aim solely at covering the abdominal content have been abandoned in most hospitals. Although these techniques may still be used in resource-poor countries, they should no longer be used in modern critical care. Towel clip closure is no longer acceptable because of the high incidence of ACS and skin necrosis. The Bogotá bag, first described in 1984, was designed to contain the abdominal contents using a large plastic, cut-up 3 L urology irrigation bag sewn to the skin. When it was introduced, the Bogotá bag was an innovative technique to improve abdominal wall compliance and reduce intraabdominal pressure (IAP).

Subsequently, different methods of TAC have been developed to protect the open abdomen and reduce these complications [5]. Unfortunately there are no randomized controlled trials (RCTs) comparing one form of closure to another. This is due to the heterogeneity of the population and the inability to establish a proper control technique. One commonly used TAC is the vacuum pack technique, i. e., the Barker Vac-Pac technique [6]. This is a 'home-made' device that involves placing a plastic covering over the bowel and suction drains in gauze or surgical towels and applying the system to wall suction. This has the advantage of removing fluid from the abdomen and improving closure rates. In 2000, Barker et al. reported closure rates of 55% using this technique; the enteric fistula rate was 4% [6]. In 2004, Miller et al. reported the successful use of a similar technique of abdominal closure after open abdomen [7]. They concluded that use of the vacuum pack technique resulted in significantly higher fascial closure rates, obviating the need for subsequent hernia repair in most patients.

This technique appeared to be the most effective way of covering the abdomen and controlling fluid losses until the application of negative pressure wound therapy (NPWT) to the open abdomen. This technique was also recommended in the latest clinical practice guidelines from the WSACS [3]. NPWT had been used for some time in peripheral chronic wound care, but application in the open abdomen revolutionized the care for these patients. NPWT is more effective in actively draining abdominal fluids and, most importantly, has resulted in superior primary fascial closure rates compared to the older TAC techniques. In particular, the combination of NPWT and synthetic mesh, and the progressive approximation of the fascial edges, as developed by Petersson et al. [8] – the so-called mesh-mediated NPWT – has proved a superior strategy in several studies [9–13].

From these observations, it can be concluded that the most appropriate method for TAC in 2015 is mesh-mediated NPWT. Occasionally, other techniques can be used as a first-line strategy in emergency situations where the operating team is unfamiliar with open abdomen treatment – closing the abdomen in these situations is probably a worse option. In these cases, patients should be scheduled for re-intervention after stabilization, and a more appropriate TAC technique should be used.

Goals of Open Abdomen Management

Abdominal cover and avoiding damage to the bowel were the primary goals when open abdomen treatment was introduced, but the goals of open abdomen management have changed significantly over the years. Fluid control and facilitation of abdominal closure are two new goals that are now key in achieving a good patient outcome (Box 2).

Box 2. Goals of temporary abdominal closure

1. Abdominal cover
- Avoid injury to intestines and abdominal organs
- Prevent infection of peritoneal cavity

2. Fluid control
- Evacuate postoperative fluids
- Decrease bowel edema
- Avoid recurrent IAH

3. Facilitation of fascial closure
- Avoid lateralization of the abdominal wall musculature and fascia
- Progressive approximation of the fascial edges
- Avoid adhesion between bowel loops and parietal peritoneum

IAH: intra-abdominal hypertension

Fluid control, which prevents recurrent increases in IAP and avoids accumulation of postoperative collections, may lead to lower superinfection and intra-abdominal abscess rates. NPWT may, as such, help to reduce disease severity by further reducing IAP and dampening systemic inflammation, although the latter effect has so far only been documented in animal models [14]. Intra-abdominal fluid collections are common and rich in cytokines with pro-inflammatory properties. Removal of abdominal fluid via NPWT resulted in a decrease in peritoneal and plasma levels of tumor necrosis factor (TNF)-α, interleukin (IL)-1β, IL-6 and IL-12 in the above-mentioned animal study [14].

Whereas previously an open abdomen was often impossible to close, and a giant hernia was taken for granted, early abdominal closure should be the target for both the surgeon and the critical care team. In this context, all open abdomens should be considered temporary and early closure the goal. Fascial retraction, or the lateral retraction of the abdominal muscles is a major hurdle to achieving early closure. Recent studies demonstrate, however, that early closure is a realistic possibility with primary abdominal closure rates of 80–90%. Another major obstacle in this context is the occurrence of an intestinal fistula; this should be a rarity, however, with modern open abdomen treatment.

Throughout the course, IAH management remains important, and factors contributing to IAH and ACS should be carefully monitored. IAP should also be monitored throughout and after open abdomen treatment, because IAH persists in most patients and ACS may relapse. In this situation, it may indicate intra-abdominal bleeding or other new intra-abdominal complications. Most importantly, fluid administration, which is among the main iatrogenic factors for IAH in the critically ill, should be judiciously used in this setting. In this respect, it is important to emphasize that ACS is a syndrome and not a disease: ACS is in fact a symptom of a disease [15]

The main goal in open abdomen treatment remains abdominal closure. Critical care management should also be focused on achieving this goal as soon as possible, as delays are associated with increased complication rates (Box 3).

Box 3. Key issues in open abdomen management in the ICU.

- Regular IAP monitoring
- Restrictive fluid management
- Maintain visceral perfusion
- Early enteral nutrition – think of protein losses and consider replacement
- Timely respiratory weaning
- Optimize wound care
- Early mobilization
- Daily evaluation with surgical team aiming for early closure

IAP: intra-abdominal pressure

Fluid Management and Open Abdomen

Fluid accumulation in the abdomen – ascites or bowel edema – will have contributed to the development of ACS in most patients [16] and, therefore, fluid administration should be carefully considered in open abdomen treatment patients. Maintaining a negative fluid balance may be difficult as often oligo-anuria is present and ongoing third spacing may lead to intravascular fluid depletion requiring more fluids [17]. NPWT may, however, be a powerful tool to remove accumulated fluid.

Achieving a negative fluid balance was associated with increased primary fascial closure rates in a study by Stone et al. [18]. In its recent update of the consensus definitions and clinical practice guidelines, the WSACS suggested using a protocol to try and avoid a positive cumulative fluid balance in the critically ill or injured patient with, or at risk of, IAH/ACS after acute resuscitation has been completed and the inciting issues have been addressed [3]. This suggestion is probably even more relevant in the setting of open abdomen treatment. This is a relatively data-poor area and research in this field is urgently needed.

Respiratory Support in Open Abdomen Patients

Respiratory insufficiency is one of the early clinical signs of ACS, and many of these patients will be receiving mechanical ventilation. Once the abdomen is left open, abdominal wall compliance will be better and there is no formal reason to continue the mechanical ventilation when the abdomen is open. When appropriately applied, the TAC should allow spontaneous breathing and weaning should not be deferred. When a mesh is used to reinforce the fascia (as in mesh-mediated NPWT), the risk of inefficient breathing is greatly reduced and this seems to be the best setting for expedited weaning in these patients.

Nutrition in the Open Abdomen

Nutrition has been identified as an important aspect of care in patients with abdominal conditions. Whereas intuitively a restrictive approach to enteral nutrition may be logical in open abdomen patients, there is no evidence to deny these patients enteral nutrition, and the benefits associated with enteral nutrition may be even more relevant in open abdomen patients [19]. Several reports found that early enteral nutrition was a safe strategy in open abdomen patients [20, 21].

When intestinal integrity is preserved, the nutritional strategy should not be different from that used in other critically ill patients. Burlew et al. found that enteral nutrition was associated with increased fascial closure rates, decreased complication rates, and decreased mortality in patients with an open abdomen and no bowel injury [22]. It is not necessary to wait for the presence of peristalsis (which may be visibly checked in some patients!).

When a fistula is present, the approach may be different depending on the location of the fistula. When it is proximal and has a high output then absorption might be impaired. Nutritional strategies should be decided on a patient-to-patient basis, taking into account the physiology of the patient and the abdominal anatomy and intestinal integrity. Often a combination of enteral and parenteral nutrition may be the solution. If patients with enteric fistula can be fed enterally early (within the first 14 days after injury), outcomes are better [23].

One particular nutritional aspect of patients with open abdomen is the protein loss in the abdominal fluid. Wade et al. found that on average 2.9 g/dl protein was lost in abdominal fluids in patients treated with NPWT; this translated to a mean protein loss of 25 ± 17 g per day [24]. This confirms earlier findings of Cheatham et al. who concluded that failure to account for this loss in nutritional calculations may lead to underfeeding and inadequate nutritional support with a direct effect on patient outcome [25].

Nursing Issues

Wound Care

Caring for an open abdomen patient used to be one of the biggest challenges in the surgical ICU from a nursing perspective. Modern open abdomen management has revolutionized the care of these patients. Specific issues in patients who are treated with a Bogota bag or moist gauze to cover the abdomen relate to fluid loss, which can be very high. Blood loss, postoperative fluid or ascites loss can be as high as several liters per day leaving the skin moist and prone to damage – often on top of systemic hypoperfusion – and skin ulceration and necrosis. Fluid balances are very unreliable even if the fluid evacuated from the wound is estimated by weighing the gauze that is being replaced. Apart from this, evaporation through the open wound adds to the unreliability of fluid balances in this context. The risk of infection is also considerable in these patients as it is almost impossible to replace the wound gauze and safeguard sterility throughout the care of the patient. When a vacuum pack is used fluid losses can be better controlled and skin care is also much easier. Nevertheless, fluid accumulation under the adhesive drape is possible, which may macerate the skin and lead to leakages.

From a nursing perspective, NPWT is the most convenient system as fluid problems are non-existent, wound care is done in the operating room (although this procedure can be done at the bedside as well if no intra-abdominal complications are expected) on a regular basis and basic nursing care is easy. Technical problems may arise however, and loss of negative pressure is probably the most common problem – often skin folds in or around the groin are responsible and can be managed by applying additional adhesive drapes in the suspected area or stoma paste in the skin fold.

Fistula Care

Fistula formation has been one of the most dreaded complications of open abdomen management, and contrary to what is often suggested, incidence of fistula in NPWT is not higher compared to other forms of TAC. Reported fistula rates are around 5% depending on the type of patient and underlying conditions that contributed to the need for open abdomen treatment. Fistulas are most likely to occur in case of inadequate resuscitation, visceral malperfusion or incorrect TAC management.

Recent studies suggest that TAC is not the culprit [26]. In fact, when a fistula is present, NPWT may offer an elegant solution to manage the open wound. Rather than letting the fistula drain into the laparostomy and applying a wound manager, several home-made solutions have been introduced and excellent outcomes have been reported. The basic concept of this approach is to either exteriorize using drains (Fig. 1) or to isolate the fistula with adhesive paste or stoma plates and allow

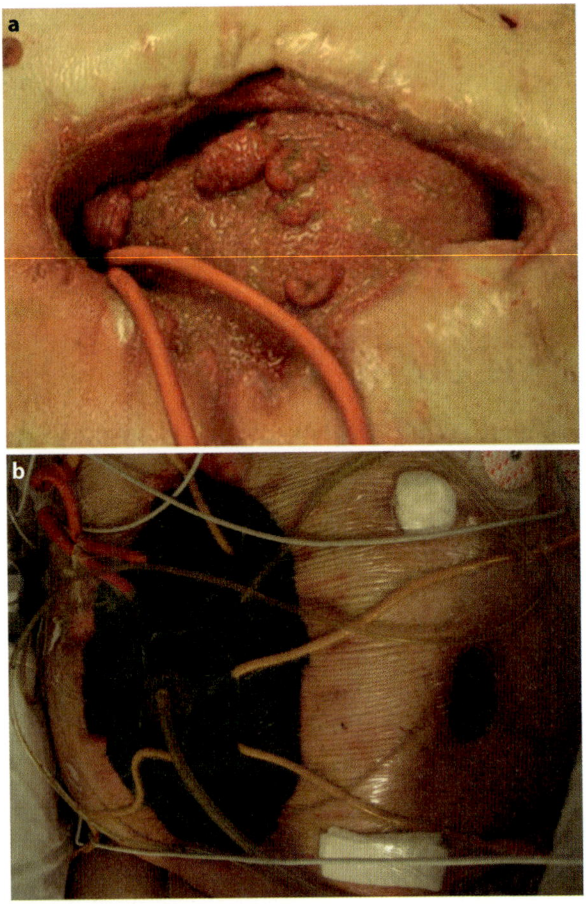

Fig. 1 Grade 4 open abdomen with multiple fistulas. Panel **a**: Before NPWT; Panel **b**: After application of NPWT and fistula isolation

NPWT around the fistula. This allows healing of the open wound around the fistula that can then be converted into a regular stoma. When the fistula is small and has a low output, spontaneous closure may occur as the granulating skin grows and covers the fistula.

Mobilizing the Patient

Whereas fear of evisceration through the abdominal wound is often a reason to keep the open abdomen patient fully sedated and even paralyzed, there is no evidence in the literature to support this. Open abdomen patients could benefit from early mobilization even more than other patients and should, therefore, not be left immobilized in their bed. Contrary to what many think, early mobilization is feasible with appropriately applied TAC. Specifically when a mesh-mediated NPWT strategy is used, full mobilization should not be delayed.

Conclusion

Open abdomen management is increasingly used in several severe abdominal conditions either as a prophylactic measure or as therapy for abdominal compartment syndrome. Critical care management is crucial in reaching the primary goal of early abdominal closure as this avoids a protracted clinical course. Judicious fluid management, proper wound care, early respiratory weaning and mobilization and timely nutritional support are key issues for success. Daily evaluation with the surgical team to evaluate the patient for abdominal closure is paramount.

References

1. Malbrain ML, Chiumello D, Pelosi P et al (2005) Incidence and prognosis of intraabdominal hypertension in a mixed population of critically ill patients: A multiple-center epidemiological study. Crit Care Med 33:315–322
2. Malbrain ML, Chiumello D, Cesana BM et al (2014) A systematic review and individual patient data meta-analysis on intra-abdominal hypertension in critically ill patients: the wake-up project. World initiative on Abdominal Hypertension Epidemiology, a Unifying Project (WAKE-Up!). Minerva Anestesiol 80:293–306
3. Kirkpatrick AW, Roberts DJ, De Waele J et al (2013) Intra-abdominal hypertension and the abdominal compartment syndrome: updated consensus definitions and clinical practice guidelines from the World Society of the Abdominal Compartment Syndrome. Intensive Care Med 39:1190–1206
4. Bjorck M, Bruhin A, Cheatham M et al (2009) Classification – important step to improve management of patients with an open abdomen. World J Surg 33:1154–1157
5. De Waele JJ, Leppaniemi AK (2011) Temporary abdominal closure techniques. Am Surg 77(Suppl 1):S46–S50
6. Barker DE, Kaufman HJ, Smith LA, Ciraulo DL, Richart CL, Burns RP (2000) Vacuum pack technique of temporary abdominal closure: a 7-year experience with 112 patients. J Trauma 48:201–206

7. Miller PR, Meredith JW, Johnson JC, Chang MC (2004) Prospective evaluation of vacuum-assisted fascial closure after open abdomen: planned ventral hernia rate is substantially reduced. Ann Surg 239:608–614
8. Petersson U, Acosta S, Bjorck M (2007) Vacuum-assisted wound closure and mesh-mediated fascial traction-a novel technique for late closure of the open abdomen. World J Surg 31:2133–2137
9. Willms A, Gusgen C, Schaaf S et al (2014) Management of the open abdomen using vacuum-assisted wound closure and mesh-mediated fascial traction. Langenbecks Arch Surg (in press)
10. Liapis CD, Moulakakis KG (2013) Vacuum and mesh-mediated fascial traction for closure of the open abdomen after abdominal aortic aneurysm repair. Eur J Vasc Endovasc Surg 45:595
11. Bjarnason T, Montgomery A, Ekberg O et al (2013) One-year follow-up after open abdomen therapy with vacuum-assisted wound closure and mesh-mediated fascial traction. World J Surg 37:2031–2038
12. Rasilainen SK, Mentula PJ, Leppäniemi AK (2012) Vacuum and mesh-mediated fascial traction for primary closure of the open abdomen in critically ill surgical patients. Br J Surg 99:1725–1732
13. Acosta S, Bjarnason T, Petersson U et al (2011) Multicentre prospective study of fascial closure rate after open abdomen with vacuum and mesh-mediated fascial traction. Br J Surg 98:735–743
14. Kubiak BD, Albert SP, Gatto LA et al (2010) Peritoneal negative pressure therapy prevents multiple organ injury in a chronic porcine sepsis and ischemia/reperfusion model. Shock 34:525–534
15. Malbrain ML, De Iaet IE (2009) Intra-abdominal hypertension: evolving concepts. Clin Chest Med 30:45–70
16. McNelis J, Marini CP, Jurkiewicz A et al (2002) Predictive factors associated with the development of abdominal compartment syndrome in the surgical intensive care unit. Arch Surg 137:133–136
17. Cordemans C, De Laet I, Van Regenmortel N et al (2012) Fluid management in critically ill patients: the role of extravascular lung water, abdominal hypertension, capillary leak, and fluid balance. Ann Intensive Care 2(Suppl 1):S1
18. Stone PA, Hass SM, Flaherty SK, DeLuca JA, Lucente FC, Kusminsky RE (2004) Vacuum-assisted fascial closure for patients with abdominal trauma. J Trauma 57:1082–1086
19. Collier B, Guillamondegui O, Cotton B et al (2007) Feeding the open abdomen. JPEN J Parenter Enteral Nutr 31:410–415
20. Byrnes MC, Reicks P, Irwin E (2010) Early enteral nutrition can be successfully implemented in trauma patients with an "open abdomen". Am J Surg 199:359–362
21. Dissanaike S, Pham T, Shalhub S et al (2008) Effect of immediate enteral feeding on trauma patients with an open abdomen: protection from nosocomial infections. J Am Coll Surg 207:690–697
22. Burlew CC, Moore EE, Cuschieri J et al (2012) Who should we feed? A Western Trauma Association multi-institutional study of enteral nutrition in the open abdomen after injury. J Trauma Acute Care Surg 73:1380–1388
23. Yuan Y, Ren J, Gu G, Chen J, Li J (2011) Early enteral nutrition improves outcomes of open abdomen in gastrointestinal fistula patients complicated with severe sepsis. Nutr Clin Pract 26:688–694
24. Wade C, Wolf SE, Salinas R et al (2010) Loss of protein, immunoglobulins, and electrolytes in exudates from negative pressure wound therapy. Nutr Clin Pract 25:510–516
25. Cheatham ML, Safcsak K, Brzezinski SJ, Lube MW (2007) Nitrogen balance, protein loss, and the open abdomen. Crit Care Med 35:127–131
26. Shaikh IA, Ballard-Wilson A, Yalamarthi S, Amin AI (2010) Use of topical negative pressure in assisted abdominal closure does not lead to high incidence of enteric fistulae. Colorectal Dis 12:931–934

Part X
Nutrition

Protein Intake in Critical Illness

O. Rooyackers and J. Wernerman

Introduction

Can nutrition influence outcome in critical illness? This is a highly controversial question with a large number of controversial issues involved, for each of which there is insufficient evidence. Over all, the aim of nutrition is to improve outcome by supplying energy and by preserving body proteins. The controversial questions are: When to start, what route of administration to use, how to determine energy need, how to determine protein need, how to consider degree of malnutrition? This chapter will focus on protein intake during critical illness and how it should be assessed and evaluated in this group of patients.

Present Recommendations and the Background Evidence

In the World Health Organization (WHO) nutrition guidelines for healthy adult subjects, a protein intake of 0.8 g/kg/day is recommended [1, 2]. In nutritional guidelines for critically ill patients, the recommendation is upgraded to 1.2–3.0 g/kg/day, with considerable variation between publications [3–5]. This variation reflects the insufficient level of evidence that exists, together with the difficulty assessing the efficacy of protein intake. Ideally, patients should be fed according to energy expenditure and randomized to different levels of protein intake and evaluated by a composite outcome measure of survival and quality of life. However, such studies do not exist and, in addition, when nutritional support should be started is controversial.

The literature contains a few randomized studies using a surrogate endpoint of nitrogen balance, together with observational studies relating protein intake to out-

O. Rooyackers · J. Wernerman ✉
Department of Anesthesia and Intensive Care Medicine, Karolinska University Hospital Huddinge and Karolinska Institute, Stockholm, Sweden
e-mail: jan.wernerman@karolinska.se

J.-L. Vincent (ed.), *Annual Update in Intensive Care and Emergency Medicine 2015*,
DOI 10.1007/978-3-319-13761-2_33

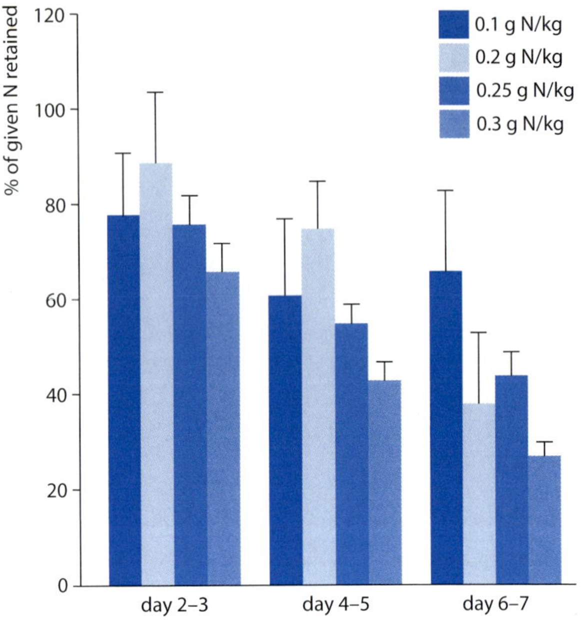

Fig. 1 Fractional nitrogen (N) retention over time in critically ill patients fed isocaloric parenteral nutrition but randomized to different protein intakes. The figure illustrates the need to be fully adapted to a certain level of intake before adequate comparisons are meaningful. Data calculated from [6]

come. Nitrogen balance has been the gold standard when evaluating the efficacy of protein intake. It gives reliable and reproducible results when applied to non-malnourished subjects adapted to a certain level of energy and protein intake over a period of time not less than 2 weeks, comparing different protein compositions. When deviating from these conditions, the reliability of nitrogen balance to evaluate protein intake becomes increasingly problematic.

The most cited and best controlled randomized study of protein intake in critical illness, is a study including patients with long bone fractures or moderate size burns given iso-caloric parenteral nutrition with variable protein content for 1 week [6]. The results showed an improvement in nitrogen balance with protein content up to approximately 1.5 g/kg/day, but no further improvement above that level. In Fig. 1, the fractional nitrogen retention was calculated for each study day, illustrating the difference in nitrogen retention related to the level of protein intake. This example shows the importance of the prerequisite being adapted to the level of protein intake for comparison of nitrogen balance results [7]. The interpretation by the authors of the study and the majority of guideline authors citing this study, is that optimal protein intake in critical illness should be at least 1.5 g/kg/day.

The other existing evidence comes from observational case series. A working group in Auckland, New Zealand has had access to a neutron activation instrument allowing for determination of body composition in the critically ill. The working group has published a number of key studies. In an observational case series of critically ill patients, their results indicate a maximum body cell mass preservation at a protein intake dose of 1.5 g/kg/day [8]. In a more recent observational case series from Copenhagen, Denmark, the dose of protein intake was compared to mortality outcome, and a statistical relation between the dose of protein administered and survival was observed [9]. These types of case series provide important hypothesis-generating observations, but the limitations involved must always be kept in mind. There is no information about the subjects not included in the series, and there is no information about why the individual subjects were given the dose of protein actually administered.

This illustrates the evidence behind the recommendation of 1.2–1.5 g/kg/day given in guidelines for the critically ill [10, 11]. Lately, databases from studies designed for other purposes have been used for *post hoc* analyses of the relationship between given dose of protein and outcomes. A working group in Amsterdam reported a better mortality outcome in patients given both calories and protein according to guidelines as compared to calories only or nutrition below the level recommended in the guidelines [12]. This association attained statistical significance for female patients in this particular study. Similar results are also reported from pooled data from several international studies, indicating that nutrition supply in accord with guidelines both concerning calories and protein was statistically associated with a better outcome [13]. On the other hand, a working group in Leuven reported no beneficial effect of either calories or protein content in the early phase of critical illness; for protein there was rather a tendency in the other direction [14].

It is obvious that selection of patients and selection of the time-point during critical illness strongly influence the effect of nutrition support. Cited studies often contain mixtures of patients with variable lengths of intensive care unit (ICU) stay, variable numbers and severities of co-morbidities, variable severities of acute illness, and variable success of feeding. Such differences between studies most likely explain a large part of the difference in results.

A second obvious difficulty is the outcome measure used. The ultimate outcome is of course survival and a high quality of life. This must, however, be related to the functional level and quality of life before the acute illness, something that is not always easy to define. The distance between nutritional therapy and survival/quality of life outcome is considerable. Therefore, the initial assumption is that preservation of body proteins or attenuation of body protein loss is a relevant outcome substitute. The use of imaging, such as neutron activation, magnetic resonance, computed tomography (CT) scanning, and ultrasound may be used in this context [15], but the sensitivity of imaging will only enable detection of differences after some time, usually weeks, in particular when differences between two treatments are to be discovered.

Whole Body Protein Turnover as a Surrogate Measure

Due to the difficulties described above, biochemical proxy endpoints may still be of value to enable detection of differences over shorter periods of time with sufficient accuracy. There are two fundamental demands on a biochemical proxy: (i) to accurately reflect changes in body protein status (indirectly survival/quality of life); and (ii) to enable comparisons between measurements that are relevant and interpretable. The traditional gold standard has been nitrogen balance as discussed above. Although the imperfection of the results obtained is generally recognized, nothing better has been available. The use of whole body protein turnover employing amino acids labeled with stable isotopes is now evolving as the future gold standard.

Just as for measurements of nitrogen balance, there are a number of underlying assumptions to consider when performing studies of whole body protein turnover [16]. The subject studied should be in a metabolic steady state during the measurement period and there should also be an isotopic steady state during measurement. If two measurements are to be compared, the metabolic steady states for the two periods need to be comparable. Authors need to define how these types of requirements are met in their study protocol. In addition, there should be a control over input of isotopic label and of the related unlabeled substance during the study period. If the amino acid used is metabolized, this should be quantified. If the unlabeled substance is supplied or lost, this should also be quantified.

Another underlying assumption is that the sampling pool (usually plasma) is in equilibrium with the whole body pool and also representative of the whole body pool. This means that recycling of an amino acid from protein degradation to protein *de novo* synthesis without leaving the cell (or organ) will not be reflected in the measurement. Another consequence is that the perfect control of amino acid supply given as parenteral nutrition intravenously is different and subject to much less control when enteral nutrition is administered. The best and only way to handle this problem is to combine enteral nutrition with a second label of the same amino acid, to reflect the enteral uptake combined with the first pass elimination through the splanchnic organs.

Whole Body Protein Turnover in the Critically Ill

When using whole body protein turnover measurements, it is possible to measure and/or calculate the rate of labeled amino acid appearance, disappearance, and oxidation. If an essential amino acid is used, the rate of appearance corresponds to protein degradation, the rate of disappearance to protein synthesis, and oxidation to the net balance, with the carbon skeleton becoming expired CO_2 and the nitrogen forming urea. Quantification of oxidation provides information to calculate all aspects of protein turnover. When studying the effect of protein feeding, a positive effect on protein balance is obtained by either increasing synthesis and/or decreasing breakdown while simultaneously a minimum of extra amino acid/protein is oxidized. The measurement of protein oxidation opens up the possibility of assessing utilization of the protein supply. Is it utilized in protein turnover or is it directly oxidized? This should give an indication as to whether or not an increase in protein supplementation will become a metabolic burden. When a measurement is performed in healthy subjects in the postabsorptive state, they are in a slight negative protein balance, as illustrated in Fig. 2 [17]. When given parenteral nutrition,

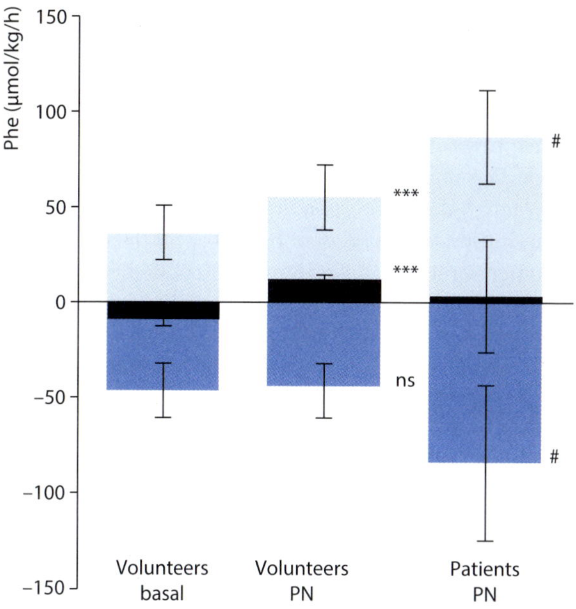

Fig. 2 Whole body protein turnover in volunteers and critically ill patients in the basal state and during parenteral feeding. The light blue bars illustrate protein synthesis, the dark blue bars protein degradation and the black bars protein balance. The volunteers are in negative balance in the basal state, moving into a positive balance in the fed state. The critically ill patients have higher synthesis and degradation; furthermore, they are in a negative protein balance although they are being fed. ***: statistically different from basal state, $p<0.001$; #: statistically different from volunteers during parenteral nutrition delivery, $p>0.05$; ns: not significant. Reproduced from [17] with permission

there is a stimulation of whole body synthesis *and* degradation, synthesis to a larger degree than degradation, resulting in a positive whole body protein balance. When critically ill patients are given the same amount of nutrition (calories and protein), they are still in a slightly negative balance. The big difference, as compared to the healthy subjects, is that both whole body synthesis and whole body degradation are enhanced 2 to 3 fold (or sometimes more).

It must be emphasized that this stimulation of protein turnover in the critically ill is not uniformly distributed between organs. In some organs, like skeletal muscle, degradation overrides synthesis resulting in a substantial net protein loss [18]. In other organs, like the liver and in immune cells, synthesis and export of proteins are stimulated, resulting in a net positive balance [19–22]. Whole body protein turnover measurements will not differentiate between the individual organs, but the technique can be expanded to study individual organs or individual proteins.

Whole Body Protein Turnover and Feeding in the Critically Ill

In the study cited above, the critically ill patients were not fed uniformly. When studied as a case series relating protein intake to net protein balance, a positive statistical relationship was found as illustrated in Fig. 3. This may be regarded as a hypothesis-generating observation suggesting that the relationship between protein intake and protein balance be more systematically studied. In another study, our working group in Stockholm studied patients with head trauma or intracranial hemorrhage receiving parenteral nutrition in the neurosurgical ICU [23]. Patients were given calories according to their energy expenditure by a commercially available all-in-one formulation with a fixed protein to calorie ratio corresponding to a protein intake of approximately 1.07 g/kg/day. Whole body protein turnover was measured during full nutrition as described and compared to measurements taken after 24 hours of a 50% supply, containing 50% of calories and 0.53 g/kg/day of protein. As illustrated in Fig. 4 the net protein balance increased during the full caloric support combined with a higher protein supply (panel a), whereas amino acid oxidation did not change significantly, indicative of unaltered urea production (panel b). These data also indicate a relationship between a higher protein intake and a less negative protein balance. There are, however, several limitations of the study; the 50% feeding was hypocaloric, both groups were fed less protein than recommended in guidelines, and parenteral nutrition was used (related to deep sedation as part of treatment for high intracranial pressure [ICP]). In this study, the result suggests a better protein balance when more protein is supplied, and the results should encourage us and others to further explore this possibility, taking into consideration the unaltered protein oxidation when employing this level of protein intake.

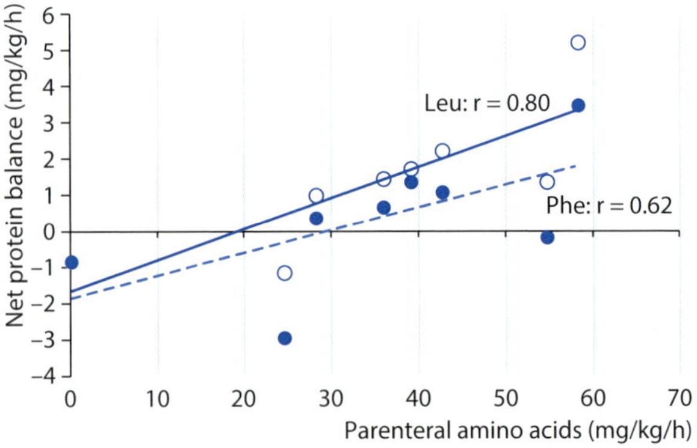

Fig. 3 Net whole body protein balance in critically ill patients during parenteral feeding. The feeding regimen was not uniform in terms of either calories or protein. Still, as a hypothesis-generating exercise, whole body protein balance is related to protein (amino acid) intake, suggestive of a positive relationship to be further explored. The open symbols represent the use of 13 C-leucine (Leu) and the filled symbols d5-phenylalanine (Phe) as isotopic tracer. Correlation coefficients for both tracers are suggestive of a covariation. Data calculated from [17]

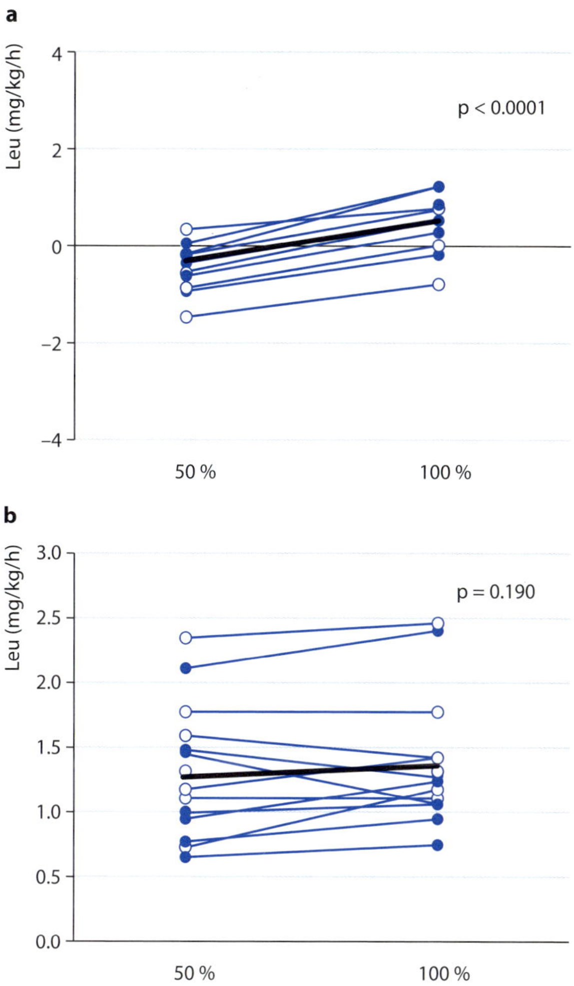

Fig. 4 Whole body protein turnover in critically ill patients with head trauma and/or intracranial bleeding during parenteral feeding. Measurements during full nutrition according to measured energy expenditure were compared to measurements during hypocaloric (50%) and low protein intake. Patients were randomized to be given normocaloric before hypocaloric (*filled symbols*), or hypocaloric before normocaloric (*open symbols*); medians are given in *black*. Panel **a** illustrates whole body protein balance, which becomes positive at an intake of 1.06 g/kg/day as compared to an intake of 0.53 g/kg/day. Panel **b** illustrates that protein oxidation is unaltered, which indicates that the higher intake is not immediately wasted, but utilized in protein turnover. Reproduced from ref [23] with permission

In parallel, a working group in Houston, Texas, studied adolescent septic patients receiving parenteral nutrition employing a similar study protocol comparing isocaloric parenteral nutrition with protein contents of 1.5 and 3.0 g/kg/day: A better protein balance was reported with the higher protein intake [24]. These authors also suggested the correct level of protein intake to titrate by dose-response studies. A limitation of this particular study is of course the group of adolescent patients, not directly representative of adults. Historically, patients with extensive burn injury were studied using a similar technique in a more stable phase of critical illness still being fed with isocaloric parenteral nutrition [25, 26]. Protein intakes of 1.4 and 2.2 g/kg/day were compared and no difference in protein turnover was seen. The authors concluded that the underlying alterations in protein metabolism were not related to the level of protein intake. The limitation of this study is of course the particular form of critical illness in burn injury, and the relative late phase of critical illness studied, which both limit the generalizability.

Having a clearcut hypothesis and a technique to study whole body protein turnover, there are a few other concerns to sort out: How to make measurement during enteral nutrition reliable and are repetitive measurements in the early phase of critical illness reproducible? To investigate the handling of enterally-supplied labeled amino acids, 13 C-leucine labeled milk proteins were used [27]. When giving a small initial dose, the first pass elimination is high: 80% for healthy volunteers and 93% for critically ill patients. Others have studied higher protein doses, reporting a lower level of first pass elimination [28]. When the isotopically-labeled milk protein is combined with a free labeled amino acid, when stabilized a similar representation in plasma of the two labeled amino acids is seen as indicated in Fig. 5 (unpublished data).

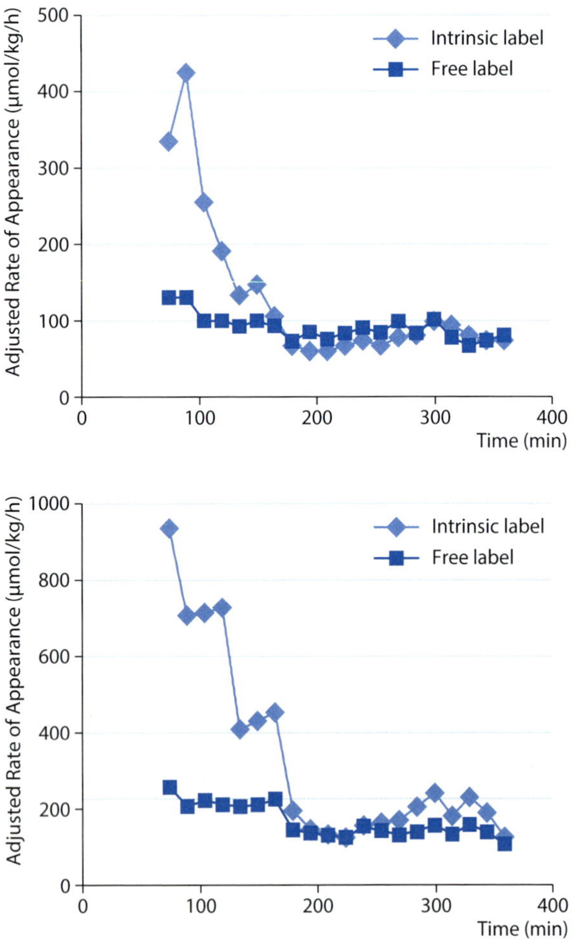

Fig. 5 The adjusted rate of appearance of phenylalanine into the plasma pool calculated from measurements of two differently labeled phenylalanine molecules: One free and one incorporated into milk protein (intrinsic label) in two individual critically ill patients (unpublished data)

In a recent study, mechanically ventilated patients in the ICU were studied by measuring whole body protein turnover on two occasions during the initial week of ICU stay (unpublished data). Preliminary results show that within that time period of ICU stay, whole body protein turnover did not change, and the response to extra protein intake was not altered. During both measurement periods, extra parenteral amino acid supplementation improved protein balance without increasing protein oxidation. Enteral nutrition was not standardized, but kept constant during the measurement period. During the later part of the measurement period, 1.0 extra gram of protein per kg and day was added in the form of an intravenous infusion of a complete amino acid solution (Glavamin, Fresenius). The relation between protein intake and protein balance under these condition is obvious. What are the limitations of this study? It included a short treatment period, which may be associated with artifacts. To overcome this limitation, a longer (at least 24 h) treatment period will be needed. The variability in energy intake, in absolute terms as well as in relation to energy expenditure, is more difficult to overcome, because if only fully fed patients can be included, we will be studying a sub-set of patients with limited generalizability.

Conclusion

To test the hypothesis that a higher protein intake may improve outcomes in critical illness, future studies must consider when to start nutrition, the degree of malnutrition and co-morbidities in included patients, the level of energy intake, and nutrition in the post-ICU period, before randomizing patients to different levels of intake. The technique discussed to measure whole body protein turnover should be helpful in titrating correct doses of protein and in identifying possible hazards of overdosing, which may relate to co-morbidities, degree of illness, or time-course of illness.

References

1. World Health Organization (2007) Protein and amino acid requirements in human nutrition. http://whqlibdoc.who.int/trs/WHO_TRS_935_eng.pdf?ua=1. Accessed Nov 2014
2. Stein J, Boehles HJ, Blumenstein I, Goeters C, Schulz R (2009) Amino acids – Guidelines on Parenteral Nutrition, Chapter 4. Ger Med Sci 7:1–8
3. Sauerwein HP, Serlie MJ (2010) Optimal nutrition and its potential effect on survival in critically ill patients. Neth J Med 68:119–122
4. Dickerson RN, Pitts SL, Maish GO 3rd et al (2012) A reappraisal of nitrogen requirements for patients with critical illness and trauma. J Trauma Acute Care Surg 73:549–557
5. Hoffer LJ, Bistrian BR (2012) Appropriate protein provision in critical illness: a systematic and narrative review. Am J Clin Nutr 96:591–600
6. Larsson J, Lennmarken C, Martensson J, Sandstedt S, Vinnars E (1990) Nitrogen requirements in severely injured patients. Br J Surg 77:413–416
7. Young VR (1986) Nutritional balance studies: indicators of human requirements or of adaptive mechanisms? J Nutr 116:700–703
8. Ishibashi N, Plank LD, Sando K, Hill GL (1998) Optimal protein requirements during the first 2 weeks after the onset of critical illness. Crit Care Med 26:1529–1535

9. Allingstrup MJ, Esmailzadeh N, Wilkens Knudsen A et al (2012) Provision of protein and energy in relation to measured requirements in intensive care patients. Clin Nutr 31:462–468
10. Kreymann KG, Berger MM, Deutz NE et al (2006) ESPEN Guidelines on Enteral Nutrition: Intensive care. Clin Nutr 25:210–223
11. Singer P, Berger MM, Van den Berghe G et al (2009) ESPEN Guidelines on Parenteral Nutrition: intensive care. Clin Nutr 28:387–400
12. Strack van Schijndel RJ, Weijs PJ, Koopmans RH, Sauerwein HP, Beishuizen A, Girbes AR (2009) Optimal nutrition during the period of mechanical ventilation decreases mortality in critically ill, long-term acute female patients: a prospective observational cohort study. Crit Care 13:R132
13. Elke G, Wang M, Weiler N, Day AG, Heyland DK (2014) Close to recommended caloric and protein intake by enteral nutrition is associated with better clinical outcome of critically ill septic patients: secondary analysis of a large international nutrition database. Crit Care 18:R29
14. Casaer MP, Wilmer A, Hermans G, Wouters PJ, Mesotten D, Van den Berghe G (2013) Role of disease and macronutrient dose in the randomized controlled EPaNIC trial: a post hoc analysis. Am J Respir Crit Care Med 187:247–255
15. Rooyackers O, Wernerman J (2014) Imaging opens possibilities both to target and to evaluate nutrition in critical illness. Crit Care 18:144
16. Wolfe RR, Chinkes DL (2005) Isotopic Tracers In Metabolic Research – Principles And Practice Of Kinetic Analysis. Wiley, Chichester
17. Rooyackers O, Kouchek-Zadeh R, Tjader I, Norberg A, Klaude M, Wernerman J (2015) Whole body protein turnover in critically ill patients with multiple organ failure. Clin Nutr (in press)
18. Klaude M, Mori M, Tjader I, Gustafsson T, Wernerman J, Rooyackers O (2012) Protein metabolism and gene expression in skeletal muscle of critically ill patients with sepsis. Clin Sci (Lond) 122:133–142
19. Barle H, Hammarqvist F, Westman B et al (2006) Synthesis rates of total liver protein and albumin are both increased in patients with an acute inflammatory response. Clin Sci (Lond) 110:93–99
20. Barle H, Januszkiewicz A, Hallstrom L et al (2002) Albumin synthesis in humans increases immediately following the administration of endotoxin. Clin Sci (Lond) 103:525–531
21. Essen P, McNurlan MA, Gamrin L et al (1998) Tissue protein synthesis rates in critically ill patients. Crit Care Med 26:92–100
22. Januszkiewicz J, Klaude M, Loré K et al (2005) In vivo protein synthesis in immune cells of ICU patients. Clin Nutr 24:575
23. Berg A, Rooyackers O, Bellander BM, Wernerman J (2013) Whole body protein kinetics during hypocaloric and normocaloric feeding in critically ill patients. Crit Care 17:R158
24. Verbruggen SC, Coss-Bu J, Wu M et al (2011) Current recommended parenteral protein intakes do not support protein synthesis in critically ill septic, insulin-resistant adolescents with tight glucose control. Crit Care Med 39:2518–2525
25. Wolfe RR, Goodenough RD, Burke JF, Wolfe MH (1983) Response of protein and urea kinetics in burn patients to different levels of protein intake. Ann Surg 197:163–171
26. Wolfe RR, Goodenough RD, Wolfe MH (1983) Isotopic approaches to the estimation of protein requirements in burn patients. Adv Shock Res 9:81–98
27. Liebau F, Rooyackers O, van Loon LJ, Werneman J (2013) Handling of dietary protein in critically ill patients. Crit Care 17(Suppl 2):P243
28. Pennings B, Groen B, de Lange A et al (2012) Amino acid absorption and subsequent muscle protein accretion following graded intakes of whey protein in elderly men. Am J Physiol Endocrinol Metab 302:E992–E999

Part XI

Trauma and Massive Bleeding

Rational and Timely Use of Coagulation Factor Concentrates in Massive Bleeding Without Point-of-Care Coagulation Monitoring

O. Grottke, D. R. Spahn, and R. Rossaint

Introduction

In this chapter, we describe our approach to emergency hemostatic management in severely bleeding patients when diagnostic information from point-of-care coag-

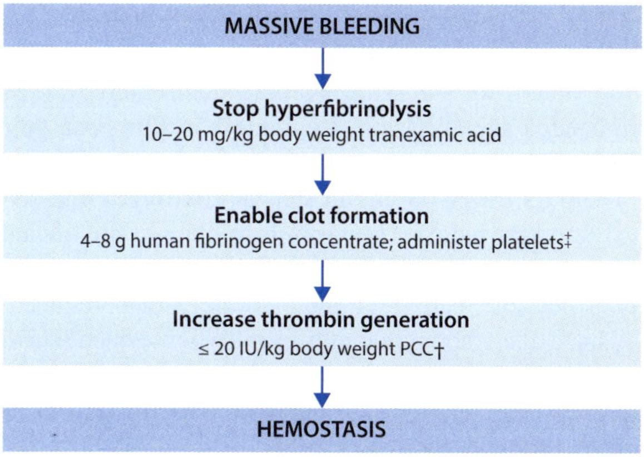

Fig. 1 Possible stepwise approach for rational and timely hemostatic therapy in patients with massive bleeding when point-of-care coagulation monitoring is unavailable. PCC: prothrombin complex concentrate; rFVIIa: recombinant human activated factor VII. ‡ Transfusion of platelets should be considered if platelet count is < 50,000–100,000/µl [1]. † If first-line treatment with a combination of surgical approaches and best-practice use of hemostatic therapy fails to control bleeding, administration of rFVIIa to enhance thrombin generation, or FXIII to increase clot stability has been considered in the literature [45]

O. Grottke ✉ · R. Rossaint
Department of Anesthesiology, RWTH Aachen University Hospital, Aachen, Germany
e-mail: ogrottke@ukaachen.de

D. R. Spahn
Institute of Anesthesiology, University Hospital Zurich, Zurich, Switzerland

J.-L. Vincent (ed.), *Annual Update in Intensive Care and Emergency Medicine 2015*,
DOI 10.1007/978-3-319-13761-2_34

ulation monitoring (thromboelastometry [ROTEM], thrombelastography [TEG]) is unavailable. We firmly believe that ROTEM/TEG-guided algorithms for hemostatic treatment represent the optimal approach, consistent with their inclusion in recent guidelines [1, 2], as coagulation diagnostics with these devices offer a number of advantages over conventional laboratory based coagulation tests [3]. However, where ROTEM/TEG measurements are not unavailable, which remains the reality in many emergency/operating rooms, it is imperative that a rational and timely strategy exists for effective hemostatic therapy in order to avoid detrimental outcomes. Here, we outline a stepwise approach that could be considered for this purpose (Fig. 1). We do not offer recommendations, guidance, or a systematic review of the literature, but instead aim to start debate about improving care for the massively bleeding patient in urgent need of effective hemostatic therapy when bedside monitoring is not possible.

Hemostatic Therapy: A Stepwise Approach

Stopping Hyperfibrinolysis

Hyperfibrinolysis (pathological clot breakdown) can develop following trauma or massive bleeding and predicts trauma-related mortality [4]. Hyperfibrinolysis should be addressed early, because it exacerbates bleeding, and antifibrinolytics can provide a foundation for subsequent procoagulant therapy. Tranexamic acid (TXA) is recommended as antifibrinolytic therapy in European guidelines [2, 5]. TXA has been demonstrated to have an acceptable safety profile, with the weight of evidence favoring its use as an initial step in controlling massive hemorrhage [6]. The Clinical Randomisation of an Antifibrinolytic in Significant Hemorrhage (CRASH)-2 study involved > 20,000 trauma patients and found that administration of TXA as early as possible, but within the first three hours, reduced mortality [7]. Multiple studies have also shown that antifibrinolytics reduce bleeding in cardiac surgery [1], though TXA has been associated with an increased risk of seizures and mortality in open-heart surgery [8]. Optimal TXA dosing has not been established and regimens vary widely (1–10 g total dose). In massive bleeding, the risk–benefit profile of TXA supports its use even in the absence of clinically diagnosed hyperfibrinolysis.

Enabling Clot Formation

As the precursor of fibrin, fibrinogen is essential for clot formation. During massive bleeding, fibrinogen reaches critically low levels (hypofibrinogenemia) before platelets and other coagulation factors [9]. Hypofibrinogenemia and impaired fibrin formation/polymerization contribute to dilutional coagulopathy following volume resuscitation. Patients with hypofibrinogenemia have a higher risk of poor clinical outcomes, and hypofibrinogenemia has been shown to independently predict mortality in trauma [10]. Additionally, in pediatric and adult patients undergoing cardiac surgery, decreased plasma fibrinogen levels have been associated with increased blood loss [11, 12]. We consider fibrinogen supplementation to be a key early step in managing coagulopathic bleeding.

Fibrinogen supplementation therapies include cryoprecipitate, fresh frozen plasma (FFP), and purified human fibrinogen concentrate. However, there have been safety concerns surrounding cryoprecipitate and FFP [13, 14]. The prophylactic and therapeutic benefits of FFP remain unproven in most settings [15]. Moreover, FFP contains relatively low levels of fibrinogen, although the exact amount in each bag is unknown. Thus, large volumes of FFP administered over a long period of time might be needed to achieve a meaningful increase in plasma fibrinogen level. In comparison, fibrinogen concentrate allows rapid, small-volume administration and more precise fibrinogen dosing. Data from randomized, controlled trials, mostly conducted in cardiac surgery settings, have shown that fibrinogen concentrate therapy can reduce perioperative transfusion requirements and blood loss, and improves plasma fibrinogen levels and fibrin-based clotting [16–18]. Observational studies have shown that fibrinogen concentrate is associated with benefits and a favorable survival rate when used as first-line hemostatic therapy in trauma patients [19, 20]. Prospective safety studies of fibrinogen concentrate are required – in the meantime, preclinical and pharmacosurveillance data suggest that fibrinogen concentrate is well tolerated, with a low thrombogenic potential and a low risk of thromboembolic events [21].

We believe that the lack of access to ROTEM/TEG testing to rapidly measure fibrinogen-based clotting need not prevent appropriate fibrinogen supplementation therapy in the massively bleeding patient. Hemoglobin and base excess are routinely tested laboratory parameters with very short turnaround times and have both been shown to correlate strongly with plasma fibrinogen levels [22]. As such, these tests may potentially inform, or at least alert, on the need for fibrinogen supplementation, if point-of-care coagulation monitoring is unavailable and urgent hemostatic intervention is necessary. If, however, bleeding is not acute and time is not a critical factor, plasma fibrinogen concentration should be measured to guide fibrinogen supplementation therapy, in the absence of viscoelastic testing. Current guidelines recommend a trigger of 1.5–2.0 g/l for fibrinogen replacement in severely bleeding patients [1, 2]. One study found that administration of 3 g fibrinogen concentrate increased plasma fibrinogen by approximately 1 g/l in a 70-kg patient [23]. The European Core Summaries of Product Characteristics, as well as the package insert of the fibrinogen concentrate used in our institutions, propose a dose between 4 and 8 g in case of severe hemorrhage. Whatever individual dose is chosen, it should reflect the clinical situation and extent of bleeding.

Administering Platelets

Effective clot formation involves thrombin generation, fibrinogen, platelets, and factor XIII. Low platelet count (thrombocytopenia) and platelet dysfunction can compromise this process. Thrombocytopenia has multiple causes, including blood loss, hemodilution, and prolonged cardiopulmonary bypass (CPB).

Fibrinogen supplementation may partially compensate for thrombocytopenia [24], but severe thrombocytopenia may impair clot formation even if fibrinogen levels and thrombin generation are adequate. Thus, platelet therapy may be required in addition to factor concentrate-based hemostatic therapy. Platelet therapy typically involves transfusion with apheresis platelet concentrate, but platelet transfusion carries a risk of adverse events [25].

Given the uncertain risk–benefit profile of platelet transfusion, we believe that therapy should be administered only if the patient bleeds continuously following fibrinogen supplementation and has a clear platelet count deficit. Platelet count can be obtained in a reasonable timeframe while priority therapies are administered. Guidelines in surgery and trauma suggest platelet transfusion when platelet count is $<50{,}000$–$100{,}000/\mu l$ [1, 2, 26]. An important consideration is whether the patient is receiving antiplatelet therapy, which compromises platelet function. Indeed, antiplatelet therapy is not always discontinued in surgical patients (e. g., cardiac surgery), varying on a case-by-case basis [27]. In severely bleeding patients receiving dual antiplatelet therapy, platelet transfusion may be appropriate before platelet count is available.

Increasing Thrombin Generation

Bleeding that continues despite fibrinogen supplementation and adequate platelet count may be due to insufficient thrombin generation, which is itself a predictor of mortality in trauma-induced coagulopathy [28]. One option for increasing thrombin generation is four-factor human prothrombin complex concentrate (PCC), containing the vitamin K-dependent coagulation factors II, VII, IX and X. Three-factor PCCs are available, but are considered less effective than four-factor PCCs due to their lower content of FVII [29]. Compared with FFP, PCC facilitates more rapid and predictable increases in coagulation factor activity [30].

PCC is indicated for congenital or acquired deficiencies of coagulation factors II, VII, IX, and X, and is widely used for emergency reversal of vitamin K antagonist-induced anticoagulation. In non-anticoagulant-associated bleeding, the best available evidence of PCC efficacy comes from observational studies in which PCC infusion arrested hemorrhage in cardiac surgery [31, 32]. PCC is also a component of POC-guided algorithms for goal-directed management of traumatic or perioperative bleeding [33, 34]. However, robust safety data on PCC are lacking. A meta-analysis has indicated a low but quantifiable thromboembolic risk associated with PCC for anticoagulant reversal [35]. However, a recent review did not identify an increase in thromboembolic events with the use of PCC [36]. Modern PCCs have an improved balance of coagulation inhibitors versus prothrombin content [37], and we suggest that the potential thromboembolic risks may be outweighed by the poor prognosis of continuing hemorrhage. Prospective studies are needed to investigate the efficacy and safety of PCC in non-anticoagulated bleeding patients.

Reported use of PCC in massive bleeding is limited and non-POC-guided triggers for PCC infusion have not been established. The International Normalized Ratio (INR), used to guide PCC therapy in anticoagulant reversal, has limited value in emergency settings because it is not a reliable surrogate marker for bleeding and turnaround times for laboratory-based measurement are too long [38]. However, if viscoelastic testing is unavailable, point-of-care INR measurement may be considered, in order to avoid potential unguided PCC administration or to avoid therapy delay due to long turn-around time of standard laboratory tests. Irrespective of the assay used, diagnosing thrombin deficit and determining appropriate PCC dosing remains challenging. Avoiding high and repeated PCC doses may potentially reduce thromboembolic risks. The Summary of Product Characteristics for one PCC states that antithrombin III substitution may be considered before treatment with PCC [39], although little evidence supports this approach. We suggest administering the lowest possible dose of PCC, $\leq$ 20 IU/kg bodyweight.

We consider PCC to be first-line therapy for thrombin deficit correction in massive bleeding. If PCC is unavailable, off-label treatment with recombinant activated factor VII (rFVIIa) may be an option for patients whose bleeding is unresponsive to other hemostatic therapies. Some reports suggest benefits of rFVIIa therapy in surgery and trauma-related bleeding [40, 41]. However, increased thromboembolic risks are associated with use of rFVIIa off-label (i. e., outside hemophilia) [42, 43].

Guidelines suggest that rFVIIa is a treatment option for bleeding following blunt trauma, though benefits in penetrating trauma are unclear [2]. A review of 13 randomized, controlled trials concluded that rFVIIa should be considered only if conventional options (including correction of acidosis, hypothermia, and hypocalcemia, antifibrinolytics, fibrinogen, best practice use of blood products, and surgical intervention) are unsuccessful [44]. One meta-analysis suggested that 60 μg/kg bodyweight is the minimum effective dose. In the absence of tests to monitor global hemostasis, it is important to note that administration of PCC *and* rFVIIa in the same patient is inappropriate and not recommended.

Considerations

Hemostatic therapy for massive bleeding often involves FFP, platelets, and/or cryoprecipitate, and potentially off-label rFVIIa. As whole blood or blood components might not be readily available, and can exacerbate coagulopathy, we believe this approach needs reconsideration. In our experience, optimal management of massive bleeding makes use of point-of-care coagulation monitoring to guide factor concentrate administration. Where ROTEM/TEG devices are not yet available, we believe that factor concentrate-based therapy represents a more rational and timely strategy than empiric blood component transfusion. Further high-quality studies are warranted and we await these with interest.

As a minimum requirement, we submit that all trauma and operating rooms should stock TXA and fibrinogen concentrate. In centers routinely treating patients with major bleeding, an organizational structure enabling timely administration of hemostatic therapy is crucial. Appropriate dosing of coagulation factor concentrates may be achieved more rapidly when the extent of the coagulopathy can be diagnosed by ROTEM/TEG. However, even in the absence of this information, effective supplementation of coagulation factors can still be achieved more quickly with factor concentrates than with blood component transfusion. Coagulation factor replacement may be guided by degree of blood loss, which may indicate critical coagulation factor levels. When plasma-poor red blood cells (RBCs) and colloid plasma substitutes were used to replace major blood loss, fibrinogen was the first factor to reach critically low levels (1.0 g/l) at a calculated blood volume loss of 142 %, compared with 201 % for prothrombin and 230 % for platelets [9].

Of note, some of the therapies we describe are not available in all countries or are not yet approved for hemorrhage with acquired coagulopathy. Where factor concentrates are not available, cryoprecipitate may be an option for supplementing fibrinogen (though it has been withdrawn in most European countries for safety reasons), and newer-generation blood products (e. g., solvent/detergent-treated, prethawed, or freeze-dried plasma) should be considered.

Conclusion

Our approach is based largely on mechanistic and observational data, complemented by our clinical experience; more data are needed to better define transfusion triggers and target levels. Further prospective clinical data are needed, which focus on the safety of fibrinogen concentrate and the safety and efficacy of PCC in massive bleeding. Nonetheless, by questioning the appropriateness of traditional strategies for managing massive bleeding, and by presenting an alternative, rational, stepwise approach, we hope to encourage debate aimed at raising the standard of emergency care for severely bleeding patients.

Acknowledgements

We would like to thank Michael Makris, Marco Ranucci, Jeffry Kashuk and Jerrold Levy for their input during the preparation of the manuscript, and Meridian HealthComms for editorial assistance, financially supported by CSL Behring.

References

1. Kozek-Langenecker SA, Afshari A, Albaladejo P et al (2013) Management of severe perioperative bleeding: guidelines from the European Society of Anaesthesiology. Eur J Anaesthesiol 30:270–382
2. Spahn DR, Bouillon B, Cerny V et al (2013) Management of bleeding and coagulopathy following major trauma: an updated European guideline. Crit Care 17:R76
3. Kozek-Langenecker SA (2010) Perioperative coagulation monitoring. Best Pract Res Clin Anaesthesiol 24:27–40

4. Kashuk JL, Moore EE, Sawyer M et al (2010) Primary fibrinolysis is integral in the pathogenesis of the acute coagulopathy of trauma. Ann Surg 252:434–442
5. Liumbruno GM, Bennardello F, Lattanzio A et al (2011) Recommendations for the transfusion management of patients in the peri-operative period. II. The intra-operative period. Blood Transfus 9:189–217
6. Cap AP, Baer DG, Orman JA et al (2011) Tranexamic acid for trauma patients: a critical review of the literature. J Trauma 71:9–14
7. Roberts I, Shakur H, Coats T et al (2013) The CRASH-2 trial: a randomised controlled trial and economic evaluation of the effects of tranexamic acid on death, vascular occlusive events and transfusion requirement in bleeding trauma patients. Health Technol Assess 17:1–79
8. Koster A, Borgermann J, Zittermann A et al (2013) Moderate dosage of tranexamic acid during cardiac surgery with cardiopulmonary bypass and convulsive seizures: incidence and clinical outcome. Br J Anaesth 110:34–40
9. Hiippala ST, Myllyla GJ, Vahtera EM (1995) Hemostatic factors and replacement of major blood loss with plasma-poor red cell concentrates. Anesth Analg 81:360–365
10. Rourke C, Curry N, Khan S et al (2012) Fibrinogen levels during trauma hemorrhage, response to replacement therapy, and association with patient outcomes. J Thromb Haemost 10:1342–1351
11. Faraoni D, Willems A, Savan V et al (2014) Plasma fibrinogen concentration is correlated with postoperative blood loss in children undergoing cardiac surgery. A retrospective review. Eur J Anaesthesiol 31:317–326
12. Kindo M, Hoang Minh T, Gerelli S et al (2014) Plasma fibrinogen level on admission to the intensive care unit is a powerful predictor of postoperative bleeding after cardiac surgery with cardiopulmonary bypass. Thromb Res 134:360–368
13. Sorensen B, Bevan D (2010) A critical evaluation of cryoprecipitate for replacement of fibrinogen. Br J Haematol 149:834–843
14. Kor DJ, Stubbs JR, Gajic O (2010) Perioperative coagulation management – fresh frozen plasma. Best Pract Res Clin Anaesthesiol 24:51–64
15. Yang L, Stanworth S, Hopewell S et al (2012) Is fresh-frozen plasma clinically effective? An update of a systematic review of randomized controlled trials. Transfusion 52:1673–1686
16. Fenger-Eriksen C, Jensen TM, Kristensen BS et al (2009) Fibrinogen substitution improves whole blood clot firmness after dilution with hydroxyethyl starch in bleeding patients undergoing radical cystectomy: a randomized, placebo-controlled clinical trial. J Thromb Haemost 7:795–802
17. Karlsson M, Ternstrom L, Hyllner M et al (2009) Prophylactic fibrinogen infusion reduces bleeding after coronary artery bypass surgery. A prospective randomised pilot study. Thromb Haemost 102:137–144
18. Rahe-Meyer N, Solomon C, Hanke A et al (2013) Effects of fibrinogen concentrate as first-line therapy during major aortic replacement surgery: a randomized, placebo-controlled trial. Anesthesiology 118:40–50
19. Danes AF, Cuenca LG, Bueno SR et al (2008) Efficacy and tolerability of human fibrinogen concentrate administration to patients with acquired fibrinogen deficiency and active or in high-risk severe bleeding. Vox Sang 94:221–226
20. Schochl H, Nienaber U, Maegele M et al (2011) Transfusion in trauma: thromboelastometry-guided coagulation factor concentrate-based therapy versus standard fresh frozen plasma-based therapy. Crit Care 15:R83
21. Dickneite G, Pragst I, Joch C et al (2009) Animal model and clinical evidence indicating low thrombogenic potential of fibrinogen concentrate (Haemocomplettan P). Blood Coagul Fibrinolysis 20:535–540
22. Schlimp CJ, Voelckel W, Inaba K et al (2013) Estimation of plasma fibrinogen levels based on hemoglobin, base excess and Injury Severity Score upon emergency room admission. Crit Care 17:R137

23. Solomon C, Pichlmaier U, Schoechl H et al (2010) Recovery of fibrinogen after administration of fibrinogen concentrate to patients with severe bleeding after cardiopulmonary bypass surgery. Br J Anaesth 104:555–562
24. Velik-Salchner C, Haas T, Innerhofer P et al (2007) The effect of fibrinogen concentrate on thrombocytopenia. J Thromb Haemost 5:1019–1025
25. Siegenthaler MA, Schneider P, Vu DH et al (2005) Haemovigilance in a general university hospital: need for a more comprehensive classification and a codification of transfusion-related events. Vox Sang 88:22–30
26. Kozek-Langenecker S, Sorensen B, Hess J et al (2011) Emotional or evidence-based medicine – is there a moral tragedy in haemostatic therapy? Crit Care 15:462
27. Bertrand M (2008) When and how to discontinue antiplatelet therapy. Eur Heart J 10(Suppl):A35–A41
28. Kashuk JL, Moore EE, Wohlauer M et al (2012) Initial experiences with point-of-care rapid thrombelastography for management of life-threatening postinjury coagulopathy. Transfusion 52:23–33
29. Holland L, Warkentin TE, Refaai M et al (2009) Suboptimal effect of a three-factor prothrombin complex concentrate (Profilnine-SD) in correcting supratherapeutic international normalized ratio due to warfarin overdose. Transfusion 49:1171–1177
30. Demeyere R, Gillardin S, Arnout J et al (2010) Comparison of fresh frozen plasma and prothrombin complex concentrate for the reversal of oral anticoagulants in patients undergoing cardiopulmonary bypass surgery: a randomized study. Vox Sang 99:251–260
31. Arnekian V, Camous J, Fattal S et al (2012) Use of prothrombin complex concentrate for excessive bleeding after cardiac surgery. Interact Cardiovasc Thorac Surg 15:382–389
32. Schick KS, Fertmann JM, Jauch KW et al (2009) Prothrombin complex concentrate in surgical patients: retrospective evaluation of vitamin K antagonist reversal and treatment of severe bleeding. Crit Care 13:R191
33. Weber CF, Gorlinger K, Meininger D et al (2012) Point-of-care testing: a prospective, randomized clinical trial of efficacy in coagulopathic cardiac surgery patients. Anesthesiology 117:531–547
34. Gorlinger K, Fries D, Dirkmann D et al (2012) Reduction of fresh frozen plasma requirements by perioperative point-of-care coagulation management with early calculated goal-directed therapy. Transfus Med Hemother 39:104–113
35. Dentali F, Marchesi C, Pierfranceschi MG et al (2011) Safety of prothrombin complex concentrates for rapid anticoagulation reversal of vitamin K antagonists. A meta-analysis. Thromb Haemost 106:429–438
36. Sorensen B, Spahn DR, Innerhofer P et al (2011) Clinical review: Prothrombin complex concentrates – evaluation of safety and thrombogenicity. Crit Care 15:201
37. Rodgers GM (2012) Prothrombin complex concentrates in emergency bleeding disorders. Am J Hematol 87:898–902
38. Haas T, Fries D, Tanaka KA et al (2015) Usefulness of standard plasma coagulation tests in the management of perioperative coagulopathic bleeding: is there any evidence? Br J Aanesth (in press)
39. Behring C (2011) Summary of product characteristics: Beriplex P/N 250 & 500 IU
40. Ranucci M, Isgro G, Soro G et al (2008) Efficacy and safety of recombinant activated factor vii in major surgical procedures: systematic review and meta-analysis of randomized clinical trials. Arch Surg 143:296–304
41. von Heymann C, Jonas S, Spies C et al (2008) Recombinant activated factor VIIa for the treatment of bleeding in major abdominal surgery including vascular and urological surgery: a review and meta-analysis of published data. Crit Care 12:R14
42. Ponschab M, Landoni G, Biondi-Zoccai G et al (2011) Recombinant activated factor VII increases stroke in cardiac surgery: a meta-analysis. J Cardiothorac Vasc Anesth 25:804–810
43. Yuan ZH, Jiang JK, Huang WD et al (2010) A meta-analysis of the efficacy and safety of recombinant activated factor VII for patients with acute intracerebral hemorrhage without hemophilia. J Clin Neurosci 17:685–693

44. Moltzan CJ, Anderson DA, Callum J et al (2008) The evidence for the use of recombinant factor VIIa in massive bleeding: development of a transfusion policy framework. Transfus Med 18:112–120
45. Levi M, Fries D, Gombotz H et al (2011) Prevention and treatment of coagulopathy in patients receiving massive transfusions. Vox Sang 101:154–174

Optimal Temperature Management in Trauma: Warm, Cool or In-between?

M. C. Reade and M. Lumsden-Steel

Introduction

The optimal approach to temperature management in trauma is unclear. Observational studies have found that trauma patients with hypothermia on admission to hospital have greater blood transfusion requirements and a higher mortality when compared to normothermic patients [1, 2]. However, this is not necessarily cause and effect, as severity of illness confounds the relationship between temperature and trauma outcome (Fig. 1). Statistical techniques to adjust for severity of illness are imperfect, in part because of the difficulty of quantifying severity of injury. Postulated adverse effects of spontaneous hypothermia in trauma (such as coagulopathy, 'wasted' energy expenditure, and peripheral vasoconstriction leading to poor wound healing) remain largely speculative. Even if spontaneous hypothermia does cause adverse outcomes in trauma, whether warming such a patient reverses these negative effects is unclear. Despite this uncertainty, most major trauma protocols prioritize active warming – in some cases using quite extreme measures, such as the US military protocol that warms operating rooms to 42 °C [3] – which may also have adverse effects. There has only ever been one controlled trial rewarming spontaneously hypothermic trauma patients. This trial randomized patients to either "standard" rewarming techniques or to standard techniques plus continuous arteriovenous rewarming, with apparent short-term benefit but no statistically significant increase in long-term survival [4]. Conversely, there are case reports of trauma patients with extreme environmental hypothermia who have unexpectedly survived. There is extensive animal evidence that therapeutic hypothermia is beneficial in

M. C. Reade ✉
Royal Australian Army Medical Corps, Joint Health Command, Australian Defense Force, University of Queensland Health Sciences Building, Royal Brisbane & Women's Hospital, Brisbane, Queensland, Australia
e-mail: michael.reade@defence.gov.au

M. Lumsden-Steel
Royal Australian Air Force, Australian Defense Force, Royal Australian Air Force Base Amberley, Queensland, Australia

J.-L. Vincent (ed.), *Annual Update in Intensive Care and Emergency Medicine 2015*,
DOI 10.1007/978-3-319-13761-2_35

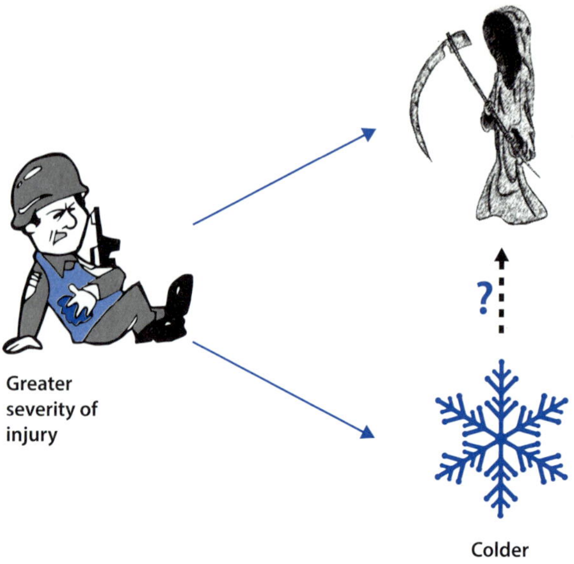

Fig. 1 Association does not necessarily equal causation in the relationship between hypothermia and outcome after trauma. Further, even if this association is causative, this does not necessarily imply that correction of hypothermia (once established) will be therapeutic

trauma [5]. This chapter reviews the surprising paucity of evidence for temperature management in trauma, makes recommendations based on the best available evidence, and defines areas in which equipoise exists for future clinical trials.

Trauma Management: If it Isn't Broken, Don't Fix it?

Improvements in trauma management have significantly reduced mortality from trauma in many systems in the last 10–15 years [6, 7]. Contributions to these improvements include protocoled pre-surgical trauma management (such as the Advance Trauma Life Support guidelines) [8], the development of pre-hospital trauma systems that deliver the 'right patient to the right hospital at the right time', and the evolution of trauma teams and trauma centers which together provide effective 'bundles of care'. Central to clinical teaching in this period of improvement has been effort to preserve body temperature and to rewarm patients who have become hypothermic. Temperature is taught as one component of the 'triad of death' in trauma (hypothermia, acidosis, and coagulopathy). There are ample observational studies showing that cold patients fare worse. For example, Shafi et al. [1] compared 3,267 hypothermic (temperature < 35 °C, 8.5% of presentations) with 35,283 normothermic adult patients (temperature ≥ 35 °C) in the American College of Surgeons Committee on Trauma National Trauma Data Bank 1994–2002. Hypothermic patients (mean temperature 34 ± 1 °C) had a higher mortality (20%) than patients with the same severity of injury who remained normothermic (1%), and hypothermic patients were more likely (25% vs 11%) to have complications including infections, renal failure, acute respiratory distress syndrome (ARDS), venous thromboembolism, coagulopathy and cardiac arrest. In multivariable analysis, hypothermia was an independent (albeit weak) predictor of mortality (odds ratio [OR] 1.19 [95% CI 1.05–1.35]). Similarly, Martin et al. [2] analyzed 701,491 patients in the National Trauma Data Bank for the period 1993 to 2004. Using body temperature at hospital admission and excluding patients with known environmental exposure causing hypothermia, comparison of 11,206 hypothermic (temperature < 35 °C) and 689,278 normothermic (temperature ≥ 35 °C) patients found that hypothermia on admission was associated with significantly higher mortality (25.5% vs. 3.0%, $p < 0.001$). Amongst survivors, admission hypothermia was also associated with longer requirement for mechanical ventilation and longer ICU and hospital stays. As expected, higher injury severity score (ISS) and base deficit were associated with hypothermia. In multivariable regression, hypothermia was the strongest predictor of mortality (OR 1.54, 95% CI 1.40–1.71), eclipsing even ISS, base deficit and Glasgow Coma Scale (GCS) score components as a poor prognostic marker. Critically, Martin et al. missed the opportunity to compare these outcomes with those of 1,187 patients with hypothermia due to environmental exposure. Perhaps the best evidence for an independent effect of trauma comes from the Prospective Observational Multicenter Major Trauma Transfusion (PROMMTT) study [9], which examined coagulation in 1,198 patients and adjusted for ISS, prehospital crystalloid administration, GCS, heart rate, systolic blood pressure, pH and base deficit, finding temperature remained a significant independent predictor of coagulopathy (e. g., as quantified by international normalized ratio [INR] >1.3: OR 0.842, $p = 0.03$). However, an INR of 1.3 is of questionable clinical significance. Furthermore, the mean temperature in the coagulopathic group was 35.8 ± 1.2 °C and in the non-coagulopathic group 36.1 ± 0.9 °C – a statistically significant but clinically meaningless distinction.

The simplistic interpretation of the above evidence is that "cold is bad, warm is good, and systems that prioritize maintaining or restoring normothermia have improved trauma outcomes. Therefore, aggressive warming should be standard of care in trauma". Regrettably, this interpretation is not necessarily correct.

Hypothermia and Trauma: Confounded by Severity of Injury?

Not all observational studies find an independent association between hypothermia and adverse outcome in trauma. For example, Steinemann et al. [10] found that stratification by physiologic and anatomic indices of injury severity removed the apparent association of hypothermia and mortality in 173 trauma patients. In a retrospective cohort of 604 trauma patients who received a massive transfusion, Reynolds et al. [11] found that in four temperature strata (> 36 °C, 35.1–36 °C, 34–35 °C and < 34 °C), only profound hypothermia (temperature of < 34 °C) was independently associated with mortality (OR 1.87, 95% CI 1.18–3.0). Further, noting significant improvements in baseline mortality between the study periods 2003–2006 and 2007–2010, Reynolds et al. only found an independent association of hypothermia with mortality in the earlier time period.

The major problem in any observational study of trauma patients is separating the effect of any putative predictor of mortality from that of severity of injury. Severity of injury (and therefore mortality prediction) is more difficult in severe trauma than in other forms of critical illness. A systematic review of anatomic (e. g., ISS and New Injury Severity Score [NISS]), physiologic (e. g., Revised Trauma Score [RTS]), and combined scores (e. g., Trauma Revised Injury Severity Score [TRISS]) [12] found 64 studies reporting receiver-operator characteristic curve (ROC) areas between around 0.7 to 0.9, but concluded that drawing generalized conclusions was impossible due to study heterogeneity and the dependence of results on the mortality rate of the sample. In comparison, mortality prediction in general critical illness using substantially more complex models (incorporating more detailed physiological parameters along with information on diagnosis and co-morbidity) reliably has ROC areas of greater than 0.9 [13]. Unfortunately, these general critical illness models perform less well in trauma, especially with increasingly infrequent deaths beyond 24 h [14]. Therefore, the 'independent' (of severity of illness) associations between temperature and mortality reported in the above studies are highly likely to be the subject of residual confounding.

There are several potential approaches to resolving the problem of residual confounding. One would be to develop a better risk-adjustment method, but an adequate model has eluded trauma researchers since the Abbreviated Injury Scale was published in 1969. Another might be to compare patients who are hypothermic because of environmental conditions (an 'induced' hypothermia) with those who become 'spontaneously' hypothermic due to their injury alone. Demarcating such groups would be difficult and, except perhaps in very cold climates, the numbers of environmental-hypothermia patients would be too low to facilitate effective comparisons – as was presumably true in the Martin study [2] quoted above. Most definitively, trauma patients could be randomized to a clinical trial of induced or permissive hypothermia vs. normothermia. Equipoise for such a trial would be difficult in the current prevailing context that prioritizes patient warming. Re-examination of the evidence underlying current teaching, such as the arguments advanced in this chapter, may be the first step towards such a trial.

Postulated Adverse Effects of Hypothermia in Trauma

There are several plausible hypothetical adverse effects of hypothermia in trauma, including coagulopathy, impaired immunity leading to infection, vasoconstriction leading to impaired wound healing, increased energy expenditure due to shivering, and altered drug metabolism leading to unpredictable drug effects. However, within the temperature range commonly encountered in clinical practice, temperature has substantially less effect on these systems than is commonly believed.

The first part of an improved understanding of the effect of hypothermia on coagulation in trauma is to understand the range of core patient temperatures commonly encountered. Luna et al. [15] reported on 94 patients treated in an urban trauma center in 1985–86, before many of the modern interventions directed at temperature management were commonplace. The mean initial temperature on hospital arrival was 35 °C; 22% were "severely" hypothermic, defined as <34 °C. In contrast, more modern studies report far fewer severely hypothermic patients. Of 2,848 military (80% penetrating) trauma patients with an overall mortality of 5%, 82% were normothermic (>36 °C), 16% were mildly hypothermic (34–36 °C), 2% were moderately hypothermic (<34 °C), and only 0.2% were profoundly hypothermic (<32 °C) [16]. In the study by Martin et al. of 700,304-patient National Trauma Data Bank patients [2], only 1.5% of trauma patients had a temperature <35 °C at the time of hospital arrival, and only 0.11% were profoundly hypothermic (<32 °C). While many of the adverse effects of hypothermia may indeed be present at very low temperatures, such profound hypothermia appears quite rare.

Contrary to popular belief, patient core temperatures commonly encountered in severe trauma cause little, if any, coagulopathy. In a series of *in vitro* experiments, Wolberg et al. [17] found that coagulation enzyme activity was essentially unchanged at 33 °C compared to 37 °C. Activated partial thromboplastin time (aPTT) was not significantly prolonged from baseline until 29 °C was reached. Platelet function was impaired by *in vitro* hypothermia to a greater degree: For example, adhesion to a surface under simulated blood flow conditions at 33 °C was reduced by 33% compared to at 37 °C. Whether this is a clinically significant reduction is unclear. Indeed, whether it even occurs *in vivo* is uncertain: Scharbert et al. [18] found that hypothermia (down to 30 °C) increased platelet aggregation in response to adenosine diphosphate. A 112-patient study of patients with ISS >9 found mildly impaired coagulation with core temperatures <34 °C, but hypercoagulability (measured by thromboelastography) at higher (but still hypothermic) temperatures [19]. Review of the available literature found no consistent independent effect of temperature in animal models or clinical practice [20]. Admittedly these are small *in vitro* and *ex vivo* studies, compared to a very large number of observational clinical studies in surgery and trauma reporting greater blood loss with hypothermia [21]. However, these observational studies must be examined in the light of the possibility of residual confounding by severity of illness or injury outlined above.

Prolonged hypothermia alters inflammatory and immune responses [22] and causes vasoconstriction and possibly ischemia, potentially predisposing to infection and impaired wound healing. Elective surgical patients randomized to aggressive intraoperative temperature maintenance, compared to those with mild hypothermia (mean intraoperative core temperature 34.7 °C), had fewer wound infections (6% vs. 19%, $p = 0.002$) [23]. However, others have failed to demonstrate this benefit. A retrospective analysis of 1,472 patients undergoing bowel surgery found a lower intraoperative temperature nadir was protective against surgical site infection [24]. Pneumonia may be more common in patients treated with therapeutic hypothermia following head injury, although the effect, if real, is small [25]. Extensive study in patients treated with therapeutic hypothermia (targeting 33 °C) after cardiac arrest shows no overall risk of increased infection [26]. Therefore, there is equivocal evidence that hypothermia is anything but a marker of injury severity, and it is this rather than temperature *per se,* that drives the association with infectious complications.

Shivering is the body's main defense against hypothermia. Increased energy expenditure and oxygen utilization through shivering is another theoretical cost of permissive or therapeutic hypothermia. In healthy patients exposed to environmental cold, shivering is maximal at 35 °C and ceases when the core temperature falls to 30–33 °C. However, trauma patients are not 'healthy'; indeed part of why they become hypothermic is that they tend not to shiver. Stoner [27] found that injured rats did not shiver at temperatures down to 31 °C, whereas healthy rats began shivering between 34.8–36.4 °C. Only one of 82 severely injured hypothermic patients in one case series was noted to shiver [27]. Some have even suggested that hypothermia, occasioned by a resetting of the hypothalamic-driven set-point for thermogenesis, may have evolved as a protective mechanism in trauma [22].

Hypothermia certainly alters drug metabolism, especially for drugs metabolized by the hepatic cytochrome p450 enzyme system [20]. This could indeed result in adverse outcomes for patients treated by unwary physicians. However, most medications administered during critical illness are titrated to effect (sedatives, inotropes, analgesics), commonly have plasma levels measured (certain antibiotics e. g., vancomycin and aminoglycosides), or have a wide therapeutic window (e. g., beta-lactam antibiotics). The widespread and safe introduction of therapeutic hypothermic for patients after cardiac arrest suggests that altered drug metabolism due to hypothermia in trauma is a spurious concern.

Rewarming in Trauma: Closing the Door After the Horse has Bolted?

Even if hypothermia in trauma is causally related to adverse outcome, it does not necessarily follow that rewarming a patient who has been allowed to cool will be therapeutic. At a simplistic level, rewarming devices (such as those listed below) may have detrimental effects – such as vasodilation (with redistribution of a reduced blood volume to the muscles and skin, with consequent hypotension) and thermal injury to ischemic skin. Moreover, hypothermia may induce pathophysiological changes that restoration of normal temperature may not reverse. An obvious example is the hypothesized mechanism of acute traumatic coagulopathy [28]. *If* hypothermia contributes to coagulopathy by causing peripheral vasoconstriction, hypoperfusion, thrombomodulin expression and activation of protein C (with consequent de-activation of factors Va and VIIIa and release of inhibition of fibrinolysis), it does not necessarily follow that restoring temperature/perfusion will return activated protein C and factor levels to their optimal levels. On this point, advocates and septics of active warming in trauma must surely agree (albeit for different reasons) – preservation of temperature is better than any effort to restore normothermia once a patient has become cold.

Methods of Rewarming in Trauma: Ineffective Interventions Chasing an Inappropriate Target?

Advocates of temperature preservation and rewarming in trauma are have a difficult battle – as has also been demonstrated in elective surgery, where virtually all studies show a reduction in core temperature during prolonged surgical operations [29, 30]. Despite prioritization of temperature management in major guidelines [3, 31, 32], mild to moderate hypothermia remains a frequent accompaniment of severe trauma. Active warming is certainly superior to passive methods, both prehospital (using chemical warmers [33]) and in hospital (using either cotton blankets or reflective 'space' blankets [34]). Table 1 demonstrates the theoretical rates of heat transfer achieved by various clinical active warming devices [35]. Of these, only the forced air warming blanket is in common use in trauma patients. The quoted heat transfer figure assumes optimal patient coverage by the warming blanket, but in multi-trauma patients this is rarely possible. Much more common is a patient exposed from chest to pelvis, with a blanket applied to head and arms and perhaps another over the legs – that is, the least effective positions for heat transfer to the core. Under-patient heating had similar efficacy (or lack thereof) in comparison to forced air warming in a trial of elective hip surgery patients [29]. Presumably the two techniques are additive, although this has not been well-studied. In elective surgery, prewarming patients with active or passive blankets reduces the central-to-peripheral temperature gradient and, therefore, reduces the fall in core temperature due to vasodilation upon induction of anesthesia. This is no doubt relevant in some trauma patients, but many arrive in the operating room already intubated, requiring little sedation, and with marked peripheral vasoconstriction. Warmed intravenous fluid is an effective method of heat preservation (compared to using cold or room-temperature fluids), but is relevant only if a patient requires large volumes of fluid resuscitation. Lavage of the abdomen or thorax with warmed fluid achieves heat transfer twice as effectively as optimal forced air warming (Table 1) – suggesting the 'blame' apportioned to anesthesiologists when trauma patients arrive cold in the intensive care unit (ICU) might better be directed at the surgical team.

The most noticeable change occasioned by contemporary 'warm the patient' dogma has been the increase in the ambient temperature of resuscitation bays and operating rooms. UK guidelines from 2008 suggest the ambient operating room temperature should be 21 °C unless forced air warming is used. In contrast, 2013 US

Table 1 Heat transfer efficiency of various clinical techniques [35]

Rewarming technique	Heat transfer (kcal/h)
Airway warming	8–12
Overhead radiant warmer	17
Forced air warming blanket	20
Body cavity lavage	36
Continuous arteriovenous circuit	92–139
Cardiopulmonary bypass	710

military guidelines recommend the operating room be kept "as warm as possible; ideally 108 °F (42 °C)" [3]. This intuitively attractive approach also has something of an emotional appeal – the operative team may feel they are suffering sometimes marked discomfort for the benefit of the patient. Postulated patient benefits are placed above the known detrimental effects of high ambient temperature on human performance [36]: For example, vigilance is degraded by high temperatures [37], as are cognitive [38] and visual-motor performance [39]. Furthermore, increased ambient temperature increases the chance of infection: Sweat from surgeons either directly [40] or through operating gowns [41] is more likely to contaminate microorganisms into the operative field at higher operating room temperatures. However, evidence for the postulated benefit of high operating room temperature is tenuous. Two studies from the 1970s [42, 43] found that ambient operating room temperature significantly influenced patient core temperature, concluding the optimal range to be 21–24 °C. These studies are recalled more often than an earlier study that found no such association [44]. The strategy of using a high ambient operating room temperature to maintain or restore patient core temperature was most recently tested in a prospective observational study of 118 emergency surgery patients [45]. Unlike earlier studies, all patients received the warming interventions that are now standard practice, including warmed intravenous fluids and forced air warming blankets on the upper and lower body. A substantial minority (29.7%) of patients developed intraoperative hypothermia (<35 °C). Ambient operating room temperature varied between 17.9 and 29 °C. The mean operating room temperature was 22.5 °C in the 39% of patients whose core temperature fell, and in the 61% whose temperature was maintained. Ambient operating room temperature (within these ranges) had no effect on patient core temperature. In the context of the known detrimental effects of high ambient temperatures on the performance of surgical teams, this study is compelling evidence supporting equipoise for a trial of operating room temperature in trauma and acute surgery.

Clinical Trial Evidence for Active Rewarming

There has only been one randomized controlled trial of an effective method of raising core temperature in trauma patients [4]. This trial randomized 57 hypothermic (temperature ≤ 34.5 °C) trauma patients to either standard care (involving warmed intravenous fluids, airway rewarming, a forced-air warming blanket and an insulating hat) or to continuous arterio-venous rewarming (CAVR) using a modified 'Level 1' (Smiths Medical, USA) rapid infusion device that incorporates a heat exchanger. CAVR patients rewarmed significantly faster than the control group. Unadjusted survival analysis to 110 hours post-admission showed a strong trend to benefit ($p = 0.059$) that reached statistical significance when adjusted for injury type (HR 0.41; $p = 0.047$). However, survival to hospital discharge (55% control vs. 66% CAVR) was not significantly different ($p = 0.24$). Interestingly (in the context of the lack of evidence for temperature-mediated correction of coagulopathy), partial thromboplastin time and prothrombin time were similar in each group. This trial represents the total evidence supporting any strategy of active rewarming of hypothermic trauma patients; it required an extracorporeal warming circulation to show barely detectable patient benefit. In summary, the evidence for active temperature management aimed at restoring normothermia in trauma is very tenuous.

Case Reports of Survival with Extreme Induced Hypothermia

In contrast to prevailing orthodoxy, there are several case reports and anecdotes of trauma patients surviving what were anticipated to be fatal injuries as a result of profound accidental hypothermia. Amongst these are the British casualties during the Falklands War who were not recovered until the morning after battles having spent the night in exposed freezing conditions. Anecdotally, their core temperatures had fallen to the point of slowing metabolism and oxygen consumption and presumably neuroprotection [46]. Regrettably, but understandably given the difficulty of recording data whilst in combat, the details of these cases have not been published. Vijayasekaran et al. [47] described the case of a 24-year old multi-trauma victim ejected from his vehicle in the Southern Arizona desert. The patient had an estimated 7 hours exposure at 3 °C before being found with a tympanic temperature of 28.1 °C, GCS 5, and blood pressure of 46/36 mmHg. The lowest intraoperative temperature was 26.9 °C. Warming was achieved by conventional means and by abdominal lavage. A shattered right kidney was removed, and the patient returned to normothermia after nine hours. He subsequently made a complete recovery. There are even historical examples: As noted by Harbinson [48], "(Sir William) Harvey was present at the Battle of Edgehill (1642). According to Aubrey: 'He told me that Sir Adrian Scrope was dangerously wounded there, and left for dead amongst the dead men, stript; which happened to be the saving of his life. It was cold clear weather, and a frost that night; which staunched his bleeding, and at about midnight, or some hours after his hurte, he awaked, and was faine to draw a dead body upon him for warmth-sake.'"

Experimental Evidence for Therapeutic Hypothermia in Animal Models of Trauma

In contrast to the lack of comparative trial evidence in human trauma, there is ample and largely congruent experimental evidence in animal models that induced mild (34 °C) to moderate (30–32 °C) hypothermia is beneficial [5]. A striking example is that of a pig model of hemorrhagic shock induced by controlled bleeding and splenic injury [49]. Induction of hypothermia (34 °C), compared to normothermia, resulted in better survival at 24 h (75% vs. 25%, $p < 0.01$). Hypothermia was not associated with measurable coagulopathy or greater blood loss. Other models have found induced hypothermia to be associated with better cardiac function and less damage to liver and skeletal muscle [5]. The hypothesized mechanism of hypothermia benefit relates to the reduced metabolic demands of cells, which reduces the requirement for adenosine triphosphate (ATP) production and, therefore, reduces oxygen consumption and metabolic waste production. This protective effect seems to occur most markedly in tissues with relatively normal oxygen tension and normal ATP levels at the time of hypothermia induction. Therapeutic hypothermia is routine practice in other areas of clinical practice: For example, in deep hypothermic cardiac arrest for complex aortic surgery, in milder hypothermia during cardiopulmonary bypass, and (at least until recently, and still in many centers) in the post-resuscitation care of comatose survivors of cardiac arrest. Neither excessive bleeding nor any of the other putative adverse effects of hypothermia in trauma appear common in these patients.

Clinical Trial Evidence for Therapeutic Hypothermia in Trauma

There are no clinical trials of induced hypothermia in trauma. However, one case series of six patients subjected to therapeutic hypothermia after traumatic cardiac arrest found much better than expected outcomes: Only one patient died; two were left dependent on skilled nursing care due to neurological disability, but three made good neurological recoveries [50]. An extension of therapeutic hypothermia in extreme trauma cases is the Emergency Preservation and Resuscitation for Cardiac Arrest from Trauma (EPR-CAT) trial (ClinicalTrials.gov Identifier: NCT01042015), currently underway. EPR-CAT enrolls penetrating trauma patients within five minutes of cardiac arrest, who do not respond to emergency room thoracotomy, to receive percutaneous extracorporeal membrane oxygenation with rapid cooling to 15 °C. Following correction of major organ and vessel anatomical disruption, the patient is rewarmed and resuscitated with extracorporeal cardiorespiratory support.

Conclusion

This review has demonstrated that the evidence supporting active warming and rewarming of trauma patients is not as strong as many clinicians believe. Active warming devices in common use are relatively ineffective at raising core temperature, but even aggressive rewarming using an extracorporeal circuit has marginal (if any) benefit. Conversely, there is weak evidence that spontaneous hypothermia is associated with worse trauma outcomes. The mechanism for this association is unclear, but it is plausible that maintaining core temperature (rather than attempting to correct hypothermia) is of therapeutic benefit. While therapeutic hypothermia may help at least some trauma patients, there is currently insufficient trial evidence to recommend this practice in all but (possibly) survivors of traumatic cardiac arrest. For now, the best pragmatic clinical advice is to attempt to preserve core temperature using the most effective practical means. There is evidence that increasing ambient temperature in operating rooms is ineffective when other measures are instituted. However, a key message of this review is that any particular temperature strategy in trauma is supported by tenuous and often contradictory evidence. Clinicians should view clinical trials of temperature management in trauma with equipoise.

References

1. Shafi S, Elliott AC, Gentilello L (2005) Is hypothermia simply a marker of shock and injury severity or an independent risk factor for mortality in trauma patients? Analysis of a large national trauma registry. J Trauma 59:1081–1085
2. Martin RS, Kilgo PD, Miller PR, Hoth JJ, Meredith JW, Chang MC (2005) Injury-associated hypothermia: an analysis of the 2004 National Trauma Data Bank. Shock 24:114–118
3. United States Army Institute of Surgical Research Damage control surgery at level IIb/III treatment facilities. http://www.usaisr.amedd.army.mil/assets/cpgs/Damage%20Control%20Resuscitation%20-%201%20Feb%202013.pdf. Accessed 17/11/14
4. Gentilello LM, Jurkovich GJ, Stark MS, Hassantash SA, O'Keefe GE (1997) Is hypothermia in the victim of major trauma protective or harmful? A randomized, prospective study. AnnSurg 226:439–447
5. Tisherman SA (2004) Hypothermia and injury. Curr Opin Crit Care 10:512–519
6. Cameron P, Gabbe B, McNeil J Victorian State Trauma Outcomes Registry (VSTORM). http://www.med.monash.edu.au/epidemiology/traumaepi/traumareg.html. Accessed 17/11/14
7. Bailey JA, Morrison JJ, Rasmussen TE (2013) Military trauma system in Afghanistan: lessons for civil systems? Curr Opin Crit Care 19:569–577
8. Mohammad A, Branicki F, Abu-Zidan FM (2014) Educational and clinical impact of Advanced Trauma Life Support (ATLS) courses: a systematic review. World J Surg 38:322–329
9. Cohen MJ, Kutcher M, Redick B et al (2013) Clinical and mechanistic drivers of acute traumatic coagulopathy. J Trauma Acute Care Surg 75:S40–S47
10. Steinemann S, Shackford SR, Davis JW (1990) Implications of admission hypothermia in trauma patients. JTrauma 30:200–202
11. Reynolds BR, Forsythe RM, Harbrecht BG et al (2012) Hypothermia in massive transfusion: have we been paying enough attention to it? J Trauma Acute Care Surg 73:486–491
12. Tohira H, Jacobs I, Mountain D, Gibson N, Yeo A (2012) Systematic review of predictive performance of injury severity scoring tools. Scand J Trauma Resusc Emerg Med 20:63
13. Paul E, Bailey M, Pilcher D (2013) Risk prediction of hospital mortality for adult patients admitted to Australian and New Zealand intensive care units: development and validation of the Australian and New Zealand Risk of Death model. J Crit Care 28:935–941
14. Gunst M, Ghaemmaghami V, Gruszecki A, Urban J, Frankel H, Shafi S (2010) Changing epidemiology of trauma deaths leads to a bimodal distribution. Proc (Bayl Univ Med Cent) 23:349–354
15. Luna GK, Maier RV, Pavlin EG, Anardi D, Copass MK, Oreskovich MR (1987) Incidence and effect of hypothermia in seriously injured patients. J Trauma 27:1014–1018
16. Arthurs Z, Cuadrado D, Beekley A et al (2006) The impact of hypothermia on trauma care at the 31st combat support hospital. Am J Surg 191:610–614
17. Wolberg AS, Meng ZH, Monroe DM 3rd, Hoffman M (2004) A systematic evaluation of the effect of temperature on coagulation enzyme activity and platelet function. J Trauma 56:1221–1228
18. Scharbert G, Kalb ML, Essmeister R, Kozek-Langenecker SA (2010) Mild and moderate hypothermia increases platelet aggregation induced by various agonists: a whole blood in vitro study. Platelets 21:44–48
19. Watts DD, Trask A, Soeken K, Perdue P, Dols S, Kaufmann C (1998) Hypothermic coagulopathy in trauma: effect of varying levels of hypothermia on enzyme speed, platelet function, and fibrinolytic activity. J Trauma 44:846–854
20. Alam HB (2012) Translational barriers and opportunities for emergency preservation and resuscitation in severe injuries. Br J Surg 99(Suppl 1):29–39
21. Rajagopalan S, Mascha E, Na J, Sessler DI (2008) The effects of mild perioperative hypothermia on blood loss and transfusion requirement. Anesthesiology 108:71–77
22. Hildebrand F, Giannoudis PV, van Griensven M, Chawda M, Pape HC (2004) Pathophysiologic changes and effects of hypothermia on outcome in elective surgery and trauma patients. Am J Surg 187:363–371

23. Kurz A, Sessler DI, Lenhardt R (1996) Perioperative normothermia to reduce the incidence of surgical-wound infection and shorten hospitalization. Study of Wound Infection and Temperature Group. N Engl J Med 334:1209–1215
24. Walz JM, Paterson CA, Seligowski JM, Heard SO (2006) Surgical site infection following bowel surgery: a retrospective analysis of 1446 patients. Arch Surg 141:1014–1018
25. Sydenham E, Roberts I, Alderson P (2009) Hypothermia for traumatic head injury. Cochrane Database Syst Rev CD001048
26. Kuchena A, Merkel MJ, Hutchens MP (2014) Postcardiac arrest temperature management: infectious risks. Curr Opin Crit Care 20:507–515
27. Stoner HB (1972) Effect of injury on the responses to thermal stimulation of the hypothalamus. J Appl Physiol 33:665–671
28. Brohi K, Cohen MJ, Ganter MT, Matthay MA, Mackersie RC, Pittet JF (2007) Acute traumatic coagulopathy: initiated by hypoperfusion: modulated through the protein C pathway? Ann Surg 245:812–818
29. Fanelli A, Danelli G, Ghisi D, Ortu A, Moschini E, Fanelli G (2009) The efficacy of a resistive heating under-patient blanket versus a forced-air warming system: a randomized controlled trial. Anesth Analg 108:199–201
30. De Witte JL, Demeyer C, Vandemaele E (2010) Resistive-heating or forced-air warming for the prevention of redistribution hypothermia. Anesth Analg 110:829–833
31. Spahn DR, Bouillon B, Cerny V et al (2013) Management of bleeding and coagulopathy following major trauma: an updated European guideline. Crit Care 17:R76
32. National Institute for Health and Care Excellence (2008) Inadvertent perioperative hypothermia: The management of inadvertent perioperative hypothermia in adults. https://www.nice.org.uk/guidance/cg65. Accessed 17/11/14
33. Allen PB, Salyer SW, Dubick MA, Holcomb JB, Blackbourne LH (2010) Preventing hypothermia: comparison of current devices used by the US Army in an in vitro warmed fluid model. J Trauma 69(Suppl 1):S154–S161
34. Ng KF, Cheung CW, Lee Y, Leung SW (2011) Low-dose desmopressin improves hypothermia-induced impairment of primary haemostasis in healthy volunteers. Anaesthesia 66:999–1005
35. Gentilello LM (1994) Practical approaches to hypothermia. In: Maull K, Cleveland HC, Feliciano DV et al (eds) Advances in Trauma and Critical Care. Mosby Inc., St Louis, pp 39–79
36. Pilcher JJ, Nadler E, Busch C (2002) Effects of hot and cold temperature exposure on performance: a meta-analytic review. Ergonomics 45:682–698
37. Hancock PA (1984) Effect of environmental temperature on display monitoring performance: an overview with practical implications. Am Ind Hyg Assoc J 45:122–126
38. Hancock PA, Vasmatzidis I (2003) Effects of heat stress on cognitive performance: the current state of knowledge. Int J Hyperthermia 19:355–372
39. Teichner WH, Wherkamp RF (1954) Visual-motor performance as a function of short-duration ambient temperature. J Exp Psychol 47:447–450
40. Mills SJ, Holland DJ, Hardy AE (2000) Operative field contamination by the sweating surgeon. Aust N Z J Surg 70:837–839
41. Hamilton HW, Booth AD, Lone FJ, Clark N (1979) Penetration of gown material by organisms from the surgical team. Clin Orthop Relat Res Jun:237–246
42. Morris RH, Wilkey BR (1970) The effects of ambient temperature on patient temperature during surgery not involving body cavities. Anesthesiology 32:102–107
43. Morris RH (1971) Operating room temperature and the anesthetized, paralyzed patient. Arch Surg 102:95–97
44. Goldberg MJ, Roe CF (1966) Temperature changes during anesthesia and operations. Arch Surg 93:365–369
45. Inaba K, Berg R, Barmparas G et al (2012) Prospective evaluation of ambient operating room temperature on the core temperature of injured patients undergoing emergent surgery. J Trauma Acute Care Surg 73:1478–1483

46. Smith J (2007) Commentary on military cold injury. J R Army Med Corps 153:89–96
47. Vijayasekaran A, Wynne J, O'Keefe T, Friese R, Joseph B, Rhee P (2012) Hypothermia (26.9 C) in a polytrauma patient: case report of survival and review of science. Emergency Medicine S2:001
48. Harbinson MJ (1999) William harvey, hypothermia, and battle injuries. BMJ 319:1561
49. Wu X, Kochanek PM, Cochran K et al (2005) Mild hypothermia improves survival after prolonged, traumatic hemorrhagic shock in pigs. J Trauma 59:291–299
50. Tuma MA, Stansbury LG, Stein DM, McQuillan KA, Scalea TM (2011) Induced hypothermia after cardiac arrest in trauma patients: a case series. J Trauma 71:1524–1527

Detection of Consciousness in the Severely Injured Brain

J. Stender, A. Gjedde, and S. Laureys

Introduction

Improvements in neurosurgical and neurological intensive care have led to increased numbers of survivors from severe traumatic brain injury (TBI). Following coma, some patients undergo transition into prolonged disorders of consciousness, including minimally conscious state (MCS) and the unresponsive wakefulness syndrome (UWS) [1]. The clinical hallmarks of consciousness are arousal and awareness. In chronic disorders of consciousness, patients commonly reestablish subcortical functions of arousal, but with decline or absence of cortical functions, leading to loss of awareness. Whereas UWS patients show no responsiveness at the bedside, MCS patients elicit fluctuating but reproducible signs of awareness of their surroundings. By convention, emergence from MCS occurs when the patient regains a capacity for functional communication or object use. Long-term recovery of consciousness from UWS remains uncertain, but progression into MCS is an important indicator of better prognosis.

As the states of MCS and UWS occupy a border zone between awareness and unconsciousness, the distinction has important ethical and therapeutic implications. For example, MCS patients may feel pain or suffering [2], and retain capacity for emotional reactions to salient stimuli, such as hearing voices or seeing faces of

J. Stender ✉
Cyclotron Research Center and Neurology Department, University and University Hospital of Liège, Liège, Belgium
Department of Neuroscience and Pharmacology, University of Copenhagen, Copenhagen, Denmark
e-mail: johanstender@gmail.com

A. Gjedde
Department of Neuroscience and Pharmacology, University of Copenhagen, Copenhagen, Denmark

S. Laureys
Cyclotron Research Center and Neurology Department, University and University Hospital of Liège, Liège, Belgium

J.-L. Vincent (ed.), *Annual Update in Intensive Care and Emergency Medicine 2015*,
DOI 10.1007/978-3-319-13761-2_36

family members [3]. Truly unconscious individuals likely do neither. Patients with disorders of consciousness frequently suffer from painful effects of immobilization, such as spasticity or decubitus, and risk social neglect by relatives and therapists [4]. The minimally conscious patients may thus benefit from interventions aimed at improving their quality of life, such as analgesic or anxiolytic treatment, physiotherapy and social care.

The prognosis of patients in MCS is dramatically better than that of patients in enduring UWS, with long-term recovery occurring in approximately 33% of MCS patients [5] and 0–12% of UWS patients [6]. Neurostimulant treatment to improve responsiveness also appears more effective in MCS than UWS patients. A recent double-blind sham-controlled study with transcranial direct current stimulation produced lasting increases in responsiveness in 43% of the patients in MCS, and 8% of the patients in UWS [7]. Deep brain stimulation with electrode placement in the thalamic intralaminar nuclei was also shown to induce systematic behavioral improvements in one MCS patient [8]. No such effect has yet been shown in unresponsive patients. Importantly, legal precedence in several countries has established the right of physicians to interrupt artificial life support from patients in persistent UWS, while withdrawal of treatment from patients in MCS remains controversial [9]. Precise diagnosis of the patient's level of consciousness is, therefore, important.

While behavioral improvements are often seen within the first few months after injury, a state of UWS is usually regarded as chronic at 3 months post-injury for non-traumatic causes such as anoxia or stroke, and at 1 year for traumatic injuries [6]. This makes differential diagnosis valuable, even in the relatively early phases of the patient's condition, for prognostication and planning of long-term therapeutic needs.

The differential diagnosis commonly rests on the results of clinical examination. Incongruence of clinical presentation and residual cerebral functionality is common nonetheless, rendering behavioral assessment imprecise. The frequency of misdiagnosis of UWS or MCS by clinical methods is high. Use of non-standard clinical consensus methods fails to detect MCS in many patients, with rates of misdiagnosis ranging from 33 to 43% [10, 11]. The error rate can be improved to some extent by means of standardized scoring systems, such as the Coma Recovery Scale-Revised (CRS-R) [12].

The CRS-R is considered to be the most sensitive tool for discriminating very low degrees of awareness [13, 14]. The CRS-R has six subscales: Auditory, visual, motor and oromotor/verbal functions, communication, and level of arousal. The 23 items are ordered by degree of complexity, ranging from reflexive to cognitively mediated behaviors. A status of MCS is associated with specific observations of outward responsiveness, such as reproducible motor or oral response to command, or visual tracking. As fluctuations of consciousness are common in MCS, the CRS-R assessment should ideally be conducted serially over several days, with the best outcome determining the diagnosis. Still, the physiological significance of several signs is contentious – visual fixation for example, may be reflexive [15], and consistent visual pursuit may depend on the specific object used, and its path across the visual field [16]. In addition, the existence of paralyzed, but fully conscious patients, such as those with the 'locked-in' syndrome, demonstrates that unresponsive patients may also be aware. Therefore, neuroimaging tools are being developed to complement the bedside diagnosis of consciousness.

Detection of Consciousness with Neuroimaging

Activation-based Neuroimaging Protocols

Severely brain injured patients may retain capacity for covert cognition, without overt responsiveness. Investigations by Owen and colleagues demonstrated that clinically diagnosed patients with UWS may retain capacity for higher order cognition. In a seminal study from 2006, a patient had similar cortical activation as healthy subjects during functional magnetic resonance imaging (fMRI) when asked to imagine playing tennis or walking through their own home [17]. Similar activations were later established in 5 out of 56 patients suffering from MCS or UWS. As an extension of these studies, simple communication could subsequently be established with one patient, using these mental imagery paradigms during fMRI as cues for 'yes' or 'no' [18]. With this communication method, another patient in UWS for 13 years demonstrated knowledge of her primary caregiver's name and her own hospitalization [19]. More recently, the same team observed complex activations in the executive networks in a patient believed unconscious for 16 years, in response to watching a Hitchcock movie [20]. These studies convincingly demonstrate that behaviorally unresponsive patients may retain awareness, volitional thought, and formation of memories after their injury.

Observations of this kind in patients perceived as unconscious fundamentally alter their ethical, legal, and therapeutic status. Yet, activation-based neuroimaging tests often rely on intact language comprehension, ability to focus attention for longer intervals, and intact sensory apparatus. Therefore, many patients fail to respond to tasks, despite showing clear signs of consciousness at the bedside [10]. This means that the prevalence of patients with complete dissociation of behavioral and mental responsiveness is unknown.

Methods of examination that discriminate between conscious and unconscious patients by means of neurophysiological correlates of consciousness are needed. To circumvent the issues of activation-based examination, the tests must reliably detect neural activity associated with consciousness, independent of the patient's voluntary cooperation and sustained attention.

Assessment of Cerebral Glucose Metabolism with FDG-PET

The cerebral metabolic rate of glucose reflects the depolarizations associated with neuronal firing. Lowered glucose metabolism, therefore, identifies damaged or dysfunctional brain areas [21]. Positron emission tomography with fluorodeoxyglucose (FDG-PET) is the method commonly used to assess whole-brain and regional glucose metabolism. Studies have shown that conscious awareness is supported by activity within specific brain areas, encompassing the frontoparietal and midline cortex and the thalamus [22]. These areas are thought to constitute a "global workspace" of consciousness [23]. States of diminished consciousness, such as coma, UWS, MCS and anesthesia, are consistently associated with a decline in metabolic activity within the global workspace areas [24].

Of particular interest for the differential diagnosis of brain injured patients, MCS patients appear to have partially preserved metabolic activity within the frontoparietal cortex and precuneus, whereas UWS patients have uniformly low metabolism across the frontoparietal and midline cortical areas. Using these characteristics as diagnostic criteria in a cohort of 122 patients, metabolic patterns after global mean normalization of FDG-uptake distinguished MCS from UWS patients with 85% accuracy [10]. Importantly, 32% of the patients with a clinical diagnosis of UWS were found to retain brain metabolism compatible with MCS. Of these patients, 75% recovered responsiveness within a year after the assessment, whereas no UWS patients with uniformly low metabolic rate of the frontoparietal cortex improved their condition. Although these findings cannot be taken as definitive proof of awareness in the UWS patients with preserved metabolism, the high recovery rate suggests that they were already at the time of scanning in, or progressing towards, MCS.

Further studies of quantitative cerebral metabolic differences among the disorders of consciousness demonstrated that patients in MCS retain higher average global metabolic activity compared to patients in UWS (Fig. 1).

A cortical metabolic rate of above 45% of normal appeared to be a necessary precondition for the increase in awareness in brain injured patients (Fig. 2) [25]. A correct diagnostic classification rate of 82% could be achieved based on mean cortical metabolic levels within the frontoparietal cortex. The probability of MCS increased dramatically with metabolic levels rising above 50% of normal, suggesting that a physiological phase transition enabling consciousness takes place at this threshold of metabolism.

Animal studies have shown that neuronal communication in low-metabolic states (<50% normal cerebral energy turnover) is dominated by slow-firing neuronal ensembles, and absence of long-range connectivity. As cerebral metabolism increases, so does the neuronal firing rate and brain-wide connectivity [26]. As unconsciousness is consistently associated with breakdown of cortical connectivity, it is reasonable to assume that preserved energy metabolism in awareness-supporting networks is a necessary precondition for the increase in conscious awareness. Examinations that combine regional and quantitative metabolic measures may serve as tools that potentially are indicative of consciousness in brain injured patients.

Electrical Signatures of Consciousness Measured with EEG

As with the above findings, direct measures of brain electric activity potentially can be used to screen for conscious awareness. Neuronal activity elicits electrical signatures that can be recorded from the scalp with electroencephalography (EEG). The

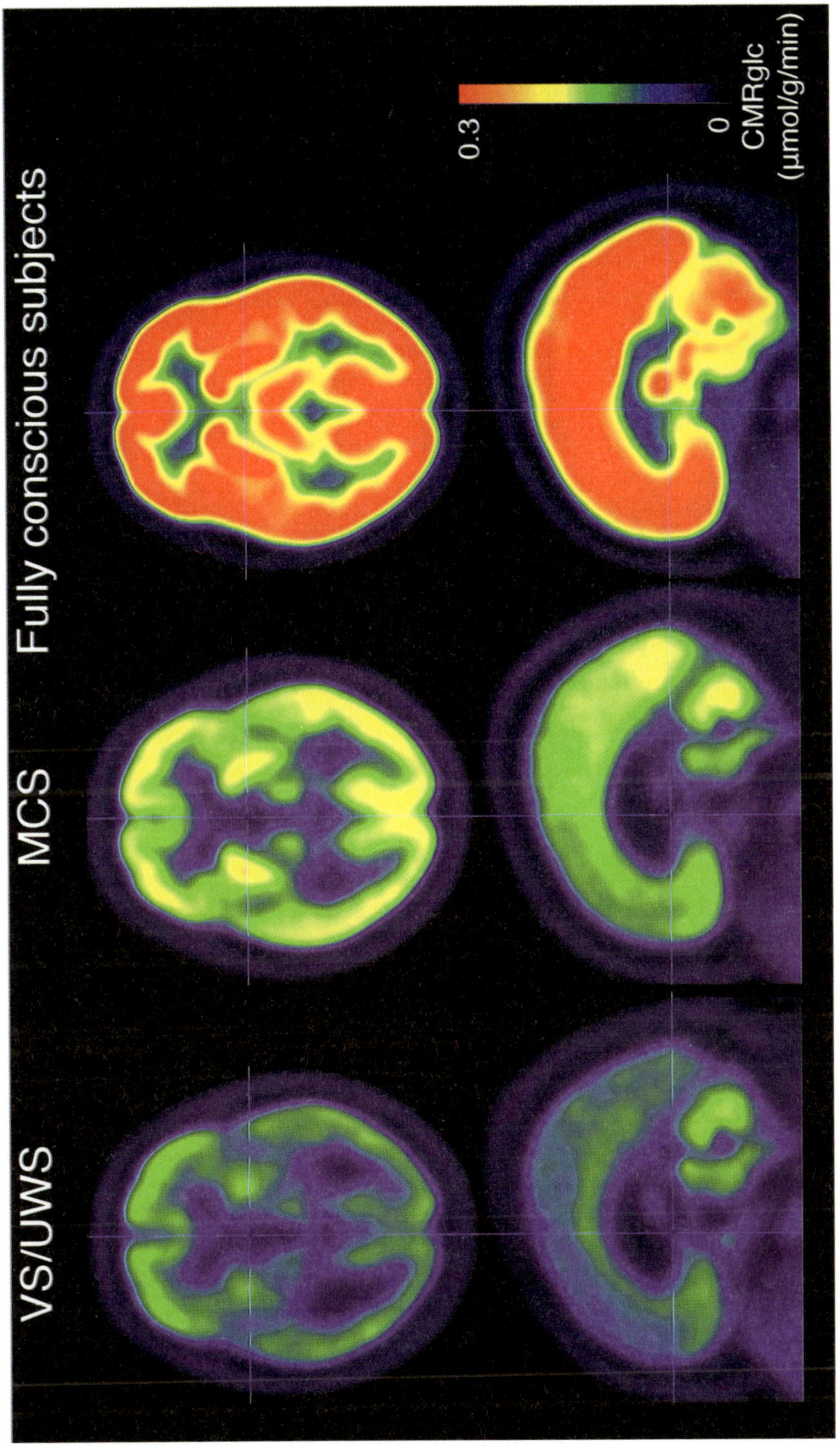

Fig. 1 Brain metabolism in disorders of consciousness. Average cerebral metabolic rate of glucose (μmol/g/min) according to condition (14 patients in vegetative state/unresponsive wakefulness syndrome [UWS], 21 patients in minimally conscious state [MCS] and 29 fully conscious controls) From [25]

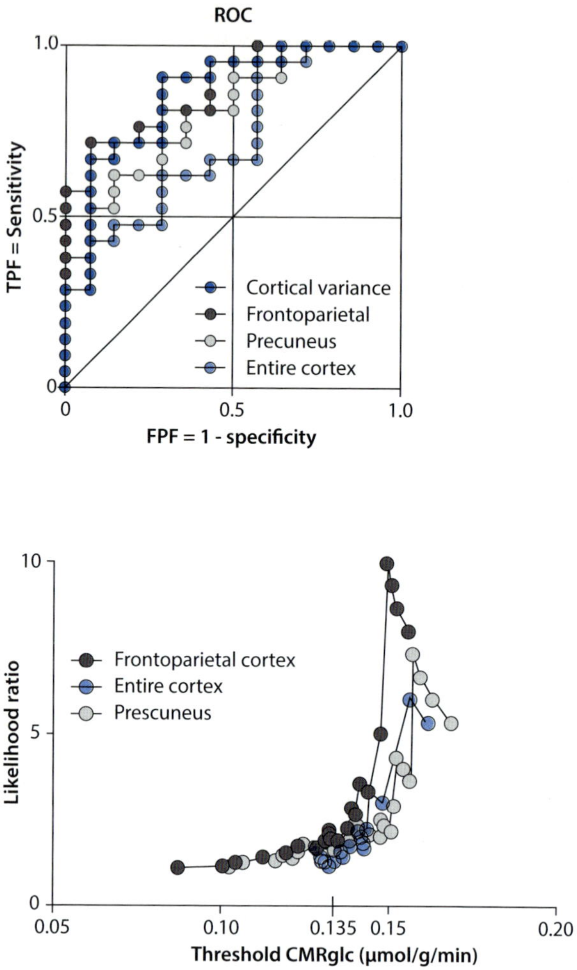

Fig. 2 Diagnostic accuracy of fluorodeoxyglucose positron emission tomography (FDG-PET): The ability to differentiate unresponsive wakefulness syndrome (UWS) from minimally conscious state (MCS), based on regional cerebral metabolic rate of glucose (CMRglc) and cortical variance. *Top*: Receiver operating characteristics (ROC) plots of metabolism within the entire cortex, precuneus, frontoparietal cortex, and the cortical variance. True positive fraction (TPF) = sensitivity to MCS, false positive fraction (FPF) = 1-specificity to MCS. *Bottom*: Likelihood ratio of having MCS rather than vegetative state (VS)/UWS at increasing metabolic thresholds. A gradual increase is seen above 0.135 μmol/g/min for all regions, corresponding to 45% of normal cortical CMRglc. From [25]

amplitude of specific EEG frequency bands has been shown to correlate strongly with CRS-R scores, with UWS patients showing dominance of slow wave delta activity, whereas MCS patients show higher amplitudes in higher frequency alpha and theta [27].

A recent investigation used support-vector-based machine-learning to identify specific characteristics of high-density EEG recordings in 181 MCS and UWS patients. The results from this automated data-mining approach largely corroborated the previous findings. Alpha and theta amplitudes were significantly lowered in UWS compared to MCS patients, whereas activity in the delta frequency band was higher in UWS patients [28]. Although the UWS patients retained relatively consistent activity, the neuronal firing rate of patients in MCS fluctuated significantly, corresponding to their inconsistent behavioral responsiveness. Consistent with this fluctuation, the EEG activity of MCS patients was more complex than that in UWS patients.

Monotonous delta frequency activity is classically observed in coma and deep sleep, supporting the view that this activity pattern is incompatible with conscious awareness. Thus, a stable state of high delta power, but reduced activity in higher-frequency bands, appears to be a robust discriminator of unconscious from conscious patients. Accordingly, in the previous study, an automatic classification algorithm based on the EEG-signal differentiated between MCS and UWS patients with 78% accuracy. Moreover, the misclassified UWS patients showed better prognosis than the patients correctly identified by the classifier to be unconscious [28].

TMS-EEG: A Perturbational Method for Investigation of Neuronal Communication

The dynamic core model of Tononi [29] stipulates that a certain level of complexity in neuronal communication is required to maintain consciousness. According to this theory, the conscious experience is encoded by shifting neuronal ensembles, where the state of the system at any point in time determines the specific conscious content, from a vast repertoire of potential conscious states. By inference, a rich and differentiated conscious experience requires both complex and highly integrated neuronal communication avenues across the brain.

By combining transcranial magnetic stimulation (TMS) with high density EEG recordings to measure the spread of the neural activation after the magnetic impulse, Casali et al. [30] employed a calculated measure of complexity and integration of the neural response, the perturbational complexity index. The perturbational complexity index was shown to accurately stratify levels of consciousness across a range of conditions with altered awareness, such as sleep, anesthesia, UWS, and MCS. Importantly, the perturbational complexity index of six UWS patients was consistently within the range of patients in deep sleep and anesthesia, while 12 patients in MCS or emergence from MCS demonstrated a perturbational complexity index midway between those and the fully conscious subjects [30]. This test represents the first credible attempt to quantify level of consciousness, and appears to reliably identify conscious patients in a brain injured population. Larger scale testing is needed to verify these results.

Assessment of Diagnostic Accuracy: The Problem of the Gold Standard

The studies cited above demonstrate that both activation-based neuroimaging methods and neurophysiological assessment can be used to screen for residual consciousness in brain-injured patients. The transfer of such methods from scientific to clinical use poses several challenges, however: The test must be reliable, provide an accurate diagnosis, and be practically feasible in a clinical setting. Validation of the diagnostic accuracy is particularly challenging [31].

In the absence of well-established quantitative neuronal measures of consciousness, the differential diagnosis in the brain-injured population can be considered in a binary context: The patient is either conscious or not. The reduction of the complex phenomenon of consciousness to a dichotomy is not without problems and poses a risk of logical circularity. Correct assessment of diagnostic accuracy requires a reliable 'gold' standard of reference. The only commonly accepted test of phenomenal awareness is behavioral responsiveness. In order to assess the reliability of neuroimaging tests of consciousness, the results can be weighed against the detection of clinical signs of consciousness in the same population. Outward behavioral response is an inadequate reference, as unresponsiveness is not necessarily associated with unconsciousness. It is possible to determine whether a test result is associated with *presence* of consciousness, but there is no conceptually solid way of determining whether a test reliably measures *absence* of consciousness in a given individual. The fact that any population of patients with disorders of consciousness may include patients who are clinically in UWS, but retain high levels of consciousness, renders this a critical issue.

The most commonly used measures of diagnostic accuracy are sensitivity and specificity; i. e., the ability of the test to detect or rule out the existence of a pathological condition. These measures are often used to describe disease detection rates against a healthy reference population. The measures can be adapted to suit the dichotomy of consciousness diagnosis in severely brain-injured patients. In a recent study, *sensitivity* to MCS was defined as the ability of the test to detect awareness in patients with disorders of consciousness, while *specificity* of MCS was defined as the ability of the test to rule out consciousness [10]. Sensitivity to MCS thus corresponds to the specificity of UWS and vice-versa (Table 1).

The lack of a reliable gold standard for absence of consciousness makes it clear that only sensitivity to MCS can be assessed reliably as the sum of positive test results in all clinically responsive patients. As specificity refers to the number of negative test results in all clinically unresponsive patients, this measure will be biased by the presence of patients with clinical appearance of UWS, but residual brain activity compatible with MCS. Similarly, the false-negative detection rate in MCS patients can be assessed, while the false positive detection rate of consciousness in unresponsive patients cannot be calculated.

Table 1 Measures of specificity and sensitivity

	Reference standard status (behavioral diagnosis)	
Test outcome	Awareness present (MCS)	Awareness absent (UWS)
Evidence of awareness (MCS)	True positive (TP)	False positive (FP)
No evidence of awareness (UWS)	False negative (FN)	True negative (TN)
	Sensitivity to MCS or specificity to UWS = n(TP)/n(TP) + n(FN)	Specificity to MCS or sensitivity to UWS = n(TN)/n(FP) + n(TN)

To address this problem, long-term outcome of the patients can be included as a secondary test reference. As MCS patients tend to have fluctuating responsiveness, it is probable that a conscious, but unresponsive patient at some point after the neuroimaging test will show signs of consciousness. Also, as the chance of further recovery is significantly better in MCS patients, the population recovery rates of patients determined to be in MCS or in UWS on a neuroimaging test can provide an indication of the test accuracy [10, 31].

The validation has significant limitations. It is difficult to differentiate between direct correlates of phenomenal (un)consciousness and other neural conditions following the brain injury, such as diminished cognitive capacity. Similarly, it is impossible to determine whether a purported neurophysiological correlate of consciousness is a direct measure of consciousness at the time of examination, or merely a necessary precondition for the rise in consciousness at a later stage.

It is also important to note that a binary framework for assessment of consciousness is likely to be an over-simplification. The rise in consciousness may be a gradual process, or entail periodic fluctuations between states, before stability in one or the other condition is achieved. With the dichotomy currently applied clinically, any patient who shows recurrent signs of consciousness, however brief, is considered to be suffering from MCS. Clearly, whether a patient dimly or fully perceives the situation, and whether the patient is consistently aware, or only enjoys brief flickers of consciousness interceded by long periods of unconsciousness, has important implications for palliative therapy and the ethics of clinical care options.

To fully resolve these issues, more nuanced assessment parameters should be introduced. To accurately monitor the transition between conscious states, a convincing theoretically-based index of consciousness should be established and validated across a range of conditions, including various degrees of anesthesia, sleep states, and epileptic seizures, as well as loss of consciousness due to acute and chronic brain injuries. If the preliminary results hold, the perturbational complexity index may fulfill this role, and subsequently could serve as reference or gold standard for the development of more wieldy clinical tools.

Practical Challenges in Neuroimaging

The use of neuroimaging to discriminate between MCS and UWS also presents a range of practical issues that may impede the transition into clinical use. Image acquisition and statistical analysis is complex and may not be possible outside of facilities with neuroscientific expertise. Perhaps more importantly, the assessment is practically demanding, and some imaging assessments may not be feasible in an intensive care unit (ICU). For example, the presence of metal implants, such as after certain cranial surgeries, rules out MRI. Epilepsy is a common complication from brain injuries that may bias examination results negatively and prohibit assessment with neural perturbation methods, such as TMS. Also, the detection of consciousness may be impeded by the use of sedative treatment; ideally, a patient should be awake for the duration of the examination. Spontaneous movement during the scanning may make the imaging assessment impossible, and restless patients may require sedation for successful image acquisition. These conflicting demands are challenges to the complex image acquisition protocols.

Clinical Implementation

Neuroimaging is challenging and usually adds no differential diagnostic information in behaviorally responsive patients. In the primary diagnostic process, functional neuroimaging may thus serve to screen for covert consciousness in unresponsive patients. As behavioral methods are insensitive to conscious but unresponsive patients, the clinical diagnosis could be balanced by the addition of a neuroimaging test with high sensitivity to MCS. Repeated testing with the CRS-R augmented with cerebral FDG-PET, high-density EEG, or TMS-EEG, could constitute such a protocol. In the chronic phase, assessment of residual cognitive capacity with activation-based fMRI tests may prove to be an invaluable tool. To address the problem of false test responses, more than one paraclinical examination method can be completed. Converging results from several examination modalities would strengthen the credibility of the findings, especially when the available methods are relatively nascent, and have not been tested on larger scales [31].

Conclusion

With increasing numbers of survivors from acute coma, chronic disorders of consciousness become more prevalent. New evidence of retained cognition and emotions in severely brain-injured individuals makes this patient group an important clinical and ethical challenge. Neuroimaging protocols are being developed that detect covert cognition or preserved consciousness, and with the rapid development of research in the field, they will soon reach a level of advance where clinical implementation is feasible. Considering the gravity of these disorders, and the difficult choices faced by relatives and therapists, such examinations should become part of the diagnostic routine as soon as possible.

References

1. Giacino JT (2004) The vegetative and minimally conscious states: consensus-based criteria for establishing diagnosis and prognosis. NeuroRehabilitation 19:293–298
2. Boly M, Faymonville ME, Schnakers C et al (2008) Perception of pain in the minimally conscious state with PET activation: an observational study. Lancet Neurol 7:1013–1020
3. Bekinschtein T, Leiguarda R, Armony J et al (2004) Emotion processing in the minimally conscious state. J Neurol Neurosurg Psychiatr 75:788
4. Chatelle C, Thibaut A, Whyte J, De Val MD, Laureys S, Schnakers C (2014) Pain issues in disorders of consciousness. Brain Injury 28:1202–1208

5. Luauté J, Maucort-Boulch D, Tell L et al (2010) Long-term outcomes of chronic minimally conscious and vegetative states. Neurology 75:246–252
6. Estraneo A, Moretta P, Loreto V, Lanzillo B, Santoro L, Trojano L (2010) Late recovery after traumatic, anoxic, or hemorrhagic long-lasting vegetative state. Neurology 75:239–245
7. Thibaut A, Bruno M-A, Ledoux D, Demertzi A, Laureys S (2014) tDCS in patients with disorders of consciousness: sham-controlled randomized double-blind study. Neurology 82:1112–1118
8. Schiff ND, Giacino JT, Kalmar K et al (2007) Behavioural improvements with thalamic stimulation after severe traumatic brain injury. Nature 448:600–603
9. Manning J (2012) Withdrawal of life-sustaining treatment from a patient in a minimally conscious state. J Law Med 19:430–435
10. Stender J, Gosseries O, Bruno MA et al (2014) Diagnostic precision of PET imaging and functional MRI in disorders of consciousness: a clinical validation study. Lancet 384:514–522
11. Schnakers C, Vanhaudenhuyse A, Giacino J et al (2009) Diagnostic accuracy of the vegetative and minimally conscious state: clinical consensus versus standardized neurobehavioral assessment. BMC Neurol 9:35
12. Giacino JT, Kalmar K, Whyte J (2004) The JFK Coma Recovery Scale-Revised: measurement characteristics and diagnostic utility. Arch Phys Med Rehab 85:2020–2029
13. Kalmar K, Giacino JT (2005) The JFK Coma Recovery Scale-Revised. Neuropsychol Rehabil 15:454–460
14. Seel RT, Sherer M, Whyte J et al (2010) Assessment scales for disorders of consciousness: evidence-based recommendations for clinical practice and research. Arch Phys Med Rehab 91:1795–1813
15. Bruno M-A, Vanhaudenhuyse A, Schnakers C et al (2010) Visual fixation in the vegetative state: an observational case series PET study. BMC Neurol 10:35
16. Thonnard M, Wannez S, Keen S et al (2014) Detection of visual pursuit in patients in minimally conscious state: a matter of stimuli and visual plane? Brain Injury 28:1164–1170
17. Owen AM, Coleman MR, Boly M, Davis MH, Laureys S, Pickard JD (2006) Detecting awareness in the vegetative state. Science 313:1402
18. Monti MM, Vanhaudenhuyse A, Coleman MR et al (2010) Willful modulation of brain activity in disorders of consciousness. N Engl J Med 362:579–589
19. Naci L, Owen AM (2013) Making every word count for nonresponsive patients. JAMA Neurol 70:1235–1241
20. Naci L, Cusack R, Anello M, Owen AM (2014) A common neural code for similar conscious experiences in different individuals. 2014. Proc Natl Acad Sci USA 111:14277–14288
21. Shulman RG, Hyder F, Rothman DL (2009) Baseline brain energy supports the state of consciousness. Proc Natl Acad Sci USA 106:11096–11101
22. Laureys S, Owen AM, Schiff ND (2004) Brain function in coma, vegetative state, and related disorders. Lancet Neurol 3:537–546
23. Dehaene S, Changeux JP (2011) Experimental and theoretical approaches to conscious processing. Neuron 70:200–227
24. Baars BJ (2005) Global workspace theory of consciousness: toward a cognitive neuroscience of human experience. Prog Brain Res 150:45–53
25. Stender J, Kupers R, Rodell A et al (2015) Quantitative rates of brain glucose metabolism distinguish minimally conscious from vegetative state patients. J Cereb Blood Flow Metab (in press)
26. Maandag NJG, Coman D, Sanganahalli BG et al (2007) Energetics of neuronal signaling and fMRI activity. Proc Natl Acad Sci USA 104:20546–20551
27. Lechinger J, Bothe K, Pichler G et al (2013) CRS-R score in disorders of consciousness is strongly related to spectral EEG at rest. J Neurol 260:2348–2356
28. Sitt JD, King J-R, Karoui El I et al (2014) Large scale screening of neural signatures of consciousness in patients in a vegetative or minimally conscious state. Brain 137:2258–2270

29. Tononi G (2008) Consciousness as integrated information: a provisional manifesto. Biol Bull 215:216–242
30. Casali AG, Gosseries O, Rosanova M et al (2013) A theoretically based index of consciousness independent of sensory processing and behavior. Sci Transl Med 5:198–105
31. Cruse D, Gantner I, Soddu A, Owen AM (2014) Lies, damned lies and diagnoses: Estimating the clinical utility of assessments of covert awareness in the vegetative state. Brain Injury 28:1197–1201

Part XII
Neuromuscular Considerations

The Role of Local and Systemic Inflammation in the Pathogenesis of Intensive Care Unit-acquired Weakness

E. Witteveen, M. J. Schultz, and J. Horn

Introduction

A previously healthy 47-year old woman was admitted to the intensive care unit (ICU) with severe pneumosepsis. She received antimicrobial therapy and supportive care consisting of fluid resuscitation, inotropes and vasopressors, and lung-protective ventilation. She developed kidney failure for which continuous venovenous hemofiltration was initiated. She recovered within several days, but after cessation of sedatives it became apparent that she was very weak and could hardly move her limbs. She was clinically diagnosed with ICU-acquired weakness. After a period of intense rehabilitation she was discharged home, but a year later she still complained of severe impairments in physical functioning. She wondered how a pulmonary infection could have led to extreme weakness of the limbs. You realize that the pathophysiology of ICU-acquired weakness is far from understood, but there are suggestions that ICU-acquired weakness develops in response to a strong and uncontrolled inflammatory response, as seen with sepsis.

In this chapter, building on a recently published translational review [1], we aim to provide an overview of studies on local and systemic inflammation in animal models of ICU-acquired weakness and in critically ill patients with ICU-acquired weakness, and discuss immune-modulating strategies that could benefit patients at risk for or with ICU-acquired weakness.

E. Witteveen ✉ · M. J. Schultz · J. Horn
Department of Intensive Care Medicine, and Laboratory of Experimental Intensive Care and Anesthesiology (L·E·I·C·A), Academic Medical Center, University of Amsterdam, Amsterdam, Netherlands
e-mail: e.witteveen@amc.nl

J.-L. Vincent (ed.), *Annual Update in Intensive Care and Emergency Medicine 2015*,
DOI 10.1007/978-3-319-13761-2_37

Intensive Care Unit-acquired Weakness

In ICU-acquired weakness, a generalized, symmetrical weakness develops, probably already shortly after the onset of a critical illness [2]. It can involve nerves (referred to as critical illness polyneuropathy, CIP), muscles (critical illness myopathy, CIM), or both (critical illness neuromyopathy, CINM) [2]. Differentiation between these three entities requires additional invasive investigations, such as electrophysiological investigations or muscle biopsy [3]. This is usually omitted, since so far, it has no clinical consequences: Treatment for ICU-acquired weakness is merely supportive.

ICU-acquired weakness is a very frequent complication of critical illness. A systematic review in 2007 [4], including 24 studies, reported a median incidence of ICU-acquired weakness of 57% in patients with sepsis, multiple organ dysfunction syndrome (MODS) or prolonged mechanical ventilation. The incidence of ICU-acquired weakness, though, depends on the patient case mix and the diagnostic criteria used. Incidences up to 100% have been reported in patients with moderate to severe MODS along with sepsis or the systemic inflammatory response syndrome (SIRS) [5]. Since survival rates from severe sepsis are improving [6, 7], it is likely that the incidence of ICU-acquired weakness will increase as patients who would have died in the past, now survive and present with ICU-acquired weakness.

The main and consistently identified risk factors for ICU-acquired weakness are SIRS, sepsis, and MODS [3, 4]. Multivariable analyses suggested that SIRS and MODS are independently associated with ICU-acquired weakness [4, 8], but this was not confirmed in other studies. This finding may be because SIRS, sepsis and MODS are highly correlated and some studies only recruited patients with (severe) sepsis. The strong association between MODS and ICU-acquired weakness suggests that muscle and nerve dysfunction can be seen as 'another failing organ', and that MODS and ICU-acquired weakness have a common cause. An exaggerated and imbalanced systemic inflammatory response is frequently proposed to play a role in the pathogenesis of MODS [9]. Thus, one could hypothesize that an exaggerated and uncontrolled inflammatory response is responsible for the muscle and nerve damage in critically ill patients.

ICU-acquired Weakness and Systemic Inflammation

In SIRS and sepsis, multiple inflammatory pathways are activated, involving inflammatory mediators, complement cascades, acute phase protein release and activation of inflammatory cells and vascular endothelium [10]. While several investigators suggest a role of systemic inflammatory mediators in the pathophysiology of ICU-acquired weakness, this has not been studied extensively.

Some studies show at best a possible correlation between elevated plasma cytokine levels (interleukin [IL]-6 and IL-2 receptor) and development of ICU-acquired weakness [11, 12]. High serum acute phase protein levels [11–14] and plasma complement products [11] do not correlate with the presence of ICU-acquired weakness.

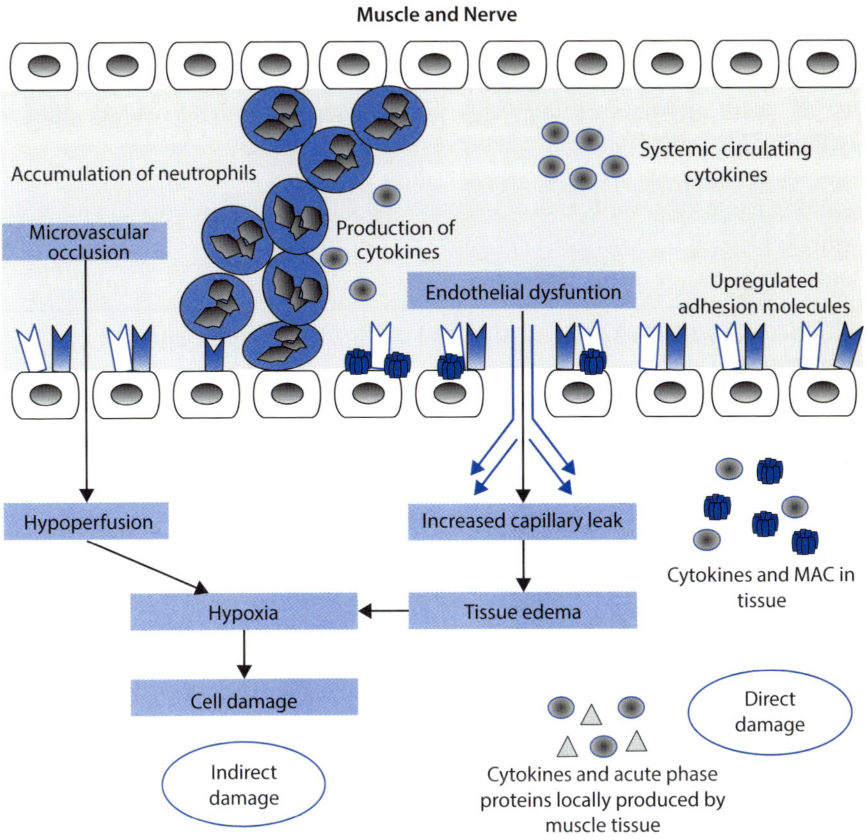

Fig. 1 Inflammatory mediators found in muscle or nerve tissue in ICU-acquired weakness and supposed mechanisms of damage (*blue boxes*). MAC: membrane attack complex

The vascular endothelium may be involved in the pathogenesis of ICU-acquired weakness, since cytokines, complement membrane attack complex (MAC) and antigen presenting molecules are found on the vascular endothelium in ICU-acquired weakness [1]. Along with the presence of adhesion molecules, this indicates endothelial cell activation. Endothelial cell activation and dysfunction are thought to play an important role in the pathogenesis of MODS [15]. Cytokines and other inflammatory mediators induce an increased permeability of vascular endothelium. Due to increased capillary leak, edema forms, impairing tissue oxygenation. Tissue oxygenation is further impaired by microvascular occlusions of neutrophils adhering to the capillary wall by adhesion molecules, causing hypoperfusion and hypoxia. Organ damage in MODS is considered to be a consequence of this indirect damage. These inflammatory mechanisms on the vascular endothelium might also play a role in muscle and nerve tissue in patients with ICU-acquired weakness (see Fig. 1), but this is highly speculative.

While in lung tissue, a massive infiltration of neutrophils causes direct tissue damage by the production of harmful factors, in other organs in MODS, the neutrophils do not enter the tissue [15]. This is in accordance with the finding that in ICU-acquired weakness, neutrophils do not infiltrate muscle or nerve tissue, further establishing the idea of muscle and nerve damage in the light of MODS.

It is also suggested that by increased endothelial permeability, a neurotoxic factor in serum might enter the nerves of patients with CIP, but such a factor has not been found [16].

ICU-acquired Weakness and Local Inflammation in Muscle and Nerve Tissue

Muscle Inflammation

While cellular infiltrates in muscle tissue have been found in animal models of ICU-acquired weakness, these are often absent in muscle biopsies from patients with ICU-acquired weakness [1]. The absence of cellular infiltrates differentiates ICU-acquired weakness from inflammatory myopathies, like polymyositis and dermatomyositis [17]. Other signs of local inflammation are frequently present, including cytokines, complement factors, antigen presenting molecules and adhesion molecules [1]. The absence of inflammatory cells but presence of these inflammatory mediators suggests that muscle tissue damage may be more a result of locally active inflammatory mediators then of destructive inflammatory cells. It could be that these inflammatory mediators are produced locally, as skeletal muscle can serve as an exocrine organ expressing and releasing so-called myokines (muscle cytokines) into muscle tissue and blood [18]. In this way, muscle inflammation might even contribute to systemic inflammation.

Notably, elevated cytokine levels in muscle tissue have also been found in ICU patients who do not have ICU-acquired weakness [14]. This suggests that the expression of inflammatory mediators in muscle might be common in ICU patients and not specific for ICU-acquired weakness.

Nerve Inflammation

There are no animal studies that have investigated local inflammation of nerve tissue in models of ICU-acquired weakness, and studies in patients with ICU-acquired weakness are scarce. Cellular infiltrates are rarely seen in nerve biopsies of patients with ICU-acquired weakness [1]. In one study, high levels of tumor necrosis factor (TNF)-α and adhesion molecules were found in the superficial peroneal nerve of patients with ICU-acquired weakness [19]. Nerve biopsies of ICU patients without ICU-acquired weakness were not performed.

Inflammatory Mediators in ICU-acquired Weakness

Acute Phase Proteins

Elevated plasma C-reactive protein (CRP) levels have been investigated in patients with ICU-acquired weakness, but were not associated with ICU-acquired weakness [11–13]. Plasma serum amyloid A (SAA) levels were lower in patients with CIM compared to ICU patients without CIM [14].

Increases in SAA1 and SAA4 expression and SAA1 accumulation in muscle were associated with CIM development. This suggests that SAA is synthesized in the skeletal muscle [14].

Cytokines

The association between plasma cytokines and development of ICU-acquired weakness has been investigated in a few small studies. Increased IL-6 plasma levels (collected 3–7 days and 8–10 days after ICU admission) were an independent risk factor for ICU-acquired weakness [12]. This study was hampered by the methodology used. ICU-acquired weakness was only defined by an abnormal muscle membrane excitability and the sample size was small (22 patients with ICU-acquired weakness and 18 without). Moreover, the effect of IL-6 plasma levels was small (hazard ratio of 1.006). Plasma IL-10, insulin-like growth factor (IGF)-1, insulin-like growth factor binding protein-1 (IGFBP)-I and IGFBP-III levels were not independently associated with ICU-acquired weakness. In an earlier study, plasma IL-6 and TNF-α levels measured in ICU patients after a diagnosis of ICU-acquired weakness were not different from control ICU patients (in whom plasma was measured during the first or second week of ICU-admission) [20]. A correlation between plasma IL-2 receptors and reduction in the amplitude of the compound motor action potential (CMAP) in the median and tibial nerves was found in another study [11]. This correlation was not found for IL-2, IL-6 or IL-10.

Cytokines have also been investigated in muscle and nerve tissue of patients with ICU-acquired weakness. In muscle tissue, both the anti-inflammatory cytokine IL-10 and pro-inflammatory cytokines (IL-1β, IL-12, interferon [IFN]-γ and TNF-α-receptor) were found [21]. Cytokines were present on vascular endothelium and in the cytoplasm of muscle fibers of patients with ICU-acquired weakness and were absent in two control biopsies of ICU patients without ICU-acquired weakness [21]. In nerve tissue from patients with ICU-acquired weakness, expression of TNF-α was described in the cytoplasm of endoneurial cell types and in vascular endothelium [19].

Complement

Plasma C3 and C4 levels did not correlate with CMAP amplitudes of the median, tibial and peroneal nerves [11]. Moreover, complement activation products (C3b/c, C4b/c and C5a) in plasma were not associated with ICU-acquired weakness (unpublished data).

In muscle tissue, only MAC (C5b9) has been studied. It was found in a majority of patients with ICU-acquired weakness [21–23], mainly on vascular endothelium and on necrotic muscle fibers [21,23]. MAC was absent in two control biopsies in ICU patients without ICU-acquired weakness [21].

Adhesion Molecules

Positive staining of intercellular adhesion molecules (ICAMs) and vascular cell adhesion molecules (VCAMs) was found in more than 50% of muscle biopsies from patients with ICU-acquired weakness [21]. These adhesion molecules were also found in 1 of 2 muscle biopsies of ICU patients without ICU-acquired weakness [21]. Therefore, the pathophysiological significance is unknown. E-selectin was not expressed in muscles of patients with ICU-acquired weakness or control patients without ICU-acquired weakness [21].

In nerve biopsies of patients with ICU-acquired weakness, E-selectin expression was present in 68% (15/22) of biopsies [19]. E-selectin was expressed in the endothelium of epineurial and endoneurial vessels. VCAM-1 and ICAM-1 were present in respectively 100% (22/22) and 77% (17/22) of nerve biopsies. While VCAM-1 and ICAM-1 are expressed under basal conditions, expression of E-selectin in nerves indicates endothelial cell activation.

Antigen Presenting Molecules

Antigen presenting molecules are frequently found in muscle biopsies of patients with ICU-acquired weakness [21–23]. A strong upregulation of both major histocompatibility complex (MHC)-I molecules (human leucocyte antigen [HLA]-1) [21–23] and MHC-II molecules (HLA-DR) [21] has been found. HLA-DR was expressed on muscle fibers, vascular endothelium and on macrophages in infiltrates. Positive staining for HLA-1 was also seen, as a secondary phenomenon, on atrophic and necrotic muscle fibers [21,23]. HLA-1 was also present in two muscle biopsies from ICU patients without ICU-acquired weakness [21].

Immunomodulatory Therapies Against ICU-acquired Weakness

So far, only intravenous immunoglobulin (IVIG) has been studied as an immunomodulatory therapy to prevent or mitigate ICU-acquired weakness, in one preclinical study and three clinical trials.

In a rat model, IgM-enriched IVIG was given within the first hour after induction of septic peritonitis [24]. Nerve conduction velocity decreased significantly in the untreated group, whereas it did not change in the sham surgery and IVIG group. However, decreased nerve conduction velocity is not typical for ICU-acquired weakness.

In a prospective randomized controlled trial, patients with MODS, SIRS or sepsis, and early clinical signs of ICU-acquired weakness were randomized to receive IgM-enriched IVIG (0.25 g/kg/day for 3 consecutive days) or placebo (human albumin) [25]. The primary outcome in this study was a severity score, consisting of a combination of results of electrophysiological studies and muscle biopsy (and not muscle strength), on day 0 and day 14 after start of treatment. The severity scores deteriorated in both the IVIG and placebo groups. Since no differences in severity scores were found during the interim analysis, this trial was terminated prematurely, after enrolment of 38 patients. The secondary outcomes (28-day mortality and length of ICU stay) were also similar in the two groups.

In a pilot-study in which three patients with an established clinical and electrophysiological diagnosis of ICU-acquired weakness were treated with IVIG (0.4 g/kg/day for 5–10 days), patients did not show an improvement in mobilization shortly after immunoglobulin administration [26]. No control patients were included.

Finally, IgM-enriched IVIG was investigated in a prospective cohort study of patients who survived MODS following multiple trauma and, thereafter, developed sepsis due to a nosocomial infection [27]. In eight patients, IVIG (0.3 g/kg/day for 3 days) was given within 24 h after the diagnosis of sepsis. Retrospective chart analysis showed that none of these patients developed ICU-acquired weakness (diagnosed by electrophysiological examination at the time of ICU-discharge). Eight other patients did not receive IVIG because they were transferred from another hospital or had a delayed diagnosis of sepsis. These patients were used as control patients and ICU-acquired weakness was diagnosed in seven of them. Based on these results, the authors suggested that IVIG administration may have prevented the development of ICU-acquired weakness.

The effects of blocking various immune mediators on the development of ICU-acquired weakness should be further investigated, either by using specific blocking agents or knock-out animals. The advances in anti-inflammatory therapies are promising, since more selective immunomodulatory drugs, which target a specific component of the immune system, have been developed [28].

Challenges and Future Perspectives

Little is known about inflammation in muscle or nerve tissue of ICU patients without ICU-acquired weakness, because most studies concerning inflammation in ICU-acquired weakness are case series or cohort studies without biopsies of control patients. Therefore, the findings described in this overview might not be specific for ICU-acquired weakness but may be seen in all ICU patients. Further research is needed to investigate whether the inflammatory response differs in patients with and patients without ICU-acquired weakness.

Furthermore, comparisons between study results are hampered by the different inclusion criteria used and different diagnostic criteria for ICU-acquired weakness. Future research should use the current diagnostic criteria for ICU-acquired weakness [2], in which the diagnosis of ICU-acquired weakness is primarily based on measurement of manual muscle strength and not on electrophysiological parameters.

As ICU-acquired weakness may be as important as other organ failures, such as kidney failure, it deserves far more attention on the ICU. Investigation and documentation of weakness on the ICU according to the present recommendations [2, 29] should be part of standard care. In the search for a better understanding of the pathophysiology of ICU-acquired weakness and possible therapies, increased awareness of ICU-acquired weakness is crucial.

Conclusion

Although the established association of ICU-acquired weakness with sepsis, SIRS and MODS suggests a role for inflammation, this has not been extensively studied and results so far are inconclusive. Inflammatory mediators have been found in plasma, and muscle and nerve tissue of patients with ICU-acquired weakness, and the vascular endothelium seems to be involved. Muscle and nerve injury in ICU-acquired weakness may be caused by indirect damage (caused by endothelial dysfunction, as in MODS) and by direct damage by locally produced inflammatory mediators, but this is still speculative. Dysfunction and damage of muscles and nerves in ICU-acquired weakness can be seen as failing organs in the spectrum of MODS.

References

1. Witteveen E, Wieske L, Verhamme C, Schultz MJ, van Schaik IN, Horn J (2014) Muscle and nerve inflammation in intensive care unit-acquired weakness: A systematic translational review. J Neurol Sci 345:15–25
2. Stevens RD, Marshall SA, Cornblath DR et al (2009) A framework for diagnosing and classifying intensive care unit-acquired weakness. Crit Care Med 37:S299–S308
3. Kress JP, Hall JB (2014) ICU-acquired weakness and recovery from critical illness. N Engl J Med 370:1626–1635

4. Stevens RD, Dowdy DW, Michaels RK, Mendez-Tellez PA, Pronovost PJ, Needham DM (2007) Neuromuscular dysfunction acquired in critical illness: a systematic review. Intensive Care Med 33:1876–1891
5. Tennilä A, Salmi T, Pettilä V, Roine RO, Varpula T, Takkunen O (2000) Early signs of critical illness polyneuropathy in ICU patients with systemic inflammatory response syndrome or sepsis. Intensive Care Med 26:1360–1363
6. Kaukonen K-M, Bailey M, Suzuki S, Pilcher D, Bellomo R (2014) Mortality related to severe sepsis and septic shock among critically ill patients in Australia and New Zealand, 2000–2012. JAMA 311:1308–1316
7. Stevenson EK, Rubenstein AR, Radin GT, Wiener RS, Walkey AJ (2014) Two decades of mortality trends among patients with severe sepsis: a comparative meta-analysis. Crit Care Med 42:625–631
8. De Letter MACJ, Schmitz PIM, Visser LH et al (2001) Risk factors for the development of polyneuropathy and myopathy in critically ill patients. Crit Care Med 29:2281–2286
9. Marshall JC (2001) Inflammation, coagulopathy, and the pathogenesis of multiple organ dysfunction syndrome. Crit Care Med 29:S99–S106
10. De Jong HK, van der Poll T, Wiersinga WJ (2010) The systemic pro-inflammatory response in sepsis. J Innate Immun 2:422–430
11. Mohammadi B, Schedel I, Graf K et al (2008) Role of endotoxin in the pathogenesis of critical illness polyneuropathy. J Neurol 255:265–272
12. Weber-Carstens S, Deja M, Koch M et al (2010) Risk factors in critical illness myopathy during the early course of critical illness: a prospective observational study. Crit Care 14:R119
13. Hermans G, Wilmer A, Meersseman W et al (2007) Impact of intensive insulin therapy on neuromuscular complications and ventilator dependency in the medical intensive care unit. Am J Respir Crit Care Med 175:480–489
14. Langhans C, Weber-Carstens S, Schmidt F et al (2014) Inflammation-induced acute phase response in skeletal muscle and critical illness myopathy. PLoS One 9:e92048
15. Brown KA, Brain SD, Pearson JD, Edgeworth JD, Lewis SM, Treacher DF (2006) Neutrophils in development of multiple organ failure in sepsis. Lancet 368:157–169
16. Druschky A, Herkert M, Radespiel-Tröger M et al (2001) Critical illness polyneuropathy: clinical findings and cell culture assay of neurotoxicity assessed by a prospective study. Intensive Care Med 27:686–693
17. Hewer E, Goebel HH (2008) Myopathology of non-infectious inflammatory myopathies – The current status. Pathol Res Pract 204:609–623
18. Pedersen BK, Febbraio MA (2008) Muscle as an endocrine organ: focus on muscle-derived interleukin-6. Physiol Rev 88:1379–1406
19. Fenzi F, Latronico N, Refatti N, Rizzuto N (2003) Enhanced expression of E-selectin on the vascular endothelium of peripheral nerve in critically ill patients with neuromuscular disorders. Acta Neuropathol 106:75–82
20. Verheul GAM, de Jongh-Leuvenink J, Op de Coul AAW, van Landeghem AAJ, van Puyenbroek MJE (1994) Tumor necrosis factor and interleukin-6 in critical illness polyneuromyopathy. Clin Neurol Neurosurg 96:300–304
21. De Letter MACJ, van Doorn PA, Savelkoul HFJ et al (2000) Critical illness polyneuropathy and myopathy (CIPNM): evidence for local immune activation by cytokine-expression in the muscle tissue. J Neuroimmunol 106:206–213
22. Bednarik J, Lukas Z, Vondracek P (2003) Critical illness polyneuromyopathy: the electrophysiological components of a complex entity. Intensive Care Med 29:1505–1514
23. Bazzi P, Moggio M, Prelle A et al (1999) Critically ill patients: immunological evidence of inflammation in muscle biopsy. Clin Neuropathol 18:23–30
24. Cankayali I, Doğan YH, Solak İ, Erİş O, Demİrgören S, Moral AR (2010) Effects of IgM-enriched immunoglobulin and fluid replacement on nerve conduction velocity in experimental sepsis. Turkish J Trauma Emerg Med 16:9–14

25. Brunner R, Rinner W, Haberler C et al (2013) Early treatment with IgM-enriched intravenous immunoglobulin does not mitigate critical illness polyneuropathy and/or myopathy in patients with multiple organ failure and SIRS/sepsis: a prospective, randomized, placebo-controlled, double-blinded trial. Crit Care 17:R213
26. Wijdicks EFM, Fulgham JR (1994) Failure of high dose intravenous immunoglobulins to alter the clinical course of critical illness polyneuropathy. Muscle Nerve 17:1494–1495
27. Mohr M, Englisch L, Roth A, Burchardi H, Zielmann S (1997) Effects of early treatment with immunoglobulin on critical illness polyneuropathy following multiple organ failure and gram-negative sepsis. Intensive Care Med 23:1144–1149
28. Kovarik J (2013) From immunosuppression to immunomodulation: current principles and future strategies. Pathobiology 80:275–281
29. Sharshar T, Citerio G, Andrews PJD et al (2014) Neurological examination of critically ill patients: a pragmatic approach. Report of an ESICM expert panel. Intensive Care Med 40:484–495

Critical Illness is Top Sport

M. Suker, C. Ince, and C. van Eijck

Introduction

Extreme exercise has been used to study how normal physiology responds to states that resemble critical illness, such as hypoxemia and hypovolemia. Studies of the Extreme Everest Research Group have shown that the body can tolerate hypoxemia by using adaptation mechanisms. One of these mechanisms was found in lowlanders who climbed Mount Everest, mirroring the hypoxemia in critical illness. There was an increase in nitric oxide (NO) in the blood in response to the hypoxic environment. These enhanced NO levels were associated with changes in microcirculatory blood flow, which may affect local tissue oxygen delivery (DO_2) [1]. Indeed extreme exercise can protect the body by adapting to cope with the hypoxic environment. This is seen in skeletal muscle function, with high altitude hypoxia inducing skeletal muscle atrophy despite unchanged exercise metabolites [2]. Another adaptation is seen in gluco-insular regulation, in which, despite an increase in insulin resistance in sustained hypoxia, glucose levels remain stable [3]. From these considerations, it can be concluded that lessons can be learned, which may be relevant to critically ill patients who need to cope with tissue hypoxia. Indeed, fitness and exercise might even hold potential lessons on how to 'train' patients to cope with surgery and critical illness. This chapter explores this idea and speculates on how such insight might benefit patients in need of surgery and at risk for critical illness.

Surgical procedures induce a significant stress on the body. The body responds to surgical stress in different ways [4]. This surgical stress response can be divided into three categories: Nervous, endocrine and immunological. The overall result of this systemic response is a catabolic effect with substrate release for energy production

M. Suker · C. van Eijck
Department of Surgery, Erasmus Medical Center, Rotterdam, Netherlands

C. Ince ✉
Department of Intensive Care, Erasmus Medical Center, Rotterdam, Netherlands
e-mail: c.ince@erasmusmc.nl

J.-L. Vincent (ed.), *Annual Update in Intensive Care and Emergency Medicine 2015*,
DOI 10.1007/978-3-319-13761-2_38

and retention of salt and water. The activation of the sympathetic nervous system leads to catecholamine release, which induces tachycardia, hypertension and an increase in the plasma glucose levels. The endocrine system produces corticotrophin which enhances the production of glucocorticoids, reduces insulin production and increases the insulin resistance. This all leads to persistent hyperglycemia. Furthermore the endocrine system activates the renin-angiotensin-aldosterone system, which promotes salt and fluid retention. The immunological system is activated by surgery with increased release of interleukin (IL)-1 and IL-6, tumor necrosis factor (TNF)-α and granulocytosis. Additionally, inflammatory cells produce reactive oxygen species (ROS) that enter damaged tissue after surgical trauma. The purpose of these inflammatory cells is to destroy invading organisms and damaged tissue. Despite this beneficial effect, the overwhelming oxidative potential can result in additional tissue destruction [5].

The control of the surgical stress response is considered an important therapeutic target to reduce postoperative morbidity and mortality [6]. A potential counteract to this stress is the pre-habilitation of the patient's fitness by preoperative training [7]. The hypothesis is that by improving physiological reserve with preoperative physical intervention, postoperative recovery will be enhanced [8]. The possible reduction in perioperative mortality and morbidity by physical training is not only potentially favorable for short-term outcomes, but also potentially for long-term ones. Prolonged postoperative morbidity was related with a higher risk for mortality in the first two years after surgery [9].

The critical illness stress response is not as well understood as the surgical stress response. Critically ill patients have a very diverse presentation and a wide range of stress factors and usually these exist in an acute situation [10]. Overall, the critical illness stress response consists of two categories: The endocrine and the neurological response. The endocrine response to critical illness is induced by increased cortisol levels, which lead to a ready supply of energy source for use by vital organs. Glucose mobilization and synthesis are enhanced to provide energy and this leads to an osmotic change that temporarily shifts volume from the intracellular to the extracellular space. A subsequent increased release of anti-diuretic hormone results in water retention. Release of catecholamines increases to cause vasoconstriction and to liberate free fatty acids to energize the heart, the skeletal muscles and hepatic gluconeogenesis. The body only can suffer this endocrine response for a limited time, otherwise it will result in an untenable loss of structural and muscle proteins, which can lead to atrophy and wasting. Furthermore, unbalanced stress metabolism leads to hyperglycemia, which directly affects the immune and neurological systems. The main neurological stress response in critical illness is an increase in catecholamine release into the blood circulation via a cascade reaction of neurological signals. This release of catecholamines further enhances the endocrine response [11].

In this chapter, we will review the current understanding of the assessment of the pre-habilitation of a patient's physical status. The physical parameters and tests known to stratify the risk for postoperative complications are discussed as well as exercise regimens known to improve postoperative outcome. Exercise intervention trials applied to critically ill patients will then be reviewed. Finally, the potential parameters and exercise regimens that could be implemented in elective surgery patients will be addressed in view of future (randomized) trials.

Parameters

In sports medicine, parameters to measure the aerobic fitness of athletes have been used for decades. The most commonly used parameters are maximal oxygen consumption (VO_{2Max}) and maximal power output (P_{Max}) reached during cardiopulmonary exercise testing (CPET). Over the last three decades, these parameters have been augmented with the addition of the submaximal fitness parameters of athletes by estimating the anaerobic threshold during ergometric testing, i. e., when ventilatory carbon dioxide (VCO_2) increases disproportionately to ventilatory oxygen consumption (VO_2). While these parameters are used in sports medicine to determine the endurance performance of athletes, there have been suggestions over the years that these parameters may also be a good tool to assess patient fitness [12]. Indeed, a prospective blinded observational study showed that CPET parameters used in sports medicine were associated with postoperative morbidity after major colonic surgery. Independently, VO_2 at anaerobic threshold, ventilator equivalent for CO_2 (V_E/VCO_2) at anaerobic threshold, and VO_{2Peak} were significantly associated with day 5 postoperative morbidity [13]. Another study showed that a preoperative anaerobic threshold < 11 ml/min/kg was associated with significantly increased cardiovascular mortality from 0.8% to 18% after major abdominal surgery [14]. The same preoperative anaerobic threshold value was identified in another study that included patients > 55 years old who underwent major colorectal surgery, radical nephrectomy or cystectomy. An anaerobic threshold < 11 ml/kg/min combined with a $V_E/VCO_2 \geq 34$ had a sensitivity of 88% and specificity of 47% for hospital mortality [15]. An anaerobic threshold < 10.1 ml/kg/min was found to be the optimum cut-off value for preoperative risk stratification for major abdominal surgery, with a sensitivity of 88% and specificity of 79% [16]. Another approach was use of an anaerobic threshold < 75% of predicted value for risk stratification, which had a sensitivity of 88% and specificity of 79% in patients undergoing major intra-abdominal surgery [17].

In upper gastrointestinal surgery, a relationship was found between preoperative VO_{2Max} and postoperative cardiopulmonary complication rate: A complication rate of 86% was found for patients with a preoperative VO_{2Max} < 699 ml/m^2/min [18]. A meta-analysis of 14 studies highlighted this relationship between VO_{2Peak} and postoperative complications in patients who underwent esophagectomy [19]. In thoracic surgery, a low VO_{2Max} and VO_{2Max} as a percentage of predicted were associated with a significantly higher level of postopcrative complications [20]. A review on this topic showed that preoperative VO_{2Max} was indeed a good predictor for postoperative morbidity after a lung resection: A value of VO_{2Max} < 10 ml/kg/min was identified as being associated with a high morbidity (71%) and mortality (28%) rate [21]. In contrast to this finding, another prospective study showed that although the actual VO_{2Peak} was not related to higher mortality, the VO_{2Peak} percentage of predicted VO_2 was. Predicted VO_2 is calculated with a standard formula based on the subject's age, height, weight and sex. A threshold of $VO_{2Peak} < 50\%$ of predicted value gave a 33% mortality rate [22]. Additionally, a study showed a threshold of $VO_{2Max} > 75\%$ of predicted value was 90% accurate in predicting an uneventful postoperative course in lung resection patients [23].

In vascular surgery, there are several studies that identified CPET parameters as being good predictors for postoperative complications. A retrospective cohort study showed that an anaerobic threshold > 11 ml/kg/min was the best predictor for reduced perioperative mortality in elective infra-renal abdominal aortic aneurysm (AAA) open surgery patients. Furthermore, the study showed that the same threshold value gave a reduced length of stay (LOS) and inpatient cost for open and endovascular repair in the same study population [24]. In addition, two other prospective cohort studies identified that the anaerobic threshold was the best predictive tool for long-term mortality in elective AAA repair patients [25, 26]. In addition to the use of CPET, other methods to estimate patient fitness have been described. The American College of Cardiology/American Heart Association (ACC/AHA) have suggested the use of predictor models for perioperative non-cardiac surgery [27]. Their last guideline advises use of one of the following risk-prediction tools: Revised Cardiac Risk Index (RCRI), American College of Surgeons National Surgical Quality Improvement Program (NSQIP) Myocardial Infarction and Cardiac Arrest (MICA), and/or American College of Surgeons NSQIP Surgical Risk Calculator. The NSQIP MICA and NSQIP Surgical Risk Calculator are two patient specific questionnaires, which have been proposed as a tool for predicting complication risk for the patient. Unfortunately, a predictive test called "Timed Up and Go" was not included in the guideline. This test is taken preoperatively and involves the patient standing up from a chair, then walking for ten feet (3 meters) and returning to the chair. This test was evaluated in patients > 65 years who underwent colorectal or cardiac surgery with the cohort being divided into groups based on their time performance. It had a superior predictive value than the NSQIP Surgical Risk Cal-

Table 1 Cardiopulmonary exercise testing parameters and their definition

Parameter	Definition
VO_2	The amount of oxygen extracted from inspired gas, usually expressed in ml/min/kg
VO_{2Max}	The maximal oxygen uptake plateau during a single maximum exercise test, usually expressed in ml/min/kg
VO_{2Peak}	The highest amount of oxygen uptake achieved during a single maximal exercise test, usually expressed in ml/min/kg
V_E/VCO_2	Ratio of the amount of air ventilated (l/min) to carbon dioxide produced (l/min)
VCO_2	The exhaled carbon dioxide amount, usually expressed in ml/min/kg
AT	The anaerobic threshold is the moment at which lactate begins to accumulate in blood. Usually the moment is expressed in ml/min/kg of VO_2
P_{Max}	The maximal work output during exercise, usually expressed in Watts

culator [28]. Other methods which are discussed in the ACC/AHA guideline are the 12-lead electrocardiogram (EKG), assessment of left ventricular function, exercise stress testing for myocardial ischemia and functional capacity, pharmacological stress testing and preoperative coronary angiography. The ACC/AHA recommends all of these tests in specific situations but not for all patients. A discussion of these tests is beyond the scope of this review. All the CPET parameters discussed above are shown in Table 1.

Preoperative Exercise

Pre-habilitation is defined as a regimen of physical activities whose main purpose is to improve postoperative outcome. Several trials have been conducted to investigate whether a preoperative exercise regimen can improve postoperative outcomes. A wide range of patient groups and types of exercise have been described in the literature. Most of the studies, however, have been performed in cardiac surgery patients. A randomized controlled trial (RCT) was conducted in which patients awaiting colorectal surgery were randomized to either a structured bike and strengthening regimen or just a simple walking and breathing regimen. The study outcome was perioperative complications, LOS and VO_{2Max}. Surprisingly, this study found no significant difference between the two randomized arms [29]. These results were in agreement with another trial that randomized patients awaiting elective colon surgery to a short-term intensive therapeutic exercise to improve muscle strength, aerobic capacity, and functional activities, given in the outpatient department or to home-based exercise advice [30]. These authors also found no significant differences in postoperative complications or LOS. Of note, they did report a significant relationship between daily (>4000 steps) walking and reduced postoperative pulmonary complications independent of the randomization arm [30]. Vascular surgery trials had the same results. A pilot RCT, which only included patients awaiting elective AAA surgery, showed that inspiratory muscle training did not significantly reduce postoperative pulmonary complications [31]. In contrast, cardiothoracic prehabilitation trials have been more fruitful. A Cochrane review of all the trials related to postoperative outcome associated with an exercise intervention prior to elective cardiac surgery has been conducted [32]. Eight studies were included in the review. One study randomized patients awaiting elective coronary artery bypass graft (CABG) surgery to either aerobic exercise training with education and reinforcement or usual care. This study showed a significant decrease in hospital LOS and stay in the intensive care unit (ICU) but not in mortality rates [33]. Another randomized trial included patients scheduled for CABG and/or valve surgery [34]. The authors randomized patients to receive either exercise sessions with a mental stress reduction program or usual care. This study showed no significant reduction in LOS. Another randomized trial used breathing exercises as the intervention for patients with chronic obstructive pulmonary disease (COPD) awaiting elective CABG [35]. The results showed that postoperative complications and LOS were significantly lower in the intervention group than in the control arm. The five other trials

Table 2 Preoperative exercise

Type of exercise intervention	Definition
Bike and strengthening regimen [29]	Start at 50% of the MHR, increased by 10%/week. • Cycling: A stationary cycle for 20 min, increasing to 30 min/day. • Strengthening: Weight lifting, push-ups, sit-ups and standing strides
Intensive therapeutic exercise program [30]	• Resistance training of the LL extensors. • Inspiratory muscle training: patients breathed against a variable resistance (10–60% of the MIP) for about 15 minutes. • Aerobic training: training to 55–75% of MHR or perceived exertion for 20–30 minutes. • Functional training: Functional activities according to the patient's capabilities and interest
Inspiratory muscle training [31, 36–40]	• With a threshold loading device. • Starting with 15–40% of MIP. • Repeating the starting pressure daily or with an incremental increase in the pressure
Aerobic exercise training with education and reinforcement [33]	• Individualized, prescribed exercise training twice a week with education and reinforcement • Monthly nurse-initiated telephone calls to answer questions and provide reassurance
Exercise sessions with mental stress reduction program [34]	• Once a week 15 min stationary cycling and 15 min treadmill walking with maximal 60% of MHR • Once a week 40 min of cycle ergometry, treadmill walking and arm ergometry • 4 times mental stress reduction therapy session

MHR: maximal heart rate; LL: lower limb; MIP: maximal inspiratory pressure.

that were included in the Cochrane review all used inspiratory muscle training as a preoperative intervention. Four trials included patients awaiting CABG [36–39] and one trial included CABG or valvuloplasty surgery [40]. Three of the trials showed a significant decrease in postoperative pulmonary complications in patients who received preoperative inspiratory muscle training [36–38], whereas the two other trials did not show this relation [39, 40]. The exercise interventions discussed in this chapter are shown in Table 2.

Physical Therapy in the ICU

In recent years, there has been a shift from measuring the quality of critical care only by mortality outcome to that of functional status and health-related quality of life. Recent studies have shown that survivors of critical illness experience poor physical, functional, and cognitive outcomes often lasting for years [41]. Focusing on the physical status of patients, a prospective study showed that CPET could be a practical method to asses exercise capacity in ICU survivors in the first 6 weeks after discharge. This study showed that ICU survivors had a VO_{2Peak} of 56% of predicted value and an aerobic threshold 41% of predicted value. Furthermore,

Table 3 Physical therapy in the ICU

Type of exercise intervention	Definition
Electrical muscle stimulation [44]	To LL, 55 min/day at frequency of 45 Hz
Electrical muscle stimulation with active limb mobilization [45]	ALM and EMS to LL (frequency 8–35 Hz) to LL 5 days/week for 4 weeks
Exercise and mobilization [46]	PLM and ALM Transfers Bed mobility Ambulation Mobilization Gait training Activities of daily living
Physical training [47]	5/week for 6 weeks Limb strengthening Diaphragmatic exercises Bed mobility Transfers Ambulation
General physiotherapy with arm ergometer [48]	Chest therapy PLM and ALM Mobilization Ambulation Upper limb cycling for 15 sessions of 20 min/day
General physiotherapy with cycle ergometer [49]	PLM and ALM Ambulation Bedside cycling on ergometer 20 min/day
General physiotherapy with cycle ergometer and walking treadmill [50]	PLM and ALM Cough education Respiratory muscle training with threshold device 2 ×/day for 10 min Cycling on ergometer 20 min/day Climbing 25 stairs 5 ×/day Treadmill walking 30 min/day (if patient completed all the above)

EMS: electrical muscle stimulation; UL: upper limb; LL: lower limb; PLM: passive limb mobilization; ALM: active limb mobilization.

the study showed that there was a significant decrease in aerobic threshold and VO_{2Peak} in patients who received > 14 days ventilation compared to patients ventilated for 5–14 days [42]. Subsequently, much research has been done on exercise interventions during ICU admission. An excellent systematic review has described these intervention studies with their most important outcomes [43]. This systematic review included 10 trials, seven of which included critically ill patients and three elective surgery patients who were admitted to the ICU. As this section focuses on critically ill patients, we will only discuss the seven trials that included these patients. The type of exercise intervention varied considerably among these trials. One trial gave ICU admitted patients daily electrical muscle stimulation (EMS) of the lower limbs as an exercise intervention. The study found a significant increase in ventilator-free days and a decrease in weaning period in the intervention arm compared to the control group [44]. The second trial tried the same EMS in combination with active limb mobilization (AML) in bed-bound COPD patients. Patients were randomly assigned to receive AML or AML plus EMS. The study showed better muscle strength in the AML plus EMS group, but no clinical improvement [45]. The third study included in the review randomized sedated ICU patients who were on mechanical ventilation < 72 hours to exercise and mobilization versus therapy as ordered by the primary care team. The exercise and mobilization arm received passive range of motion (PROM), active range of motion (AROM), postural training, activities of daily living, bed mobility, sit up, sit to stand, gait training and early mobilization. This resulted in a significantly decreased duration of delirium, increase in ventilator-free days and increased functional independence [46]. The fourth study focused on patients with prolonged mechanical ventilation (> 14 days) and randomized patients to receive verbal encouragement for mobilization or limb strengthening, diaphragmatic exercises, bed mobility, transfers, standing and ambulation. The main result was that there was an increased functional independence in the exercise group versus the control group [47]. The last three trials randomized patients between standard medical care and physiotherapy or general physiotherapy with aerobic exercise. The aerobic exercise was an in-bed arm ergometer [48], a bedside cycle ergometer [49] and a bedside cycle ergometer and if possible treadmill walking [50]. All three trials showed an improvement in the endurance and exercise capacity of patients but did not include or show improvement in clinical outcomes. The exercise interventions that have been discussed are shown in Table 3.

Conclusion

The surgical stress response has a great impact on the human body. Pre-habilitation has been suggested to help the body overcome the adverse events of the surgical stress response, by arming the body with an extra physical reserve. To use the right kind of pre-habilitation a risk stratification tool should be adapted to predict the risk of surgery. Many parameters have been introduced to identify patients who are at-risk for the surgical intervention. Overall, it seems that the aerobic threshold is one of the strongest tools to identify surgical patients at high risk. Another effective tool, but unfortunately not validated in many of the trials, is the Timed Up and Go test. Exercise regimens have been examined in a wide range of patient groups. The group that has been most widely studied is cardiac surgery patients. Exercise regimens associated with the greatest improvements in clinical postoperative outcomes were inspiratory muscle training and aerobic exercise with an ergometer. Although strong links between the physical status of a patient and their illness have been shown in ICU patients, this is a difficult group on which to perform rehabilitation programs. There are preliminary signs that a full package of early physical therapy is beneficial to clinical outcome. In conclusion, critical illness is top sport. Like athletes training for a big competitive event, patients should train to undergo an illness event. Identification of the different patient groups and of optimal exercise regimens should be increasingly targeted by randomized trials.

References

1. Levett DZ, Fernandez BO, Riley HL et al (2011) The role of nitrogen oxides in human adaptation to hypoxia. Sci Rep 1:109
2. Edwards LM, Murray AJ, Tyler DJ et al (2010) The effect of high-altitude on human skeletal muscle energetics: P-MRS results from the Caudwell Xtreme Everest expedition. PLoS One 5:e10681
3. Siervo M, Riley HL, Fernandez BO et al (2014) Effects of prolonged exposure to hypobaric hypoxia on oxidative stress, inflammation and gluco-insular regulation: the not-so-sweet price for good regulation. PLoS One 9:e94915
4. Desborough JP (2000) The stress response to trauma and surgery. Br J Anaesth 85:109–117
5. van Rossen ME, Sluiter W, Bonthuis F, Jeekel H, Marquet RL, van Eijck CH (2000) Scavenging of reactive oxygen species leads to diminished peritoneal tumor recurrence. Cancer Res 60:5625–5629
6. Kehlet H (2011) Fast-track surgery-an update on physiological care principles to enhance recovery. Langenbecks Arch Surg 396:585–590
7. Jack S, West M, Grocott MP (2011) Perioperative exercise training in elderly subjects. Best Pract Res Clin Anaesthesiol 25:461–472
8. Carli F, Zavorsky GS (2005) Optimizing functional exercise capacity in the elderly surgical population. Curr Opin Clin Nutr Metab Care 8:23–32
9. Moonesinghe SR, Harris S, Mythen MG et al (2014) Survival after postoperative morbidity: a longitudinal observational cohort studydagger. Br J Anaesth 113:977–984
10. Epstein J, Breslow MJ (1999) The stress response of critical illness. Crit Care Clin 15:17–33
11. Santos L (2013) Stress response in critical illness. Curr Probl Pediatr Adolesc Health Care 43:264–272
12. Meyer T, Lucia A, Earnest CP, Kindermann W (2005) A conceptual framework for performance diagnosis and training prescription from submaximal gas exchange parameters–theory and application. Int J Sports Med 26 (Suppl 1):S38–S48
13. West MA, Lythgoe D, Barben CP et al (2014) Cardiopulmonary exercise variables are associated with postoperative morbidity after major colonic surgery: a prospective blinded observational study. Br J Anaesth 112:665–671
14. Older P, Smith R, Courtney P, Hone R (1993) Preoperative evaluation of cardiac failure and ischemia in elderly patients by cardiopulmonary exercise testing. Chest 104:701–704
15. Wilson RJ, Davies S, Yates D, Redman J, Stone M (2010) Impaired functional capacity is associated with all-cause mortality after major elective intra-abdominal surgery. Br J Anaesth 105:297–303
16. Snowden CP, Prentis JM, Anderson HL et al (2010) Submaximal cardiopulmonary exercise testing predicts complications and hospital length of stay in patients undergoing major elective surgery. Ann Surg 251:535–541
17. Hightower CE, Riedel BJ, Feig BW et al (2010) A pilot study evaluating predictors of postoperative outcomes after major abdominal surgery: Physiological capacity compared with the ASA physical status classification system. Br J Anaesth 104:465–471
18. Nagamatsu Y, Shima I, Yamana H, Fujita H, Shirouzu K, Ishitake T (2001) Preoperative evaluation of cardiopulmonary reserve with the use of expired gas analysis during exercise testing in patients with squamous cell carcinoma of the thoracic esophagus. J Thorac Cardiovasc Surg 121:1064–1068

19. Forshaw MJ, Strauss DC, Davies AR et al (2008) Is cardiopulmonary exercise testing a useful test before esophagectomy? Ann Thorac Surg 85:294–299
20. Benzo R, Kelley GA, Recchi L, Hofman A, Sciurba F (2007) Complications of lung resection and exercise capacity: a meta-analysis. Respir Med 101:1790–1797
21. Burke JR, Duarte IG, Thourani VH, Miller JI Jr (2003) Preoperative risk assessment for marginal patients requiring pulmonary resection. Ann Thorac Surg 76:1767–1773
22. Win T, Jackson A, Sharples L et al (2005) Cardiopulmonary exercise tests and lung cancer surgical outcome. Chest 127:1159–1165
23. Bolliger CT, Jordan P, Soler M et al (1995) Exercise capacity as a predictor of postoperative complications in lung resection candidates. Am J Respir Crit Care Med 151:1472–1480
24. Goodyear SJ, Yow H, Saedon M et al (2013) Risk stratification by pre-operative cardiopulmonary exercise testing improves outcomes following elective abdominal aortic aneurysm surgery: a cohort study. Perioper Med (Lond) 2:10
25. Thompson AR, Peters N, Lovegrove RE et al (2011) Cardiopulmonary exercise testing provides a predictive tool for early and late outcomes in abdominal aortic aneurysm patients. Ann R Coll Surg Engl 93:474–481
26. Becher G, Kinsella J (2007) Mid-term survival after abdominal aortic aneurysm surgery predicted by cardiopulmonary exercise testing. Br J Surg 94:966–969
27. Fleisher LA, Fleischmann KE, Auerbach AD et al (2014) 2014 ACC/AHA Guideline on Perioperative Cardiovascular Evaluation and Management of Patients Undergoing Noncardiac Surgery: A Report of the American College of Cardiology/American Heart Association Task Force on Practice Guidelines. J Am Coll Cardiol 64:e77–e137
28. Robinson TN, Wu DS, Sauaia A et al (2013) Slower walking speed forecasts increased postoperative morbidity and 1-year mortality across surgical specialties. Ann Surg 258:582–590
29. Carli F, Charlebois P, Stein B et al (2010) Randomized clinical trial of prehabilitation in colorectal surgery. Br J Surg 97:1187–1197
30. Dronkers JJ, Lamberts H, Reutelingsperger IM et al (2010) Preoperative therapeutic programme for elderly patients scheduled for elective abdominal oncological surgery: a randomized controlled pilot study. Clin Rehabil 24:614–622
31. Dronkers J, Veldman A, Hoberg E, van der Waal C, van Meeteren N (2008) Prevention of pulmonary complications after upper abdominal surgery by preoperative intensive inspiratory muscle training: a randomized controlled pilot study. Clin Rehabil 22:134–142
32. Hulzebos EH, Smit Y, Helders PP, van Meeteren NL (2012) Preoperative physical therapy for elective cardiac surgery patients. Cochrane Database Syst Rev 11:CD010118
33. Arthur HM, Daniels C, McKelvie R, Hirsh J, Rush B (2000) Effect of a preoperative intervention on preoperative and postoperative outcomes in low-risk patients awaiting elective coronary artery bypass graft surgery. A randomized, controlled trial. Ann Intern Med 133:253–262
34. Rosenfeldt F, Braun L, Spitzer O et al (2011) Physical conditioning and mental stress reduction–a randomised trial in patients undergoing cardiac surgery. BMC Complement Altern Med 11:20
35. Rajendran AJ, Pandurangi UM, Murali R, Gomathi S, Vijayan VK, Cherian KM (1998) Preoperative short-term pulmonary rehabilitation for patients of chronic obstructive pulmonary disease undergoing coronary artery bypass graft surgery. Indian Heart J 50:531–534
36. Carvalho T, Bonorino KC, Panigas TF (2011) Preoperative respiratory muscle training reduces complications in coronary artery bypass surgery. Eur Heart J 32:P2309 (abst)
37. Hulzebos EH, van Meeteren NL, van den Buijs BJ, de Bie RJ, Brutel de la Riviere A, Helders PJ (2006) Feasibility of preoperative inspiratory muscle training in patients undergoing coronary artery bypass surgery with a high risk of postoperative pulmonary complications: a randomized controlled pilot study. Clin Rehabil 20:949–959
38. Hulzebos EH, Helders PJ, Favie NJ, De Bie RA, Brutel de la Riviere A, Van Meeteren NL (2006) Preoperative intensive inspiratory muscle training to prevent postoperative pulmonary complications in high-risk patients undergoing CABG surgery: a randomized clinical trial. JAMA 296:1851–1857

39. Weiner P, Zeidan F, Zamir D et al (1998) Prophylactic inspiratory muscle training in patients undergoing coronary artery bypass graft. World J Surg 22:427–431
40. Ferreira PE, Rodrigues AJ, Evora PR (2009) Effects of an inspiratory muscle rehabilitation program in the postoperative period of cardiac surgery. Arq Bras Cardiol 92:275–282
41. Desai SV, Law TJ, Needham DM (2011) Long-term complications of critical care. Crit Care Med 39:371–379
42. Benington S, McWilliams D, Eddleston J, Atkinson D (2012) Exercise testing in survivors of intensive care–is there a role for cardiopulmonary exercise testing? J Crit Care 27:89–94
43. Kayambu G, Boots R, Paratz J (2013) Physical therapy for the critically ill in the ICU: a systematic review and meta-analysis. Crit Care Med 41:1543–1554
44. Routsi C, Gerovasili V, Vasileiadis I et al (2010) Electrical muscle stimulation prevents critical illness polyneuromyopathy: a randomized parallel intervention trial. Crit Care 14:R74
45. Zanotti E, Felicetti G, Maini M, Fracchia C (2003) Peripheral muscle strength training in bed-bound patients with COPD receiving mechanical ventilation: effect of electrical stimulation. Chest 124:292–296
46. Schweickert WD, Pohlman MC, Pohlman AS et al (2009) Early physical and occupational therapy in mechanically ventilated, critically ill patients: a randomised controlled trial. Lancet 373:1874–1882
47. Chiang LL, Wang LY, Wu CP, Wu HD, Wu YT (2006) Effects of physical training on functional status in patients with prolonged mechanical ventilation. Phys Ther 86:1271–1281
48. Porta R, Vitacca M, Gile LS et al (2005) Supported arm training in patients recently weaned from mechanical ventilation. Chest 128:2511–2520
49. Burtin C, Clerckx B, Robbeets C et al (2009) Early exercise in critically ill patients enhances short-term functional recovery. Crit Care Med 37:2499–2505
50. Nava S (1998) Rehabilitation of patients admitted to a respiratory intensive care unit. Arch Phys Med Rehabil 79:849–854

Part XIII
Rapid Response Teams

Vital Signs: From Monitoring to Prevention of Deterioration in General Wards

M. Cardona-Morrell, M. Nicholson, and K. Hillman

Introduction

Vital sign measurement is at the core of our care for hospitalized patients. Together with other observations, such as seizures, airway obstruction or a decrease in the level of consciousness, changes in vital signs can describe patients who are at serious risk of deterioration [1]. They form the basis of the criteria for medical emergency teams (METs) or, as they are also known, rapid response systems [1]. Sudden or gradual changes in vital signs can indicate life-threatening clinical states requiring urgent intervention and sometimes triage to a higher level of care. Interestingly, patients in an intensive care environment rarely die or have a cardiac arrest unexpectedly. The majority of deaths are as a result of withdrawing and/or withholding active management [2]. The reason is simple: Patients in intensive care are continuously monitored and are under the care of well-trained staff. Rapid response systems can now provide an urgent response by appropriately trained staff outside the intensive care unit (ICU) setting. However, general ward staff must be able to identify patients who are at-risk and, when appropriate, escalate care [3]. This is difficult when patients on general wards are monitored intermittently in much the same way they have been for over a century. Much can happen to a patient's clinical state in the hours between vital sign recordings, often taken at 8 to 24-hour intervals. Unfortunately this low frequency of observations has little or no evidence base and may be inappropriate, especially for the current hospital population, which is older, more vulnerable as a result of chronic illness, and is having more complex

M. Cardona-Morrell ✉
South Western Sydney Clinical School, University of New South Wales, Sydney, Australia
e-mail: m.cardona-morrell@unsw.edu.au

M. Nicholson
Intensive Care Unit, Liverpool Hospital, Sydney, Australia

K. Hillman
South Western Sydney Clinical School, University of New South Wales, Sydney, Australia
Intensive Care Unit, Liverpool Hospital, Sydney, Australia

J.-L. Vincent (ed.), *Annual Update in Intensive Care and Emergency Medicine 2015*,
DOI 10.1007/978-3-319-13761-2_39

procedures with higher rates of complications. The frequency of vital sign observations has been based on tradition, [4] and usually is not changed unless obvious deterioration is detected or higher frequency is recommended by doctors [5].

In this chapter, we describe the history of vital signs monitoring as a routine part of hospital care; discuss implications for identifying and managing patient deterioration; broadly summarize technological options for more accurate or frequent observations; and propose additional roles for ICU staff in preventing escalation of care on the general ward and subsequent unplanned ICU admissions.

History of Vital Signs Monitoring

The history of monitoring of vital signs in health services illustrates that it took centuries to evolve from a physician-dominated duty of manually checking parameters to the routine nurse-led multi-parameter activity we take for granted today, spanning ancient times to the early 20th century (Fig. 1); and how new parameters and technology were progressively introduced to improve the quality of hospital care. Four parameters: Pulse, temperature, respiratory rate and blood pressure constitute the minimal set used since the beginning of the 20th century.

Today's routine suite of vital signs in ward care includes the 'core' four, along with level of consciousness and, sometimes, pulse oximetry [6]. On some wards, this is supplemented with other clinical observations, such as spirometry, urinary output, pain levels and seizures, which may indicate deterioration [7], although their addition was based on limited research or expert opinion rather than high level evidence of effectiveness [8].

Despite technological advances, the measurement of some vital signs, such as respiratory rate, still exhibits poor inter-rater reliability [9], whether measured manually or electronically [10]. Although oxygen saturation monitoring with pulse oximetry is convenient and reduces the need for frequent arterial gas tests, there is evidence that it can be misleading in the presence of deficient peripheral perfusion and anemia [7]. Nonetheless, the importance of monitoring vital signs has been well established as confirmation of serious illness or physiological derange-

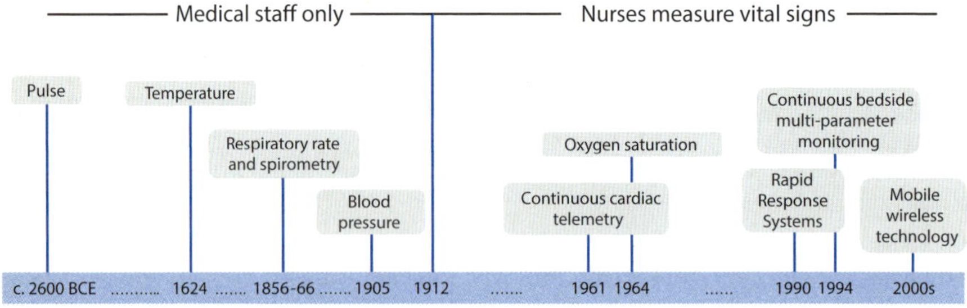

Fig. 1 Illustrated history of vital signs monitoring

ment and continues to be essential in the prediction of poor patient outcomes during hospitalization [3, 6].

Bedside continuous monitoring of heart rate and electrocardiogram (EKG) was introduced over 50 years ago, mainly in coronary care units (CCU), followed by pulse oximetry in the 1970s for monitoring in operating rooms and ICUs, and to monitor progress in chronic respiratory disease wards. Pulse oximetry is now used in the general wards of hospitals. Measures of level of consciousness, such as the Glasgow Coma Scale score, and indicators of urinary output were added later. In environments such as ICUs, continuous monitoring has been used since the 1960s, often employing invasive techniques, such as blood pressure monitoring using arterial lines, central venous pressures, monitoring of intracranial pressures and intra-abdominal pressures. [11]

More recently, non-invasive devices with sensors for multiple concurrent parameters, display monitors, wireless communications, automated early warning scoring and clinical decision support tools are being developed and refined. Conceivably, these will provide safer care and save time in clinical response to changes in vital signs. It is early days and their accuracy in identifying instability, or demonstrating cost-effectiveness, is yet to be determined or verified.

Evolution of Hospitals

It is not surprising that with the evolution of medical technology, societal expectation and demand for access to life-prolonging care has also grown. Consequently hospitals now admit older and more complex patients receiving concurrent management by several specialists, unintentionally increasing the need for higher levels of critical care skills on general wards [12]. Hospital resources for rapid response to deterioration have not necessarily increased with demand [13]. Despite the increased workload associated with caring for more complex patients, there has not been an increase in staff/patient ratios, particularly at night and on weekends, with the obvious consequence of reduction in the quality and frequency of vital signs recording and ability to respond to their changes. Respiratory rate and temperature are most often overlooked [14], even in the resuscitation room [15]. Pulse and blood pressure measurement are also commonly reported as not being recorded in 50% of cases within the 8–24 hours prior to an 'unexpected' adverse event, such as death, cardiac arrest or admission to the ICU [16]. Elderly and postoperative patients on general wards may have seemingly less dangerous vital sign profiles and symptoms but because of their increased vulnerability the signs may not always reflect the seriousness of their illness [17]. A higher level of awareness may be necessary for these patients.

Impact of Low Frequency and Poor Quality Vital Signs Monitoring

The main concern stemming from inappropriate frequency, incompleteness or absence of vital signs monitoring is the failure to detect the deteriorating patient [5] and the delay of definitive resuscitation [1]. Physiological changes and compensatory mechanisms can go undetected if observations are inconsistently taken or interpreted without considering the individual patient context, i. e., not taking into account age, underlying comorbidities, medication regimens [18], oxygen therapy, frailty or mental status [17]. To enhance this recognition, consensus has been reached on the core signs and symptoms necessary to trigger an urgent response to patients on general wards [6].

The 'calling criteria' for triggering a rapid response system generally consist of a hospital-wide standardized list of vital sign thresholds for all patients, for example an oxygen saturation < 90%, a respiratory rate of > 36, a heart rate of < 40, or systolic blood pressure of < 90 mmHg [16]. The concept of using severe vital sign abnormalities for triggering an urgent rapid response system call is widely accepted. Within the overall concept there are many minor variations on the thresholds across different countries and even within hospitals in the same country [19]. Awareness that increased monitoring may impose an increased workload on already busy staff [20] has led to multiple investigations on the use and effect of continuous monitoring technology including bedside, mobile, patient-worn, wired and wireless devices.

It is surprising that after more than a century of using vital sign monitoring in acute hospitals there is little research or sound evidence as to the most appropriate ways of measuring vital signs, nor the frequency at which the signs should be measured [21].

Many versions of 'standard' frequencies of observations for stable patients are used in hospital policies. The frequency of vital signs monitoring ranges from every 15 minutes to every 30 minutes during blood transfusions; 4 hourly following surgery [3]; to 3 times per day on general wards [5]; and down to once daily in stable patients after several days of hospitalization [22]. These frequencies may be based on nursing discretion but almost always are historically determined by 'custom' or pre-existing policy without evidence [3, 8].

A logical argument is that recommendations on frequency of observations are best decided on the basis of the individual patient's diagnosis and disease stage, acuity of underlying conditions, intensity of treatment currently administered and overall assessment of health status [18]. While this may be underpinned by logic, there is little in the way of evidence-based guidelines to make it of any practical use in the clinical situation. The tradition of monitoring based on administrative hospital policy is probably not safe or consistent with the patients' clinical needs. The implementation of rapid response systems in the early 1990s prompted an examination of the underlying purpose for measuring vital signs, and the frequency needed, to safely detect seriously ill and deteriorating patients [16].

Detecting Deteriorating Patients on the General Floors of Hospitals: Rapid Response Systems

It has long been recognized that increasing signs and symptoms of instability, such as hypotension and a fall in level of consciousness, precedes 'unexpected' cardiac arrests by several hours [23]. It follows that responding early to these patients with appropriately skilled clinicians makes sense [6]. The rapid response system was established to close the disconnection between monitoring and action. The failure to seek urgent assistance is related to entrenched professional chains of command in hospitals, where, for example, junior nurses at the frontline of observation-taking are not empowered to initiate remedial action or request higher-level consultations from staff with appropriate skills and experience. The past two decades have seen a proliferation of rapid response system teams, and a variety of models has been employed to suit local needs and resources.

The physician-led MET is widespread in Australia and operates 24/7. The team usually consists of ICU medical and nursing staff with appropriate expertise in resuscitation. There are variations in team composition that may impact on response appropriateness and outcomes [24].

The nurse-led Critical Care Outreach model is prevalent in the UK [25] and New Zealand [26], and operates either on a part-time or 24-hour basis. Nurses with high dependency and intensive care experience play a key role in supporting ward staff in patient physical assessment, including adjusting the frequency of vital sign measurement, advising medical staff on changes to medication, titration of oxygen therapy and tracheostomy for patients discharged from the ICU [25, 26].

In the US, the Rapid Response Team can usually be triggered by any health worker, bypassing the typical hierarchy [27]. The composition of the rapid response team varies but often comprises an intensivist or physician assistant and an ICU nurse. Their functions are mainly rapid assessment and critical intervention and often operate in parallel with the Blue Code team, which is still called for cardiac arrests.

The concept of a rapid response system makes intuitive sense and is widely implemented around the world [1]. However, a decade after the first description of the concept, a large multicenter study reported that half of all deaths, cardiac arrests and ICU admissions of inpatients still did not have vital sign measurements documented within the 24 hours before the event [16]. As recently as three years ago, patients with vital signs derangement in the 24 hours prior to an adverse event did not receive rapid response team attendance because nurses failed to recognize deterioration or did not adhere to the early call for response [21]. Low frequency of observations [5], poor knowledge of the meaning of signs and symptoms of instability, inability to identify vital sign trends and failure to seek advice are largely responsible for these avoidable sequelae.

The burden of undetected deterioration on general wards continues to be experienced at all levels of hospital care [28]. At the same time, the annual numbers of rapid response system attendances have escalated over the years, which may or may not be effectively funded. Associated with the lack of adequate funding may be poor availability of specialized assistance [29] and a low capacity for nurses and junior medical staff to respond to an emergency on the wards.

Approximately one in ten serious incidents in UK hospitals are related to three aspects of patient deterioration, potentially remedied through staff education [30]:

- prolonged periods where no vital observations are checked and, therefore, changes in a patient's vital signs go undetected;
- lack of recognition of the signs of deterioration and/or lack of response other than recording of observations, without regard to crossing of vital sign thresholds or trends indicating deterioration;
- delays in the provision of medical care, despite deterioration being detected and recognized.

Rapid Response System Achievements and Departures from the Original Purpose

The introduction of rapid response teams meant that nursing staff could summon help by trained clinicians at any time without being subject to historical and cultural imperatives [13]. Prior to this, a Code Blue team could be called only after the patient's heart had stopped or when breathing ceased. Under that system, nurses could only document the patient's condition while they slowly died. Essentially, the historical nature of the way hospitals operated trumped patient care. There was a dangerous disconnect between nurses documenting vital signs and the triggering of an appropriate response. When there was a response, it was often hierarchical, with attending staff not formally trained in the care of the seriously ill. With the introduction of the MET/rapid response team, nurses could call for assistance using predetermined calling criteria or when they were worried about a patient in their care even if the patient had not formally met the calling criteria [31]. As a result, nurses were empowered to be genuine advocates for their patients.

The implementation of an organization-wide deteriorating patient response system has uncovered other deficits in the way hospitals operate. For example, almost one third of all rapid response system calls were for patients with end of life issues [32]. This means that clinicians in acute hospitals often have difficulty in distinguishing those dying patients with little or no chance of recovery from those dying unnecessarily. Becoming the surrogate end-of-life team was not one of the planned functions of the rapid response system. Just as the function of a rapid response system is to empower nursing staff to prevent deterioration, the system also allows clinicians to care for patients at the end of life in a more appropriate way [33].

The evidence for effectiveness of the MET/rapid response team in reducing mortality has been mixed [1]. A meta-analysis of 11 adult studies in 2010 [34] indicated a decline in the relative risk for cardiopulmonary arrests in half the studies but only two studies found significant reductions in overall in-hospital mortality. The Medical Early Response, Intervention and Therapy (MERIT) study did not show improvement in rates of cardiac arrest or unplanned ICU admission [16], but did demonstrate a reduction in fatality rates in those hospitals with an MET system [35]. Another study, of over 80 hospitals, showed a significant reduction in cardiac arrest and mortality rates as hospitals implemented rapid response systems [36]. The same study reported that improvements in mortality from hospital cardiac arrest rates were related to their prevention and not to improvements in cardiopulmonary resuscitation (CPR) techniques. It has been postulated that further improvements may not be possible [37], and that greater impacts cannot be expected unless continuous monitoring also becomes integral to ward care [38].

Review of the Evidence for More Frequent or Continuous Monitoring

The measurement of vital signs on the general wards of acute hospitals is still mainly performed and entered manually. Even when there is an electronic patient record system, vital sign data are still based mainly on manual measurement. The change in frequency of vital sign measurement usually follows medical recommendation but often is up to the discretion of individual nurses at the bedside. However, nurses are still largely confined to measuring and recording vital signs, not trained to interpret or empowered to act on them [39].

The next steps in the operation of rapid response systems will probably involve improvement in the way we monitor patients on the general ward. This may involve the use of innovative technology to assist usual ward care in documenting trends, identifying pre-defined abnormalities, alerting staff, and issuing clinical decision support prompts. It is early days as yet and the available evidence is mostly based on small sample sizes and on study designs at the lower level of the evidence pyramid, as seen in the examples in Table 1.

Current research and development includes evaluation of continuous or more frequently measured intermittent monitoring at the bedside. Other options have used mobile monitoring devices, both wired or wireless versions. Some incorporate warning scores or clinical decision prompts, which have the potential to add performance value to ward care, especially in busy and understaffed hospitals. Their error rates, cost-effectiveness and alarm burden for patient and staff are yet to be determined. Obviously, e-monitoring does not substitute for the skills and clinical assessment conducted by trained staff, such as examination of a patient's level of consciousness, urinary output or cognitive status [6]. Instead, they are aimed at complementing the clinical skills of bedside nursing staff and improving patient care.

Table 1 Selected examples of electronic approaches to continuous vital signs monitoring

Technology functionality and study type	Findings	Author/date
Retrospective review of vital signs using a PDA with bar-code technology enabling wireless capture and transmission of data directly from the vital sign monitor into the EMR	The system reduced documentation error rate to less than 1% through automated capture and data upload	Smith et al. 2009 [48]
Observational study comparing a clinical documentation system with "computers on wheels" workstation outside the patient's room, and a clinical documentation system with a Tablet PC affixed to the vital signs monitor versus usual paper-based recording of observations	Providing care technicians with a Tablet PC affixed to the vital signs monitor can improve timeliness and quality of documentation	Wager et al. 2010 [49]
Study of bedside electronic recording of patient observations, with historical controls, linked to a computer system that calculates patient risk and then issues automatic graded alerts	The system can improve clinical attendance to general medical ward patients with critical early warning scores and reduce length of hospital stay	Jones et al. 2011 [47]
Controlled trial of automated advisory vital signs monitors to assist in the acquisition of vital signs and calculation of early warning scores on general wards	Use of this technology was associated with improved RRS team calls triggered by respiratory criteria, increased survival of patients receiving RRS services, and decreased time required for vital signs measurement and recording	Bellomo et al. 2012 [46]
Non-interventional prospective study with retrospective data analysis of an innovative monitoring device under the patient's mattress	Continuous monitoring of RR and HR provides low alert frequency and is theoretically promising in accurately predicting patient deterioration	Zimlichman et al. 2012 [50]

PDA: palm-held digital assistant; EMR: electronic medical record; RR: respiratory rate; HR: heart rate; RRS: rapid response system.

Implications for Practice

Variations have been noted in the reproducibility and effectiveness of early-warning scores for different outcomes in various settings, and research on post-discharge survival for recipients of rapid response system responses is not as yet available. A recent ecological study of a decade of hospital fatality rates does suggest that the gradual uptake of rapid response systems is associated with a reduction in in-hospital cardiac arrest and hospital fatality overall [36]. While not all saved lives can be attributed directly to the rapid response system actions, the mortality decline may have been related to increased staff awareness of deterioration resulting in better management and less need to activate the rapid response system. Likewise in the US, this down-trend in-hospital mortality was also observed for several years before the introduction of rapid response systems, so the decline could not be unambiguously attributed to the introduction of rapid response systems [40]. Thus rapid response systems appear to have evolved as a formalized implementation and extension of this awareness. Unfortunately, due to the high uptake of rapid response systems, it would be difficult to design randomized controlled trials to compare effects of rapid response system intervention to no rapid response system intervention.

Two decades after the introduction of the first organized rapid response system, many lessons have been learnt about how a rapid response system has empowered general ward staff to challenge the doctor-nurse divide when instability is recognized [13]. Calling the admitting team even earlier in an attempt to reduce the number of rapid response calls has had no beneficial effect [37]. In an era of increasing specialization it would be difficult, and extremely expensive, to train all members of the admitting teams in skills, such as tracheal intubation, ventilation and central venous cannulation. Moreover, even if the techniques and associated knowledge were taught, they would need to be used on a regular basis to maintain those skills. Furthermore, ongoing educational activities would be required to incorporate recent advances in acute medicine and resuscitation technique. Just as intensivists may have diminishing skills in performing surgery or diagnosing dermatological disorders, the staff on the general wards of hospitals will never be able to maintain the knowledge, skills and experience of those who have undergone formal training and are continuously working in that area. However, it is crucial that the admitting team and general ward nursing staff understand the importance of vital signs, that they recognize at-risk patients early and are able to trigger an immediate response by appropriate staff to care for their patient [41].

As yet, there is no general agreement on the exact sensitivity and specificity of the calling criteria. It could be that the exact numbers, or thresholds, are less important than the fact that the rapid response system has changed the culture of an organization to one of increased awareness that there are seriously ill patients in a hospital and that urgent assistance is available at all times. However, there may be a need to adjust the thresholds according to the clinical context. For example, patients with chronic respiratory failure often have low oxygen saturation ($SatO_2$), even when in the community. The $SatO_2$ levels consequently would need to be adjusted for those patients to prevent alarm fatigue. Patients with traumatic brain injury (TBI) may need readjusting of systolic blood pressure alarms to higher levels to prevent secondary brain insults, as traditional targets of <90 mmHg may fail to prevent these adverse events [42]. There may be other examples where staff need to adjust calling criteria according to clinical context, such as patients on beta-blockers but there is no evidence that multiple versions of charts or software programs to calculate risk improve the process or outcome.

The important factor is the cultural change to a more rational and planned approach to escalation of care where appropriate [13]. Changing hospital culture is a slow process that must include the combined efforts of hospital policy supporting the culture change; a comprehensive educational program; managers supporting and coordinating the support and funding for the implementation and maintenance of an effective RRS; and the use of relevant outcome indicators to monitor the effectiveness of the system as a basis for continuous improvement activities [1].

Future Directions

As well as triggering an urgent response to seriously ill patients, the concept of a rapid response system has facilitated the use of nursing staff, often with intensive care experience, to work with ward nurses to increase their awareness of at-risk patients. One such system is the outreach program. Intensive care personnel can play a role in supporting ward staff by facilitating ICU discharge and follow up instructions to prevent ICU re-admission [43]. The practice of thorough ICU discharge planning with a focus on communication is fundamental to the care to be provided in the less resourced environment of general wards [44]. This is particularly relevant for elderly patients who experience recurrent clinical deterioration episodes in general wards and consequent repeat emergency team activations [45]. Detailed communication between the two environments is intuitively important to prevent subsequent unexpected adverse events.

Vital signs are increasingly being used to identify not only patients who are deteriorating with an underlying potentially preventable cause, but also patients who are at the end of life who need to be managed in a more appropriate way [32]. The implementation of rapid response systems could facilitate more appropriate ways of identifying and managing these patients. Vital signs could be used together with other information, such as age, level of frailty and underlying clinical condition to identify patients at the end of life earlier as a basis for a more appropriate care pathway. It also appears inevitable that patients in hospital general wards will require more advanced ways of monitoring vital signs to enable more timely detection of instability. The variety and scope of automated non-invasive systems being developed is increasing rapidly [46–50]. However, before any widespread implementation occurs it is important that future research and evaluation builds evidence of their clinical effectiveness, workload burden and cost-effectiveness. Hospitals would welcome new and more intensive ways of monitoring if evidence demonstrates that those tools improve patient care over and above what clinicians are already achieving with the intermittent monitoring and rapid response systems.

Conclusion

The long-standing practice of vital signs measurement is at the heart of caring for hospitalized patients. However, we have much to learn about the most appropriate measures and the frequency with which we should be measuring them. Nor do we have adequate awareness of the contexts in which we make these measurements and their variations according to the type of patient. Perhaps, as in operating rooms, emergency departments and ICUs, we will need to continuously monitor all patients in an acute hospital as we can never be sure which patients will suffer a life-threatening adverse event. This argument is stronger when we consider the changing nature of a hospital's population over the last 20 years. Patients are now older, with more co-morbidities and are undergoing more complex procedures. As a result of empowering them, ward nurses may be more actively involved in developing escalation policies and education initiatives. Further evaluation of accuracy, efficacy, timeliness of alarms and determining the cost-effectiveness of improved general ward monitoring should be integral to its deployment in general wards. A combined approach of training and technological assistance with more frequent automated monitoring may have potential to greatly improve patient safety in our hospitals.

References

1. Jones DA, DeVita MA, Bellomo R (2011) Rapid-response teams. N Engl J Med 365:139–146
2. Seymour JE (2000) Negotiating natural death in intensive care. Soc Sci Med 51:1241–1252
3. Lockwood C, Conroy-Hiller T, Page T (2004) Vital signs. Systematic review. JBI Reports 2:207–230
4. Zeitz K, McCutcheon H (2006) Observations and vital signs: ritual or vital for the monitoring of postoperative patients? Appl Nurs Res 19:204–211
5. Van Leuvan CH, Mitchell I (2008) Missed opportunities? An observational study of vital sign measurements. Crit Care Resusc 10:111–115
6. DeVita MA, Smith GB, Adam SK et al (2010) Identifying the hospitalised patient in crisis – A consensus conference on the afferent limb of Rapid Response Systems. Resusc 81:375–382
7. Elliott M, Coventry A (2012) Critical care: the eight vital signs of patient monitoring. Br J Nurs 21:621–625
8. Evans D, Hodgkinson B, Berry J (2001) Vital signs in hospital patients: a systematic review. Int J Nurs Studies 38:643–650
9. Edmonds ZV, Mower WR, Lovato LM, Lomeli R (2002) The reliability of vital sign measurements. Ann Emerg Med 39:233–237
10. Lovett PB, Buchwald JM, Sturmann K, Bijur P (2005) The vexatious vital: neither clinical measurements by nurses nor an electronic monitor provides accurate measurements of respiratory rate in triage. Ann Emerg Med 45:68–76
11. Puri N, Puri V, Dellinger RP (2009) History of technology in the intensive care unit. Crit Care Clin 1:185–200
12. Massey D, Aitken LM, Chaboyer W (2009) What factors influence suboptimal ward care in the acutely ill ward patient? Intensive Crit Care Nurs 25:169–180
13. Benin AL, Borgstrom CP, Jenq GY, Roumanis SA, Horwitz LI (2012) Defining impact of a rapid response team: qualitative study with nurses, physicians and hospital administrators. BMJ Qual Saf 21:391–398
14. Cretikos MA, Bellomo R, Hillman K, Chen J, Finfer S, Flabouris A (2008) Respiratory rate: the neglected vital sign. Med J Aust 188:657–659
15. Smith JJ, Bland SA, Mullett S (2005) Temperature – the forgotten vital sign. Accid Emerg Nurs 13:247–250
16. Hillman K, Chen J, Cretikos M et al (2005) Introduction of the medical emergency team (MET) system: a cluster-randomised controlled trial. Lancet 24:2091–2097
17. Wolf L (2007) How normal are "normal vital signs"? Effective triage of the older patient. J Emerg Nurs 33(6):587–589
18. Schulman CS, Staul L (2010) Standards for frequency of measurement and documentation of vital signs and physical assessments. Critical Care Nurse 30:74–76
19. Hravnak M, Devita MA, Clontz A, Edwards L, Valenta C, Pinsky MR (2011) Cardiorespiratory instability before and after implementing an integrated monitoring system. Crit Care Med 39:65–72
20. Cox H, James J, Hunt J (2006) The experiences of trained nurses caring for critically ill patients within a general ward setting. Intensive Crit Care Nurs 22:283–293

21. De Meester K, van Bogaert P, Clarke PS, Bossaert L (2013) In-hospital mortality after serious adverse events on medical and surgical nursing units: a mixed methods study. J Clin Nursing 22:2308–2317
22. New South Wales Health Ministry, Clinical Excellence Commission (2013) Recognition and Management of Patients who are Clinically Deteriorating – Policy Directive. http://www0.health.nsw.gov.au/policies/pd/2013/pdf/PD2013_049.pdf. Accessed Nov 2014
23. Kause J, Smith G, Prytherch D, Parr M, Flabouris A, Hillman K (2004) A comparison of antecedents to cardiac arrests, deaths and emergency intensive care admissions in Australia and New Zealand, and the United Kingdom – the ACADEMIA study. Resuscitation 62:275–282
24. ANZICS-CORE dose Investigators (2012) Rapid Response Team composition, resourcing and calling criteria in Australia. Resusc 83:563–567
25. Marsh S, Pittard A (2012) Outreach: 'the past, present, and future'. Contin Educ Anaesth Crit Care Pain 12:78–81
26. Pedersen A, Psirides A, Coombs M (2015) Models and activities of critical care outreach in New Zealand hospitals: results of a national census. Nurs Crit Care (in press)
27. Gould D (2007) Promoting patient safety: The rapid medical response team. T Perm J 11:26–34
28. Donaldson LJ, Panesar SS, Darzi A (2014) Patient-safety-related hospital deaths in England: thematic analysis of incidents reported to a national database, 2010–2012. PLoS Med 11:e1001667
29. National Patient Safety Agency, Thomson R, Luettel D, Healey F, Scobie S (2007) Safer care for the acutely ill patient: learning from serious incidents. http://psnet.ahrq.gov/resource.aspx?resourceID=6065. Accessed September 2014
30. NHS National Patient Safety Agency (2007) Recognising and responding appropriately to early signs of deterioration in hospitalised patients. http://www.nrls.npsa.nhs.uk/resources/?entryid45=59834. Accessed September 2014
31. Santiano N, Young L, Hillman K et al (2009) Analysis of Medical Emergency Team calls comparing subjective to "objective" call criteria. Resuscutation 80:44–49
32. Jones D, Moran J, Winters B, Welch J (2013) The rapid response system and end-of-life care. Curr Opin Crit Care 19:616–623
33. Hillman KM (2014) Failure to recognise patients at the end of life in acute hospitals. Acta Anaesthesiol Scand 58:1–2
34. Chan PS, Jain R, Nallmothu BK, Berg RA, Sasson C (2010) Rapid response teams: A systematic review and meta-analysis. Arch Intern Med 170:18–26
35. Chen J, Bellomo R, Flabouris A, Hillman K, Finfer S, Study Investigators (2009) The relationship between early emergency team calls and serious adverse events. Crit Care Med 37:148–153
36. Chen J, Ou L, Hillman KM et al (2014) Cardiopulmonary arrest and mortality trends, and their association with rapid response system expansion. Med J Aust 201:167–170
37. Herod R, Frost SA, Parr M, Hillman K, Aneman A (2014) Long term trends in medical emergency team activations and outcomes. Resuscitation 85:1083–1087
38. Sarani B (2014) Identifying the ICU recidivist in the hospital. Crit Care Med 42(7):1725–1726
39. Odell M, Victor C, Oliver D (2009) Nurses' role in detecting deterioration in ward patients: systematic literature review. J Adv Nurs 65:1992–2006
40. Salvatierra G, Bindler RC, Corbett C, Roll J, Daratha KB (2014) Rapid response team implementation and in-hospital mortality. Crit Care Med 42:2001–2006
41. Nurmi J, Harjola VP, Nolan J, Castrén M (2005) Observations and warning signs prior to cardiac arrest. Should a medical emergency team intervene earlier? Acta Anaesthesiol Scand 49:702–706
42. Brenner M, Stein DM, Hu PF, Aarabi B, Sheth K, Scalea TM (2012) Traditional systolic blood pressure targets underestimate hypotension-induced secondary brain injury. J Trauma Acute Care Surg 72:1135–1139

43. Odell M, Adam S (2011) Critical care outreach. In: Nimmo GR, Singer M (eds) ABC of Intensive Care, 2nd edn. ABC Series, vol 180. John Wiley & Sons, Chichester, pp 66–70
44. Cognet S, Coyer F (2014) Discharge practices for the intensive care patient: A qualitative exploration in the general ward setting. Intensive Crit Care Nurs 30:292–300
45. Stelfox HT, Bagshaw SM, Gao S (2014) Characteristics and outcomes for hospitalized patients with recurrent clinical deterioration and repeat medical emergency team activation. Crit Care Med 42:1601–1609
46. Bellomo R, Ackerman M, Bailey M et al (2012) A controlled trial of electronic automated advisory vital signs monitoring in general hospital wards. Crit Care Med 40:2349–2361
47. Jones S, Mullally M, Ingleby S, Buist M, Bailey M, Eddleston JM (2011) Bedside electronic capture of clinical observations and automated clinical alerts to improve compliance with an Early Warning Score protocol. Crit Care Resusc 13:83–88
48. Smith LB, Banner L, Lozano D, Olney CM, Friedman B (2009) Connected care: reducing errors through automated vital signs data upload. Comput Inform Nurs 27:318–323
49. Wager KA, Schaffner MJ, Foulois B, Swanson Kazley A, Parker C, Walo H (2010) Comparison of the quality and timeliness of vital signs data using three different data-entry devices. Comput Inform Nurs 28:205–212
50. Zimlichman E, Szyper-Kravitz M, Shinar Z et al (2012) Early recognition of acutely deteriorating patients in non-intensive care units: assessment of an innovative monitoring technology. J Hosp Med 7:628–633

Rapid Response Systems: Are they Really Effective?

C. Sandroni, S. D'Arrigo, and M. Antonelli

Introduction

Despite the immediate availability of qualified life support, the outcome of in-hospital cardiac arrest (IHCA) remains poor, with survival to discharge rarely exceeding 20% [1]. However, more than half of all cardiopulmonary arrests are preceded by deterioration in vital signs [2, 3], which are often not appropriately evaluated, suggesting that many of these adverse events could be prevented by early identification and treatment [4].

In-hospital rapid response systems have been established to manage unstable patients in general wards, with the aim of preventing further deterioration leading to cardiac arrest [5]. Implementation of a rapid response system includes education of the ward staff (the afferent limb of the system) to systematically detect signs of physiological instability and identify patients needing urgent evaluation by a medical emergency team (MET). The MET (the efferent limb of the system) includes medical doctors and/or nurses experienced in management of critical patients; it is activated by ward staff in patients fulfilling specific criteria or in response to staff concerns, and its roles are to stabilize the patient in the ward or move the patient to a higher level of care.

Although the theory underlying MET systems is compelling, there is no definite evidence that their implementation improves patient outcome [6]. In effect, whereas a series of before-and-after, single center studies demonstrated benefit, the only multicenter randomized trial (RCT) conducted so far, the Medical Emergency Response, Intervention and Therapy (MERIT) study [7], did not show any significant change in the composite outcome of cardiac arrest, unexpected death, or unplanned intensive care unit (ICU) admission in the hospitals where MET was implemented. This and other results [6] have raised questions about the effectiveness of rapid response systems.

C. Sandroni · S. D'Arrigo · M. Antonelli ✉
Department of Anaesthesiology and Intensive Care, A. Gemelli University Hospital, Catholic University of the Sacred Heart, Rome, Italy
e-mail: m.antonelli@rm.unicatt.it

J.-L. Vincent (ed.), *Annual Update in Intensive Care and Emergency Medicine 2015*,
DOI 10.1007/978-3-319-13761-2_40

Table 1 Characteristics of interventional studies on rapid response systems

Author, year	Country	Outcomes	Adjusted for
Bristow, 2000 [13]	Australia	IHCA, hospital mortality, unplanned ICU admission	CC, D
Buist, 2002 [8]	Australia	IHCA, hospital mortality, unplanned ICU admission	CM
Bellomo, 2003 [17]	Australia	IHCA, hospital mortality	no adj.
DeVita, 2004 [37]	US	IHCA	CM
Kenward, 2004 [9]	UK	IHCA, hospital mortality	no adj.
Priestley, 2004 [38]	UK	Hospital mortality	CM, RCT
Hillman, 2005 [7]	Australia	IHCA, hospital mortality, unplanned ICU admission	CM, RCT
Jones, 2005 [29]	Australia	IHCA, hospital mortality	no adj.
Dacey, 2007 [24]	US	IHCA, hospital mortality, unplanned ICU admission	no adj.
Jolley, 2007 [26]	US	IHCA, hospital mortality	N/A
Baxter, 2008 [25]	Canada	IHCA, hospital mortality, unplanned ICU admission	no adj.
Chan, 2008 [11]	US	Non-ICU cardiac arrest, hospital mortality	D, CM, T
Campello, 2009 [27]	Portugal	IHCA, hospital mortality	C, D
Hatler, 2009 [30]	US	Non-ICU cardiac arrest	no adj.
Konrad, 2010 [18]	Sweden	IHCA	C, D, LOS
Lighthall, 2010 [28]	US	IHCA, hospital mortality	S, CCI
Santamaria, 2010 [19]	Australia	IHCA, hospital mortality, unplanned ICU admission	C, CM, D
Beitler, 2011 [20]	US	IHCA, hospital mortality	T
Laurens, 2011 [21]	Australia	IHCA, hospital mortality, unplanned ICU admission	no adj.
Sarani, 2011 [31]	US	Non-ICU cardiac arrest, hospital mortality	no adj.
Shah, 2011 [39]	US	IHCA, hospital mortality	T
Howell, 2012 [40]	US	Hospital mortality	CCI, CM, D, S, ICUBC
Simmes, 2012 [16]	The Netherlands	IHCA, unexpected mortality, unplanned ICU admission	D, ASA
Tobin, 2012 [22]	Australia	Hospital mortality	Year
Al-Qahtani, 2013 [14]	Saudi Arabia	IHCA, hospital mortality	no adj.
Chen, 2014 [23]	Australia	IHCA, hospital mortality	D, year

ASA: American Society of Anesthesiologists classification; C: comorbidities; CC: concurrent controls; CCI: Charlson Comorbidity Index; CM: case-mix severity; D: demographics; ICU: intensive care unit; ICUBC: intensive care unit bed capacity; IHCA: in-hospital cardiac arrest; LOS: length of stay; RCT: randomized clinical trial; S: seasonality; T: time trends; US: United States; UK: United Kingdom.

Measures of Effectiveness

A key issue when evaluating the effectiveness of rapid response systems is the choice of the relevant outcome variables used for the measurement (Table 1). The main three outcome measures that have been employed are the rates of unexpected cardiac arrest, the rate of unplanned ICU admission, and the hospital mortality.

Rates of Unexpected Cardiac Arrest

The earliest endpoint in the clinical course for a study addressing the effectiveness of rapid response systems is the rate of unexpected cardiac arrests occurring outside ICUs, i. e., the rates of cardiac arrest occurring in ward patients who have no do-not-attempt-resuscitation (DNAR) order.

Results of available studies almost consistently indicate that introduction of rapid response systems is associated with a significant reduction of in-hospital cardiac arrest rates (pooled risk ratio [RR] 0.64 [0.55–0.73]; $p < 0.0001$) (Fig. 1). This endpoint, however, is potentially biased by the fact that part of the observed reduction

Study name	Statistics for each study				
	Risk ratio	Lower limit	Upper limit	Z-Value	p-Value
Bristow, 2000 (1) [13]	0.880	0.625	1.239	−0.731	0.464
Bristow, 2000 (2) [13]	1.000	0.730	1.370	0.000	1.000
Buist, 2002 [8]	0.500	0.349	0.717	−3.767	0.000
Bellomo, 2003 [17]	0.350	0.217	0.563	−4.323	0.000
DeVita, 2004 [37]	0.810	0.708	0.927	−3.060	0.002
Kenward, 2004 [9]	0.920	0.722	1.173	−0.673	0.501
Jones, 2005 [29]	0.470	0.353	0.626	-5.176	0.000
Hillman, 2005 [7]	0.940	0.786	1.124	−0.678	0.498
Dacey, 2007 [24]	0.390	0.261	0.582	−4.600	0.000
Jolley, 2007 [26]	0.860	0.687	1.076	−1.320	0.187
Baxter, 2008 [25]	0.610	0.396	0.940	−2.240	0.025
Chan, 2008 [11]	0.590	0.396	0.880	−2.586	0.010
Campello, 2009 [27]	0.730	0.542	0.983	−2.070	0.038
Hatler, 2009 [30]	0.680	0.361	1.282	−1.192	0.233
Konrad, 2010 [18]	0.740	0.554	0.988	−2.043	0.041
Santamaria, 2010 [19]	0.250	0.155	0.403	−5.687	0.000
Beitler, 2011 [20]	0.490	0.397	0.605	−6.626	0.000
Sarani, 2011 [31]	0.570	0.470	0.691	−5.739	0.000
Shah, 2011 [39]	0.970	0.719	1.308	−0.199	0.842
Simmes, 2012 [16]	0.489	0.165	1.452	−1.288	0.198
Al-Qahtani, 2013 [14]	0.680	0.534	0.866	−3.123	0.002
Chen, 2014 [23]	0.480	0.419	0.549	−10.669	0.000
	0.637	0.554	0.733	−6.317	0.000

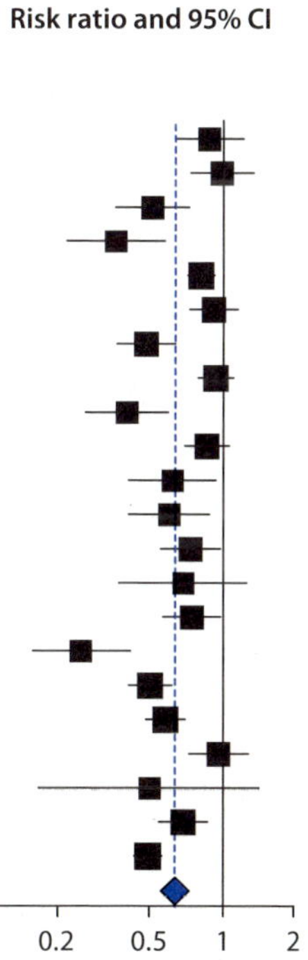

Fig. 1 Pooled risk ratio of adult in-hospital cardiopulmonary arrest after rapid response system implementation

Table 2 The percentage of MET interventions resulting in placement of a DNAR order

Author, year	DNAR/MET calls (%)
Buist, 2002 [8]	17/152 (11.2)
Bellomo, 2003 [17]	2/99 (2)
Kenward, 2004 [9]	32/130 (24.6)
Hillman, 2005 [7]	106/1319 (8)
Jones, 2005 [29]	18/327 (5.5)
Chan, 2008 [11]	73/376 (19.4)
Lighthall, 2010 [28]	10/378 (2.6)
Beitler, 2011 [20]	96/855 (11.2)
Laurens, 2011 [21]	55/296 (18.5)
Al-Qahtani, 2013 [14]	269/2879 (9.3)

in the rate of *unexpected* cardiac arrest observed after the implementation of a rapid response system may be due to a parallel increase in the fraction of *expected* cardiac arrests due to placement of a DNAR order. One of the tasks of METs in several institutions is to identify ward patients for whom resuscitation would be inappropriate. In these cases, calls to the MET result in discussion with the doctor who is in charge of the patient and in a decision to place a DNAR order or treatment limitations. For example, in a well-known study from Buist et al. [8], the MET calls resulted in placement of a DNAR order for 17/124 patients (14%), 13 of whom died. After the implementation of a rapid response system, the number of unexpected cardiac arrests decreased from 73 to 47 and the relevant mortality from 56/73 (76.7%) to 26/47 (55.3%) ($p = 0.024$). However, in the absence of a DNAR from the MET, the additional 13 deaths would have become unexpected cardiac arrests, potentially increasing mortality to 39/60 ($p = 0.2$). The percentage of MET interventions resulting in placement of a DNAR order is even higher in other studies, up to 24.6% [9] (Table 2).

On the other hand, placement of a DNAR order does not necessarily prevent MET intervention or the escalation of therapy. In a recent study [10], 45 ward patients with a DNR order in place were reviewed by the MET and 18 (40%) were transferred to the ICU after MET activation.

Rates of Unplanned ICU Admission

Another endpoint for measuring rapid response system effectiveness is reduction in the rate of unplanned ICU admissions. The rationale is that the introduction of a rapid response system should increase the number of ICU admissions that are planned early, before further deterioration occurs, and decrease those occurring as emergencies, such as after resuscitation from cardiac arrest. This model has been indirectly investigated for ICU admissions from the emergency room [4], where an earlier transfer to the ICU has been demonstrated to decrease both ICU and hospital mortality. However, this is not always the case with rapid response systems. In a large American before-and-after study [11], in which 41.2% of the MET interventions resulted in ICU admission, implementation of the rapid response system was followed by a significant reduction in non-ICU codes (from 6.08 pre-intervention to 3.08 post-intervention; $p < 0.001$) but this did not translate into a reduction in hospital-wide mortality rates per 100 admissions (from 3.22 pre-intervention to 3.09 post-intervention; $p = 0.41$). In that study, mortality in patients transferred from ward to ICU was relatively high (43/155; 28%), and issues in patient selection, appropriateness and timeliness of ICU transfer have been advocated to explain those results [12].

Moreover, although some studies demonstrated a decrease in the rate of unplanned ICU admissions [13, 14] after the implementation of an in-hospital rapid response system, others [7, 15] showed no effect, and in a recent cohort study [16] rapid response system implementation was paradoxically followed by a significant increase in unplanned admissions to the ICU (from 34/1376 [2.47%] to 100/2410 [4.15%]; OR 1.66, CI 1.07–2.55). Since the percentage of cardiac arrests in the study period decreased, although not significantly (from 4/1367 [0.29%] to 3/2410 [0.12%]; OR 0.38, CI 0.09–1.73), this result was explained by the authors as an increase in ICU referrals for unstable patients in the ward. However, it is worth noting that the median APACHE II score at unplanned ICU admission was unchanged in that study, indicating that ICU referrals were apparently not done at an earlier stage of illness in the ward.

Hospital Mortality

A reduction in hospital mortality represents the most comprehensive and important outcome measure for rapid response systems. In fact, the achievement of intermediate endpoints, such as the rates of unexpected cardiac arrests outside ICU or unplanned ICU admission, is of limited benefit, if the patient's final outcome does not change.

Results of earlier studies in terms of hospital mortality were conflicting, with several studies [8, 14, 17–23] showing a reduction and others [9, 11, 13, 24–28] showing no change or even an increase [29] in hospital mortality following rapid response system implementation. A systematic review and meta-analysis from Chan et al. [11] did not demonstrate any overall benefit from rapid response systems in terms of hospital mortality (pooled $RR = 0.96$ [0.84–1.09]) with a significant heterogeneity of results ($I^2 = 90.3\%$; $p < 0.001$). However, a meta-analysis including more recent evidence showed an overall significant reduction in hospital mortality associated with the introduction of rapid response systems (pooled $RR = 0.88$ [0.83–0.93] (Fig. 2) even though heterogeneity remained significant ($I^2 = 89.4$; $p < 0.001$).

Study name	Statistics for each study				
	Risk ratio	Lower limit	Upper limit	Z-Value	p-Value
Bristow, 2000 (1) [13]	0.930	0.771	1.122	−0.759	0.448
Bristow, 2000 (2) [13]	1.200	1.003	1.435	1.998	0.046
Buist, 2002 [8]	0.870	0.755	1.003	−1.920	0.055
Bellomo, 2003 [17]	0.740	0.697	0.786	−9.758	0.000
Kenward, 2004 [9]	0.990	0.913	1.074	−0.243	0.808
Priestley, 2004 [38]	0.520	0.319	0.847	−2.624	0.009
Hillman, 2005 [7]	1.030	0.834	1.271	0.275	0.783
Dacey, 2007 [24]	1.070	0.874	1.310	0.654	0.513
Jones, 2005 [29]	1.180	1.098	1.268	4.515	0.000
Baxter, 2008 [25]	0.990	0.852	1.150	−0.132	0.895
Chan, 2008 [11]	0.950	0.812	1.112	−0.638	0.523
Jolley, 2007 [26]	1.000	0.738	1.356	0.000	1.000
Campello, 2009 [27]	0.830	0.642	1.073	−1.421	0.155
Konrad, 2010 [18]	0.900	0.838	0.967	−2.870	0.004
Lighthall, 2010 [28]	0.820	0.618	1.087	−1.379	0.168
Santamaria, 2010 [19]	0.480	0.411	0.561	−9.228	0.000
Beitler, 2011 [20]	0.890	0.818	0.968	−2.719	0.007
Laurens, 2011 [21]	0.760	0.662	0.873	−3.894	0.000
Sarani, 2011 (Med) [31]	0.740	0.682	0.803	−7.263	0.000
Sarani, 2011 (Surg) [31]	0.920	0.803	1.054	−1.202	0.229
Shah, 2011 [39]	0.890	0.791	1.001	−1.938	0.053
Howell, 2012 [40]	0.910	0.820	1.010	−1.774	0.076
Tobin, 2012 [22]	0.900	0.880	0.920	−9.291	0.000
Al-Qahtani, 2013 [14]	0.900	0.851	0.951	−3.713	0.000
Chen, 2014 [23]	0.770	0.711	0.833	−6.472	0.000
	0.880	0.830	0.933	−4.271	0.000

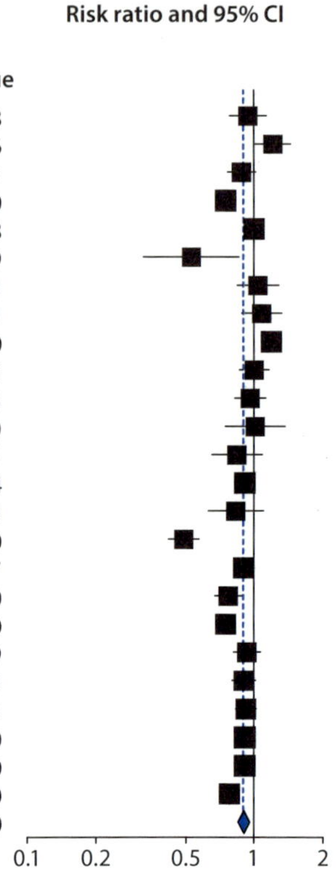

Fig. 2 Pooled risk ratio of adult hospital mortality after rapid response system implementation

Quality of Evidence

In general, the quality of evidence of observational studies on rapid response systems is low. Most of these investigations assessed the in-hospital cardiac arrest rate without distinguishing the location of the event. Only a few studies [8, 11, 14, 20, 24, 30, 31] limited the analysis to cardiac arrests outside the ICU and none of these studies conducted any blinded outcome assessment.

Almost all studies on rapid response systems have a before-and-after design, which makes them prone to bias. Indeed, in this kind of study, the reduction in hospital mortality observed during the study periods may be part of the secular trend started before the intervention and due to factors unrelated to rapid response system implementation, such as a change in the hospital case mix. In some of these studies, the adjustment for bias implicit in the study design has been made using multivariate models, including severity of illness or comorbidities, and autocorrelation (Table 1).

Randomized trials would represent the ideal solution to control for confounders in studies assessing rapid response system effectiveness. However, these trials have ethical and implementation issues. Patients cannot be randomized at individual level and cluster randomization should rather be used. On the other hand, in cluster randomization there is a high risk of contamination between the study arms because the study intervention cannot be blinded. This has been a major issue in the only multicenter randomized trial on rapid response systems conducted so far, the MERIT study [7], whose results were neutral. Although the authors of that study made every effort to prevent contamination, so that no specific training in the recognition of patients at risk had been made in hospitals in the control group, hospital safety issues in general and the benefits of the MET system in particular were largely reported in the media during the study period, which could have affected personnel behavior in the control hospitals. This is consistent with the fact that in the MERIT study the rates of in-hospital cardiac arrest decreased more in the hospitals of the control group than in those of the interventional group between the two study periods (from 2.61 to 1.64 [$p=0.004$] vs. 1.60 to 1.31 [$p=0.171$]).

Implementation Issues

Another major implementation issue in the MERIT trial, as in general for rapid response systems, was an afferent limb failure [32], i. e., absent or delayed MET activation by the ward staff in patients fulfilling MET calling criteria, due to an incomplete compliance of the ward personnel with the MET calling procedure. In the MERIT study, among 313 patients who had documented MET calling criteria more than 15 min before an unplanned ICU admission, the MET was actually called by the ward staff in only 95 cases (30%). With such a low utilization rate, any potential benefit from the rapid response system would have been difficult to identify. Moreover, there is evidence that MET activation from the ward staff is often delayed, which is associated with increased hospital mortality [33, 34]. Reasons for this afferent limb failure include adherence to the traditional system of calling the covering medical staff, a fear of creating false alarms, or disagreement with the MET calling criteria. Continuous education of the ward staff, review of the episodes of MET activation and feedback from MET users may help reduce those barriers and increase compliance with the rapid response system [19].

Long-term Effectiveness of Rapid Response Systems

The inconsistent results observed in studies on rapid response system effectiveness may also be due to insufficient time allowed for the evaluation of the study endpoint. One Australian study [19] showed that reduction in cardiac arrest rates achieved statistical significance at two years and reduction in hospital mortality at four years after the implementation of a rapid response system. Buist et al. [35] specifically examined rapid response system performance over time and found that the proportion of patients with delayed MET activation decreased as the rapid response system matured and that six years after MET implementation the MET calls had increased by 46% and the IHCA per 1,000 hospital admissions decreased by 24% a year (from 2.4 in 2000 to 0.66 in 2005). Similarly, a recent comparative study [36] showed that hospitals with mature rapid response systems performed better than similar hospitals where rapid response systems were recently implemented.

Reproducibility

A final issue for evaluating rapid response system effectiveness is reproducibility. The vast majority of studies is single-center and has been conducted in U.S. or Australian healthcare systems, while only a minority of studies has been conducted in the UK or in continental Europe. The effectiveness of a rapid response system depends on the nature and the quantity of the urgent, unmet patients' needs in general wards. This model may, therefore, not necessarily work in places where the severity of ward patients, the education of the ward personnel or the availability of human resources is different from those of places where this model was developed. International multicenter studies will be needed to ensure reproducibility of results.

Conclusion

There are different ways of measuring the effectiveness of rapid response systems. The major endpnoits include the rate of unexpected cardiac arrests outside the ICU, the rate of unplanned ICU admissions, and hospital mortality. All these outcome metrics have limitations and are prone to bias. The level of evidence supporting the effectiveness of rapid response systems is relatively low and almost all studies have a before-and-after design. Supporting evidence comes from a limited number of countries and needs to be reproduced in different hospital systems and organizations. Despite the ethical and implementation difficulties, high-quality randomized trials are warranted to reliably assess the effectiveness of rapid response systems.

References

1. Sandroni C, Nolan J, Cavallaro F, Antonelli M (2007) In-hospital cardiac arrest: incidence, prognosis and possible measures to improve survival. Intensive Care Med 33:237–245
2. Schein RM, Hazday N, Pena M, Ruben BH, Sprung CL (1990) Clinical antecedents to in-hospital cardiopulmonary arrest. Chest 98:1388–1392
3. Hillman KM, Bristow PJ, Chey T et al (2001) Antecedents to hospital deaths. Intern Med J 31:343–348
4. Chalfin DB, Trzeciak S, Likourezos A, Baumann BM, Dellinger RP (2007) Impact of delayed transfer of critically ill patients from the emergency department to the intensive care unit. Crit Care Med 35:1477–1483
5. DeVita MA, Smith GB, Adam SK et al (2010) "Identifying the hospitalised patient in crisis" – a consensus conference on the afferent limb of rapid response systems. Resuscitation 81:375–382
6. Chan PS, Jain R, Nallmothu BK, Berg RA, Sasson C (2010) Rapid response teams: A systematic review and meta-analysis. Arch Intern Med 170:18–26

7. Hillman K, Chen J, Cretikos M et al (2005) Introduction of the medical emergency team (MET) system: a cluster-randomised controlled trial. Lancet 365:2091–2097
8. Buist MD, Moore GE, Bernard SA, Waxman BP, Anderson JN, Nguyen TV (2002) Effects of a medical emergency team on reduction of incidence of and mortality from unexpected cardiac arrests in hospital: preliminary study. BMJ 324:387–390
9. Kenward G, Castle N, Hodgetts T, Shaikh L (2004) Evaluation of a medical emergency team one year after implementation. Resuscitation 61:257–263
10. Smith RL, Hayashi VN, Lee YI, Navarro-Mariazeta L, Felner K (2014) The medical emergency team call: a sentinel event that triggers goals of care discussion. Crit Care Med 42:322–327
11. Chan PS, Khalid A, Longmore LS, Berg RA, Kosiborod M, Spertus JA (2008) Hospital-wide code rates and mortality before and after implementation of a rapid response team. JAMA 300:2506–2513
12. Sherner JH (2009) Rapid response team implementation and hospital mortality rates. JAMA 301:1658–1659
13. Bristow PJ, Hillman KM, Chey T et al (2000) Rates of in-hospital arrests, deaths and intensive care admissions: the effect of a medical emergency team. Med J Aust 173:236–240
14. Al-Qahtani S, Al-Dorzi HM, Tamim HM et al (2013) Impact of an intensivist-led multidisciplinary extended rapid response team on hospital-wide cardiopulmonary arrests and mortality. Crit Care Med 41:506–517
15. Subbe CP, Davies RG, Williams E, Rutherford P, Gemmell L (2003) Effect of introducing the Modified Early Warning score on clinical outcomes, cardio-pulmonary arrests and intensive care utilisation in acute medical admissions. Anaesthesia 58:797–802
16. Simmes FM, Schoonhoven L, Mintjes J, Fikkers BG, van der Hoeven JG (2012) Incidence of cardiac arrests and unexpected deaths in surgical patients before and after implementation of a rapid response system. Ann Intensive Care 2:20
17. Bellomo R, Goldsmith D, Uchino S et al (2003) A prospective before-and-after trial of a medical emergency team. Med J Aust 179:283–287
18. Konrad D, Jaderling G, Bell M, Granath F, Ekbom A, Martling CR (2010) Reducing in-hospital cardiac arrests and hospital mortality by introducing a medical emergency team. Intensive Care Med 36:100–106
19. Santamaria J, Tobin A, Holmes J (2010) Changing cardiac arrest and hospital mortality rates through a medical emergency team takes time and constant review. Crit Care Med 38:445–450
20. Beitler JR, Link N, Bails DB, Hurdle K, Chong DH (2011) Reduction in hospital-wide mortality after implementation of a rapid response team: a long-term cohort study. Crit Care 15:R269
21. Laurens N, Dwyer T (2011) The impact of medical emergency teams on ICU admission rates, cardiopulmonary arrests and mortality in a regional hospital. Resuscitation 82:707–712
22. Tobin AE, Santamaria JD (2012) Medical emergency teams are associated with reduced mortality across a major metropolitan health network after two years service: a retrospective study using government administrative data. Crit Care 16:R210
23. Chen J, Ou L, Hillman KM et al (2014) Cardiopulmonary arrest and mortality trends, and their association with rapid response system expansion. Med J Aust 201:167–170
24. Dacey MJ, Mirza ER, Wilcox V et al (2007) The effect of a rapid response team on major clinical outcome measures in a community hospital. Crit Care Med 35:2076–2082
25. Baxter AD, Cardinal P, Hooper J, Patel R (2008) Medical emergency teams at The Ottawa Hospital: the first two years. Can J Anaesth 55:223–231
26. Jolley J, Bendyk H, Holaday B, Lombardozzi KA, Harmon C (2007) Rapid response teams: do they make a difference? Dimens Crit Care Nurs 26:253–260
27. Campello G, Granja C, Carvalho F, Dias C, Azevedo LF, Costa-Pereira A (2009) Immediate and long-term impact of medical emergency teams on cardiac arrest prevalence and mortality: a plea for periodic basic life-support training programs. Crit Care Med 37:3054–3061
28. Lighthall GK, Parast LM, Rapoport L, Wagner TH (2010) Introduction of a rapid response system at a United States veterans affairs hospital reduced cardiac arrests. Anesth Analg 111:679–686

29. Jones D, Bellomo R, Bates S et al (2005) Long term effect of a medical emergency team on cardiac arrests in a teaching hospital. Crit Care 9:R808–R815
30. Hatler C, Mast D, Bedker D et al (2009) Implementing a rapid response team to decrease emergencies outside the ICU: one hospital's experience. Medsurg Nurs 18:84–90
31. Sarani B, Palilonis E, Sonnad S et al (2011) Clinical emergencies and outcomes in patients admitted to a surgical versus medical service. Resuscitation 82:415–418
32. Sandroni C, Cavallaro F (2011) Failure of the afferent limb: a persistent problem in rapid response systems. Resuscitation 82:797–798
33. Trinkle RM, Flabouris A (2011) Documenting Rapid Response System afferent limb failure and associated patient outcomes. Resuscitation 82:810–814
34. Calzavacca P, Licari E, Tee A et al (2010) The impact of Rapid Response System on delayed emergency team activation patient characteristics and outcomes – a follow-up study. Resuscitation 81:31–35
35. Buist M, Harrison J, Abaloz E, Van Dyke S (2007) Six year audit of cardiac arrests and medical emergency team calls in an Australian outer metropolitan teaching hospital. BMJ 335:1210–1212
36. Chen J, Ou L, Hillman K et al (2014) The impact of implementing a rapid response system: A comparison of cardiopulmonary arrests and mortality among four teaching hospitals in Australia. Resuscitation 85:1275–1281
37. DeVita MA, Braithwaite RS, Mahidhara R, Stuart S, Foraida M, Simmons RL (2004) Use of medical emergency team responses to reduce hospital cardiopulmonary arrests. Qual Saf Health Care 13:251–254
38. Priestley G, Watson W, Rashidian A et al (2004) Introducing Critical Care Outreach: a ward-randomised trial of phased introduction in a general hospital. Intensive Care Med 30:1398–1404
39. Shah SK, Cardenas VJ, Jr., Kuo YF, Sharma G (2011) Rapid response team in an academic institution: does it make a difference? Chest 139:1361–1367
40. Howell MD, Ngo L, Folcarelli P et al (2012) Substained effectiveness of a primary-team-based rapid response system. Crit Care Med 40:2562–2568

Severe Sepsis Beyond the Emergency Department and ICU: Targeting Early Identification and Treatment on the Hospital Floor

C. A. Schorr, J. Sebastien, and R. P. Dellinger

Introduction

The Surviving Sepsis Campaign (SSC) was created in 2002 with the intent to decrease mortality in severe sepsis through educating the public/influencing public policy (Phase I), defining best practice though the creation of guidelines (Phase II), and improving patient management with the development of a sepsis performance improvement program (Phase III). Phase I included introduction of the Campaign at several major international critical care medicine conferences, beginning with the European Society of Intensive Care Medicine (ESICM) meeting in Barcelona, Spain, in 2002. Phase II was designed to create evidence-based guidelines for managing severe sepsis and septic shock through an international consensus committee, including representation from scientific organizations with interest and expertise in sepsis. Phase III included a performance improvement program designed to measure severe sepsis management and outcomes with focus on diagnosis and management in the emergency department (ED) and the intensive care unit (ICU).

The first SSC sepsis management guidelines were published in 2004, with revisions in 2008 and most recently in 2013 [1–6]. The Campaign has continued to evolve over the past 12 years and is now moving forward in 2014 to Phase IV, early identification and management on the hospital floors. This initiative is sponsored by an unrestricted grant from the Gordon and Betty Moore Foundation.

History of the Surviving Sepsis Campaign

In 2002, the SSC announced a goal of reducing mortality in severe sepsis by 25%, laudable given that mortality from severe sepsis was reported to range from 40–

C. A. Schorr ✉ · J. Sebastien · R. P. Dellinger
Division of Critical Care Medicine, Dept of Medicine, Cooper University Hospital, Camden, USA
e-mail: Schorr-christa@cooperhealth.edu

J.-L. Vincent (ed.), *Annual Update in Intensive Care and Emergency Medicine 2015*,
DOI 10.1007/978-3-319-13761-2_41

80% [7, 8]. The SSC leaders developed a volunteer program in 2005 for hospitals throughout the world to participate in the severe sepsis performance improvement initiative. The program provided web-based resources to participating hospitals to include help in identification of administrative and unit-based healthcare provider champions, severe sepsis education tools, methodology to apply the severe sepsis bundles to clinical practice, and the electronic means (SSC software program) developed to capture data on severe sepsis management and outcomes. Participating sites electronically collected data on compliance with the severe sepsis quality indicators. The database was designed to track compliance with the then 6-hour (resuscitation) and 24-hour (management) performance improvement bundles. The de-identified data were submitted to a central repository housed at the Society of Critical Care Medicine (SCCM). Patients included in the database were admitted to the ICU with severe sepsis or septic shock or were in the ICU for a diagnosis other than severe sepsis and subsequently developed severe sepsis or septic shock during their ICU stay. Patients were classified into one of three categories based on their origin at the time of presentation: Presenting to the ICU from the ED; presenting to the ICU from an area other than the ED (floors/wards); previously admitted to the ICU for a diagnosis other than sepsis and subsequently developed severe sepsis during their ICU stay. The primary champions for the Phase III performance improvement program were physicians and nurses from the ED and the ICU.

Phase III Reveals Poor Outcome when Severe Sepsis Develops on the General Floor

The results of the SSC performance-improvement program revealed a sustained improvement in compliance with both the 6- and 24-hour quality indicators with longer participation in the campaign [9, 10]. A significant decrease in mortality was also observed. Interestingly, the mortality for patients presenting to the ICU from the ED was 27% compared to 44.3% for those presenting to the ICU from the wards. Despite the association with an overall observed decrease in mortality, the SSC leadership realized that the primary efforts in Phase III focused on the ED and the ICU. Noteworthy, was that although the group of patients admitted from the floors accounted for only 34.8% of patients, the mortality was close to 2-fold that of those admitted from the ED [9, 10]. The Campaign is now choosing to focus on patients on the hospital floors in hope of further improving survival. The SSC Phase IV program is created to draw attention to early identification of severe sepsis on hospital floors, hopefully driving the initiation of more timely management and resulting in improved outcomes.

Efforts Targeting Hospital Floors

The hospital floors initiative is called Phase IV and is currently underway with close to 60 hospitals participating in collaborative groups in four regions across the United States. The Phase IV effort includes application of the new 3- and 6-hour severe sepsis bundles based on the most recent SSC guidelines (Box 1) and built into the long-established SSC performance improvement program. The focus of the floors initiative is the 3-hour bundle, which includes obtaining a serum lactate, obtaining blood cultures before administration of antibiotics, administration of broad-spectrum antibiotics and administration of 30 ml/kg crystalloid in those patients with a lactate $\geq$ 4 mmol/l and/or hypotension. The 6-hour bundle may be started on the hospital floors, but typically requires transfer to a higher level of care to accomplish.

Box 1. Surviving Sepsis Campaign Sepsis Bundles
To be completed within 3 and 6 hours of time of presentation to emergency department or diagnosis on floors or in ICU.

3 hours:
1. Measure lactate level
2. Obtain blood cultures prior to administration of antibiotics
3. Administer broad spectrum antibiotics
4. Administer 30 ml/kg crystalloid for hypotension or lactate $\geq$ 4 mmol/l (36 mg/dl)

6 hours:
5. Apply vasopressors (for hypotension that does not respond to initial fluid resuscitation to maintain a mean arterial pressure (MAP) $\geq$ 65 mmHg)
6. In the event of persistent arterial hypotension despite volume resuscitation (septic shock) or initial lactate $\geq$ 4 mmol/l (36 mg/dl):
   - Measure central venous pressure (CVP)
   - Measure central venous oxygen saturation ($ScvO_2$)
7. Re-measure lactate if initially elevated

The Phase IV initiative is concentrating on hospital floors, with an emphasis on severe sepsis screening (minimum of twice daily and labelled "every patient, every shift"), focused communication for early identification and initiation of timely management of severe sepsis. Nurse and physician champions from hospital floors are encouraged to work with their ED and ICU counterparts jointly to facilitate promotion and support of the program. Similar to Phase III, this program provides tools to facilitate educational sessions with nursing and physician staff (focus on early identification of severe sepsis), including evaluation for presence of active or newly suspected infection, systemic manifestations of infection, and presence of new organ dysfunction. When patients are identified as meeting the criteria for severe sepsis, data are reviewed and confirmed with the clinical team (time zero or T_0) in an expedited manner with focus on implementation of the 3-hour bundle indicators and facilitation of entry into the 6-hour bundle if indicated.

Possible Reasons Patients Admitted to the ICU from Hospital Floors Have a Worse Prognosis

There are several potential reasons for a worse prognosis in severe sepsis patients presenting to the ICU from the floors. One possible reason may be that patients are admitted from the ED to the floor with severe sepsis but without it being identified in the ED, e. g., organ dysfunction or tissue hypoperfusion that was not recognized until deterioration occurs on the floor. A second possible reason may be that patients can present to the ED with severe sepsis and may be determined by the ED clinician to be stable for the floor (not require an ICU bed) but over time clinical status declines and then the patient is transferred to the ICU. In a single center study of 1,853 patients admitted to the hospital with severe sepsis over a 5 year period, 45% were initially admitted to a non-ICU setting [11]. Adverse outcomes in this group of patients were linked to older age, higher burden of comorbid conditions, an oncology diagnosis, and a do-not-resuscitate order at admission, and the patients were more severely ill, described as an initial serum lactate > 4 mmol/l and a higher APACHE II score [11]. Patients with severe sepsis admitted to a non-ICU setting commonly experience a new functional disability, regardless of their baseline functional status [12]. In severe sepsis patients requiring ICU care, 37.5% were discharged home compared to 54.2% of those not requiring ICU care; 37.5% died compared to 4.2% [12].

In a study of 22 inpatient wards in Scotland, Marwick and colleagues sought to improve time to antibiotic administration within 4 hours of sepsis onset [13]. Prior to the intervention, 241 episodes of sepsis with antibiotic administration were reviewed. The mean time between sepsis onset and receipt of antibiotics was 11 hours with a median of 6 hours. Analysis of the steps involved in antibiotic delivery revealed a significant delay from medical review to prescription of antibiotics with little delay from antibiotic prescription to administration. The intervention focused attention on junior doctors' decision making. The number of sepsis cases was infrequent with a median of 2 (range 0–6) across general medical wards, 4 (0–10) across general surgical wards and 1 (0–3) on orthopedic wards. The low number of cases made feedback a challenge. Also studied was a questionnaire to assess physician knowledge on sepsis identification. Doctors who were confident that they could determine when a patient had severe sepsis were no more likely than those who were not confident to correctly identify which clinical features would or would not indicate severe sepsis. The conclusion was that sepsis is not recognized and treated early [13].

Physicians may be reluctant to diagnosis sepsis as it would dictate treatment in the presence of antibiotic restrictions in place to reduce *Clostridium difficile* infection. Additionally, some may be hesitant to order antibiotics unless cultures return a positive result despite the patient displaying systemic manifestation of sepsis and infection [13]. It is unlikely that one or two doses of antibiotics, while in search of a non-infectious etiology of organ dysfunction will increase antibiotic burden significantly.

Initiating Support for a Hospital Floor Sepsis Performance Improvement Program

Respected leadership through designated champions is crucial to enable a hospital floors sepsis program to gain administrative attention, and is needed to drive support from frontline caregivers. Administrative support facilitates educational requirements, information technology support and data collection needs. A viable Phase IV severe sepsis program requires support on multiple levels in order to facilitate change in clinical behavior. This includes twice daily nurse screening, development of a script for staff to communicate findings supporting severe sepsis, and potentially developing an order set for severe sepsis. Initiatives to help move the early identification process forward may include 24/7 severe sepsis surveillance via the electronic medical record (alerts) using a modified electronic warning system (score to alert clinicians of a change in clinical status). A sepsis response team may also be deployed (discussion to follow). The early inclusion of nursing staff and hospitalists in the planning of this program is essential. Additional members of the team should include medical informatics, pharmacy, critical care and emergency medicine providers, unit-based medical technicians and if applicable a sepsis response team leader.

The significance of administrative backing early in the program can help to facilitate downstream needs for clinical, information technology (IT) and data collection support. Support may include allowing the program leadership time away from their clinical responsibilities to provide educational sessions and serve as a resource for frontline staff. IT support may include the development of a screening tool in the electronic medical record (EMR) and in the creation of a sepsis alert. Data collection is essential for success of this performance improvement program, allowing for reporting compliance with the bundle indicators and outcomes as well as providing feedback to the clinical team.

Engaging Frontline Caregivers

Methods to streamline procedures geared toward patient identification and implementation of a severe sepsis protocol are needed. During the planning process, institutions may choose to use standardized improvement methodologies (e. g., Lean Six Sigma or plan-do-study-act [PDSA] cycle) [14, 15]. The process owners (unit-based champions) for the program should be a nurse and a physician leader both with a vested interest in the floor units involved in the performance improvement program. Key members of the floor severe sepsis program should walk through the steps (workout) on how to identify a severe sepsis patient using a formal protocol. The intervention should focus on plotting out the steps necessary to identify areas that work well (e. g., medical technician obtains vital signs every shift within 1 hour of arrival of all admitted patients), require clarification (e. g., when in the process is the physician notified) or need a more efficient method to perform a specified task (e. g., administer antibiotics). Findings from the workout can provide information to help the team simplify the overall process and potentially eliminate areas where inefficiencies may occur.

Education is essential when starting any new program but the odds of retaining the information over time remains minimal. Even in the presence of a strong foundation in medicine, diagnosing sepsis is not an easy task for most clinicians. Often the systemic manifestations of sepsis may go unnoticed or when recognized may not appear to need urgent intervention, often influenced by individual physician diagnostic capability and workload. The systemic manifestations of sepsis that should raise awareness for physicians may be overlooked or managed from a distance. Even when notified by nursing staff, physicians in training may not recognize the physiologic changes that can lead to a more severe infectious process [16].

Nursing engagement may be key to improving sepsis survival, especially if educated and resourced with the capability to recognize systemic physiologic changes in patients early, leading to early intervention and reduced organ dysfunction with improvement in outcomes. Floor nurses have a patient load that may range from 4–8 patients depending on the type of unit and hospital size. Caring for an average of 6 patients requires a great deal of organizational skill. A full assessment in these 6 patients is generally completed at the start of each shift. Incorporating a sepsis screening tool alongside the daily shift assessment may be an efficient and effective method to identify sepsis early. Unlike the emergency department where patients are assessed soon after arrival by a triage nurse, nurses practicing in units outside the ED may not get to the assessment of all of their assigned patients until 2–3 hours into the shift. Built-in electronic record warning systems to alert the nurses to which patients should receive priority evaluation may facilitate early identification and initiation of treatment.

Screening Methods

Screening for severe sepsis may be achieved with a paper screening tool, an electronic sepsis alert, or a hybrid of paper and electronic screening. Although somewhat easy to complete, paper data collection has limitations in that another staff member typically confirms that the screening was positive and data collection is required for feedback to the team. Electronic severe sepsis screening may be accomplished through 24/7 automated surveillance of electronic data capture including vital signs and laboratory data [17]. The surveillance method requires that specified parameters be written so that the screening method is consistent. This automated process may be linked to a sepsis alert in which the 24/7 electronic surveillance triggers an alert message to the nurse indicting that the patient may have sepsis. This may be done via a message to a smart device or a pop-up alert on the EMR for the specific patient. Although there is a sense of efficiency with electronic surveillance, it is equally important to include the clinician assessment and confirmation of sepsis criteria. Once the assessment for infection is completed, the surveillance system can be designed to review blood pressure readings and laboratory data to determine if organ dysfunction is present. The clinicians should review the information and determine whether the organ dysfunction is chronic or if it is related to the infection. Once confirmed that the organ dysfunction is new and related to the infection, proceeding with confirmation and implementation of the severe sepsis bundles should follow.

Although not specific to sepsis, the use of modified early warning signs may be incorporated into the daily care plan to help the clinician determine if there has been a significant change in clinical condition based on specified criteria, primarily vital signs and laboratory data. The changes in clinical condition may or may not be due to sepsis but can aid with early identification.

Effective Clinician Communication

Nurse-to-physician communication can be a challenge, as nurses are trained to communicate in a narrative style whereas physicians are taught to report in brief bullet type points. Effective communication creates a more effective work environment in addition to building a safe quality environment [18]. Basic to any performance improvement program is mutual respect among the team members. For this program to excel, the clinical team (physicians and nurses) will need to acknowledge the competence of the nurse to identify a severe sepsis patient requiring rapid intervention. On the other hand, the nurse needs to develop appropriate skills to assess a patient for severe sepsis and communicate his/her findings to the physician.

The communication method may be scripted using situation, background, assessment and recommendation (SBAR). The SBAR technique for healthcare professionals promotes quality and patient safety through effective communication with common agreed upon expectations [19].

Example

Introduction: Dr. Jones, this is Mary Smith RN. I am calling about your patient Mr. Black.

Situation: Mr. Black is experiencing fever with chills and is complaining of severe pain in his right leg.

Background: The background information is that he was admitted yesterday with cellulitis of his right lower extremity. At 8 am today, he reported that the redness had extended 2 inches outside the markings placed on admission. His temperature is 101.5°, heart rate is 98 and respiratory rate is 24. He is complaining of severe pain.

Assessment: My assessment of the situation is that he may be experiencing a worsening of his soft tissue infection.

Recommendation: I recommend that you see him immediately and that we order a serum lactate, blood cultures and a basic metabolic panel. Do you agree?

The physician should confirm, clarify and request additional information and then work with the nurse to take appropriate action with this patient.

Incorporating Protocols and Order-Sets

A progressive next step in the sepsis performance improvement evolution is to enable the nurse to initiate a pre-approved order set. This may be completed in one of two ways, either with or without physician confirmation. In the first scenario, the nurse may initiate orders after confirmation by the clinician. Alternatively, the nurse may choose to initiate orders after his/her assessment and prior to calling the physician. In this case, the laboratory specimens may be obtained, with pending results, prior to calling the physician. Based on the order set and protocol, the nurse may elect to call the physician after the laboratory results are received using SBAR to report the recent laboratory values. Sepsis order sets when used appropriately, save time and improve patient outcomes [20, 21].

Role of Response Teams

Rapid response teams have emerged over the years for acute issues on the hospital floors that could be but are not necessarily serious. At some institutions this has evolved into sepsis response teams. The sepsis team responds to calls similar to a rapid response team. However, the sepsis response team comes equipped with antibiotics, fluids and even the potential equipment to obtain central venous access in the presence of shock. The team may also be equipped to provide respiratory support in the event that mechanical ventilation is required (similar to a rapid response team). The team may be composed of a critical care nurse, physician and a respiratory therapist. Rapid transport to the critical care area is then facilitated by the rapid response/sepsis response team when vasopressors and/or mechanical ventilation are needed. Utilization of the response team along with early initiation of therapy may improve outcome [22].

Data Collection and Feedback

In order to assess progress with performance improvement, data capture and analysis feedback to clinicians is key. Methods to capture and evaluate data may be as simple as searching discharge codes for severe sepsis and septic shock with associated mortality (administrative data). However, when evaluating process measures, such as lactate measurement, blood cultures before antibiotics and antibiotic administration, administrative data are somewhat limiting. If administering antibiotics earlier and earlier following recognition of severe sepsis improves outcomes, then capturing details of severe sepsis identification and time of antibiotic administration is crucial.

Addressing the Challenge in Sepsis Identification

Troubleshooting problems soon after they occur should be a part of any valid performance improvement program. Meaningful definitions of sepsis and severe sepsis that are easily understood by both junior and senior physicians and nurses are essential. Despite clinicians expressing understanding of sepsis, documentation review often yields a poor understanding of sepsis. In some cases, determining the source of infection can be a challenge and cause a delay in initiation of treatment. However, once a source is identified, the team needs to evaluate for source control issues. For example, if the patient develops new systemic manifestations of infection and/or new organ dysfunction, a system to review the antibiotic regimen and/or evaluate the patient for a new source of infection should be in place. Stressing the importance of differentiation between a patient with an active infection that is being treated with antibiotics versus a patient with a new or suspected infection should be an essential educational component for nurses on the medical/surgical floors. Complex patients with various chronic health conditions also present a challenge to clinicians in determining if the organ dysfunction is new versus pre-existing. Consideration should be given to infection in patients with worsening chronic organ failure.

When evaluating patients for sepsis and severe sepsis, false positive screen patients will be reported by protocol. However, circumstances will also arise wherein the clinical team does not believe the patient has sepsis despite a positive screen, but in review of the case the patient did indeed meet the criteria and should have been treated. Unfortunately, this type of patient when not identified as having sepsis and appropriately treated often progresses to develop organ dysfunction with transfer to a higher level of care.

Electronic Alert Fatigue

Alert fatigue has long been identified as problematic. It is particularly pervasive when using EMRs and may lead to a decrease in healthcare provider responsiveness to new events. Studies have shown that a substantial number of alerts are ignored by health care providers, for example, drug interaction (up to 95% in some instances) [23, 24]. This well-known phenomenon occurs because of the lack of specificity of such alerts, their lack of major impact on clinical care and their multiplicity.

Success Includes a Change in Workflow and Adoption of the Change

When we look at the entirety of running a successful hospital floor sepsis initiative there are two major issues to be addressed: The change in work flow and the willingness of health care providers to adopt that change.

Any change can be difficult. Changes in the health care system setting can be even more difficult because of the complexity of systems interactions and unantic-

Table 1 Heterogeneity of healthcare providers on medical floors

	Residents in training	Attending physician	Registered nurse	Medical assistant	Unit-based pharmacist
Years in training	8 years+	11 years+	4 years+	1 year	8 years
Patient contact	Yes	Yes	Yes	Yes	No
Schedule	24/7 8 to 10 hours overlapping shifts	24/7 12 hours overlapping sifts	24/7 12 hours non-overlapping shifts	24/7 8 hours non-overlapping shifts	8 am–4 pm No overlap
Entering medical orders	Yes need co-signature	Yes	No	No	No
Number of patients	Regulated ACGME rule	Not regulated	Regulated union contract	Institution bylaws	Unit based
Scheduled vital signs	No	No	Yes	Yes	No
Give medications	No	No	Yes	Yes	No
Monitoring of clinical plan	Yes	Yes	Yes	No	No

ACGME: Accreditation Council for Graduate Medical Education.

ipated consequences and the heterogeneity of background, people and work flow (Table 1). For example, a change in the order pattern for patients in the radiology suite could impact the throughput in the ED (upstream effect) and delay results delivered to primary care offices (downstream effect). Looking at a process in isolation may not reflect the entire complexity of a situation. Things as simple as a patient transported for a routine chest radiograph from the floor to the radiology department involves systems that include clinicians, nurses, transport, finance, informatics, maintenance, information technology. Education/awareness sessions followed by periodic feedback are needed. Projects may not be successful because following the initial education effort there was no reinforcement training sessions

Table 2 Barriers and solutions to implementing a sepsis performance improvement program on the hospital floors

Barrier	Solution
Lack of personnel engagement	Use of 'influence' methods
Lack of education and awareness	Using repeated education sessions
Personnel turnover	Using repeated education sessions
Alert fatigue	Making the alert more specific than sensitive
Complexity of medical decisions	Re-engineering of process
Unintended consequences	Close monitoring and modification as needed

to follow. Healthcare provider turnover also creates performance improvement education problems. Barriers and potential solutions relevant to this type of initiative are presented in Table 2.

Process Improvement Steps

Lessons can be learned from our hospital's experience with a hospital floors severe sepsis initiative. As described by Kotter in his seminal article, the first step was to create a burning platform [25]. The initial message was quite simple as data clearly showed that patients on our medical floors did worse than others in regards to identification and treatment of sepsis. The second step was to create a guiding coalition that would lead this effort. This led to gathering all stakeholders: Administration, nurses, physicians, medical assistants, medical informatics, quality and pharmacists. The next step was to share and communicate the vision to a broader group. Once the vision was shared, the next step was to proceed to process re-engineering.

Process Change

When it comes to change, there are two major ways process change evolves over time: Either through rapid process re-engineering or with incremental change over time. Process re-engineering is a radical quick change that may be required in certain situations. There could be a need to rapidly implement a solution, such as with new regulatory requirements. Downside effects of this method are the resource intensive aspects and need for engagement from all players which may be associated with resistance.

Incremental changes over time may be chosen with the purpose of realizing change over a longer period of time with no sudden major changes in the environment. Obviously a combination of both methodologies can also be used.

Some of the most commonly used methods for change are Lean Six Sigma or the Toyota Methods. Lean Six Sigma is a continuous process improvement methodology that aims at reducing waste (Lean method) and eliminating defects (Six Sigma). It has been used in several major companies, such as Motorola and General Electric, and over the last decade has made its way into the health care industry with major successes reported, reducing cost and improving quality of care [26].

Influence Methods

After the process has been optimized by thc stakeholders it may still not be fully embraced and adopted. In this circumstance, 'influence' methods and tactics can be very powerful tools for success. A substantial amount of work has been done in this domain by sociologists. Some of the most widely accepted methods are built on the work of Cialdini [27]. Applying sources of influence to this performance improvement program may include: Liking (selecting several champions that are well respected and liked by all providers), endorsement (peer pressure), concession (by involving all providers and tweaking the process periodically), consistency (highlighting successes and giving timely feedback to providers who did not comply) and scarcity (one of the first hospitals involved in such a project).

Conclusion

The 2005–2008 SSC performance improvement program was adopted around the world and the resulting increase in compliance with the 6-hour and 24-hour sepsis bundles' quality indicators was associated with a decrease in mortality. Analysis of the data, however, revealed that mortality was unacceptably high in patients admitted from the hospital floors to the ICU. This was particularly troubling since the 2005–2008 initiative concentrated on building ED-ICU relationships to tackle the majority of admissions with severe sepsis that came from the ED.

With the above information in hand, the SSC has embarked on a hospital floors sepsis performance improvement initiative targeting early identification and treatment of floor patients with a new diagnosis of severe sepsis. The new initiative features the new 3-hour sepsis bundle (measure lactate, blood cultures, antibiotics and give fluids for hypotension or lactate ≥ 4 mmol/l). The Moore Foundation grant-funded program spreads across 4 US hospital performance indicator collaboratives (60 + hospitals), builds on lessons learned from the earlier SSC initiative, encourages a process change methodology and hopes to decrease mortality in this patient population.

References

1. Dellinger RP, Carlet JM, Masur H et al (2004) Surviving Sepsis Campaign guidelines for management of severe sepsis and septic shock. Crit Care Med 32:858–873
2. Dellinger RP, Carlet JM, Masur H et al (2004) Surviving Sepsis Campaign guidelines for management of severe sepsis and septic shock. Intensive Care Med 30:536–555
3. Dellinger RP, Levy MM, Carlet JM et al (2008) Surviving Sepsis Campaign: international guidelines for management of severe sepsis and septic shock: 2008. Crit Care Med 36:296–327
4. Dellinger RP, Levy MM, Carlet JM et al (2008) Surviving Sepsis Campaign: international guidelines for management of severe sepsis and septic shock: 2008. Intensive Care Med 34:17–60
5. Dellinger RP, Levy MM, Rhodes A et al (2013) Surviving sepsis campaign: international guidelines for management of severe sepsis and septic shock: 2012. Crit Care Med 41:580–637
6. Dellinger RP, Levy MM, Rhodes A et al (2013) Surviving Sepsis Campaign: international guidelines for management of severe sepsis and septic shock, 2012. Intensive Care Med 39:165–228
7. Dombrovskiy VY 1, Martin AA, Sunderram J, Paz HL (2007) Rapid increase in hospitalization and mortality rates for severe sepsis in the United States: a trend analysis from 1993 to 2003. Crit Care Med 35:1244–1250

8. Friedman G, Silva E, Vincent JL (1998) Has the mortality of septic shock changed with time? Crit Care Med 26:2078–2086
9. Levy MM, Dellinger RP, Townsend SR et al (2010) The Surviving Sepsis Campaign: results of an international guideline-based performance improvement program targeting severe sepsis. Crit Care Med 38:367–374
10. Levy MM, Dellinger RP, Townsend SR et al (2010) The Surviving Sepsis Campaign: results of an international guideline-based performance improvement program targeting severe sepsis. Intensive Care Med 36:222–231
11. Whittaker SA, Fuchs BD, Gaieski DF et al (2015) Epidemiology and outcomes in patients with severe sepsis admitted to the hospital wards. J Crit Care 30:78–84
12. Odden A, Rohde JM, Bonham C et al (2013) Functional outcomes of general medical patients with severe sepsis. BMC Infect Dis 13:588
13. Marwick CA, Guthrie B, Pringle JE et al (2014) A multifaceted intervention to improve sepsis management in general hospital wards with evaluation using segmented regression of interrupted time series. BMJ Qual Saf 23:e2
14. Young TP, McClean SI (2008) A critical look at Lean thinking in healthcare. Qual Saf Health Care 17:382–386
15. Cleghorn GD, Headrick LA (1996) The PDSA cycle at the core of learning in health professions education. Jt Comm J Qual Improv 22:206–212
16. Assunção M 1, Akamine N, Cardoso GS et al (2010) Survey on physicians' knowledge of sepsis: do they recognize it promptly? J Crit Care 25:545–552
17. McRee L, Thanavaro JL, Moore K, Goldsmith M, Pasvogel A (2014) The impact of an electronic medical record surveillance program on outcomes for patients with sepsis. Heart Lung 43:546–549
18. Manojlovich M (2010) Nurse/physician communication through a sensemaking lens: shifting the paradigm to improve patient safety. Med Care 48:941–946
19. Institute for Healthcare Improvement (2014) SBAR Technique for Communication: A Situational Briefing Model. http://www.ihi.org/resources/Pages/Tools/SBARTechniqueforCommunicationASituationalBriefingModel.aspx. Accessed Nov 2014
20. Micek ST, Roubinian N, Heuring T et al (2006) Before-after study of a standardized hospital order set for the management of septic shock. Crit Care Med 34:2707–2713
21. Shorr AF, Micek ST, Jackson WL Jr, Kollef MH (2007) Economic implications of an evidence-based sepsis protocol: can we improve outcomes and lower costs? Crit Care Med 35:1257–1262
22. Funk D, Sebat F, Kumar A (2009) A systems approach to the early recognition and rapid administration of best practice therapy in sepsis and septic shock. Curr Opin Crit Care 15:301–307
23. Embi PJ, Leonard AC (2012) Evaluating alert fatigue over time to EHR-based clinical trial alerts: findings from a randomized controlled study. J Am Med Inform Ass 19:e145–e148
24. Weingart SN, Toth M, Sands DZ, Aronson MD, Davis RB, Phillips RS (2003) Physicians' decisions to override computerized drug alerts in primary care. Arch Intern Med 163:2625–2631
25. Kotter JP (1995) Leading Change: Why Transformation Efforts Fail. Harvard Business Review (March-April):1–10
26. Glasgow JM, Scott-Caziewell JR, Kaboli PJ (2010) Guiding inpatient quality improvement: a systematic review of Lean and Six Sigma. Jt Comm J Qual Patient Saf 36:533–540
27. Redelmeier DA, Cialdini RB (2002) Problems for clinical judgement: 5. Principles of influence in medical practice. CMAJ 166:1680–1684

Part XIV
Data Management

State of the Art Review: The Data Revolution in Critical Care

M. Ghassemi, L. A. Celi, and D. J. Stone

Introduction

Many recent articles highlight the data revolution in healthcare, an offshoot of the vast amount of digital medical information that has now accumulated in electronic medical records (EMRs), and present it as an opportunity to create a 'learning healthcare system'. The generally proposed vision is for a population data-driven knowledge system that generalizes from every patient's life, disease and treatment experiences to impute the best course of action for diagnosis, prognosis and treatment of future patients.

There have also been many articles focusing on the risk that naïve use of Big Data (or data in general) poses. As stated by Zak Kohane of Harvard Medical School, Big Data in healthcare cannot be a simple, blind application of black-box techniques: "You really need to know something about medicine. If statistics lie, then Big Data can lie in a very, very big way." [1]

This paper will discuss the general issue of data in critical care with a focus on the Big Data phenomenon that is sweeping healthcare. With the vast amount of digital medical information that has accumulated in EMRs, the challenge is the transformation of the copious data into usable and useful medical knowledge.

Marzyeh Ghassemi
Department of Computer Science and Electrical Engineering, Computer Science and Artificial Intelligence Laboratory, Massachusetts Institute of Technology, Cambridge, USA

L. A. Celi ✉
Harvard-MIT Division of Health Science and Technology, Division of Pulmonary, Critical Care and Sleep Medicine, Beth Israel Deaconess Medical Center, Cambridge, USA
e-mail: lceli@mit.edu

D. J. Stone
Departments of Anesthesiology and Neurological Surgery, and the Center for Wireless Health, University of Virginia, Charlottesville, USA

J.-L. Vincent (ed.), *Annual Update in Intensive Care and Emergency Medicine 2015*,
DOI 10.1007/978-3-319-13761-2_42

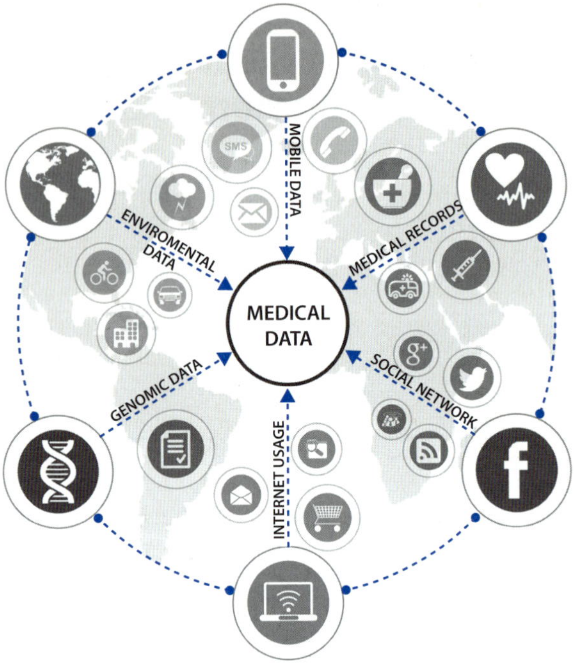

Fig. 1 Where Big Data in healthcare come from (figure courtesy of Yuan Lai)

We are experiencing a rapidly expanding collection of vast amounts of clinical data from routine practice and ambulatory monitoring. Clinicians must already make sense of a diverse variety of data input streams in order to make clinical decisions. Data from our everyday activities (financial transactions, cellphone and Internet use, social media posts), the environment, and even the local government promise to provide even more clinically relevant information (Fig. 1), but to what end? And how can increasing amounts of data be incorporated into a system of already overburdened clinicians?

The bottom line is that pertinent quality data add tremendous value, which accounts for their 'unreasonable effectiveness'. There is no way to minimize undesirable variability in practice without the data to substantiate the standardization. The volume and variety of increasingly available Big Data can allow us to interrogate clinical practice variation, personalize the risk-benefit score for every test and intervention, discover new knowledge to understand disease mechanisms, and optimize processes such as medical decision making, triage and resource allocation. Clinical data have been notorious for their variable interoperability and quality, but a holistic use of the massive data sources available (vital signs, clinical notes, laboratory results, treatments including medications and procedures) can lead to new perspectives on challenging problems. While the wetware of the human mind is a wonderful instrument for this purpose, we must design better data systems to support and improve those components of this data integration process that exceed human abilities [2].

Data in Critical Care

Critical care environments are intense by definition. Decisions in the intensive care unit (ICU) are frequently made in the setting of a high degree of uncertainty, and clinical staff may have only minutes or even seconds to make those decisions. The increasing need for intensive care has spiked the ratio of ICU beds to hospital beds as the ICU plays an expanding role in acute hospital care [3]. But the value of many treatments and interventions in the ICU is unproven, with many standard treatments being ineffective, minimally effective, questionably effective, or even harmful to the patient [4]. In a setting where the effects of every intervention are subject to patient and clinical context-specific factors, the ability to use data for decision support becomes very attractive and closer to essential as increasing complexity transcends typical cognitive capabilities.

An example of collected data being used to infer high-level information is the ICU scoring systems in use today. ICU scoring systems, such as APACHE (Acute Physiology and Chronic Health Evaluation), MPM (Mortality Probability Model), and SAPS (Simplified Acute Physiology Score), are all based on the use of physiologic and other clinical data for severity adjustment (Table 1). While these scores are primarily used to assess and compare ICU performance (e. g., by examining the ratio of actual-to-predicted outcomes) they also have use as short-hand indicators of patient acuity [5]. But scoring system value depends not only on the accuracy of the underlying data, but also on clinical trust in the reliability of the data and the predictions based on that data. In 2012, scoring systems were used in only 10% to 15% of US ICUs, despite demonstrated good discrimination and calibration [6].

In practice, clinical prediction must be motivated by the needs of clinical staff, and this must be driven in large part by perceived utility and an increase in technical comfort amongst clinicians. Some of the biggest opportunities for Big Data to make practical gains quickly are focused on the most expensive parts of current clinical practice: Reliable, predictive alerting and retrospective reporting analytics for high-cost patients, readmissions, triage, clinical decompensation, adverse events, and treatment optimization for diseases affecting multiple organ systems [7].

ICU physicians have embraced the value of collecting and storing electronic clinical records, and this has led to partnerships between industrial and academic entities. For example, the commercial APACHE Outcomes database has gathered partial physiologic and laboratory measurements from over 1 million patient records across 105 ICUs since 2010 [8]. The Philips eICU archives data from participating ICUs, and has collected an estimated database of over 1.5 million ICU stays. As an ongoing provider, the eICU adds more than 400,000 patient records per year to its stores, and these data are also commercially available to selected researchers via the eICU Research Institute [9]. In contrast to these commercial databases, the Multiparameter Intelligent Monitoring in Intensive Care (MIMIC) database is open and publicly accessible (Fig. 2). Over the past decade, the MIMIC database has collected clinical data from over 60,000 stays in Beth Israel Deaconess Medical Center ICUs, including clinical notes, physiological waveforms, laboratory measurements, and nurse-verified numerical data [10].

Table 1 A comparison of intensive care unit (ICU) scoring systems (from [47] with permission)

ICU Scoring System	Timing of data collected	Physiological values	Other required data	Total data elements required	Original reported mortality prediction performance
SAPS III	Prior to and within 1 hour of ICU admission	10	Age, six chronic health variables, ICU admission diagnosis, ICU admission source, LOS prior to ICU admission, emergency surgery, infection on admission, four variables for surgery type	26	AUC = 84.8% (n = 16,784)
APACHE IV	First ICU day (16–32 h depending on time of admission)	17	Age, six chronic health variables, ICU admission diagnosis, ICU admission source, LOS prior to ICU admission, emergency surgery, thrombolytic therapy, FiO_2, mechanical ventilation	32	AUC = 88.0% (n = 52,647)
MPM_0-III	Prior to and within 1 hour of ICU admission	3	Age, three chronic health variables, five acute diagnosis variables, admission type (e. g., medical-surgical) and emergency surgery, CPR within 1 h of ICU admission, mechanical ventilation, code status	16	AUC = 82.3% (n = 50,307)

SAPS: Simplified Acute Physiology Score; MPM: Mortality Prediction Model; APACHE: Acute Physiology and Chronic Health Evaluation; AUC: area under the curve; CPR: cardiopulmonary resuscitation; LOS: length of stay.

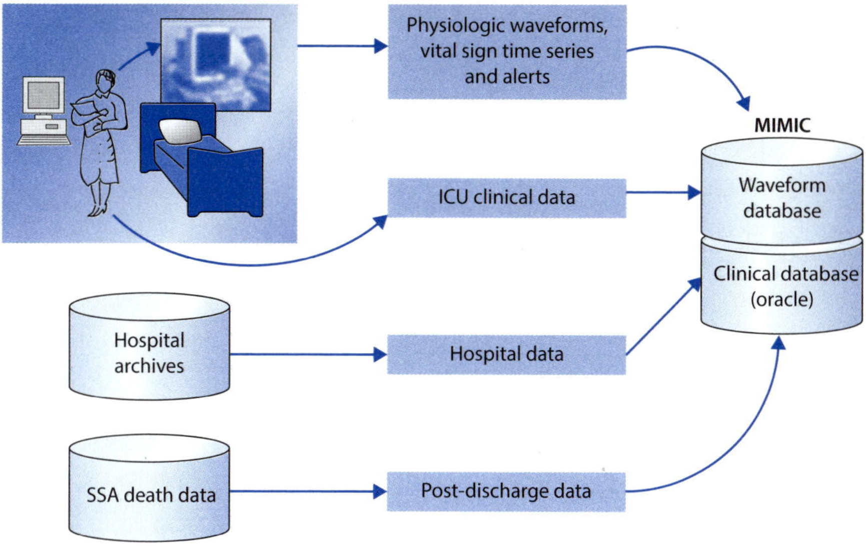

Fig. 2 The MIMIC Database. SSA: social security administration (figure courtesy of the Laboratory of Computational Physiology, Massachusetts Institute of Technology)

Establishing Knowledge

Medicine is ultimately based on knowledge, and each of the many ways to establish knowledge has certain advantages and pitfalls. Here, we focus on the randomized controlled trial (RCT), observational studies and what we have termed "dynamic clinical data mining" (DCDM) (Fig. 3).

RCTs are the gold-standard for clinical knowledge discovery. But 65 years after the first RCT was published, only 10–20% of medical decisions are based on RCT-supported evidence [11]. When examining the validity of a variety of medical interventions, about half of systematic reviews report insufficient evidence to support the intervention in question. Most treatment comparisons of clinical interest have actually never been addressed by an RCT [12]. The reality is that the exponential combinations of patients, conditions and treatments cannot be exhaustively explored by RCTs due to the large cost of adding even small numbers of patients. Furthermore, the process of performing RCTs often intentionally or inadvertently excludes groups of patients, such as those with particular co-morbidities or medications, or of certain ages or ethnic groups. Thus, when trying to make a real decision under practice conditions, the RCT conclusions may simply not be applicable to the patient and situation in hand. This was thc driver for the concept of DCDM in which the user of an EMR would be automatically presented with prior interventions and outcomes of similar patients to support what would otherwise be a completely subjective decision (see below).

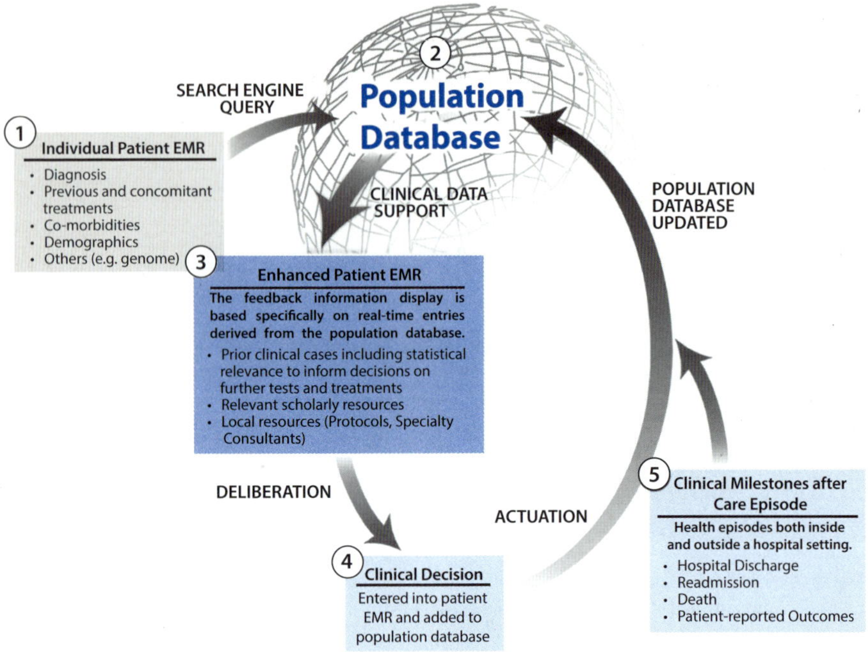

Fig. 3 Dynamic clinical data mining. EMR: electronic medical record (figure courtesy of Kai-ou Tang and Edward Moseley, from [20] with permission)

Recent observational studies on the MIMIC ICU database have yielded many interesting findings. These include the heterogeneity of treatment effect of red blood cell (RBC) transfusion [13], the impact of pre-admission selective serotonin reuptake inhibitors on mortality in the ICU [14], the interplay between clinical notes and structured data on mortality prediction [15], optimization of heparin dosing to minimize the probability of over- and under-anticoagulation [16], long-term outcomes of minor troponin elevations in the ICU [17] and the association between serum magnesium and blood pressure in the critically ill [18], to name a few. But these observations may be specific to the Beth Israel Deaconess Medical Center and need to be validated using databases from other institutions.

Others have examined institution-specific databases, and these studies have yielded findings that have been translated into practice: A recent study at Seattle Children's compared a wide range of performance metrics and translated results into prioritized departmental and enterprise-wide improvements [19].

Celi, Zimolzak and Stone described an operational vision for a digitally based, generalized decision support system that they termed "Dynamic Clinical Data Mining" [20]. The proposed system aggregates individual patient electronic health data in the course of care; queries a universal, de-identified clinical database using modified search engine technology in real time; identifies prior cases of sufficient similarity as to be instructive to the case at hand; and populates the individual

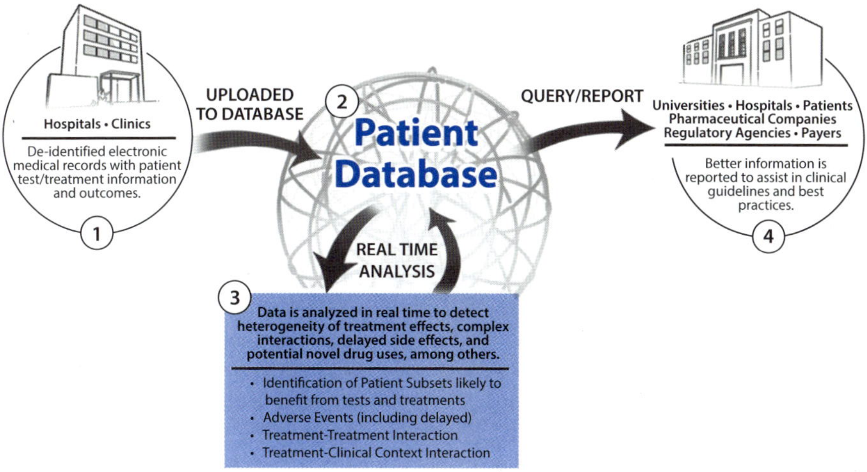

Fig. 4 Clinical care optimization: a Big Data model for efficient targeting of tests and treatments and vigilance for adverse events (figure courtesy of Kai-ou Tang and Edward Moseley, from [21] with permission)

patient's EMR with pertinent decision support material such as suggested interventions and prognosis, based on prior treatments and outcomes (Fig. 3).

Some of the most clear-cut arguments for Big Data in healthcare are in conjunction with the formulation of fully digitized prevention and pharmacovigilance processes [21] (Fig. 4). Clinicians of the future will have to work with user friendly versions of these tools to make timely and informed decisions about the drugs their patients are receiving. In a more general sense, clinicians will have to begin to consider an individual EMR as only part of a patient's record with the remainder of the record consisting of the two-way relationship of the patient's EMR with the entire population database. The essential starting point of the individual patient can be enhanced by the knowledge present in population-level databases, and the resulting information combinations and comparisons used to make informed clinical decisions. In turn, the information accumulated from individuals benefits the healthcare of the entire population.

Industry is also taking note. National pharmaceutical benefits manager, Express Scripts, can predict which patients may fail to take their medication 12 months in advance, with an accuracy rate of 98% [22]; IBM is modifying their famed Watson system (in tight collaboration with clinicians) for predicting different types of cancer [23]. 23andMe's database has already been used to find unknown genetic markers for Parkinson's disease [24] and myopia [25], and their acquisition of $1.3 million in National Institute of Health funding has shown additional confidence in their goals [26].

The Open Data Movement and Medicine

More recently, the open data movement has been quietly sweeping almost every industry, including the specialized domain of healthcare. It calls for data sharing, and by its very nature, requires a degree of accountability as well as collaboration across disciplines never seen before. At the forefront of the open data movement in healthcare is the pharmaceutical industry. In October 2012, GlaxoSmithKline (GSK) announced that it would make detailed data from its clinical trials widely available to researchers outside its own walls, stunning the scientific community [27]. For a company that spends $6.5 billion a year on research and development, it was a sharp turn away from a historic system of data secrecy. In May 2013, the company began posting its own data online. It then invited others to join ClinicalStudyDataRequest.com [28], where GSK and six other drug makers have already uploaded data from nearly 900 clinical trials. The following month, the medical device company, Medtronic, teamed up with Yale University and shared its clinical trials data through the Yale University Open Access Data (YODA) Project [29].

Other important trends in open data are crowdsourcing, data marathons and hackathons, which leverage several newly available phenomena [30]. These include combining publically available, detailed, and de-identified EMRs with crowdsourcing techniques and coordinated hackathons to capture, organize and integrate stakeholder user input from a necessary variety of input sources (Fig. 5). The traditional approach to knowledge discovery involves publication in peer-reviewed journals by a very circumscribed group of contributors. This process excluded a number of potentially valuable contributors, such as full time clinical physicians, nurses, medical trainees, and patients, among others.

Hackathons are large-scale events that contemporaneously bring together (physically and/or by teleconferencing) large groups of qualified individuals to collectively contribute their expertise towards a common problem set [31]. Crowdsourcing also focuses large groups of qualified individuals towards a common problem, but allows those individuals to do so asynchronously and in a mobile manner using phones, tablets, laptops and other devices to contribute from any location. With such tools, individual clinical encounters no longer have to be experienced in a silo-like fashion. The clinical 'crowd' can be leveraged to form a 'data substrate' available freely to clinicians and data scientists [4]. This amalgamation of individual knowledge should allow each clinician to address gaps in their knowledge, with the confidence that their decisions are supported by evidence in clinical practice.

In January 2014, the inaugural Critical Data Marathon and Conference was held at the Massachusetts Institute of Technology [30]. In the data marathon, physicians, nurses and pharmacists were paired with data scientists and engineers, and encouraged to investigate a variety of clinical questions that arise in the ICU. Over a 2-day period, more than 150 attendees began to answer questions, such as whether acetaminophen should be used to control fever in critically ill patients, and what the optimal blood pressure goal should be among patients with severe infection. This

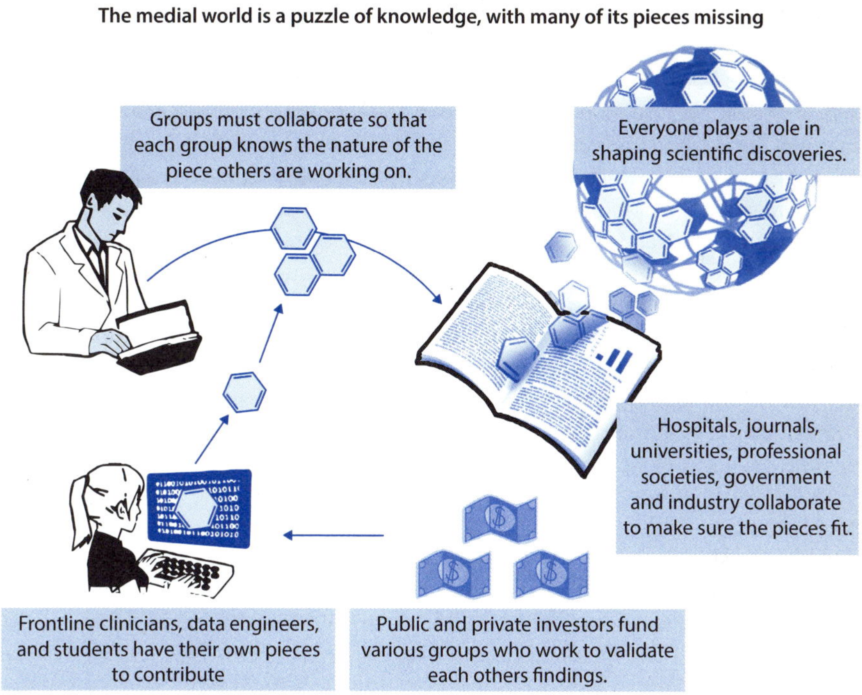

Fig. 5 Beyond open Big Data: Addressing unreliable research (figure courtesy of Kai-ou Tang)

event fostered collaboration between clinicians and data scientists that will support ongoing research in the ICU setting. The associated Critical Data Conference addressed growing concerns that Big Data will only augment the problem of unreliable research. Thought leaders from academia, government and industry across disciplines including clinical medicine, computer science, public health, informatics, biomedical research, health technology, statistics and epidemiology gathered and discussed the pitfalls and challenges of Big Data in healthcare. The consensus seemed to be that success will require systematized and fully transparent data interrogation, where data and methods are freely shared among different groups of investigators addressing the same or similar questions [30]. The added accuracy of the scientific findings is only one of the benefits of the systematization of the open data movement. Another will be the opportunity afforded to individuals of every educational level and area of expertise to contribute to science.

From a broader analysis of Big Data, we can try to understand larger patterns by comparing the strength of many signals in large populations. Larger data sets must also herald the advance of shared data sets. There is a critical need for collaborative research amongst many groups that explore similar questions. The association between data sharing and increased citation rate [32], and an increasing commitment by companies, funding agencies and investigators to more widely share clinical research data [33] point to the feasibility of this move. The prospect of using Big Data in an open environment may sound overwhelming, but there have been key steps to encourage this cultural transformation. For example, the Centers for Medicare and Medicaid Services (CMS) have begun to share data with providers and states [34]. As the largest single payer for health care in the United States, CMS has used its vast store of data to track hospital readmission rates in the Medicare program (importantly finding a rapid decline in readmission rates in 2012 and 2013), and combat Medicare fraud (in its first year the system stopped, prevented, or identified an estimated $115 million in improper payments).

As large amounts of shared data become available from different geographic and academic sources, there will be the additional benefit from the collection of data from sources with different viewpoints and biases. While individual researchers may not be aware of their own biases or assumptions that may impact reported results, shared exploration of Big Data provides us with an inherent sanity check that has been sorely lacking in many fields.

Big Data *per se*

In a recent analysis of data-driven healthcare by the MIT Technology review, the authors noted that "medicine has entered its data age" [1]. Driven by the promise of an estimated $300 to $450 billion a year [35], companies of all sizes are beginning to fight in earnest to capture and tame the data explosion. Key innovations fall into three major areas: More and more data, especially resulting from mobile monitoring; better analytics using new machine learning and other techniques; and meaningful recommendations that focus on prediction, description, and prevention of poor health outcomes (that are finally captured in an easily accessible format).

The mass of new data rests primarily in the proprietary hands of large entities like insurance companies and care providers. For example, the genomics company 23andMe is famously creating a huge database of genomic data, moving from over 700,000 records towards their goal of tens of millions [26]. Some countries with centralized healthcare systems like Denmark are also beginning to leverage that accessible data [36]. In addition, smaller companies like WellDoc [37] and Ginger.io [38] are beginning to focus on rampant cell-phone penetration to get into the health-data market. Mobile phones can now seamlessly acquire daily patient metrics on meals, exercise, call patterns and other behaviors; WellDoc uses these data to recommend personalized insulin doses based on patients' daily habits, and Ginger.io monitors patients with mental illnesses for the kinds of actions that might indicate a need for help. Other companies provide physical attachments to mobile devices that enrich the possible data types available: CellScope sells an attachment to support remote otoscopy; AliveCor provides electrocardiogram (EKG) signals; Propeller Health attaches to an inhaler to record pertinent data; and there are a slew of others for nearly every imaginable data need [39].

But bigger data require better methods, and better machine learning techniques for clinical data have been a long time in coming. The most intuitive argument

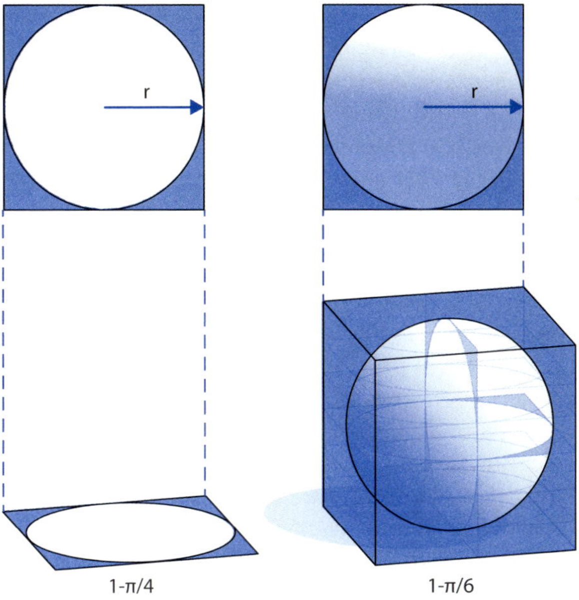

Fig. 6 The data space and corner cases (figure courtesy of Yuan Lai)

(that more data from which to learn cannot be worse, so must be better) is true: There have been empirical demonstrations that predictive models built from sparse, fine-grained data see marginal gains in predictive performance even to massive scale [40]. But there is another less intuitive argument for bigger data: Certain rare trends or behaviors simply may not be observed in sufficient numbers without employing Big Data. Dubbed the 'heavy tail' of data, these rare behaviors are even more difficult to observe as we add more features to our datasets. Intuitively, we can think of datasets as a set of samples out of a larger space; for example, a circle inscribed within a square gets most of the area, leaving only the corners out. But as we move from inscribing a circle within a square, to inscribing a sphere within a cube, the ratio of space in the corners increases [41] (Fig. 6). Repeat this to a higher dimension and most of the volume of the cube will be concentrated in its (many) corners. But it is these rare instances (sometimes appropriately referred to as 'corner cases') of behaviors or patient characteristics that machine learning cannot reliably analyze with historically available data sample sizes. The Big Data explosion is finally offering data at a scale large enough to overcome the risks of higher-dimensional spaces when working with healthcare data issues.

Along with Big Data's promise, there have been warnings of over confidence and disaster, labelled by Lazer et al. as "Big Data hubris" [42]. The warning parable told to illustrate this is Google's "Flu Trends" [43]. In 2008, Google launched its Flu Trends, which used the search terms typed into Google to track the progression of influenza epidemics over time. However, this approach was subsequently revealed to have suffered from several known data analysis pitfalls (e. g., overfitting and concept drift) so that by 2012–2013, the prevalence of flu was being greatly overestimated. Other oft-cited risks include misleading conclusions derived from spurious associations in increasingly detailed data, and biased collection of data that may make derived hypotheses difficult to validate or generalize [44].

But avoiding spurious conclusions from data analysis is not a challenge unique to Big Data. A 2012 *Nature* review of cancer research found reproducibility of findings in only 11% of 53 published papers [45]. There is concern that Big Data will only augment this noise, but using larger datasets actually tends to help with inflated significance, as the estimated effect sizes tend to be much smaller [46].

The biased collection of data is a non-trivial question. If researchers have large amounts of data that severely oversample certain populations or conditions, their derived hypotheses can be incorrect or at least understandably difficult to validate. The way that current literature is designed, generated, and published creates sequential 'statistically significant' discoveries from restricted datasets. It is not uncommon in the scientific literature to get a different story for a variable's (vitamin E, omega-3, coffee) relationship to outcome (mortality, Alzheimer's, infant birth-weight) depending on what is adjusted for, or how a population was selected. There is little meaning to exploring the impact of one variable for one outcome: it is the big picture that is meaningful.

Conclusion

The benefits of the data explosion far outweigh the risks for the careful researcher. As target populations subdivide along combinations of comorbid conditions and countless genetic polymorphisms, as diagnostic and monitoring device including wearable sensors become more ubiquitous, and as therapeutic options expand beyond the evaluation of individual interventions including drugs and procedures, it is clear that the traditional approach to knowledge discovery cannot scale to match the exponential growth of medical complexity.

Rather than taking turns hyping and disparaging Big Data, we need organizations and researchers to create methods and processes that address some of our most pressing concerns, e. g., who is in 'charge' of shared data, who 'owns' clinical data, and how do we best combine heterogeneous and superficially non-interoperable data sources? We need to use Big Data in a different way than we have traditionally used data – collaboratively. By creating a culture of transparency and reproducibility, we can turn the hype over Big Data into big findings.

References

1. MIT editors (2014) Business Report: Data-driven Health Care. MIT Technology Review 117:1–19
2. Celi LA, Csete M, Stone D (2014) Optimal data systems: the future of clinical predictions and decision support. Curr Opin Crit Care 20:573–580
3. Vincent JL (2013) Critical care-where have we been and where are we going? Crit Care 17(Suppl 1):S2

4. Celi LA, Mark RG, Stone DJ, Montgomery RA (2013) "Big data" in the intensive care unit. Closing the data loop. Am J Respir Crit Care Med 187:1157
5. Breslow MJ, Badawi O (2012) Severity scoring in the critically ill: Part 2 -Maximizing value from outcome prediction scoring systems. Chest 141:518–527
6. Breslow MJ, Badawi O (2012) Severity scoring in the critically ill: Part 1 – Interpretation and accuracy of outcome prediction scoring systems. Chest 141:245–252
7. Bates DW, Saria S, Ohno-Machado L, Shah A, Escobar G (2014) Big Data In health care: Using analytics to identify and manage high-risk and high-cost patients. Health Aff (Millwood) 33:1123–1131
8. APACHE Outcomes. Available at: https://www.cerner.com/Solutions/Hospitals_and_Health_Systems/Critical_Care/APACHE_Outcomes/Accessed Nov 2014
9. McShea M, Holl R, Badawi O, Riker R, Silfen E (2010) The eICU research institute – a collaboration between industry, health-care providers, and academia. IEEE Eng Med Biol Mag 29:18–25
10. Saeed M, Villarroel M, Reisner AT et al (2011) Multiparameter Intelligent Monitoring in Intensive Care II (MIMIC-II): a public-access intensive care unit database. Crit Care Med 39:952
11. Smith M, Saunders R, Stuckhardt L, McGinnis JM, Committee on the Learning Health Care System in America, Institute of Medicine (2013) Best Care At Lower Cost: The Path To Continuously Learning Health Care In America. National Academies Press, Washington
12. Mills EJ, Thorlund K, Ioannidis J (2013) Demystifying trial networks and network meta-analysis. BMJ 346:f2914
13. Dejam A, Malley BE, Feng M et al (2014) The effect of age and clinical circumstances on the outcome of red blood cell transfusion in the critically ill patients. Crit Care 18:487
14. Ghassemi M, Marshall J, Singh N, Stone DJ, Celi LA (2014) Leveraging a critical care database: selective serotonin reuptake inhibitor use prior to ICU admission is associated with increased hospital mortality. Chest 145:745–752
15. Ghassemi M, Naumann T, Doshi-Velez F et al (2014) Unfolding physiological state: Mortality modelling in intensive care units. KDD 2014:75–84
16. Ghassemi MM, Richter SE, Eche IM, Chen TW, Danziger J, Celi LA (2014) A data-driven approach to optimized medication dosing: a focus on heparin. Intensive Care Med 40:1332–1339
17. Velasquez A, Ghassemi M, Szolovits P et al (2014) Long-term outcomes of minor troponin elevations in the intensive care unit. Anaesth Intensive Care 42:356–364
18. Celi LA, Scott DJ, Lee J et al (2013) Association of hypermagnesemia and blood pressure in the critically ill. J Hypertension 31:2136–2141
19. Kolker E, Kolker E (2014) Healthcare analytics: Creating a prioritized improvement system with performance benchmarking. Big Data 2:50–54
20. Celi LA, Zimolzak AJ, Stone DJ (2014) Dynamic clinical data mining: search engine-based decision support. JMIR Med Inform 2:e13
21. Celi LA, Moseley E, Moses C et al (2014) From pharmacovigilance to clinical care optimization. Big Data 2:1–8
22. The Runaway Cost of Diabetes. Available from: http://lab.express-scripts.com/insights/drug-options/the-runaway-cost-of-diabetes Accessed Sept 2014
23. Edwards C (2014) Using patient data for personalized cancer treatments. Communications of the ACM 57:13–15
24. Do CB, Tung JY, Dorfman E et al (2011) Web-based genome-wide association study identifies two novel loci and a substantial genetic component for Parkinson's disease. PLoS Gen 7:e1002141
25. Kiefer AK, Tung JY, Do CB et al (2013) Genome-wide analysis points to roles for extracellular matrix remodeling, the visual cycle, and neuronal development in myopia. PLoS Gen 9:e1003299
26. 23andMe Scientists Receive Approximately $1.4 Million in Funding from the National Institutes of Health. http://mediacenter.23andme.com/press-releases/nih_grant_2014/. Accessed Sept 2014

27. GSK announces further initiatives to advance openness and collaboration to help tackle global health challenges. Available from: http://us.gsk.com/en-us/media/press-releases/2012/gsk-announces-further-initiatives-to-advance-openness-and-collaboration-to-help-tackle-global-health-challenges/ Accessed Sept 2014
28. Clinical Study Data Request Site (2014) Available from: https://clinicalstudydatarequest.com/ (accessed Nov 2014)
29. Krumholz HM, Ross JS, Gross CP et al (2013) A historic moment for open science: the Yale University Open Data Access Project and Medtronic. Ann Intern Med 158:910–911
30. Badawi O, Brennan T, Celi LA et al (2014) Making big data useful for health care: a summary of the inaugural mit critical data conference. JMIR Med Inform 2:e22
31. Celi LA, Ippolito A, Montgomery RA, Moses C, Stone DJ (2014) Crowdsourcing knowledge discovery and innovations in medicine. J Med Internet Res 16:216
32. Piwowar HA, Day RS, Fridsma DB (2007) Sharing detailed research data is associated with increased citation rate. PloS One 2:e308
33. Wilhelm EE, Oster E, Shoulson I (2014) Approaches and Costs for Sharing Clinical Research Data. JAMA 311:1201–1202
34. Brennan N, Oelschlaeger A, Cox C, Tavenner M (2014) Leveraging the big-data revolution: CMS is expanding capabilities to spur health system transformation. Health Affairs 33:1195–1202
35. Kayyali B, Knott D, Van Kuiken S (2013) The big-data revolution in US health care: Accelerating value and innovation. McKinsey & Company. http://www.mckinsey.com/insights/health_systems_and_services/the_big-data_revolution_in_us_health_care. Accessed Nov 2014
36. Saunders MK (2014) In Denmark, big data goes to work. Health Affairs 33:1245–1245
37. Quinn CC, Clough SS, Minor JM, Lender D, Okafor MC, Gruber-Baldini A (2008) WellDoc™ mobile diabetes management randomized controlled trial: change in clinical and behavioral outcomes and patient and physician satisfaction. Diabetes Technol Ther 10:160–168
38. Giles J (2012) Computational social science: Making the links. Nature 488:448–450
39. M Health Health and appiness. The Economist Magazine. http://www.economist.com/news/business/21595461-those-pouring-money-health-related-mobile-gadgets-and-apps-believe-they-can-work (Created Feb 1, 2014). Accessed Nov 2014
40. Junqué de Fortuny E, Martens D, Provost F (2013) Predictive modeling with big data: is bigger really better? Big Data 1:215–226
41. Bishop CM (2006) Pattern Recognition And Machine Learning. Springer, New York, p 740
42. Lazer D, Kennedy R, King G, Vespignani A (2014) The parable of Google flu: traps in big data analysis. Science 343:1203–1205
43. Butler D (2013) When Google got flu wrong. Nature 494:155
44. Harford T (2014) Big Data: are we making a big mistake. Financial Times Magazine. http://www.ft.com/cms/s/2/21a6e7d8-b479-11e3-a09a-00144feabdc0.html#axzz3Jvb2tbcP. Accessed Nov 2014
45. Begley CG, Ellis LM (2012) Drug development: Raise standards for preclinical cancer research. Nature 483:531–533
46. Ioannidis JP, Panagiotou OA (2011) Comparison of effect sizes associated with biomarkers reported in highly cited individual articles and in subsequent meta-analyses. JAMA 305:2200–2210
47. Mayaud L (2014) Prediction of mortality in septic patients with hypotension. PhD Thesis, Oxford University

Creating a Learning Healthcare System in the ICU

J. Yu and J. M. Kahn

Introduction

The intensive care unit (ICU) is a high-pressure, high-stakes clinical environment where patients at high risk for morbidity and mortality receive critical organ support. Patients and families are at their most vulnerable, with fates outside of their control and little experience to help guide them through the process. To provide care in this environment, ICU clinicians must rely on an uncertain evidence base, with few high quality studies to guide clinical decision making. Although we have reams of data, including vital signs, laboratory studies, clinical notes and physiological tracings, we lack the tools to quickly organize, assimilate and interpret those data in a way that makes them useful at the bedside.

These challenges are not unique to the ICU. Indeed, the same can be said about the healthcare system as a whole: Patients in need, an anemic evidence-base for decision making, and more data than can be readily interpreted [1]. One response to this challenge is to move towards what is increasingly known as the "learning healthcare system" [2]. First advanced as an ideal by the United States Institute of Medicine (IoM), a learning healthcare system is one in which "evidence is both applied and developed as a natural product of the care processes" [3]. In a learning healthcare system, the clinical enterprise and the research enterprise are integrated, rather than largely separate as they are now. Clinicians and researchers can make full use of available data to expand the evidence based for decision making in near real-time.

Achieving a learning healthcare system is a laudable goal, both in the ICU and elsewhere in medicine. Yet at present little is known about how this shift will impact the practice of critical care and how we can best move in this direction. In this chapter, we discuss the rationale for developing a learning healthcare system in the

J. Yu · J. M. Kahn ✉
Dept of Critical Care Medicine, University of Pittsburgh School of Medicine, Pittsburgh, USA
e-mail: kahnjm@upmc.edu

J.-L. Vincent (ed.), *Annual Update in Intensive Care and Emergency Medicine 2015*,
DOI 10.1007/978-3-319-13761-2_43

ICU, review some of the key barriers to creating a learning healthcare system in the ICU, and outline a roadmap through we which we can move towards this goal.

What Is Meant by a "Learning Healthcare System"?

The concept of the learning healthcare system is a response to many different problems in healthcare, but chief among these is the notion that providers lack timely and actionable evidence to inform clinical decisions. Despite enormous investments in clinical research over the last decades, few clinical decisions are informed by robust evidence [4]. Moreover, due to the slow pace of and high expense research, innovations in healthcare, both in terms of therapeutics and healthcare delivery strategies, go untested for years after their introduction, if at all [5].

The learning healthcare system addresses this problem by integrating clinical care and research through a mature electronic health record (Fig. 1) [3]. Rather than research occurring in parallel to clinical care, knowledge generation is the natural byproduct of clinical care, all patients actively and continuously contribute data for research, which can then be used to rapidly generate clinical evidence. In turn, that new evidence is directly applied in real time. Such a system would have several key elements, including a robust, interoperable electronic medical record (EMR) that can be quickly and easily mined; a culture of shared responsibility for healthcare improvement on the part of clinicians, researchers and the public, such that patients willingly participate in the generation of new knowledge as part of their role in the larger healthcare system; and alignment of incentives to rapidly generate and apply new knowledge, eliminating the disconnect between research and clinical care [3].

The Rationale for the Learning Healthcare System in Critical Care

There are several problems with current critical care systems that would directly be impacted by a learning healthcare system (Box 1).

Box 1. Rationale for the Learning Healthcare System

Research is not routinely implemented in practice
Research is not informed by clinical practice
Research is costly and time-consuming
Research paradigms do not answer the right questions

- Research is not routinely implemented in practice. The gap between clinical evidence and clinical practice is well documented in critical care [6]. For example, several studies convincingly demonstrate that patients with acute respiratory

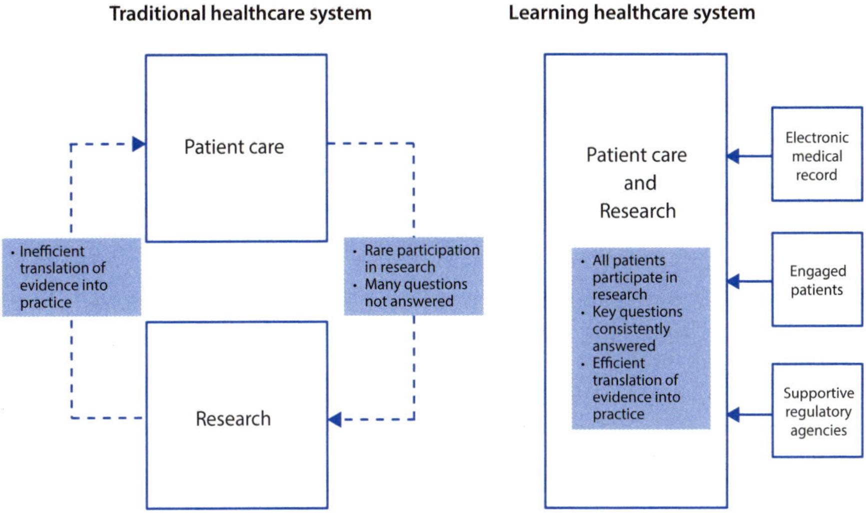

Fig. 1 A model of the current healthcare system and a learning healthcare system. In the current healthcare system, research runs in parallel to clinical care. In the learning healthcare system, research is integrated into clinical care supported by a mature electronic medical record

distress syndrome (ARDS) do not routinely receive a lung protective ventilation strategy proven to save lives [7, 8]. Moreover, patients receiving mechanical ventilation frequently do not receive evidence-based preventive care, daily interruption of continuous sedation or daily spontaneous breathing trials [9]. As a consequence there is preventable mortality among critically ill patients, with wide variation in outcomes across hospitals not accounted for by variation in case-mix [10].

- Research is not informed by clinical practice. New evidence itself is frequently not directly applicable to clinical practice. Because of the disconnect between clinicians and researchers, clinical trials and observational studies do not always answer the most important and timely research questions. For example, pharmaceutical companies generally fund only research into proprietary therapeutics with potential to generate revenue [11]. Generic medicines that lack a profit potential but have clinical potential, such as heparin in sepsis [12] and antidepressants for post-ICU depression [13], are rarely subjected to large trials. Additionally, the vast majority of patient care is wasted from a learning standpoint. Every day patients are subjection to variations in treatments, yet we have no capacity to learn from our experiences in a systematic way. We may 'learn by doing' as individual clinicians, but these experiences generate no collective knowledge that can be used to advance the field. Meanwhile, front-line clinicians with important questions about how to best deliver care have no mechanism to drive knowledge discovery, instead relying on the academic research enterprise.
- Research is costly and time-consuming. Even a small clinical trial in the ICU costs upwards of $5 million, and will ultimately answer only a relatively narrow set of research questions. Moreover, most ICU-based clinical trials take years

to complete, furthering the disconnect between evidence generation and clinical practice [14]. For example, a recent study of weaning strategies in prolonged mechanical ventilation took over 10 years to enroll 316 patients [15], and a research question that was timely over a decade ago remained unanswered until just recently. Another example can be found in the rise and fall of drotrecogin alfa for severe sepsis. It took three clinical trials conducted over nearly 15 years to assess the value of this drug, which was ultimately withdrawn from the market due to lack of efficacy [16]. Despite all these trials, reasonable doubt still exists as to whether drotrecogin alfa may still be life saving in some groups of patients, such as those with meningococcemia [17]. Many years and untold millions of dollars later, we still do not fully understand whether and when drotrecogin alfa may work.

- Research paradigms do not answer the right questions. An analogous problem is that the research enterprise itself is not set up to answer the right questions. Randomized controlled trials (RCTs), the mainstay of causal inference in biomedical research, are extremely limited in many regards. RCTs can only answer questions in highly selected patient populations that are frequently not representative of the population of interest. Thus, although RCTs often yield internally valid results, these results may be just as biased, if not more so, than the results of carefully conducted observational trials [18]. RCTs also only give results on the average treatment effects for the selected population. They cannot give other important results, such as the proportion of patients in a population who might benefit from a treatment, or whether a treatment will benefit a specific individual patient [18]. This information is arguably more important to decision makers such as clinicians, who are treating individual patients, and regulatory agencies, who are making determinations about drug approval populations rather than means [19].

How the Learning Healthcare System Would Help

A learning healthcare system in the ICU would overcome these problems in several ways. To correct the problem of research failing to inform practice, the learning healthcare system would incorporate clinical decision support and protocols at the point of care, overcoming some of the frequently cited barriers to evidence-based practice [20]. These decision support systems would not be static but would rapidly adapt to new data informing outcome probabilities with recent treatments. They could also be used to rapidly test different pragmatic treatment strategies, randomly assigning clinicians or ICUs to different permutations of the decisions support system.

To correct the problem of research failing to be informed by practice, every patient would directly contribute data to an ICU registry that could be queried to not only determine current treatment patterns but also assess treatment variation, ensuring that clinical studies answer questions of relevance to patients and clinicians.

Clinicians themselves could also query these databases, asking questions like "for patients like mine, which treatment did they most often receive, X or Y?"

To correct the problem of costly and time consuming trials, the learning healthcare system would be able to rapidly and facilely enroll large numbers of patients in clinical studies. Both patient enrollment and clinical data collection would be facilitated by an EMR that is at once complete and easily queried [21]. The recurring problem of clinical trials being underpowered because the outcome incidence is lower than anticipated would be reduced or eliminated, since researchers would always have access to recent and accurate patient-level data on disease incidence and outcomes [22].

To correct the problem that RCTs are not necessarily the gold standard for clinical decision making, the learning healthcare system would facilitate rapid observational studies as well as large-scale, effectiveness trials designed to answer questions of immediate importance to clinicians [23]. Exploiting natural variation in treatment processes, we can learn about how treatments work in the real-world instead of only relying on experimental evidence. Experiments are important, but all types of evidence will be essential for understanding treatment effects and guiding decision making.

Examples

Under a learning healthcare system in the ICU, the daily practice of critical care would be directly and tightly tied to research, and vice versa. Here we offer several examples of how this might work in practice.

Understanding Disease Burden

Investigators wishing to design a clinical trial need accurate, up-to-date information on the burden of disease. This information is necessary to assess the potential clinical value of a novel treatment, to understand the possible number of eligible patients at each center, and to perform accurate power calculations based on the incidence of the outcome of interest. Rather than look to the published literature, which is often out of date and subject to publication bias, the investigators could query the ICUs in the learning healthcare system. Using their EMRs, the ICUs could quickly return accurate and actionable data for use in planning the trial or deciding whether to go ahead with it in the first place.

Conducting a Randomized Controlled Trial

Next, the investigators could conduct the clinical trial directly in the participating ICUs making use of the EMR. The EMR could automatically screen each admitted patient for eligibility. When the EMR discovers an eligible patient, an automated notice could be sent to the physician asking for permission to enroll the patient. After enrollment, the EMR could be used to collect outcome data. Such a system would enable researchers to conduct trials of much larger scope than is currently possible, at much reduced cost. The trial could be even more powerful by directly tying randomization to real-time treatment decisions. For example, if the EMR notices that an ICU physician is prescribing a certain therapy, perhaps through computerized physician order entry (CPOE), it could embed an enrollment alert directly into the CPOE system, inquiring: "I notice that you are prescribing drug X. In similar scenarios, physicians have prescribed both X and Y. Would you consider randomizing your patient to receive either X or Y?", then acting on the physician's response. In this way, research can be directly embedded in clinical care, greatly increasing the efficiency of the research enterprise.

Assessing the Effectiveness of a Novel Therapeutic

The learning healthcare system could also be used for post-marketing surveillance of novel therapeutics based on the EMR. If unexpected side effects are encountered, these could be tracked using the EMR and fed back to a central repository quickly. As experience with the drug grows, investigators could quickly assemble a large, continually updated patient registry that could be used to perform observational studies of effectiveness, controlling for observed covariates using traditional methods like regression, and controlling for unobserved covariates using instrumental variables and other techniques for causal inference in observational data [24]. Most powerfully, with a large enough dataset the analyses could be customized for individual patients, not just populations. In this way, physicians could determine how patients like theirs responded to the drug, better informing individualized decisions at the bedside.

Barriers

Achieving a fully realized learning healthcare system faces numerous barriers (Box 2).

Box 2. Barriers to the Learning Healthcare System

Poorly functional electronic health records

Data privacy

The need for informed consent in prospective studies

Competition among providers

Poorly Functional EMRs

Most existing EMRs are poorly equipped to handle the demands of a true learning healthcare system [25]. The data exist in complex databases that are difficult to query, often requiring customized programming languages and other poorly interoperable tools to abstract data for research. Different systems use different data architectures and naming conventions, making data sharing and collaboration across health systems difficult. Alternatively, these data must be cleaned and archived prior to use, making them ineffective for real-time decision making. The human interfaces for these systems are also lacking, with alarms that are easily ignored or, perhaps more frequently, non-specific and thus more annoying than helpful [26].

Privacy and Regulatory Barriers

Data privacy and confidentiality are important concerns, particularly in the modern era of hackers and security breaches, which can occur in even the most secure systems. Yet they also pose a substantial barrier to the learning healthcare system. Many regulations, including the US Health Insurance Portability and Accountability Act, require permission to use protected health data for research if it is at all possible. This well-meaning regulation works on a small scale, but becomes infeasible and impractical on a large scale. Similarly, the learning healthcare system will still rely on randomized study designs, which, when the studies involve hundreds of thousands patients, can make informed consent a prohibitive obstacle to success [27]. Yet decades of work in the ethics of research appropriately prohibits patient-level randomization without informed consent in most biomedical research.

Competition Among Providers

A successful learning healthcare system requires collaboration across numerous healthcare providers, both within provider types (e. g., across multiple hospitals) and across provider types (e. g., across hospitals and insurers) [28]. Yet many of these stakeholders compete for patients and revenue, making large scale collaboration a challenge. Researchers also can be more competitive than collaborative. For example, when the learning healthcare system requires coordination across multiple academic medical centers, issues such as grant revenue and academic credit must be dealt with, posing a potential challenge.

Future Directions

These challenges, although large, are not insurmountable, and even at present we can take several steps toward the learning healthcare system in the ICU. First, we can work to build more useful EMRs that are designed not just as data repositories but as tools for data analysis and interpretation. The information technology already exists and is widely applied in other industries – we simply need to bring it to healthcare. EMRs can be made more interoperable by building off novel data-sharing tools such as I2B2, which facilitates collaborative data repositories [29], and SHRINE, which allows for multiple EMRs to be queried simultaneously without moving data across firewalls [30]. Search functions and natural language processing can also be incorporated into EMRs. For example, Google anticipates what users are searching for and offers suggestions based on the prior searches of the individual user and other users. Similarly, EMRs could see what other clinicians have done for similar patients and make similar suggestions.

Second, we can convene a large-scale effort to deal with the regulatory and privacy issues that go part and parcel with the learning healthcare system [31]. A first step is better engaging patients as partners in the research process. We have already accepted the notion that patients need not consent to give their records for quality improvement, since the overall goal of quality improvement is to improve individual patient health. Yet this goal is not in principle different from that of the learning healthcare system. Perhaps by working more closely with patients and informing them of the potential uses of their data we can move towards a world where personal health information can be more rapidly used to generate new knowledge. Ultimately we can create novel 'integrated consent' paradigms that give new flexibility to the learning healthcare system while offering patients important protection [32].

Conclusion

A learning healthcare system for the ICU is a laudable goal. In many ways, the ICU is a ripe area for the development of such a system, given its history as a data-rich clinical environment [33]. The idea is also catching on. Since first advanced by the IoM, the learning healthcare system has been endorsed by the US Patient Centered Outcomes Research Institute, which is working to develop a learning healthcare system in the US through its Clinical Data Research Networks [34]. Moreover, much of what we describe as the learning healthcare system is already gaining traction through other names, such as 'big data' and 'analytics' [35]. Together, these concepts underlie an essential effort to better use data to improve healthcare outcomes, not just through quality improvement but also through research and the creation of generalizable knowledge. The continuing gap between evidence and practice, and the lack of evidence for the bulk of clinical decisions, demands no less.

References

1. Riley WT, Glasgow RE, Etheredge L, Abernethy AP (2013) Rapid, responsive, relevant (R3) research: a call for a rapid learning health research enterprise. Clin Transl Med 2:10
2. Friedman CP, Wong AK, Blumenthal D (2010) Achieving a nationwide learning health system. Sci Transl Med 2:57–29
3. Olsen L, Aisner D, McGinnis JM (2007) Roundtable on Evidence-Based Medicine: The Learning Healthcare System: Workshop Summary. National Academies Press, Washington
4. Eddy DM (2005) Evidence-based medicine: a unified approach. Health Aff (Millwood) 24:9–17
5. Berwick DM (2003) Disseminating innovations in health care. JAMA 289:1969–1975
6. Kahn JM (2009) Disseminating clinical trial results in critical care. Crit Care Med 37:S147–S153
7. Cooke CR, Watkins TR, Kahn JM et al (2008) The effect of an intensive care unit staffing model on tidal volume in patients with acute lung injury. Crit Care 12:R134
8. Esteban A, Ferguson ND, Meade MO et al (2008) Evolution of mechanical ventilation in response to clinical research. Am J Respir Crit Care Med 177:170–177
9. Kahn JM, Brake H, Steinberg KP (2007) Intensivist physician staffing and the process of care in academic medical centres. Qual Saf Health Care 16:329–333
10. Chen LM, Render M, Sales A, Kennedy EH, Wiitala W, Hofer TP (2012) Intensive care unit admitting patterns in the veterans affairs health care system. Arch Intern Med 172:1220–1226
11. Angell M (2008) Industry-sponsored clinical research: a broken system. JAMA 300:1069–1071
12. Davidson BL, Geerts WH, Lensing AWA (2002) Low-dose heparin for severe sepsis. N Engl J Med 347:1036–1037
13. Weinert C, Meller W (2006) Epidemiology of depression and antidepressant therapy after acute respiratory failure. Psychosomatics 47:399–407
14. Ioannidis JP (1998) Effect of the statistical significance of results on the time to completion and publication of randomized efficacy trials. JAMA 279:281–286
15. Jubran A, Grant BJB, Duffner LA et al (2013) Effect of pressure support vs unassisted breathing through a tracheostomy collar on weaning duration in patients requiring prolonged mechanical ventilation: A randomized trial. JAMA 309:671–677

16. Wenzel RP, Edmond MB (2012) Septic shock – evaluating another failed treatment. N Engl J Med 366:2122–2124
17. Faust SN, Levin M, Harrison OB et al (2001) Dysfunction of endothelial protein C activation in severe meningococcal sepsis. N Engl J Med 345:408–416
18. Deaton A (2010) Instruments, Randomization, and Learning about Development. Journal of Economic Literature 48:424–455
19. Harris KM, Remler DK (1998) Who is the marginal patient? Understanding instrumental variables estimates of treatment effects. Health Serv Res 33:1337–1360
20. Garg AX, Adhikari NKJ, McDonald H et al (2005) Effects of computerized clinical decision support systems on practitioner performance and patient outcomes: a systematic review. JAMA 293:1223–1238
21. D'Avolio L, Ferguson R, Goryachev S et al (2012) Implementation of the Department of Veterans Affairs' first point-of-care clinical trial. J Am Med Inform Assoc 19:e170–e176
22. Halpern SD, Karlawish JHT, Berlin JA (2002) The continuing unethical conduct of underpowered clinical trials. JAMA 288:358–362
23. Dahabreh IJ, Kent DM (2014) Can the learning health care system be educated with observational data? JAMA 312:129–130
24. Iwashyna TJ, Kennedy EH (2013) Instrumental variable analyses. Exploiting natural randomness to understand causal mechanisms. Ann Am Thorac Soc 10:255–260
25. Blumenthal D, Tavenner M (2010) The "meaningful use" regulation for electronic health records. N Engl J Med 363:501–504
26. Graham KC, Cvach M (2010) Monitor alarm fatigue: standardizing use of physiological monitors and decreasing nuisance alarms. Am J Crit Care 19:28–34 (quiz 35)
27. Faden R, Kass N, Whicher D, Stewart W, Tunis S (2013) Ethics and informed consent for comparative effectiveness research with prospective electronic clinical data. Med Care 51:S53–S57
28. Fleurence RL, Beal AC, Sheridan SE, Johnson LB, Selby JV (2014) Patient-powered research networks aim to improve patient care and health research. Health Affairs 33:1212–1219
29. Murphy SN, Weber G, Mendis M et al (2010) Serving the enterprise and beyond with informatics for integrating biology and the bedside (i2b2). J Am Med Inform Assoc 17:124–130
30. McMurry AJ, Murphy SN, MacFadden D et al (2013) SHRINE: enabling nationally scalable multi-site disease studies. PLoS ONE 8:e55811
31. Faden RR, Beauchamp TL, Kass NE (2014) Informed consent, comparative effectiveness, and learning health care. N Engl J Med 370:766–768
32. Kim SYH, Miller FG (2014) Informed consent for pragmatic trials – the integrated consent model. N Engl J Med 370:769–772
33. Zimmerman JE, Kramer AA (2014) A history of outcome prediction in the ICU. Curr Opin Crit Care 20:550–556
34. Amin W, Tsui FR, Borromeo C et al (2014) PaTH: towards a learning health system in the Mid-Atlantic region. J Am Med Inform Assoc 21:633–636
35. Pinsky MR, Dubrawski A (2014) Gleaning knowledge from data in the intensive care unit. Am J Respir Crit Care Med 190:606–610

Index

J.-L. Vincent (ed.), *Annual Update in Intensive Care and Emergency Medicine 2015*,
DOI 10.1007/978-3-319-13761-2

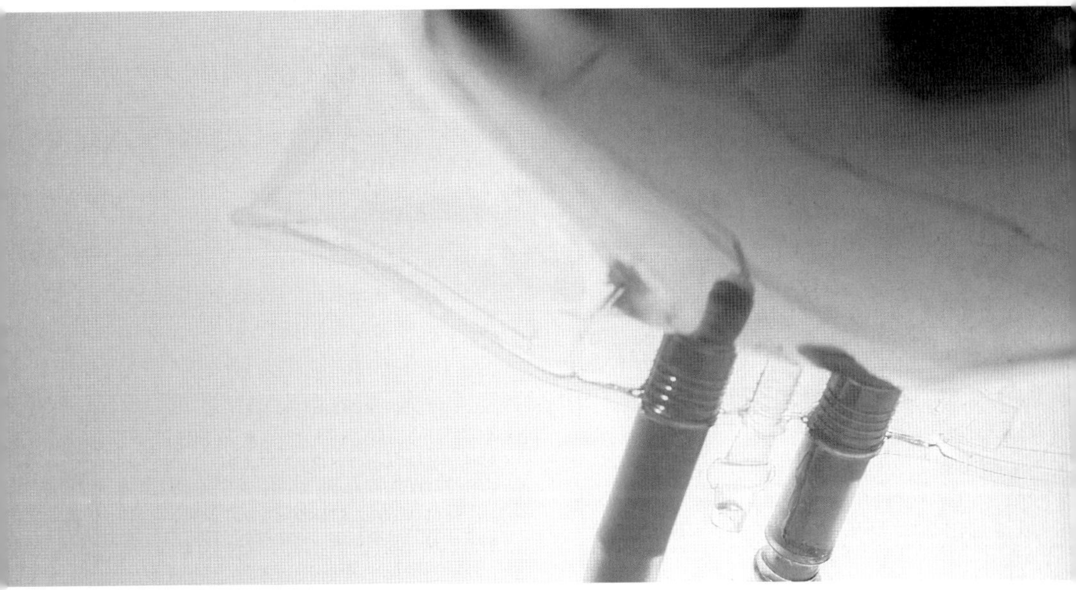

Printing: Ten Brink, Meppel, The Netherlands
Binding: Ten Brink, Meppel, The Netherlands